Handbook of Toxicogenomics

Edited by
Jürgen Borlak

Further Titles of Interest

Dev Kambhampati

Protein Microarray Technology

2003
ISBN 3-527-30597-1

Christoph W. Sensen

Essentials of Genomics and Bioinformatics

2002
ISBN 3-527-30541-1

Journal of Biochemical and Molecular Toxicology

6 Issues per year
ISSN 1095-6670

Handbook of Toxicogenomics

Strategies and Applications

Edited by
Jürgen Borlak

WILEY-VCH

WILEY-VCH Verlag GmbH & Co. KGaA

Editor

Univ.-Prof. Dr. Jürgen Borlak
Fraunhofer Institute of Toxicology
and Experimental Medicine
Drug Research and Medical Biotechnology
Nikolai-Fuchs-Strasse 1
30625 Hannover
Germany

and

Medical School of Hannover
Centre Pharmacology and Toxicology
Carl-Neuberg-Strasse 1
30625 Hannover
Germany

Library of Congress Card No.: applied for

British Library Cataloguing-in-Publication Data: A catalogue record for this book is available from the British Library.

Bibliographic information published by Die Deutsche Bibliothek
Die Deutsche Bibliothek lists this publication in the Deutsche Nationalbibliografie; detailed bibliographic data is available in the Internet at <http://dnb.ddb.de>

Printed in the Federal Republic of Germany
Printed on acid-free paper

Cover illustration: SCHULZ Grafik-Design, Fußgönheim
Composition ProSatz Unger, Weinheim
Printing betz-druck GmbH, Darmstadt
Bookbinding J. Schäffer GmbH & Co. KG, Grünstadt

ISBN-13: 978-3-527-30342-7
ISBN-10: 3-527-30342-1

To the memory of my parents

Forewords

Genome research, combinatory chemistry and high throughput screening methods yield a large number of target structures and potential pharmaceutical agents. Numerous substance candidates in the pharmaceutical industry, however, are doomed to fail during the preclinical or even clinical development phase because their toxicity is not recognized in time. Fast and economic tox screening tests which are nevertheless meaningful for humans are, therefore, urgently required, so that the substances with the most promising potential can be prioritized. Such prioritization should be accomplished as soon as possible, i. e. before entering into the costly development phase.

The German Federal State of Lower Saxony, therefore, supports the initiative of the Fraunhofer Institute of Toxicology and Experimental Medicine (ITEM) to considerably enhance its focus on Pharmaco- and Toxicogenomics, which has been successfully operated for several years by now and has recently become a center of excellence. A genome-based understanding of drug and chemical toxicity is of paramount importance and required as to develop meaningful methods for predictive toxicity testing. One core technology is based on microarrays but methods to study the proteom are essential as well. These genomic platform technologies are highly costly. The Federal State of Lower Saxony supports and fosters the development of competence clusters, spin-offs as to enable the pharmaceutical industry to equally make use of these technologies. The German Federal State of Lower Saxony has therefore provided substantial funding to enable the Fraunhofer Institute of Toxicology and Experimental Medicine to develop novel methods for predictive toxicology and to become internationally competitive in chemical and drug safety testing. Therefore, Pharmaco- and Toxicogenomic research at the Fraunhofer Institute in Hanover has become a hallmark for the capital city of Lower Saxony. Further, the German Federal Government program “Gesundheitsforschung – Forschung für den Menschen”, an initiative to promote research for human health, places the emphasis on an integration of basic and applied research and on the exploitation of the results by the industry. This is way the Fraunhofer Institute of Toxicology and Experimental Medicine in Hanover is perfectly suited to fulfill this task.

Lutz Stratmann
Minister for Science and Culture, Lower Saxony

Handbook of Toxicogenomics: Strategies and Applications. Edited by Jürgen Borlak

ISBN: 3-527-30342-1

With the advent of sequence information for the entire genome of many species, it is now possible to analyse gene expression and genetic variability on a global scale. It is therefore feasible to study gene expression profiles in entire genomes and to use this information for a mechanism based risk assessment. In conjunction with an assessment of entire proteomes it is now possible to develop early diagnostics and preventive measure particularly in at-risk populations or individuals. The Fraunhofer Institute of Toxicology and Experimental Medicine is well suited to carry out basic and applied science as to foster an understanding of chemical and drug induced toxicity. Indeed, in depth collaboration between academia and industry is of major importance to reduce attrition rates in the search for and development of new drugs and the Fraunhofer-Gesellschaft with its institutes has been practicing this principle with much success for several decades already. The creation of vast amounts of genomics and toxicogenomics data has sparked the development of novel systems as to improve predictability of drug response at toxic dose levels and the Food and Drug Administration (FDA) has recently issued a draft "Guidance for Industry" Pharmacogenomics Data Submission (FDA 2003) to account for these developments in medical sciences. Specifically, many principles in this draft apply to toxicogenomics and the newly created tool for voluntary submission of genomics data will pave the way in advancing public health and drug development based on holistic information. The Fraunhofer Institute of Toxicology and Experimental Medicine is committed to provide leadership in this field of genomic science and to develop mechanism based understanding of toxicity for an improved risk assessment of human health.

Hans-Jörg Bullinger
President of the Fraunhofer-Gesellschaft

The pharmaceutical industry is continuously facing increasing costs for developing new drugs on one hand and a high incidence of pipeline dropouts due to unexpected toxicity on the other hand. Furthermore, rare but serious adverse drug reactions still occur when new drugs are being used without being detected during development by preclinical or clinical studies. Therefore, new technologies that can predict more precisely the liabilities of drugs in early and late development are considered highly valuable. There are currently various new technologies under evaluation or even already in routine use to improve the prediction of drug-related side effects. One of these technologies is toxicogenomics, a concept which is intensively described and explained in the new "Handbook of Toxicogenomics" edited by Prof. Dr. Jürgen Borlak. This handbook provides an impressive overview of the current knowledge on the various technological platforms in the field of toxicogenomics. The topic of bioinformatics, which plays a key role in this field, is also addressed in detail. In addition, various authors from both academia and industry provide the reader with an overview of the current practical applications of toxicogenomics in fields such as hepatotoxicity, nephrotoxicity and search for biomarkers. The "Handbook of Toxicogenomics" is therefore considered to provide a comprehensive insight into the basic concepts of a new technology with the potential to positively impact human safety assessment in the near future.

Andreas Barner
Chairman of the Verband der Forschenden Arzneimittelhersteller, e.V.

Research and development in the fields of toxicology and pharmacology are currently undergoing drastic changes. New findings in the areas of molecular pharmacology/toxicology, molecular genetics, functional genomics, molecular immunology and cell biology open up new possibilities in the search for and development of pharmaceutical agents. In this context, the interdisciplinary development of pharmaceuticals has become particularly important, and the integration of the areas of genomics, molecular biology, surface technology, optics, robotics and combinatorial synthesis plays an important part in the creation of miniaturized and automated screening methods. The development of HTS (high throughput) systems, for instance, allows for millions of drug substance candidates to be evaluated within a single year in an almost completely automated laboratory. A toxicological assessment of drug substance candidates at an early stage is, however, a mandatory condition for the HTS strategy to be successful. Therefore a close interplay between academic and industrial research is of pivotal importance since for the pharmaceutical companies it is becoming increasingly impossible to cover the whole range of technologies and competences by themselves. Further, the high attrition rate in the R&D process and post launching drug failures due to adverse drug reactions requires an in-depth understanding of the mechanism of toxicity.

The Fraunhofer Institute of Toxicology and Experimental Medicine with more than 20 year experience of drug and chemical safety testing has now become a center for Pharmaco- and Toxicogenomic Research as well and the center has developed an international network of strong collaboration with academic and industrial collaborators including the National Institute of Health in the US and Japan. Undoubtedly, toxicogenomics is on the path to evolve into an independent genomic science as to enable prediction of toxicity based on a systems biology approach.

Uwe Heinrich
Chairman of the Fraunhofer Life Sciences Alliance

Preface

Toxicogenomics is a rapidly growing field of genomic science and holds promise for the identification and development of new founded knowledge in human and animal health. Basically, all major genomic platform technologies are being applied to toxicogenomic research and this includes transcriptome and proteome analysis as well as hyphenated LC-MS-NMR technology used to obtain metabolic fingerprints during intoxication and disease. Therefore, this book captures expert knowledge and provides in depth information on an application of toxicogenomics for the prediction of adverse drug reaction and for an improved understanding of the molecular basis of drug induced toxicity. There is also vision of how toxicogenomics will develop in the future and for communicating the challenges for it's application in risk assessment and to obtain regulatory acceptance. The book is divided into four major sections and starts with in-depth information on the various genomic platforms applied to toxicogenomic research. This is followed by a thorough discussion on bioinformatic tools, novel genetic algorithms and the architecture of various databases. It includes a description of the the Chemical Effects and Biological Safety database of the National Institute of Environmental Health Sciences (NIEHS of the US) and an appreciation of the various software applications used to analyse toxicogenomic data. Because of it's considerable importance a systems biology approach to toxicogenomics is described as well. In the third section the reader will be informed on fine examples of toxicogenomic research and this includes, amongst others, the prediction of hepato-, cardiovascular-, nephro- and haematotoxicity as well as endocrine disruption. One contribution focuses specifically on the application of toxicogenomics to teratogenicity studies and therefore this section highlights successful applications of toxicogenomics to predict drug induced toxicity. The fourth section gives an account of various national toxicogenomic programs and a perspective of an ICH harmonised guideline for inclusion of toxicogenomic data into the drug registration process.

In conclusion, the vast amounts of genomics and toxicogenomics data has provided novel insight into the molecular basis of drug induced toxicity. Inevitably, this knowledge will impact chemical- and drug safety testing and has initiated a fundamental shift of paradigm with the consequence of developing novel and above all better approaches for the prediction of drug induced toxicity.

Handbook of Toxicogenomics: Strategies and Applications. Edited by Jürgen Borlak

ISBN: 3-527-30342-1

I very much hope this book will become a stimulating resource for investigative toxicology with the aim to continuously improve strategies for predictions of unwanted drug effects and drug induced toxicities.

Jürgen Borlak
Hanover, January 2005

Acknowledgement

I wish to thank Susanne Steinmann for her diligence in communicating with the authors and for her help in the many editorial tasks. I further wish to thank my co-workers and colleagues at the Fraunhofer Institute of Toxicology and Experimental Medicine and particularly Uwe Heinrich for his continuous support and encouragement. Many thanks also to my colleagues at the National Centre of Toxicogenomics (NCT) of the National Institute of Environmental Health Sciences (NIEHS) US and the National Institute of Health Sciences of Japan as well as my colleagues at the Centre of Pharmacology and Toxicology of the Medical School of Hanover for the good and stimulating discussions. I am particular indebted to Christian Börger and Hans Schröder of the Ministry of Culture and Science of Lower Saxony, Germany, for their invaluable support and I wish to thank the Alexander von Humboldt foundation who supported Paul Nettesheim of the National Institute of Environmental Health Science of the US during his research sabbatical at this Institute. Indeed, this support greatly facilitated scientific exchange across the ocean and enabled joint research programs between both institutions.

Contents

Handbook of Toxicogenomics: Strategies and Applications. Edited by Jürgen Borlak

ISBN: 3-527-30342-1

List of Contributors

M. Beilmann
Boehringer Ingelheim Pharma
GmbH & Co. KG
Department of Non-Clinical
Drug Safety
Molecular and Cell Toxicology
Birkendorfer Strasse 65
88397 Biberach
Germany

Gerd Bode
Altana Pharma AG
Institut für Pathologie und Toxikologie
Friedrich-Ebert-Damm 101
22047 Hamburg
Germany

Gary Boorman
(address see Michael D. Waters)

Jürgen Borlak
Fraunhofer Institute of Toxicology and
Experimental Medicine
Drug Research and Medical Biotechnology
Nikolai-Fuchs-Strasse 1
30625 Hannover
Germany

and

Medical School of Hannover
Centre Pharmacology and Toxicology
Carl-Neuberg-Strasse 1
30625 Hannover
Germany

Andreas Bosio
Memorec Biotec GmbH
Stöckheimer Weg 1
50829 Köln
Germany

Pierre Bushel
(address see Michael D. Waters)

Katrin Buss
Memorec Biotec GmbH
Stöckheimer Weg 1
50829 Köln
Germany

Olivia Corcoran
King's College London
Department of Pharmacy
Frank Wilkins Building
150 Stamford Street
London SE1 9NH
United Kingdom

Jürgen Cox
Genedata GmbH
Lena-Christ-Strasse 50
82152 Martinsried
Germany

Michael Cunningham
(address see Michael D. Waters)

Handbook of Toxicogenomics: Strategies and Applications. Edited by Jürgen Borlak

ISBN: 3-527-30342-1

Damian G. Deavall
AstraZeneca
R&D Alderly Park
Safety Assessment UK
Mereside, Alderly Park
Macclesfield, Cheshire SK10 4TG
United Kingdom

David Finkelstein
Hartwell Center for Bioinformatics and Biotechnology
332, N. Lauderdale Street
Mail Stop 312
Memphis, TN 38015–2794
USA

Andreas Freier
Faculty of Technology
Bioinformatics Department
Bielefeld University
PO Box 100131
33501 Bielefeld
Germany

Timothy W. Gant
Medical Research Council
Toxicology Unit
University of Leicester
PO Box 138
Lancaster Road
Leicester, LE1 9HN
United Kingdom

Rodolfo Gasser
Hoffmann-La Roche Ltd.
Non-Clinical Drug Safety
Grenzacherstrasse, B69/146
4070 Basel
Switzerland

Thomas Gerloff
Institute of Clinical Pharmacology
Campus Charité Mitte
Charité – Universitätsmedizin Berlin
Schuhmannstrasse 20/21
10117 Berlin
Germany

Andreas Gescher
Medical Research Council
Toxicology Unit
University of Leicester
PO Box 138
Lancaster Road
Leicester, LE1 9HN
United Kingdom

Hans Gmünder
Genedata AG
Scientific Consulting
Maulbeerstrasse 46
4016 Basel
Switzerland

Peter Greaves
Medical Research Council
Toxicology Unit
University of Leicester
PO Box 138
Lancaster Road
Leicester, LE1 9HN
United Kingdom

Philip G. Hewitt
Merck KGaA
Institute of Toxicology
Frankfurter Strasse 250
64293 Darmstadt
Germany

Heinz Hildebrand
Bayer Health Care AG
Genetic and Molecular Toxicology
Aprather Weg 18a
42096 Wuppertal
Germany

Yoko Hirabayashi
National Institute of Health Sciences
Cellular and Molecular Toxicology Division
Kamiyoga, 1-18-1 Setagayaku
158-8501 Tokyo
Japan

Matthias Höchsmann
International NRW Graduate School
in Bioinformatics and Genome Research
Center of Biotechnology (CeBiTec)
University of Bielefeld
Universitätsstrasse 25
33501 Bielefeld
Germany

Ralf Hofestädt
Faculty of Technology
Bioinformatics Department
Bielefeld University
PO Box 100131
33501 Bielefeld
Germany

Andreas Hohn
GeneData AG
Maulbeerstrasse 46
4016 Basel
Switzerland

Earl Hubbell
Affymetrix Inc.
3380 Central Expressway
Santa Clara, CA 95051
USA

Tohru Inoue
Center for Biological Safety and Research
National Institute of Health Sciences
Kamiyoga 1-18-1, Setagayaku
Tokyo 158-8501
Japan

Rick Irwin
(address see Michael D. Waters)

Arno Kalkuhl
Boehringer Ingelheim Pharma
GmbH & Co. KG
Department of Non-Clinical Drug Safety
Molecular and Cell Toxicology
Birkendorfer Strasse 65
88397 Biberach
Germany

Alexander Kel
BIOBASE GmbH
VP Research & Development
Halchtersche Strasse 33
33804 Wolfenbüttel
Germany

Olga Kel-Margoulis
BIOBASE GmbH
VP Database Annotation
Halchtersche Strasse 33
33804 Wolfenbüttel
Germany

Jürgen Klempnauer
Medical School of Hannover
Clinic Viszeral- and Transplant Surgery
Carl-Neuberg-Strasse 1
30625 Hannover
Germany

Masatoshi Komiyama
Graduate School of Medicine
Bioenvironmental Medicine
Chiba University
Inohana 1-1, Chuoku
260-8670 Chiba
Japan

Peter-J. Kramer
Merck KGaA
Institute of Toxicology
Frankfurter Strasse 250
64293 Darmstadt
Germany

Wolf D. Lehmann
Central Spectroscopy
German Cancer Research Center (DKFZ)
Im Neuenheimer Feld 280
69120 Heidelberg
Germany

Anke Lühe
Hoffmann-La Roche Ltd.
Non-Clinical Drug Safety
Grenzacherstrasse, B90/505a
4070 Basel
Switzerland

Mark McCormick
NimbleGen Systems, Inc.
1, Science Court
Madison, WI 53711
USA

Alex Merrick
(address see Michael D. Waters)

Frauke Meyer
Altana Pharma AG
Institut of Pathology and Toxikology
Friedrich-Ebert-Damm 101
22047 Hamburg
Germany

Jonathan G. Moggs
Syngenta, Central Toxicology Laboratory
Research and Investigative Toxicology
Alderly Park
Macclesfield, Cheshire SK10 4TJ
United Kingdom

Chisato Mori
Graduate School of Medicine
Bioenvironmental Medicine
Chiba University
Inohana 1-8-1, Chuoku
260-8670 Chiba
Japan

Taku Nagao
National Institute of Health Sciences
Department of Life-Pharmaceutics
Kamiyoga 1-18-1, Setagaya-ku
Tokyo 158-8501
Japan

Monika Niehof
Fraunhofer Institute of Toxicology and
Experimental Medicine
Nikolai-Fuchs-Strasse 1
30625 Hannover
Germany

Emile F. Nuwaysir
NimbleGen Systems, Inc.
1, Science Court
Madison, WI 53711
USA

Kenneth Olden
(address see Michael D. Waters)

Björn Oleson
International NRW Graduate School
in Bioinformatics and Genome Research
Center of Biotechnology (CeBiTec)
University of Bielefeld
Universitätsstrasse 25
33501 Bielefeld
Germany

George Orphanides
Syngenta, Central Toxicology Laboratory
Research and Investigative Toxicology
Alderly Park
Macclesfield, Cheshire SK10 4TJ
United Kingdom

Martin Paul
Institute of Clinical Pharmacology
and Toxicology
Department of Toxicology
Campus Benjamin Franklin
Charité – Universitätsmedizin Berlin
Garystrasse 5
14195 Berlin
Germany

Richard Paules
(address see Michael D. Waters)

Klaus Prank
International NRW Graduate School
in Bioinformatics and Genome Research
Center of Biotechnology (CeBiTec)
University of Bielefeld
Universitätsstrasse 25
33501 Bielefeld
Germany

Uwe Rapp
Bruker Daltonik GmbH
Fahrenheitstrasse 4
28359 Bremen
Germany

Hubert Rehrauer
Genedata AG
Maulbeerstrasse 46
4016 Basel
Switzerland

Jacques Retief
Affymetrix, Inc.
Department of Genomic Collaboration
3380 Central Expressway
Santa Clara, CA 95051
USA

Ivar Roots
Institute of Clinical Pharmacology
Campus Charité Mitte
Charité – Universitätsmedizin Berlin
Schuhmannstrasse 20/21
10117 Berlin
Germany

Thomas Schmidt
International NRW Graduate School
in Bioinformatics and Genome Research
Center of Biotechnology (CeBiTec)
University of Bielefeld
Universitätsstrasse 25
33501 Bielefeld
Germany

Gilbert Schönfelder
Institute of Clinical Pharmacology
and Toxicology
Department of Toxicology
Campus Benjamin Franklin
Charité – Universitätsmedizin Berlin
Garystrasse 5
14195 Berlin
Germany

Harald Schrem
Medical School of Hannover
Clinic Viszeral- and Transplant Surgery
Carl-Neuberg-Strasse 1
30625 Hannover
Germany

Dieter Schwarz
Institute of Clinical Pharmacology
Campus Charité Mitte
Charité – Universitätsmedizin Berlin
Schuhmannstrasse 20/21
10117 Berlin
Germany

James K. Selkirk
(address see Michael D. Waters)

Andrew G. Smith
Medical Research Council
Toxicology Unit
University of Leicester
PO Box 138
Lancaster Road
Leicester, LE1 9HN
United Kingdom

Stanley Stasiewicz
(address see Michael D. Waters)

Laura Suter
Hoffmann-La Roche Ltd.
Non-Clinical Drug Safety
Grenzacherstrasse, B90/505a
4070 Basel
Switzerland

Leila Taher
International NRW Graduate School
in Bioinformatics and Genome Research
Center of Biotechnology (CeBiTec)
University of Bielefeld
Universitätsstrasse 25
33501 Bielefeld
Germany

Dimitry Tchekmenev
BIOBASE GmbH
Research & Development
Halchtersche Strasse 33
38304 Wolfenbüttel
Germany

Raymond W. Tennant
(address see Michael D. Waters)

Thomas Thum
University Hospital of Würzburg
Cardiology
Josef-Schneider-Strasse 2
97080 Würzburg
Germany

Thoralf Töpel
Faculty of Technology
Bioinformatics Department
Bielefeld University
PO Box 100131
33501 Bielefeld
Germany

Tetsuro Urushidani
National Institute of Health Sciences
Osaka Branch
Fundamental Research Laboratories
for Development of Medicine
Asagi 7-6-8, Saito, Ibaraki
Osaka 567-0085
Japan

Ben Van Houten
(address see Michael D. Waters)

Nigel Walker
(address see Michael D. Waters)

Honghui Wan
14410 Kings Crossing Boulevard
Boyds, MD 20841
USA

Michael D. Waters
National Institute of Environmental
Health Sciences
111, Alexander Drive
Research Triangle Park, NC 27709
USA

Brenda Weis
(address see Michael D. Waters)

Dion Whitehead
International NRW Graduate School
in Bioinformatics and Genome Research
Center of Biotechnology (CeBiTec)
University of Bielefeld
Universitätsstrasse 25
33501 Bielefeld
Germany

Edgar Wingender
Faculty of Medicine
Department of Bioinformatics
University of Göttingen
Goldschmidtstrasse 1
37077 Göttingen
Germany

1
Introduction

Jürgen Borlak

1.1
A Shift in Paradigm

Traditionally, toxicologists use experimental animals to identify hazardous substances for humans. These studies often require large amounts of substance, have a duration of several years, are relatively expensive and are of limited value in a mechanistic understanding of toxicity. To be able to estimate the hazard and risk for humans, additional studies on the mechanism of action, species extrapolation and effects in the low and human-relevant dose range need to follow. For reasons of cost and time, in depth investigations, in particular on environmental chemicals, are only carried out in the chemical industry, if requested by evaluating authorities, which is why risk assessments is frequently based on insufficient experimental data. Accordingly, there are substantial uncertainties in the risk assessment of chemicals. Because of the high costs, only a limited number of chemicals are investigated in detail and long-term studies including an assessment of carcinogenicity is not done routinely and does depend on production volume, e.g. >1000 t/year. In contrast, drug safety evaluation of pharmaceutical agents is somewhat more complex, as drug exposure to the human body is intentional, but mechanisms of toxicity are rarely persued, as well. These uncertaintes need to be overcome. Specifically, the knowledge gained from genome research as well as the rapid development of microarray technology offers new possibilities and in depth information. Indeed, microarray technology is by far the most cost-efficient method to detect alterations in the expression of pharmacologically and toxicologically relevant genes, or to investigate the relevance of genetic variability in drug response. Microarrays may also be used for chromosome or genome-wide investigations to reserach the circuitry of transcription factor networks based on the newly developed ChIP-chip assay. The study of protein-DNA and protein-protein interactions will thus lead to fundamental knowledge on the basic mechanism of gene regulation and it's modulation by drugs and other xenobiotics for robust prediction of drug safety.

Toxicogenomics is a major break through in toxicology and combines genome-wide mRNA expression profiling with protein expression patterns and metabolite

Handbook of Toxicogenomics: Strategies and Applications. Edited by Jürgen Borlak

ISBN: 3-527-30342-1

fingerprints using bioinformatics to understand the role of gene-drug interactions in disease and dysfunction. The use of DNA microarray technologies enables a genome wide assessment of changes in gene expression and will have a large impact on many fields, including developmental biology and molecular diagnostic. This technology will produce a paradigm shift in biology and toxicology as it allows a global perspective on how an organism responds to a specific stress, drug or toxicant. Data generated in toxicogenomic studies will provide information on cellular networks of responding genes that will help define important target molecules associated with the mechanism of toxicity, provide eventually biomarkers for clinical studies, and support the development of new toxicity screening procedures.

Specifically, experiments with microarrays will help to define the complex regulatory circuitry within a cell, tissue and organ that is responding to specific stressors. This technology is particularly important because it may be able to help pinpoint locations and time points to effectively intercede in the cascade of biochemical and molecular events perturbed by drugs and chemicals and, thus, positively modulate the cellular response in a manner reducing or preventing adverse effects. DNA microarray technology will undoubtedly become a major tool in molecular medicine, for both diagnosis/prognosis determinations for specific diseases or dysfunctions and the examination of interacting drug sensitivities and effectiveness.

DNA arrays are therefore a key technology of molecular biology. Their high degree of parallelization enables the visualization and simultaneous analysis of complex genetic alterations. Under precisely defined experimental conditions, the individual array elements yield detailed information on the expression of gene in a reference state as compared to the altered state of an organism, for instance in a healthy and a pathological tissue or organ.

For the design and fabrication of arrays, automated methods of genome analysis are indispensable. High throughput PCR's, fast purification methods as well as a robotized transfer to carrier materials on an industrial scale are essential preconditions for the production and use of DNA arrays. The analysis of DNA arrays requires new instruments and evaluation techniques, to allow for the abundant information yielded by such gene expression experiments to be properly interpreted.

A major point in analyzing the data procured by DNA microarrays is to correctly recognize and quantify the hybridization signals of the individual spots on an array. In a second step, the data are standardized and combined in functional groups prior to visualization. Software packages for image recording and analysis are necessary to allow for a efficient statistic analysis of the microarrays. Image analysis with the required software packages is, however, only the first step of the data evaluation. The development of new software tools for a further analysis and interpretation of the data obtained is mandatory, showing the increasing importance of bioinformatics in this area.

1.2 Enabling Technologies Lead to New Founded Knowledge in Genomic Science

The use of enabling genomic platform technologies leads to the generation of large amounts of data but turning data into knowledge will be a major challenge. In addition, new statistical evaluation methods for identifying relevant data sets are in need, in particular hierarchical cluster methods allowing to recognize identical or similar expression patterns within a large set of data. Hitherto, microarray technology can be used to identify toxic substances individually or as constituents of mixtures. It can be used to detect toxic effects at low doses and to identify sensitive tissue and cell types, and to extrapolate the detected effects from one species to another.

Microarrays can therefore be used to work on any problem in molecular medicine that requires a parallel identification, quantification or sequence analysis of a large number of different DNAs or RNAs. Because of the thermal instability of the hybrids, microarrays with oligonucleotides allow to discriminate fragments in which single base pairs have been replaced. Consequently, these arrays are suitable for sequencing and thus also for the detection of SNPs (single-nucleotide polymorphisms) and may be used for genotyping in general. Indeed, an important finding of the human genome project was the observed variability in the genomic sequence of coding genes. Seen from a purely statistical point of view, practically every 1,200th base exists as a variant. Only a few of the estimated 2 million nucleotide polymorphisms are functionally relevant, i.e. they trigger protein alterations resulting in changed or missing activity. It has been estimated that approximately 5–10 percent of all SNPs are disease-relevant or play a role in pharmacotherapy. Arrays allow to carry out complex SNP analyses. Today it is already possible to analyze up to –100,000 SNPs simultaneously by microarray. Besides molecular diagnostics of disease-associated nucleotide polymorphisms, SNP analyses also allow to identify biomarkers for groups of patients, enabling stratification of patient cohorts. Depending on the particular drug and indication, clinical trials have average success rates of 30–40% only. To be able to demonstrate a statistically safe therapeutic effect, several thousand patients often need to be studied over a period of several years, though not all patients will benefit from this drug treatment.

An identification of genetic biomarkers for therapy-responsive patients may become possible through array based analysis. Genetic markers suited for patient recruiting are then derived using appropriate mathematical methods. Only the "informative" sequence varaitions, i.e. those in agreement with a particular indication and patient cohort, are applied to the carrier material. Patients are then genotyped through chip-based SNP analyses and either proposed or rejected for an investigation. Likewise, this apporach may be taken in occupational medicine to identify employees at risk.

Further, the request for an evidence based medicine now forces drug companies to develop individualized pharmacotherapies. Already today, it is a recognized fact that a connection exists between undesired side effects in pharmacotherapy and SNPs of drug-metabolizing enzymes. Undesired side effects of pharmaceuticals cause each year substantial costs to health insurance companies (an estimated 5 billion US$ per year). Public and private insurance funds as well as long-term therapy patients are interested in alternative pharmacotherapies with little side effects. Genotyping of patients is done already today for high-risk patients and will be substantially enhanced in the future.

The possibility to identify and quantify nucleic acids enables the creation of expression profiles which in turn provide information on the state of the investigated tissue. In research, such gene expression profiles enable the analysis of molecular interactions, the identification of gene interactions (pathways) and of groups of genes acting together, as well as the elucidation of the function of new genes. In the clinical domain, the screening, diagnosis, monitoring and prognostic evaluation of diseases in fields such as oncology, infectiology, neurology or metabolic-cardiovascular diseases is of primary interest; in toxicology, it is the analysis of the mechanism of action of the toxicity and the kinetics of a drug, as well as the identification of new marker genes, allowing to recognize at an early stage potential toxicological or carcinogenic effects.

1.3
Translating RNAs Into Proteins

In toxicoproteomics, numerous methodological strategies are evaluated and currently validated regarding their suitability for solving a variety of biological problems.

In general, highly complex protein mixtures are first separated on SDS gels in pH-dependent electrical fields and stained in order to visualize the individual proteins. An optimal separation of protein mixtures presupposes excellent sample preparation. After the gels have been stained, the proteins are cut out with a "spotcutter" under the control of a CCD camera. The cut-out proteins are placed on a microtiter plate, where they are digested by means of proteases and subsequently spotted onto a target (e. g. a metal plate) that has been chemically prepared for target spotting. Laser treatment then leads to a release of peptide ions whose time of flight in a tube is measured. By means of protein database queries, the times of flight of experimentally obtained peptide ions are compared to reference values, thus principally allowing for an identification of proteins.

Comparable to genome wide mRNA transcript profiling, proteome mapping is done in a similar fashion, though some technical hurdles still need to be overcome. The mapping of proteoms allows to recognize toxicologically relevant expression patterns and use them for an assessment of drug action. Besides a determination of differentially expressed proteins, methods of mass spectroscopy allow to investigate posttranslational modifications, protein folding and structure, protein maturation and degradation, protein-protein interactions and alternative splice variants of ribosomally translated RNA molecules. Proteome analyses can be carried out in extracts of tissues and organs from the above mentioned animal experiments. A major objective of these proteome analyses is the reproducible identification and characterization of regulated proteins (e. g. production of new proteins or alterations in the expression of constitutively expressed proteins) upon drug exposure. The proteome mappings are stored in corresponding databases. A reference proteome database needs to be set up to enable the evaluation of drugs under development through comparative analyses.

Finally, highly complex spectroscopic methods are used with the aim to elucidate the structure of endogenous metabolites in response to drug exposure and toxicity or disease. All endogenous metabolites and their degradation products (resulting e.g. from fat, carbohydrate and protein metabolisms) may be referred to as "metabonome". In addition to MS- techniques, high-resolution NMR devices are used in the first place. Unfortunately, MS is not capable of providing all the information required for sufficient structural elucidation. Through its large experimental variety (protons, 13C or 2-dimensional spectroscopy), NMR spectroscopy allows for an unambiguous identification of compounds. A drawback of NMR spectroscopy is its relatively low sensitivity as compared to mass spectroscopy. In addition, sulphate conjugates of metabolites cannot be determined using common proton and 13C NMR spectroscopy, because sulphur nuclei are not NMR-active. Despite this minor restriction, however, NMR spectroscopy, in particular in combination with HPLC (high-pressure liquid chromatography for the separation of substance mixtures), has established itself in metabolism research for the investigation of biological matrices. Furthermore, NMR spectroscopy enables the structural elucidation of proteins, resulting in valuable synergies and a high degree of concatenation in the use of the technology platform as well as in the development of new products. The isolation of the analytes and subsequent purification for NMR spectroscopy is very time-consuming. By coupling NMR spectroscopy and HPLC, matrix components can be separated beforehand.

A major objective is the detection and characterization of metabolically derived degradation products, e.g. formation of new metabolites or quantitative shifts in individual compounds within the body, which are observed in toxicological evaluations and can be attributed to altered activities of constitutively expressed proteins. A reference database needs to be set up to enable the evaluation of drugs under development through comparative analyses. By analyzing the metabonome, alterations in the transcriptome and the proteome are recognized or confirmed, which is why the integration of the different platforms will be a highly valuable

1.4
Toxicogenomics – A Perspective

An assessment of toxicity requires a broad and interdisciplinary research and development strategy, which implies the use of numerous methods, some of them being highly complex. This book captures some of the most advanced developments in genomic platform technologies and their application to chemical and drug safety and aims to provide a snapp shot and some vision of how this field of genomic science will develop. The book is devided into major chapters on various technology platforms (Chapters 2 to 8) and bioinformatic tools in toxicogenomics including a systems biology approach (Chapters 9 to 13) followed by a large number of case studies (Chapters 14 to 24) on liver, kidney, cardiovascular, endocrine, in utero and teratogenicity. Further applications include haematotoxicity and periheral blood cell studies and investigations into the consequences of genetic variability in drug induced and idiosynchratic toxicity. A further report from the industry gives an account of how toxicogenomics guided the decision and development program of two 5-HT_6 receptor antagonists with similar pharmacological activity but different toxicity profiles. Finally, in Chapters 25 and 26 the national toxicogenomics programs of the US and Japan are being summarised and the book concludes with an outlook of how toxicogenomic guidelines can be developed and integrated in to the International Conference on Harmonisation of Technical Requirements for the Registration of Pharmaceuticals for Human Use (ICH).

Technology Platforms in Toxicogenomics

Handbook of Toxicogenomics: Strategies and Applications. Edited by Jürgen Borlak

ISBN: 3-527-30342-1

2 Expression Profiling Using SAGE and cDNA Arrays

Katrin Buss and Andreas Bosio

2.1 Introduction

Life scientists today are trying to understand and foresee the phenotypic appearance of a living system by correlating massive amounts of data about the molecular state of the underlying cells. This trend is mainly due to new techniques and technologies that enable massive parallel assessment of information as well as to the rapid development of tools for data mining and analysis. The molecular state of a cell or cell population is thought to be efficiently described when as many data as possible are gathered on the different molecules participating in the information processing. Researchers aim to set up quantitative pathway and interaction maps allowing the molecular events outlining a cell's fate to be dissected. However, starting with DNA as the ground level, the complexity of information increases rapidly when moving to RNA and finally to proteins and derived molecules. Although the genome is defined by its sequence and modifications, the transcriptome is also specified by the amount of each of the different RNA species. The proteome carries additional information that is partly imposed by the environment (e.g., pH, ionic strength) but also retained in posttranscriptional modifications and an infinity of possible molecular interactions. Currently, there is no method allowing all classes of molecules to be observed at once, but numerous attempts are being made to analyse each class of molecules. Each class of molecules bears substantial information, and it is hard to decide which one is more important. Detecting a point mutation does not allow one to directly draw a link to a cellular alteration. On the other hand, the proteome often reflects only already-integrated signals, which do not necessarily point to the underlying cause. However, budgetary restraints force researchers to select the most cost-effective methodology. Most often, analysis of the transcriptome is the method of choice, as it already reflects the actual state of a cell but is much less complex and cumbersome to analyse and to interpret than the proteome. In general, the 'omics' approaches can be arranged into so-called open systems and those that are restricted to a given matrix of information. Accordingly, and following the old question: Which came first, the experiment or the idea? the scientific community is di-

Handbook of Toxicogenomics: Strategies and Applications. Edited by Jürgen Borlak

ISBN: 3-527-30342-1

vided into believers in hypothesis-driven approaches and those who love inductive systems.

In this chapter we review two methodologies for gene expression profiling, covering both schools of thinking and in addition using two fundamentally different ways of identifying and quantifying RNAs. The first one is the serial analysis of gene expression (SAGE), the second is the PIQOR™ cDNA microarray system. Each method has its advantages and disadvantages defining which is more suited to individual experimental requirements. After describing technological aspects in detail and giving examples of the application of SAGE and PIQOR, we conclude with a proposal for the combined use of both methods.

2.2 SAGE Technology

2.2.1 Principles of SAGE Technology

The serial analysis of gene expression – SAGE – is a sequencing-based method of generating expression profiles from any given cell type or tissue. As an open system, SAGE characterizes a short segment of DNA from a defined location in each expressed gene, as a unique identifier for that gene. The ability to count many thousands of short DNA segments, called SAGE tags, allows the detection of genes that are expressed at very low levels in a high-throughput manner. From a historical point of view, SAGE is a logical progression of approaches that simply count gene transcripts, like counting plaques in a cDNA library or counting expressed sequence tags (ESTs) for a single sequence. However, SAGE has revolutionized the generation of countable, gene-specific tags and has introduced a way of rapid counting. But the basic principle of counting still plays a fundamental role in the statistics of SAGE. It is one of the major differences to technologies like microarrays, which are based on analogue results relying on measurement of signal intensities resulting from nucleic acid hybridization.

SAGE is a patented technology developed in the laboratory of Bert Vogelstein and Ken Kinzler [1], which has been used since then in many laboratories and has led to about 300 publications. SAGE has been selected by the US NCI as a method of choice for the Cancer Genome Anatomy Project (CGAP) [2].

Four principle steps underlie the SAGE technology (Figure 2.1):

1. Isolation of tags: a short DNA fragment (SAGE tag), which is unique for each mRNA species, is isolated.
2. Concatenation: tags are ligated to form large DNA molecules (concatemers).
3. Sequencing: the concatemers are sequenced.
4. Expression profiling: tags are identified, annotated, and counted. The expression profile is deduced by comparing the nature and frequency of tags within two or more libraries.

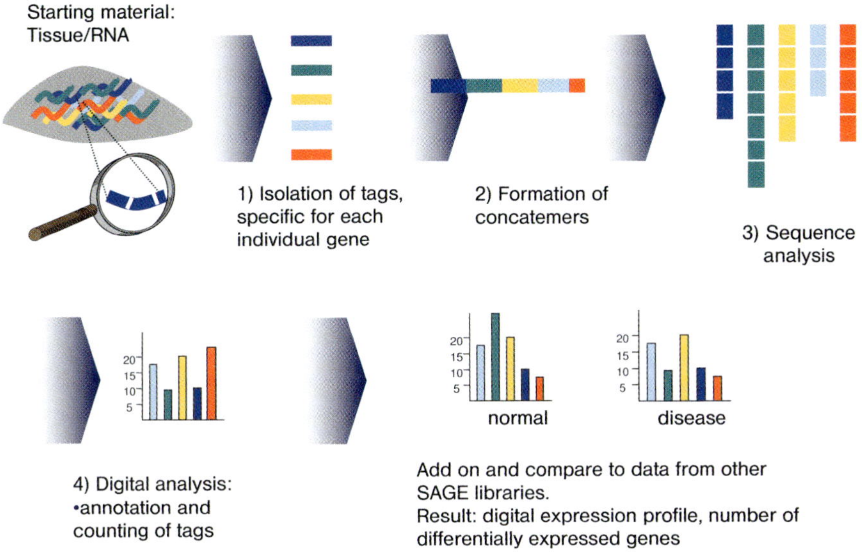

Fig. 2.1 Outline of SAGE technology.

2.2.2
Generation of SAGE Libraries

RNA is extracted from a tissue or cell culture. As in all gene expression profiling methods, both the integrity and purity of the RNA are of crucial importance. At least 1 µg of total RNA is required. The RNA is reverse-transcribed to form double-stranded cDNA using biotinylated oligo-dT for priming. The cDNA is cleaved with a restriction enzyme (4-bp cutter, *Nla*III), and only short cDNA fragments located at the 3′ end are separated from the rest using streptavidin beads. The cDNA fragments, which are – on average – 256 base pairs (bp) long, are divided into two pools and ligated to different linkers both carrying the recognition sequence for a type II restriction enzyme (*Bsm*FI) and a PCR primer sequence. The type II restriction enzyme cuts 15 bp downstream of the 4-bp recognition site, resulting in an 11-bp tag unique to the individual cDNA molecule.

The linked SAGE tags from both pools are blunt-ended using DNA polymerase, mixed together, and ligated to generate head-to-tail ditags. The ditags are PCR-amplified, and again digested with *Nla*III to release the primer adaptors. The SAGE ditags are then polymerised (concatenation) to form a series of 22-bp segments and are cloned into a plasmid vector.

Each concatemer is purified from a clone and sequenced. The better the concatenation step has been performed, the more information is yielded per sequence. At Memorec we routinely sequence about 30 to 40 tags per lane; 30 000–50 000 tags are identified and counted in a typical SAGE study. The steps described above for generating and sequencing the SAGE tags are basic molecular biology procedures. However, as the SAGE technology combines multiple enzymatic reactions, including PCR, with repeated purification procedures, it is crucial to use only the highest purity reagents and to carefully follow the protocol in each step.

2.2.3
SAGE Bioinformatics

After the concatemers have been sequenced, the bioinformatics work starts. The series of computational events is, in a way, the reverse of the molecular cloning events performed in the laboratory. First, the concatemer sequences are split into ditags. Then ditags that are present more than one time are removed. The ligation of tags to ditags prior to PCR amplification is a random event. Thus, two ditags with the same sequence are thought to be an artefact resulting from a preferential PCR amplification. By removing these ditags, which make up a negligible percentage of all ditags, PCR artefacts are discriminated. Hence, the SAGE technology, although using the benefits of PCR amplification, rules out the general pitfalls of PCR-based methodologies, such as differential display. In the next step, ditags are split to generate the appropriate SAGE tags. The process is finalized by assignment of tags to genes and counting the tags. This can be done using one of several publicly available SAGE analysis software packages (some are online, e.g., at http://www.ncbi.nlm.nih.gov/SAGE). At Memorec we have developed our own software for accurate SAGE tag mapping using an extensive proprietary tag database. It includes automatic annotation derived from EST/genomic data that takes into account several hundred manually annotated tags that are elusive to automatic annotation. SAGE artefacts and uninformative tags derive from polymorphic tags, ribosomal RNA, mitochondrial RNA, linker tags, LINE/SINE tags, and sequencing errors are removed by proprietary filtering algorithms. The software allows the comparison of two (or more) different libraries by providing tools for normalization, calculation of significance levels, and interactive graphical output. Already at this stage, SAGE results can be used to define the complete, unrestricted transcriptome of a given tissue. The level of sensitivity is determined not primarily by a labelling or detection system but by the amount of sequencing that can be carried out in a cost-effective manner. A typical SAGE analysis of 50 000 tags will identify 10 000–15 000 different transcripts in most cell types. It has been shown that, at a sufficient depth, SAGE can identify the entire set of genes represented in a cell type. A typical SAGE library contains many more tags than can be practically sequenced. This represents an inexhaustible resource when additional data is required for statistical purposes.

However, most applications of SAGE point to the identification of differentially expressed genes within two probes. This is achieved by simply comparing the number of counted tags in each of the probes. Because of the digital nature of SAGE data, it is possible to assess the differential expression analysis by statistical methods, which is not true when two microarray experiments are compared [3]:

$$p(y \mid x) = \left(\frac{N_2}{N_1}\right)^y \frac{(x+y)!}{x!y!\left(1+\frac{N_2}{N_2}\right)^{(x+y+1)}}$$

where N_1 and N_2 represent the total number of tags counted per library, x and y are the number of tags for a given gene, and p is the significance level of regulated gene expression.

As one can see, the degree of significance of differentially expressed genes depends on the number of tags counted for a given gene. The differential expression of genes with tag counts of, for example, 200 : 100 is much more significant than for genes with tag counts of 20 : 10 or even 2 : 1. Finally, sensitivity improvements are achieved by clustering multiple tags belonging to one gene and also by biological pathway analysis.

2.2.4 SAGE Applications

The SAGE technology has been used in almost every possible genomic research area, including the analyses of cardiovascular, inflammatory, neurological, and genetic diseases in *Homo sapiens* and other species, such as *Arabidopsis thaliana, Bos taurus, Medicago truncatula, Mus musculus,* and *Rattus norvegicus.* At Memorec, numerous SAGE analyses has been performed as customer services and for in-house research in drug target discovery and clinical programs. Starting with the quality control of delivered or prepared total RNA (about 1 μg of total RNA is required), a common SAGE project with two libraries and sequencing and analysis of 100 000 tags is finished within 14–16 weeks. As it is very cost-intensive to perform repeats of SAGE libraries, it is recommended to use RNA that has been extracted and pooled from different samples so as to reduce the impact of biological variation among individuals. To keep the costs as low as possible, the sequencing of SAGE tag libraries can be done in a stepwise procedure. After about 15 000 tags/library, an initial analysis is performed and repeated every 10 000 tags/library until an appropriate degree of sensitivity and statistical validity of results is achieved (for most projects done at Memorec, between 15 000 and 60 000 tags per library have been sequenced). Normally, not more than 500 genes are found to be differentially expressed with a significance level of >0.05 and fewer than 100 with $p > 0.01$. By using extensive bioinformatics tools and cross-species comparisons, most of the sequenced tags can be annotated or at least a functional prediction is achieved by using extensive proprietary libraries of domains and motifs. If 'unknown' genes are of interest, several techniques have been developed for de novo isolation of the corresponding genes. To identify marker genes or putative drug targets, genes can be selected again using bioinformatics including pathway analysis.

2.3
cDNA Arrays

2.3.1
Principles of PIQOR Technology

DNA microarrays are miniaturized devices for the parallel analysis of ribonucleic acids by hybridization. The technology essentially reverses the setup of the classical hybridization methodology originnally invented by Southern [4]. DNA microarrays are widely used for expression analysis because they require only small amounts of sample material. Since – generally speaking – microarrays consist of immobilized probes spotted on a solid substrate which allows for automation, they meet the demands for high-throughput screening: low need of sample material and the possibility to automate the process. Microarray formats differ regarding the substrates, the probe selection strategies, and the way the probes are immobilized. Several aspects of the technology are discussed in detail below.

Memorec produces low-density microarrays suitable for two-colour experiments, that is, direct comparison of treated and control samples ending in the determination of expression ratios (Figure 2.2). The PIQOR (parallel identification and quantification of mRNA) system so far comprises a cDNA collection for the human, mouse, and rat species, a set of predefined arrays for specific subjects, and the possi-

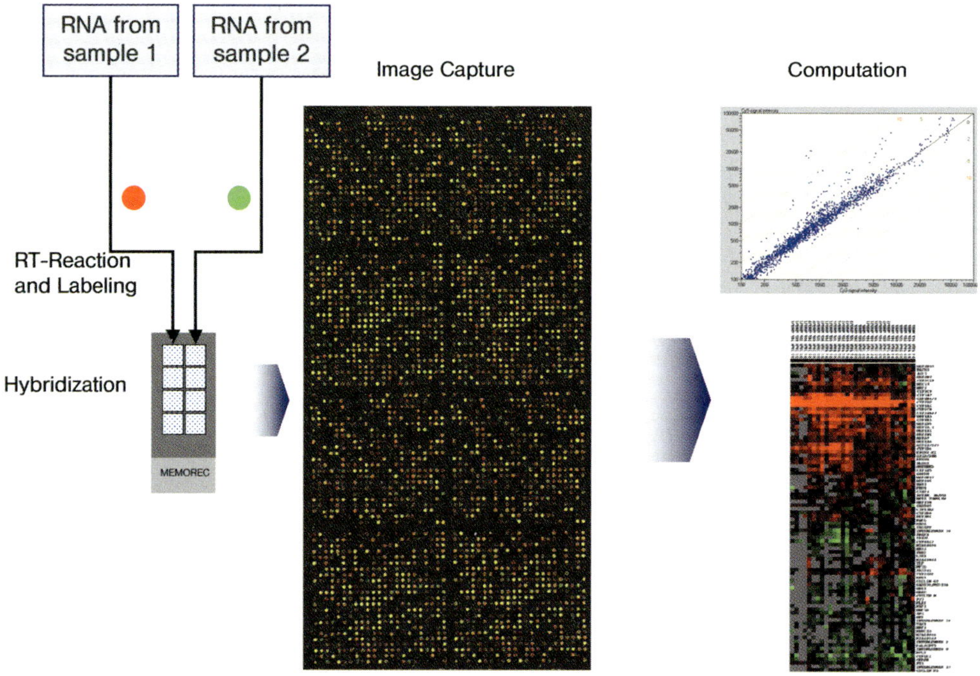

Fig. 2.2 Outline of expression profiling using cDNA microarrays.

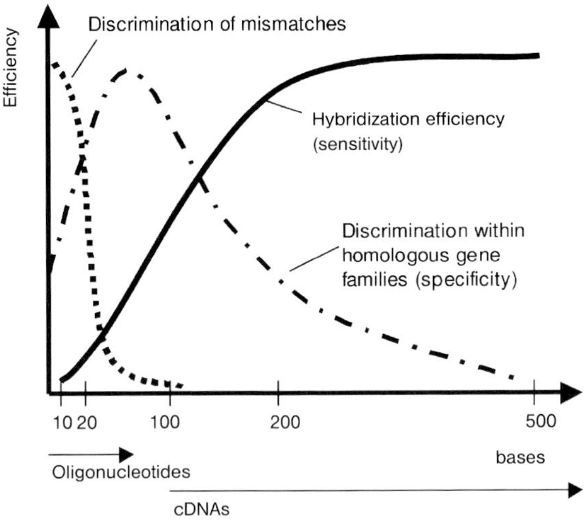

Fig. 2.3 Hybridization efficiency as a function of cDNA chain length.

bility to customize each array configuration with respect to the kind, number, and replicates of the probes. PIQOR arrays carry highly specific cDNA fragments 200–400 base pairs long, which are handpicked following complex bioinformatics methods and the amplification of suitable gene regions by PCR.

The length of the employed cDNA fragments is of particular interest regarding the robustness of the hybridization process. With increasing length of the used probes, the kinetics become more stable. The asymptotic curve (Figure 2.3) illustrates that a length of 200 bases is adequate to guarantee a stable hybridization independent of single nucleotide polymorphisms and varying GT contents of the single probes. The latter permits the hybridization conditions to be optimised for all of the probes that are hybridized in parallel. Furthermore, the sensitivity of DNA arrays increases the longer the probes are, since more labelled samples may hybridize with the matching immobilized probes. The length of the probes should be limited to a maximum of about 400 base pairs to avoid the probability of cross hybridization caused by repetitive elements and unspecific interactions. Furthermore, limitation to ~400 base pairs provides the ability to distinguish even genes from highly homologous gene families like those for the cytochrome P450 enzymes by choosing fragments from appropriate (i. e., poorly conserved) gene regions (see Section 2.3.2).

Compared to cDNA arrays, the spotting or in situ synthesis of oligonucleotides is a completely different manufacturing strategy having a deep impact on the way the results are analyzed. The arrayed oligonucleotides range from some 25 to 70 residues per probe. Depending on the length of the probes, a set of different oligonucleotides is necessary to unambiguously detect particular genes. Thus, several signals are gained for one gene, which sometimes may be contradictory due to differing hybridization kinetics or splice variants and therefore hard to interpret.

In general, the probe selection strategy for microarrays is subject to several prerequisites such as the objective of the experiment, the available sequence information regarding the organism to be investigated, and the efforts one is willing to supply in advance of the actual hybridization. If one were interested in overviewing the expression levels of as many genes as possible in a small set of experiments, it would be sufficient to spot cDNA libraries, uncharacterized ESTs, or oligonucleotides derived therefrom. This postpones in-depth sequence analysis and annotation to the point when hybridization has been performed and the resulting clones/genes of interest have been identified. This strategy reduces the expenses for prechip sequencing and bioinformatics to nothing. It may be most appropriate for high-throughput arraying projects. In contrast, if the experimental setup calls for accurate identification and quantification of particular mRNA species by hybridization, one can either buy ready-to-spot sets or go the time and effort of cloning and sequence-verifying the cDNAs oneself. However, these processes should be accompanied by extensive quality management (especially when targeting diagnostics).

2.3.2
Selection and Annotation of Suitable cDNA Fragments

Above all, the unambiguous identification of any particular gene (i. e., the prevention of false signals caused by cross hybridization events) is the goal of the probe-selection strategy. By amplification of suitable sequence regions of preselected genes, important properties such as length, orientation, and position within the mRNA can be determined. To facilitate interspecies comparisons by expression profiling, Memorec's strategy is to generate – whenever possible – fragments from the corresponding cDNA regions of orthologous genes for the three species.

Methods of probe selection and annotation have been highly refined, both because the arrays are focused on a limited number of DNA fragments and because the available sequence information for the human, mouse, and rat species allow for extensive prechip bioinformatics [5]. Below, some considerations for probe selection are discussed; the discussion can also be used as a catalogue of typical reasons for misinterpretation of array data.

Whereas cross hybridizations based on unspecific binding events can be reduced by optimizing the experimental conditions, other reasons for undesirable cross hybridizations include repetitive elements such as Alu repeats, microsatellite repeats, and SINEs or LINEs (short or long interspersed elements) within the DNA sequence. Comparing the selected sequence to those in databases such as REPBASE will give some information about this feature.

As different mRNA species may emerge from a single gene, the selection of a suitable array fragment – depending on the question to be answered by the array experiment – detect either all or specific observed splice variants of a given gene.

If alternative polyadenylation signals occur in the sequence, the 3′ untranslated end of the mRNA may be constituent or regulated – if the latter, a fragment detecting only one possible variant would bias the expression ratio of a given gene. By using information from, for example, EST databases or SAGE tags, it is possible to identify even cryptic polyA signals.

Alternative splicing (the excision of distinct exons) is another source of different mRNA species from a single gene. The consequences for the selection of array fragments are the same as for alternative polyadenylation. Since the resulting gene products serve different purposes, it may be interesting to distinguish the mRNA species. For example, the UDP-glucuronosyl transferase (UGT) 1A family is derived from one gene with alternative exons 1. In this special instance, the potential of using cDNA fragments instead of whole cDNAs is obvious, since the homology between all members of the UGT1A family is very high for the entire cDNA sequence. Hence, when using different probes spanning not only exon 1 but also some of exons 2–5, uninterpretable data would be obtained.

Most important with respect to quality management of the array production is careful documentation of the expected hybridization properties of the fragment. In addition, each fragment should be completely annotated according to all the names used in public databases such as UniGene, SwissProt, TrEMBL, and other relevant data sources. This alleviates the burden of gene selection for the customers by simultaneously avoiding redundancy caused by the probable utilization of different names for the same gene.

2.3.3 Production of Microarrays

2.3.3.1 Substrates

The production of suitable substrates is as crucial for reliable and reproducible results as the generation of probes. Several aspects have to be considered when producing solid substrates for microarrays.

When working with fluorescence-labelled samples, autofluorescence of the substrate may strikingly limit the sensitivity of hybridization experiments. Since a high background decreases the signal-to-noise ratio, a priori autofluorescence of the surface has to be decreased to a minimum. This should be accompanied by optimizing surface properties such as planarity (which is mainly influenced by the solid phase used), uniformity, mechanical and chemical stability, and the DNA-binding capacity. Other points such as control of inter- and intra-batch uniformity should be kept in mind while developing a coating protocol for array production.

Generally, substrates are composed of a solid phase and one or two layers to hydrophobize the surface and simultaneously provide reactive groups to covalently bind DNA. Most of the coatings that have been developed, e.g., silyl (reactive aldehyde), silane (reactive amino groups), or polylysine, make use of the reactivity of the nucleobases and lead to an unspecific crosslinking of DNA to the surface [6]. These interactions can reduce the conformational freedom of the cDNAs and hence their affinity for complementary molecules in solution. In contrast, we and others have developed some other surfaces suitable for covalent binding of the DNA to the surface via a specific linker attached to the 5′ or 3′ end of the DNA [7, 8]. End-specific covalent binding offers the opportunity to direct the amount of attached cDNAs to an optimal density at which enough cDNAs are present, but charge and steric effects are minimal.

2.3.3.2 Probes

After selection of appropriate cDNA fragments and the respective primers, the cDNA fragments are amplified by RT–PCR and checked for the predicted length. Subsequently, the PCR products are cloned and rechecked for the right size by restriction analysis. Having passed these steps, the clones are sequence-verified. The results of sequence analysis are BLASTed against Memorec's fragment library – a process that has been largely automated to rule out artefacts.

Sequence verification and documentation is a crucial step in quality management. Careful handling of sequencing information is essential for reliable expression profiling results. Ideally, any data that is acquired during probe generation is documented in a laboratory information management system (LIMS) or another relational database, according to any special requirements, permitting optimal quality management of the complete array-production process.

When the clones are sequence-verified, they can be used for vector PCR in which the ready-to-spot amplicons are generated. By using specific amino-linked primers, the resulting PCR products are prepared for covalent binding to the activated surface of the substrate. This step is also quality-controlled by checking for the right fragment length. After reformatting and generation of master plates for spotting, an additional quality control step should be performed, repeating several PCRs using gene-specific primers, to ensure correct positioning of the DNA fragments.

2.3.3.3 Spotting

For the manufacture of microarrays, contact- and non-contact–printing methods have been developed. Contact printing allows for very rapid production, but lacks some advantages of non-contact printing. Memorec has focused on non-contact printing following the principle of ink-jet printers. In contrast to contact-printing technologies, this allows for dispensing defined volumes of DNA solution controlled by a piezoelement placed on the nozzle. In addition, non-contact printing permits the respotting of single probes. Thus, zero-error production becomes possible. For detection with even higher reliability, especially of weakly expressed genes, probes should be spotted in replicates. To minimize the impact of probable spatial effects on the measured expression ratio, the replicates should not be located close together in the spotting area but should be uniformly distributed over the whole spotting area [9]. Hence, even in areas like the edges, which are prone to inhomogeneous hybridization conditions (e.g., by bubbles caused by degassing, etc.), no more than two of four replicates are impaired.

Since it is very laborious to determine the identity of the probes retrospectively, the spotting process should be accompanied by accurate documentation. The positioning of the genes has to be traceable unequivocally.

At Memorec, the arrays are produced in a dedicated cleanroom facility, according to anticipated GXP standards, using a proprietary, advanced, non-contact high-throughput arrayer (HTA). The HTA is equipped with 96 spotting nozzles and is able to produce up to 1000 arrays in a single lot. Seven integrated CCD cameras that generate pictures of each slide are used for in-line process controls, providing the possibility to re-spot each cDNA directly. The slides are bar-coded so that the spotting process for each slide can be documented automatically. Again, the entire processes are recorded in Memorec's LIM system.

2.3.4 Application of Microarrays

Although it may sound trivial, the first crucial step in achieving reliable gene expression results is RNA isolation. If the RNA is slightly degraded or contaminated, the results may be biased and irreproducible. Since RNA extraction protocols may influence the outcome of the expression analysis, it is worthwhile to check in advance for an appropriate protocol and to use it for all the samples that should be analyzed in one batch of experiments. For example, total RNA extracted with Trizol reagent contains the entire range of fragment lengths, whereas silica filters have a cutoff size of about 50–100 bases. Thus, for microarray applications it is often recommended to clean up total RNA that has been isolated by the Trizol method by using an appropriate kit.

The necessary amount of total RNA depends on the labelling method and the kind of array.

For application of cDNA arrays, it is recommended to use fluorescence labelling and to start with ~20 μg of total RNA (equivalent to 0.5 μg mRNA) if any direct labelling method is chosen. If the amount of available RNA is limited, e.g., when samples obtained by biopsies or microdissections are analyzed, the RNA can be subjected to linear amplification to produce aRNA [10]. Subsequently, the labelling reaction can be performed by reverse transcription, for which 1 μg of the produced aRNA should be used. cDNA arrays are suitable for two-colour experiments, i.e., samples (treated cells, pathologic tissues) and the appropriate controls (untreated cells, normal tissue) can be analyzed simultaneously. The treated samples are usually labelled with Cy5 (red) and the control sample with Cy3 (green). To assess the influence of the different fluorophores (and to check if subsequent normalization can eliminate the effects completely), dye-swap experiments can be done.

There are different ways to introduce the fluorescent dyes into the sample. In a one-step labelling method the markers are introduced by reverse transcription of the mRNA using dye-labelled dCTPs. The samples to be compared are labelled separately, and the resulting cDNAs are pooled after reverse transcription. Since direct integration of the fluorescent dyes is often problematic due to steric hindrance, two-step labelling protocols have been established which first introduce a (smaller) reactive compound into the cDNA, which is subsequently derivatized with fluorescent reagents. Some of these protocols result in increased sensitivity, so that the amount of starting material can be decreased. But on the other hand, these two-step protocols are not as highly reproducible as single-step methods, since they require more reactions (not only enzymatic but also chemical reaction) and purification steps. To monitor the labelling process, the arrays should be provided with positive controls (e.g., control RNAs) positioned at the edges of each quadrant. The respective *in vitro* transcripts can be spiked into each RNA sample so that an effective labelling reaction leads to light signals simultaneously facilitating spatial orientation on the array.

Generally, in investigations of biological repeats, the variance caused by the array experiment itself should be less than the biological variance. This can be easily assessed comparing the results obtained by repeated labelling reactions starting from the same sample and analyzing one array per sample with results obtained from repeated experiments starting from different samples.

If several control samples are accessible for one time point, the extracted RNA should be pooled before starting the labelling, since the biological variation of the control samples could mimic variations between treatments. Pooling of the controls assures that each individual treatment can be compared to an identical control and that the observed differences can be ascribed to (biological) variation of the treatments. To obtain an idea about the biological variability within the controls and to permit statistical approaches such as ANOVA, each control sample can also be hybridized against the pool.

Changes in gene expression can only be assessed against appropriate control samples. As a consequence, it is very important to choose the right control so as to gain valuable data. The best controls are obviously untreated cells or unaffected tissue from the same origin. Before starting a series of experiments, one should be assured that the control samples will be accessible throughout the whole study. If it is impossible to obtain samples of the same origin as the control samples, which may occur when dealing with human material, it would be useful to establish an artificial common reference, for example, by pooling RNA from a set of different cell lines or from a sufficient number of control samples such as normal tissue or mock-treated cell culture. The best approach depends on factors such as accessibility, reproducibility, and coverage (i. e., how many genes are detectable in the control channel). The latter should of course be determined before starting the experiments.

The most cumbersome and critical step for array applications is the hybridization step, in which the labelled target DNA and the affixed probe DNA are brought together. Therefore, this step should be automated whenever possible.

2.3.5 Array Data: Acquisition, Analysis, and Mining

2.3.5.1 Data Acquisition

This section focuses on data acquisition from hybridizations performed with fluorescence-labelled probes.

Data acquisition from microarray experiments consists of two parts: digitalizing the fluorescence signals by using scanning devices and subsequent image analysis using appropriate software packages. To generate digitalized images, two general types of scanner can be used: one approach is based on CCD cameras that generate a picture by exposing the arrays to the complete UV–visible spectrum and collecting the emitted light simultaneously. Signals derived from the respective fluorescence dyes (single channels) can be extracted afterwards. The other system is based on different lasers specific for the extinction of Cy5 or Cy3 dyes; the images for the separate channels can be generated subsequently or even simultaneously. In our experience, it is advisable to use laser-scanning devices due to better resolution in the lower range of signal intensities.

Additional scanning differences are a consequence of the way in which the arrays are scanned. Some devices scan the arrays from the bottom to utilize the refraction of the glass substrate to improve the signal-to-noise ratio. Other suppliers have decided to scan the top of the arrays to avoid problems that occur if the bottom of the slides is even slightly contaminated with dust particles (this is one reason for the appearance of ghost spots).

Depending on the technology utilized for digitalization of the fluorescence signals, the extent of the differences ranges from negligible to significant, especially for signals of lower intensities. The differences between laser scanners are usually restricted to differences in the dynamic range of the expression ratios.

In short, the use of different scanning devices may influence the quantification of spot signals and hence lead to variational ratios. Thus, when analyzing a series of arrays, a single scanner should be used to prevent additional variance.

For quantification of the fluorescence signals, appropriate image analysis software should be used. The market offers many software packages. Important quality features include the abilities to discriminate valid from unwanted signals and to flag empty and negative spots as well as spots of irregular shape or spots having other minor quality features. In addition, algorithms should be included that enable automated spot finding, which is invaluable for quickly optimizing the grid that defines the regions of interest (ROIs = spots). The data output (primary data) should include information about the standard deviation of the spot and the background signals.

2.3.5.2 **Data Analysis**

After the primary data are generated, the ratios of gene expression level have to be calculated and the resulting ratios must be normalized. To include only valid signals in subsequent analysis, several procedures should be performed before starting to calculate the expression ratios. The spot signals should be filtered according to the flags derived from image analysis – only 'good' QC spots should be considered in further analysis. Moreover, the data can be filtered according to negative controls spotted on the individual array (e. g., salmon sperm DNA and buffer), which can be used to define additional thresholds for discriminating unreliable spot signals. Another possibility is to define thresholds according to the average local background of all good QC spots. Usually, background values are subtracted from spot signal intensities to obtain the net spot signal. One method to determine the relative expression of each gene is to compute the Cy5/Cy3 ratios for each spot. These single-spot ratios are normalized following global or intensity-dependent normalization procedures (below) and using only spots for which the fluorescent intensity in one of the channels is at least x times the background signal (x should be dynamically determined for each array from the negative controls/background values). Subsequently, the resulting data for the replicates are averaged. By postponing the averaging to this point in the analysis, it is possible to indicate a coefficient of variation for each ratio. Another possibility that is often implemented in array analysis software is to first average the fluorescence intensities for each gene and then compute the ratios for the respective genes.

Several types of dye effects have to be considered for normalization. Differences occur with respect to the efficiency of integration, which may be mainly (but not solely) influenced by the different solubilities and stereochemical properties of Cy3 and Cy5. This can be accounted for by global normalization methods leading to a linear shift of all signal intensities. If applying global normalization, the median of the single-spot ratios is robust enough for normalization only if most of the detected genes are not regulated. If one is expecting nearly all of the genes to be regulated (this is of special interest when small arrays are used), a set of housekeeping genes should be included to the array configuration. These genes should be chosen carefully, since even genes defined as housekeeping genes are subject to regulation under certain conditions. Moreover, since this method tends to be affected by outliers, the set of housekeeping genes should be large enough to avoid any problems.

In addition to all the methods for global normalization, it is necessary to deal with nonlinear dye effects. Since the wavelength for extinction of Cy3 also induces fluorescence signals from other substances, including SDS, the Cy3 background is usually higher than the Cy5 background. This leads to intensity-dependent effects that may vary from array to array (due to differences in probe labelling efficiency, hybridization conditions, etc.) One efficient nonlinear normalization method is the LOWESS fit originally proposed by Cleveland [11, 12]. The iterative function in LOWESS estimates the normalized value for each spot using the positions of the vicinal spots (parameters have to be defined), weighting them according to the distance from the spot of interest.

Owing to the multiparametric nature of microarray experiments, bioinformatics and data mining represent essential tools for interpretation of the mass of numerical data produced by (series of) microarray experiments. Starting with relatively simple demands for appropriate visualization of the data, bioinformatics tools are necessary to focus on candidate genes and to indicate subtle changes in expression of many genes. Such expression patterns have predictive power but are difficult to spot.

Reliable identification of candidate genes by statistical methods often suffers from a limited number of replicate experiments. Since people are sometimes overwhelmed by the mass of data produced in even a single experiment, they ignore the basic necessity of repeated assays. Biological replicates are essential when one is dealing with expression profiling, especially if subtle changes in gene expression will be used, for example, to define disease states or to distinguish substances by means of their effects on hepatocytes. Based on an appropriate amount of data, classification can be performed by using statistical methods to identify genes characterizing experiment classes. To address this issue, a classification tool has been set up in a first approach at Memorec.

Additional bioinformatics methods, for example, cluster analysis, principal component analysis, or self-organising maps, can be used to identify groups of interesting genes (see the relevant chapters in this book). One method commonly used is hierarchical cluster analysis, by which genes and arrays can be ordered according to similarity in expression behaviour [13]. To screen these results semi-automatically, bioinformatics infrastructures can be used that integrate the knowledge stored in diverse databases, for example, those containing pathway information, genomic localisation, or protein family classification.

2.4
Integrated Approaches Using Microarrays

Changes in gene expression do not necessarily result in proportional changes at the level of protein synthesis or activity. However, there is no doubt that all changes in cellular processes are reflected by altered gene expression. Thus, the field of microarray application seems to be of endless variety. The only point to be discussed is whether (and to what extent) expression analysis should be accompanied by further 'omics' or other conventional analysis methods, which of course depends on the objective of the experiments.

In contrast to investigation of, for example, the activity or amount of different proteins, the measurement of changes in mRNA levels can be done in parallel at high standards of reliability and reproducibility, since differences in the physicochemical properties of mRNA rising from different genes are negligibly low compared to those of the respective gene products.

The actual benefit of microarrays becomes obvious when integrating them into wide approaches that combine traditional methods and gene-expression analysis with the goal of elucidating the molecular mechanisms of actions ultimately responsible for particular phenotypes. These studies may characterize the outcome of treatments or define disease states. However, additional or even new classifications of disease states become conceivable when expression-profiling methodologies are used.

Particularly concerning such integrated approaches, generating many expression profiles means that only the first part of the work is done. In addition, it is necessary to think about how to organize and understand all the data. The bare expression ratios call for scientific interpretation, which is not possible until additional information, at least about the history of each sample, is available. To provide an optimal tool to assess the meaning of the expression profiles, it is advisable to generate databases that hold both the experimental data relating to the probe collection and the hybridization results and which are linked to additional data sources (e. g., SwissProt, UniGene, CAS) in a way that allows for bidirectional queries.

It would be truly best to consider some questions about data storage in advance, since the data that is collected during probe generation (and which may be missing if one tries to collect it retrospectively) should match the needs for, e. g., statistical interpretation.

Another question often discussed in this context is the necessary number of genes per array. In contrast to Memorec's medium- to low-density arrays, some manufacturers supply so-called full-genome arrays (which have to be updated regularly). But investigating genome-wide expression using microarrays is always limited. Here, a genuinely open approach like SAGE would produce better results. Furthermore, the greater the number of genes on an array, the more difficult becomes the identification of specific expression patterns characterizing disease states or treatments. The noise caused by genes that can be measured as expressed but only slightly regulated hampers, for example, meaningful cluster analysis.

Microarrays can be used to find out more about pathophysiological processes, disease states, etc., by comparing, for example, affected tissues with the respective healthy ones. In this context, some substantial questions have to be asked in addition to the usual question regarding the necessary number of samples (which may be simply answered according to the availability of probands). Since complex tissues often consist of a number of different cell types in varying proportions, one should take steps to be assured that the measured differences in gene expression are not merely artefacts caused by comparison of inappropriately matched samples. Hence, for example, standard operating procedures for the extraction of biopsies are advantageous.

Another important application of microarrays is in the field of toxicogenomics and compound profiling [14–17]. Here, *in vitro* and *in vivo* models are used to investigate the (toxic) effects of substances on the level of gene expression. By profiling different substance classes, specific expression patterns can be related to toxic mechanisms. In addition, analysis of altered gene expression correlated with traditional toxic endpoints may help to elucidate the mechanisms of action of various (toxic) substances. The fields of *in vivo–in vitro* correlation and interspecies comparisons of the effects of (toxic) substances can especially be advanced by array applications.

2.5 Combination of Microarrays and SAGE

Recent experience in genomics research has shown that, although a multitude of different technologies are available, none of them offers both true genome coverage and high-throughput applicability. However, the combination of SAGE and PIQOR fulfils most of the requirements for the establishment of molecular disease markers and the search for drug target candidates. SAGE is an open system in which no previous information on observable genes is needed, thus covering the whole genome of every organism. Because of the digital nature of the data, absolute information on percentages of mRNAs can be calculated, simple statistics enable assessment of differentially expressed genes, and SAGE libraries generated in different laboratories can be compared very easily. These distinguishing attributes enable SAGE to be used as a primary discovery tool. On the other hand, SAGE is relatively expensive, especially if high significance is required, and therefore it is not well suited for high numbers of samples. That is where cDNA arrays fit perfectly. Although high-quality arrays are hard to implement for large numbers of genes, medium- to low-density arrays allow probes to be chosen carefully, so as to guarantee the specificity and reproducibility of the hybridization results; such arrays thus have the potential to become an inexpensive standard technology.

References

1. Velculescu, V.E., Zhang L., Vogelstein B. and Kinzler K.W. (**1995**) Serial analysis of gene expression. *Science, 270,* 484–487.
2. Lash, A.E., Tolstoshev C.M., Wagner L., Schuler G.D., Strausberg R.L., Riggins G.J. and Altschul S.F. (**2000**) SAGEmap: a public gene expression resource. *Genome Res, 10,* 1051–1060.
3. Audic, S. and Claverie J.M. (**1997**) The significance of digital gene expression profiles. *Genome Res, 7,* 986–995.
4. Southern, E.M. (**1975**) Detection of specific sequences among DNA fragments separated by gel electrophoresis. *J Mol Biol, 98,* 503–517.
5. Tomiuk, S. and Hofmann K. (**2001**) Microarray probe selection strategies. *Briefings Bioinf, 2,* 329–340.
6. Schena, M., Shalon D., Davis R.W. and Brown P.O. (**1995**) Quantitative monitoring of gene expression patterns with a complementary DNA microarray (*see* comments). *Science, 270,* 467–470.
7. Bosio, A., Stoffel W. and Stoffel M. (**1999**) Device for the parallel identification and quantification of polynucleic acids, *EP0965647.* Memorec Stoffel GmbH, Cologne, Germany.
8. O'Donnell-Maloney, M.J., Smith C.L. and Cantor C.R. (**1996**) The development of microfabricated arrays for DNA sequencing and analysis. *Trends Biotechnol, 14,* 401–407.
9. Bosio, A., Knorr C., Janssen U., Gebel S., Haussmann H.J. and Muller T. (**2002**) Kinetics of gene expression profiling in Swiss 3T3 cells exposed to aqueous extracts of cigarette smoke. *Carcinogenesis, 23,* 741–748.
10. Eberwine, J. (**1996**) Amplification of mRNA populations using aRNA generated from immobilized oligo(dT)-T7 primed cDNA. *BioTechniques, 20,* 584–591.
11. Yang, Y.H., Dudoit S., Luu P., Lin D.M., Peng V., Ngai J. and Speed T.P. (**2002**) Normalization for cDNA microarray data: a robust composite method addressing single and multiple slide systematic variation. *Nucleic Acids Res, 30,* e15.
12. Cleveland, W.S. (**1979**) Robust locally weighted regression and smoothing scatterplots. *J Am Stat Assoc, 74,* 829–836.
13. Eisen, M.B., Spellman P.T., Brown P.O. and Botstein D. (**1998**) Cluster analysis and display of genome-wide expression patterns. *Proc Natl Acad Sci USA, 95,* 14863–14868.
14. Farr, S., Dunn, R. T. II (**1999**) Gene expression applied to toxicology. *Toxicol Sci, 50,* 1–9.
15. Waring, J. F., Jolly, R. A., Ciurlionis, R., Lum, P. Y., Praestgaard, J. T., Morfitt, D. C., Buratto, B., Roberts, C., Schadt, E., and Ulrich, R. G. (**2001**) Clustering of hepatotoxins based on mechanism of toxicity using gene expression profiles. *Toxicol Appl Pharmacol, 175,* 28–42.
16. Pennie, W. D. (**2000**) Use of cDNA microarrays to probe and understand the toxicological consequences of altered gene expression. *Toxicol Lett, 12–113,* 473–477.
17. Peddada, S. D., Lobenhofer, E. K., Li, L., Afshari, C. A., Weinberg, C. R., and Umbach, D. M. (**2003**) Gene selection and clustering for time-course and dose–response microarray experiments using order-restricted inference. *Bioinformatics, 19,* 834–841.

3
Oligo Arrays, Global Transcriptome Analysis

Jacques Retief, Earl Hubbell, and David Finkelstein

3.1
Introduction to GeneChip® Microarray Technology

3.1.1
Introduction to RNA Expression Microarrays

Recent years have seen a rapid adoption of gene expression profiling in the field of toxicology – an application broadly referred to as toxicogenomics. This development comes at an opportune time, when toxicology has increasingly become a limiting step in the drug development process. By identifying successful drug candidates earlier in the drug development pipeline, toxicogenomics promises to improve the efficiency of toxicology studies and the drug development process as a whole (Nuwaysir et al. 1999; Burczynski et al. 2000; Aardema and MacGregor 2002; Ulrich and Friend 2002; Scheel et al. 2003). In the second half of this section we will discuss new DNA genotyping microarrays and the potential impact of toxicogenetics.

A critical hypothesis in toxicogenomics is that altered gene expression is one of the earliest measurable responses to a toxic challenge (Dunn and Kolaja 2003). To translate this hypothesis into an application with high quality and accuracy, we need robust experimental design and a thorough understanding of the technology. Expression microarray technologies are based on nucleotide strands attached to a substrate. These can be broadly divided into long cDNA clones or short oligonucleotides. Increasingly, oligonucleotides are seen as more specific and reliable than cDNA clones for expression profiling (Li and Johnson 2003). In this section we focus on the unique characteristics that distinguish the Affymetrix GeneChip® technology from other microarray methods.

3.1.2
GeneChip® RNA Expression Microarray Technology

A microarray is not just a chip, but part of a complete system including the array construction, assay, array design, scanner, washing station, analysis software, and functional annotation of the sequences. All these elements operate in the context of

Handbook of Toxicogenomics: Strategies and Applications. Edited by Jürgen Borlak

ISBN: 3-527-30342-1

the experimental design, quality control, and data analysis. Each component contributes to the performance of the system as a whole.

3.1.2.1 GeneChip® Microarray Construction

A detailed description of GeneChip® microarray construction is available at http://www.affymetrix.com/technology/manufacturing/(Fodor et al. 1991, 1993). The oligonucleotides synthesized on the surface of the chip are called the *probes* because they are used to interrogate or 'probe' the sample. Each probe is synthesized in many identical copies in designated regions of the array called *features*.

The light-directed synthesis is carried out in a series of chemical steps that begins with the attachment of synthetic linkers modified with photochemically removable protecting groups. Light passes through open regions of a mask where it activates or deprotects exposed linkers. A hydroxyl-protected deoxynucleoside is then flushed into the synthesis chamber and incubated with the surface. Chemical coupling of the deoxynucleoside with the linker occurs at the deprotected sites. The chemical coupling is followed by a capping step that acylates uncoupled active sites. After the capping step, the next in the series of masks is aligned, and the process is repeated until the probes are synthesized to full length. The manufacturing process ends with a comprehensive series of quality control tests.

A key feature of the synthesis is the parallel nature of the process. Within each array, up to 1.5×10^6 probes are synthesized in parallel in a small number of steps.

Implications

1. No cloning, spotting, or polymerase chain reaction (PCR) steps are required; consequently, the sequence of each probe molecule on the array is known. The synthesis is monitored by a synthesis fidelity feature that is built into the array and checked during manufacturing.
2. Due to the parallel nature of the GeneChip microarray synthesis process, the synthesis efficiency of all the probes is similar. This allows the use of a single colour stain, which simplifies experimental design, data interpretation, and evaluation of historical data (these points are further discussed in subsequent sections). In contrast, when oligonucleotides are mechanically spotted, controls are required to compensate for variation in spot deposition. These takes the form of an internal standard and two dyes, usually CY-3 and CY-5, one for a standard and one for the sample. The incorporation efficiency of the two dyes is not equivalent, so a dye-reversal experiment needs to be carried out for every sample.
3. Owing to the precision of the photolithographic process, no correction is needed for misshapen features.
4. The signal value produced by single-colour experiments is a single, not a relative, value. This is similar to typical toxicology laboratory data, which makes it easy to integrate GeneChip microarrays into standard data analysis pipelines and databases.

5. Single-colour measurements are robust against small effects that destabilize measurements of ratios. In other words, if a transcript is undetectable in the control but expressed in the experiment, it is very difficult to calculate an accurate ratio.

6. The compact size of the array allows the use of high-quality fused silica as a substrate, which substantially reduces background fluorescence and thus improves the sensitivity of detection.

7. Scanning at a single wavelength avoids problems with different fluorescence backgrounds. The wavelength at which an array is scanned produces a characteristic fluorescence background. When two wavelengths are used for scanning, two different backgrounds are produced. For accurate comparisons when two wavelengths are used, the differences in the background need to be corrected (Martinez et al. 2003).

8. Even though the synthesis efficiency is high, not all probes are completely synthesized. If a synthesis step is incomplete for a specific probe, the probe is capped. Such capped probes cannot proceed to the following synthesis steps and are therefore truncated. This reduces the potential for nonspecific hybridization.

9. Primers that are mechanically spotted and directly linked to the substrate have limited freedom to hybridize. In contrast, the *in situ* synthesized probes on GeneChip arrays are attached at the 3′ end by a linker to the substrate. This reduces steric hindrance and allows an optimum conformation for hybridization (Figure 3.1).

3.1.2.2 **Array Design**

Two core elements of the array design are the Perfect Match–Mismatch probe strategy and the use of several probes, called a probeset, to represent a single transcript.

Perfect Match–Mismatch

The Perfect Match–Mismatch probe strategy requires that, for each probe designed to match a target sequence, a partner probe is generated that is identical except for a single base mismatch in its centre. These probe pairs are called the Perfect Match probe (PM) and the Mismatch probe (MM). The MM probe is used to determine in-

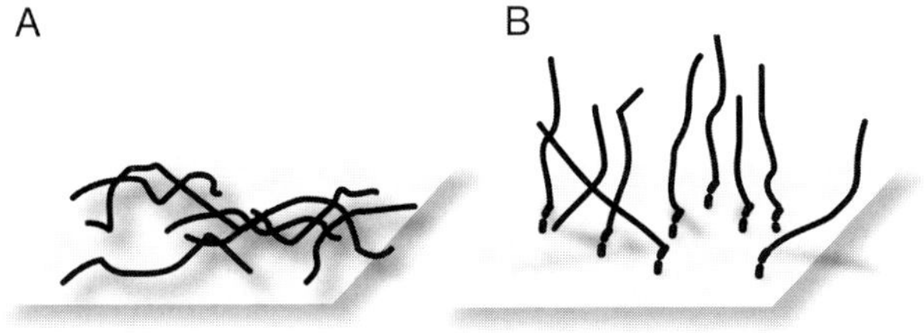

Fig. 3.1 (A) DNA probe sequences deposited on a substrate have limited freedom to hybridize. (B) *In situ* synthesized probes are bound to the substrate via a linker that prevents steric effects during the hybridization reaction.

tensity due to nonspecific cross-hybridization, which can then be subtracted from the overall intensity. The difference in hybridization signals between the partner probes, as well as their intensity ratios, serve as indicators of specific target abundance. The actual calculations are described in http://www.affymetrix.com/support/technical/whitepapers/sadd_whitepaper.pdf.

Implications

1. The benefits of the PM–MM strategy are not readily apparent in the absence of known transcript concentrations. At moderate to high transcript concentrations, the additional measurement produced by the MM probe adds noise, and the combined PM–MM measurements are slightly noisier than with PM alone. However, at low transcript concentrations using the MM probe is a significant benefit, because it allows an accurate background subtraction for each probe, which allows more accurate measurements at low concentrations. This effectively extends the dynamic range of the system (Figure 3.2).
2. The MM probes occupy approximately 50% of the area of the array, which limits the number of transcripts that can be represented on a single array. Several strategies have been published to eliminate or reduce the number of MM probes used (Irizarry et al. 2003). At present none have been widely adopted, and the PM–MM probe strategy remains the most robust and sensitive approach to determining transcript concentrations accurately at low concentration.
3. The PM–MM strategy determines the probe length, because shorter probes can be more reliably destabilized with a single-base mismatch.

Probeset Design

Each transcript is represented by 11 to 16 probe pairs. Each probe pair consists of a PM and an MM probe. The intensity values produced by each probe are combined within a probeset to produce a signal value. A description of the algorithm is available at http://www.affymetrix.com/support/technical/whitepapers/sadd_whitepaper.pdf

Implications

1. The signal value is robust against individual probe performance. Probes occasionally hybridize nonspecifically or poorly for various reasons. The signal calculation contains strategies to limit the effect of abnormally performing (outlier) probes. For example, the signal calculation is based on a median. Therefore, as long as more than half of the probe pairs behave well, the signal values are not affected significantly.

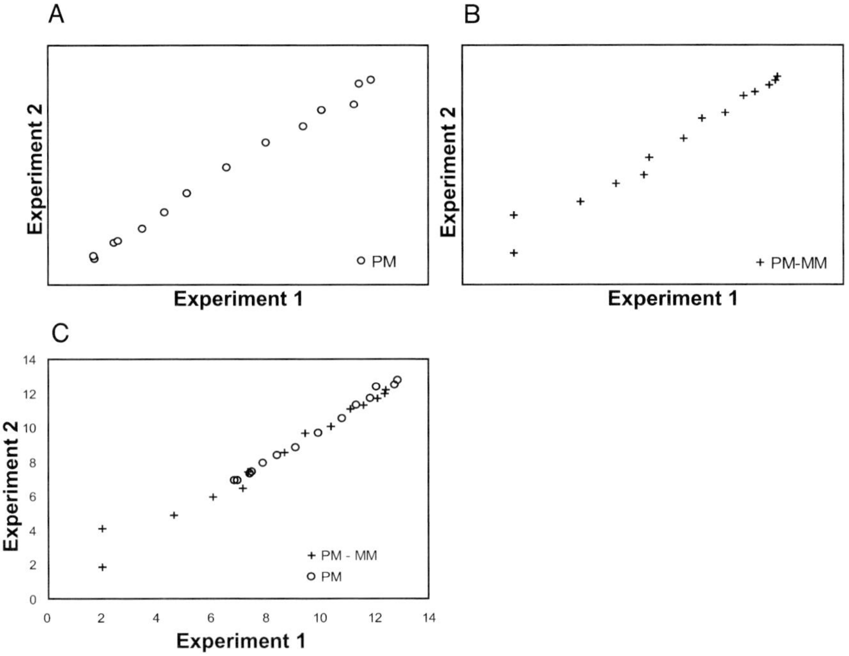

Fig. 3.2 The use of mismatch probes extends the linear range of measurements, especially at low concentrations. The use of scatter plots to display sample variation between experiments and among technologies can be misleading. These plots represent several measurements of the same gene at different concentrations on a series of HG_U95 arrays. The sample contains complex tissue as background. The gene is not detected in the tissue used, and known concentrations of the cloned gene were added to the sample. The experiment was repeated and the two experiments are compared in scatter plots. (A) Signal calculated for PM probes only and the variation between the two experiments displayed as a scatter plot. (B) Signal calculated for PM–MM probes and the variation between the two experiments displayed as a scatter plot. On the surface, it appears that PM probes behave better and have less noise than do PM–MM probes, but when the two datasets are plotted on the same scale (C) it becomes clear that the use of MM probes extends the sensitivity of the detection appreciably. However, in typical microarray experiments without known values, this effect tends to be obscured. These results are typical for human genes and for genes in other organisms that have been studied in this way. Datasets in which the concentrations of some probes are known are available at http://www.affymetrix.com/analysis/download_center2.affx and http://www.stat.berkeley.edu/users/terry/zarray/Affy/affy_index.html.

2. Detection is robust against point mutations. The probes making up a probeset are usually distributed over an approximately 600-bp region. For a mutation to disrupt the hybridization of a probe, the mutation needs to be located near the centre of the probe. This limits the number of bases within a probeset at which mutations can affect probe hybridization (Figure 3.3). In addition, due to the robust nature of the signal calculation (mentioned in point 1), hybridization of almost half of the probes must be disrupted before signal values are severely affected.

3. Detection is robust against insertions. Small insertions have very little effect on probeset performance, because at most, only one probe is affected by an insertion (Figure 3.3). However, the labelling reaction is biased towards the 3′ end of the transcript. If an insert is very large and at the 3′ end of the transcript, the 5′ end of the probeset is presumably not labelled and the performance of the probeset suffers. When clean, intact RNA is used in the labelling reaction, longer transcripts are labelled, which limits this effect.

4. Detection is highly specific. Since a single base difference can destabilize a probe, probesets can be selected to specifically distinguish between transcripts from different gene family members. This is particularly useful in toxicogenomics, where many of the toxicological responses are from very closely related gene family members, such as members of the CYP gene family. It has been demonstrated that the expression of individual genes within cytochrome P-450 gene subfamilies with up to ~90% DNA identities could be distinguished (Gerhold et al. 2001).

5. The array design can be tuned for sensitivity. By increasing or decreasing the number of probe pairs in each probeset, the confidence with which the signal value is determined can be controlled. For example, if a transcript is expressed at a high level, very few probe pairs are needed. However, if a transcript is expressed at a low level, more probe pairs enable us to reliably distinguish the low signal from noise. The number of probe pairs used in every commercial array design is selected to give the best performance over the widest range of transcript levels.

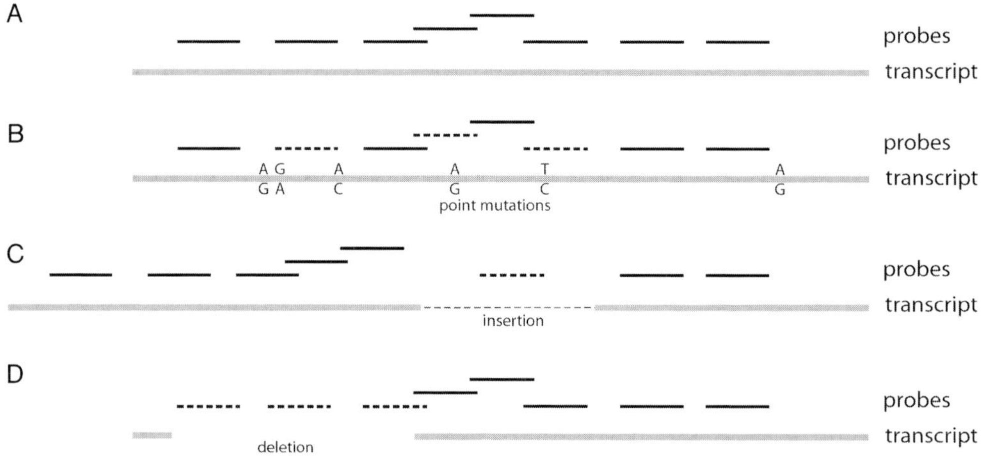

Fig. 3.3 (A) A typical probeset with probes distributed at the 3′ end of the gene. Probeset performance is stable if fewer than half of the probes are adversely affected. (B) Point mutations have little effect on the performance of the probeset. To completely corrupt the performance of a probeset, the gene must have point mutations close to the centre of the majority of probes in the probeset. (C) Small insertions have very little effect on probeset performance. (D) Deletions have very little effect on probeset performance, as long as the majority of the probes in the probeset remain.

6. Probe pairs are not adjacent on the array, but distributed, to ensure that signal values are robust against small local defects on the array.

The Labelling Reaction

The labelling reaction is described in detail in the GeneChip® Expression Analysis Technical Manual at http://www.affymetrix.com/support/technical/manual/expression_ manual.affx. This section highlights aspects that affect data analysis.

Labelling starts at the polyadenylation site at the 3′ end of the transcript. The quality of the RNA and the efficiency of the labelling reaction determine how far the labelling extends toward the 5′ end of the transcript. For many genes, the polyadenylation sites are some distance from the coding regions. In such genes a large part, or all, of the probeset is located in the 3′ untranslated region (UTR) of the gene. The 3′ bias affects array design and data analysis.

Implications

1. To ensure the best performance over a wide range of RNA qualities, the probes are selected within a 600-bp region from the polyadenylation site.
2. The polyadenylation site needs to be determined accurately. When polyadenylation sites are ambiguous or when there is evidence for more than one polyadenylation site, a probeset is synthesized for each potential site. This strategy improves detection of different polyadenylated isoforms but causes redundancy in the probesets. This redundancy should be accounted for in the data analysis, especially because it violates the statistical assumption that probesets behave independently.
3. Noncoding regions, such as UTRs, evolve relatively rapidly. Probesets that are designed against such regions may be able to distinguish between gene family members or splice variants for which the protein products are highly similar.
4. The detection is insensitive to changes at the 5′ end of the gene.
5. Mapping proteins, as opposed to transcript sequences, between different organisms or technologies may not be accurate, because the probesets do not necessarily represent the coding region of the gene.
6. Transcripts, such as mitochondrial RNA, that do not contain polyadenylation sites are not labelled by the specific labelling reaction.
7. The labelling reaction consists of a number of steps and is, next to the biology, the biggest source of variability. Establishing standard operating procedures (SOPs) within a laboratory can greatly reduce data variability due to the operator.

Sequence Selection

In situ synthesized oligonucleotide arrays can potentially represent any sequence in the genome. The challenge is therefore to organize the millions of known sequences in the public databases to accurately represent the whole transcriptome. The strategies used to curate and select the sequences affect data analysis and interpretation.

For assays of eukaryotic organisms, such as humans, mouse, and rat, expressed sequences from databases – including GenBank, RefSeq, and dbEST – are collected and clustered into groups of similar sequences. Using clusters provided by the UniGene database as a starting point, sequences are further subdivided into subclusters representing distinct transcripts. The reclustering of the UniGene sequences compensates for a known problem, that UniGene clusters sometimes contain more than one distinct gene. Clustering is also improved by using primary sequence information, when available. This categorization process involves alignment to the human genome, which reveals splicing and polyadenylation variants. The alignment also extends the annotation information supplied by the databases pinpointing low-quality sequences. These can be trimmed for the subsequent generation of high-quality consensus sequences. Alternatively, quality ranking can be used to select representative sequences, called exemplars, for probe design. The 5′ to 3′ orientation of each transcript is confirmed by identification of splice signals, polyadenylation sites, and polyadenylation signals. If the orientation cannot be determined with high confidence due to contradictory information, then the probes for both strands are generated.

Implications

1. The clustering used for probe selection is not exactly the same as in any single public source such as UniGene, but is instead based on a comprehensive set of public information. Also, the UniGene databases are constantly being updated, so the current version may not match the version used for the array design. The UniGene links provided with the data should therefore be considered as a guide and confirmed by sequence comparison. The sequences used for probe selection and those of the probes are available on the web at www.affymetrix.com.
2. There are many-to-many relationships between GenBank accession numbers and probesets. A single DNA GenBank accession number may be polycistronic and have many genes associated with it. In addition, more than one probeset may be designed to detect a single gene. This is often necessary if there are indications of more than one polyadenylation site or if the orientation of the gene is uncertain. In some instances, a single probeset may have more than one gene mapped to it, such as occurs in closely related gene families. This many-to-many relationship between probesets and accession numbers causes any simple mapping between probesets and accession numbers to miss potentially important associations. The only certain way to map between sequences and probesets is to use a sequence comparison of the sequences used to tile the probesets. A sequence search function based on BLAST is available in the NetAffx™ Analysis Center on the Internet.
3. Many statistical algorithms make the assumption that measurements are independent. When more than one probeset represent the same gene, the measurements are not truly independent. This usually leads to a very small error when considering a complete array, but may become more of an issue when smaller groups of probesets are considered. Biological processes and genes usually behave in concert; consequently, gene measurements are rarely completely independent.

Probe Selection

In addition to choosing probes based on their predicted hybridization properties, candidate sequences are selected for specificity. Their potential for cross-hybridizing with similar but unrelated sequences is evaluated. Probes are 3′-biased to match the target-generation characteristics of the sample amplification method, but they are also widely spaced to sample various regions of each transcript and to provide robustness of detection.

Implications

1. A primary criterion for probe selection is a linear response to changes in transcript concentration. Usually these probes are not the tightest binding or 'brightest'. Very 'bright' probes, usually with a higher GC content, may be desirable for determining low abundance transcripts or for RT–PCR. However, these probes tend to saturate quickly at higher transcript concentrations, which affects the specificity and linear response of the probe.
2. During the design of a whole-genome array, probes are checked for cross hybridization against the complete transcriptome. In the process, potentially useful probes may be excluded, because not all transcripts are expressed in a typical experiment. For example, we would not expect to see the expression of brain-specific genes in the liver. This conservative strategy is very effective in limiting cross hybridization in a typical experiment and protects against incorrect or incomplete prior information.

3.1.2.3 Hybridization and Wash Stations

The GeneChip system includes an automated software-controlled hybridization and wash station, called the fluidics station.

Implications

1. Controlled washing and staining are critical for achieving reproducible data.
2. The washing station processes four arrays at a time. Three runs or 12 arrays is the practical limit of the number of arrays that can be processed in one day with a single wash station. This is often the limiting step in array processing. Several washing stations can be attached to a scanner to improve throughput.

3.1.3 Biological Annotations

When expression changes in transcripts are linked to biological knowledge, it becomes valuable to the biologist. Annotations provide the links between a transcript and its associated biological processes. These associations are derived from the literature, public databases such as GenBank, and computationally derived annotations. Derived annotations are necessary for organisms such as the rat, for which directly relevant annotations are rare. Despite this, it is remarkable that an estimated equivalent of 45 000 typed pages of annotations is supplied with the rat 230A array. These annotations are available at the NetAffx™ Analysis Center, a publicly accessible website (www.NetAffx.com). The site is also linked to the Analysis Center at www.affymetrix.com. The following is not a comprehensive review of the contents of the NetAffx™ but a guide to some of its most useful functions for toxicogenomics research.

3.1.3.1 NetAffx™ Analysis Center

The NetAffx™ Analysis Center has been described in detail elsewhere (Liu et al. 2003) and extensive documentation is available at https://www.affymetrix.com/support/technical/whitepapers.affx. Functionally the databases can be divided into nucleotide and peptide databases (Figure 3.4).

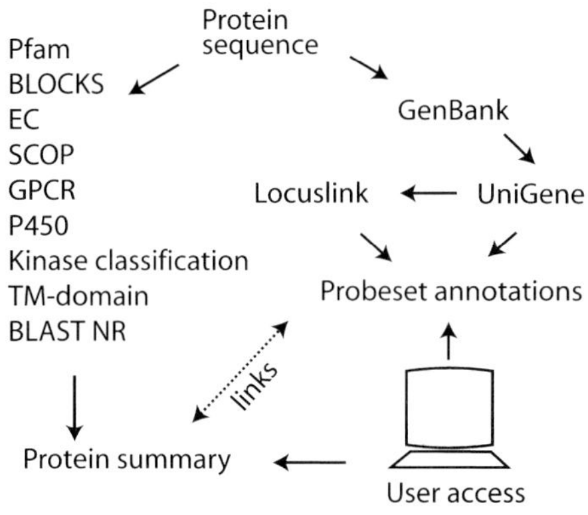

Fig. 3.4 Schematic of annotations available in the NetAffx™ Analysis Center.

Nucleotide Information

The following is a brief list of functions available from NetAffx™:

- View and download probe, target, and consensus/exemplar sequences.
- Search Affymetrix GeneChip® microarray databanks using numerous search terms – including gene names, probe set IDs, and accession numbers (Figure 3.5).
- Visualize alignment of probe sets relative to Affymetrix consensus sequences.
- Batch-query search GeneChip® arrays using gene names, probe set IDs, and accession numbers.
- Use the probe match tool to search for perfect matches between your query sequence and the probe sequences on GeneChip® arrays.
- The download centre allows you to download GeneChip® array sequence files, including probe sequences for efficient integration with your data analysis pipelines.

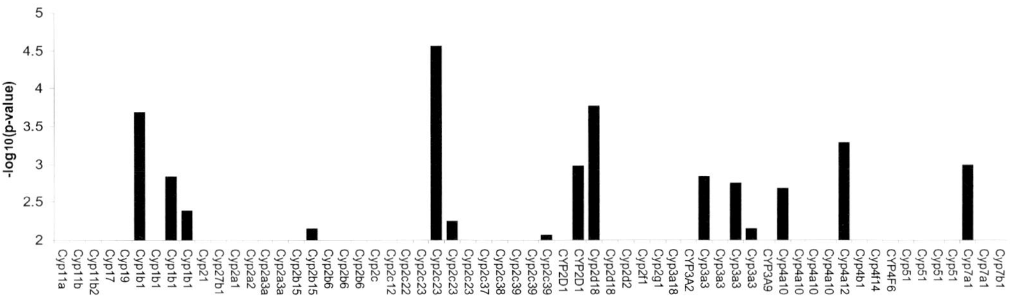

Fig. 3.5 Toxicological response of the CYP gene family on RG_U34A. The *y* axis is based on the confidence of the transcript response. The *x* axis is based on a list of probesets for which the gene name contains 'CYP'. The query was performed in NetAffx™. The appearance of multiple probesets reflects the conservative tiling strategy, where potential polyadenylation sites and splice variants are synthesized. This complex response is difficult to predict and is made evident only thanks to the data accessed from NetAffx™.

Implications

1. Probe sequences on the arrays are the only truly stable information related to the signal. All other annotations are derived from sequence matches such as BLAST searches. As more sequences are added to the databases, more matches may be discovered. Sequence errors, and increasingly frequently, splice variants may become apparent in time. Access to probe sequences is critical to validate derived annotations.
2. Access to probe sequence information makes it possible to verify transcription changes by other methods, such as RT–PCR.
3. The databases underlying the NetAffx™ Analysis Center are updated quarterly. In any long-term project a researcher should repeat searches on NetAffx™ to ensure that the information is up to date.
4. NetAffx is a web-based tool and subject to the security issues associated with the Internet. All scientific data transferred to and from the NetAffx™ Analysis Center is encrypted during transmission by the Secure Sockets Layer (SSL) communications protocol. This industry-standard Internet security protocol, using a level of encryption similar to that used for Internet banking and online credit card transactions, ensures that data is protected while in transit. If security is a concern, data can be batch downloaded for integration into your own database.

GenMAPP

The single most important contribution of genomics to toxicology is the rapid identification of mechanisms of toxicity, knowledge of which provides insight into potential drug–drug interactions. These mechanisms may also indicate which animal models and metabolic pathways should be targeted for further investigation. Deductions require links between expression profiles and functional annotations. A visualization tool is required to gain insight (Figure 3.6). The best known repository of

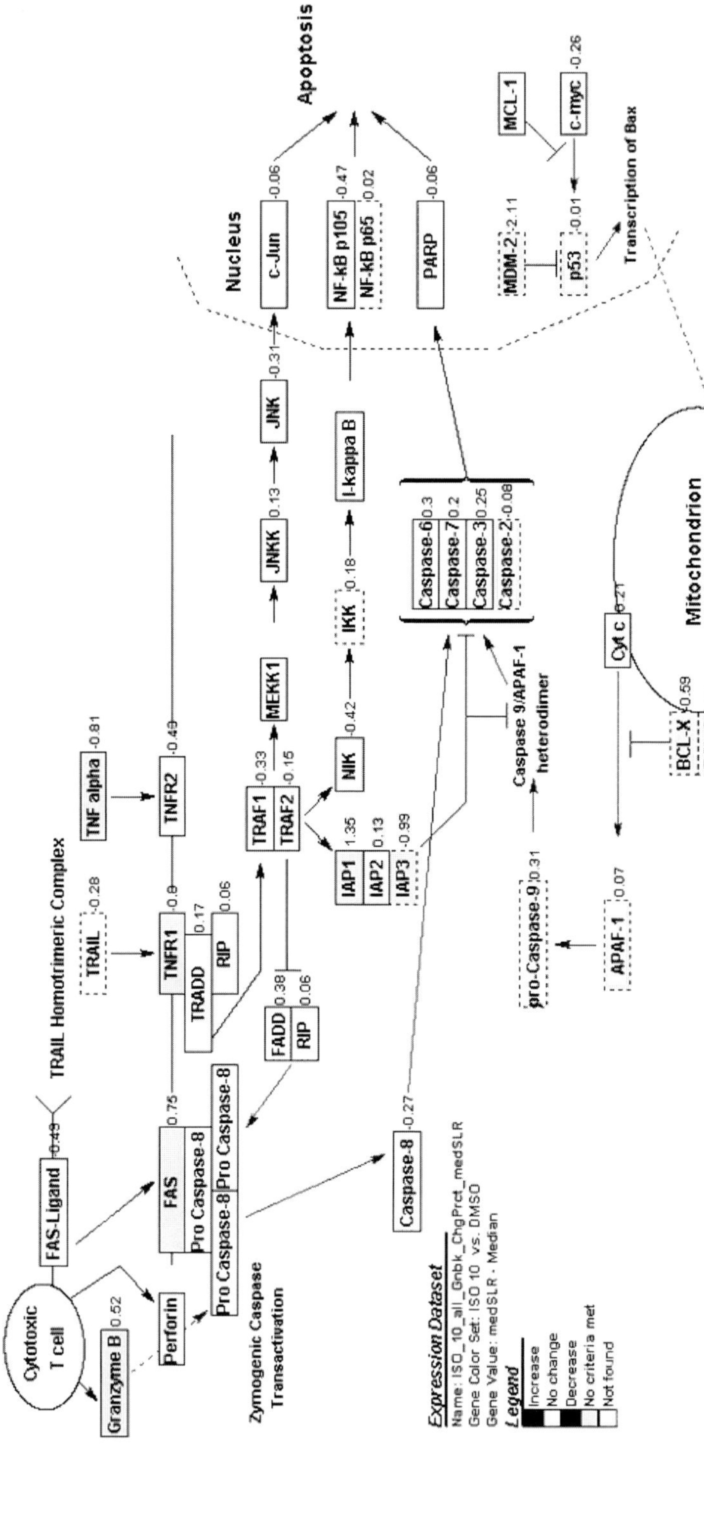

Fig. 3.6 GenMAPP provides a detailed view of the apoptosis pathway shaded according to changes in expression.

functional information is the KEGG database (Ogata et al. 1998; Nakao et al. 1999; Ogata et al. 1999; Kanehisa and Goto 2000; Kanehisa 2002; Kanehisa et al. 2002). Many of the KEGG gene functions are available in GenMAPP (Gene MicroArray Pathway Profiler), which is a computer application designed to visualize gene expression data on maps representing biological pathways and groupings of genes (www.genmapp.org) (Dahlquist et al. 2002; Doniger et al. 2003).

Implications

1. Linking expression profiles to a biological pathway that elucidates a mechanism of action is the ideal outcome of a microarray experiment.
2. Relatively few pathways are fully annotated in GenMAPP. Annotations should improve over time as more information becomes available.
3. The view of a pathway is highly focused and does not give an overview of all the reactions in the cell. Ontologies are better at providing an overview. A practical strategy for biological interpretation is to begin with a broad overview, such as an ontology, and to use the results as a guide to focus on a specific pathway.

Gene Ontologies

The use of function annotations, such as gene ontologies (GO) (Ashburner et al. 2000), provides a cohesive structure and a controlled vocabulary to extract information from an expression experiment. An ontology can be considered a summary of all prior functional knowledge about a gene. Ontologies represent more than a single pathway and provide an overview of all the processes in the cell in a single view (Figure 3.7). In toxicogenomics this characteristic is particularly valuable, because it can alert the investigator to an unexpected response. Once a response is identified, more detailed views of specific pathways, such as those provided by KEGG and GenMAPP, can be used for further investigation. Large toxicogenomic databases offer an opportunity to validate the use of ontologies. It is likely that ontologies will increasingly be used to predict off-target effects and toxic effects.

Implications

1. Side effects may be predicted based on function. In other words, we may begin to understand the mechanism of toxicity even if that mechanism is completely new and not represented in the database.
2. Annotations provide insight into mechanism of action. Once we postulate a mechanism of action we can predict potential risks. Then, by focusing on the appropriate biological models, we can confirm the mechanism and evaluate the risks. A detailed knowledge of the mechanism of action is highly desirable for regulatory approval.

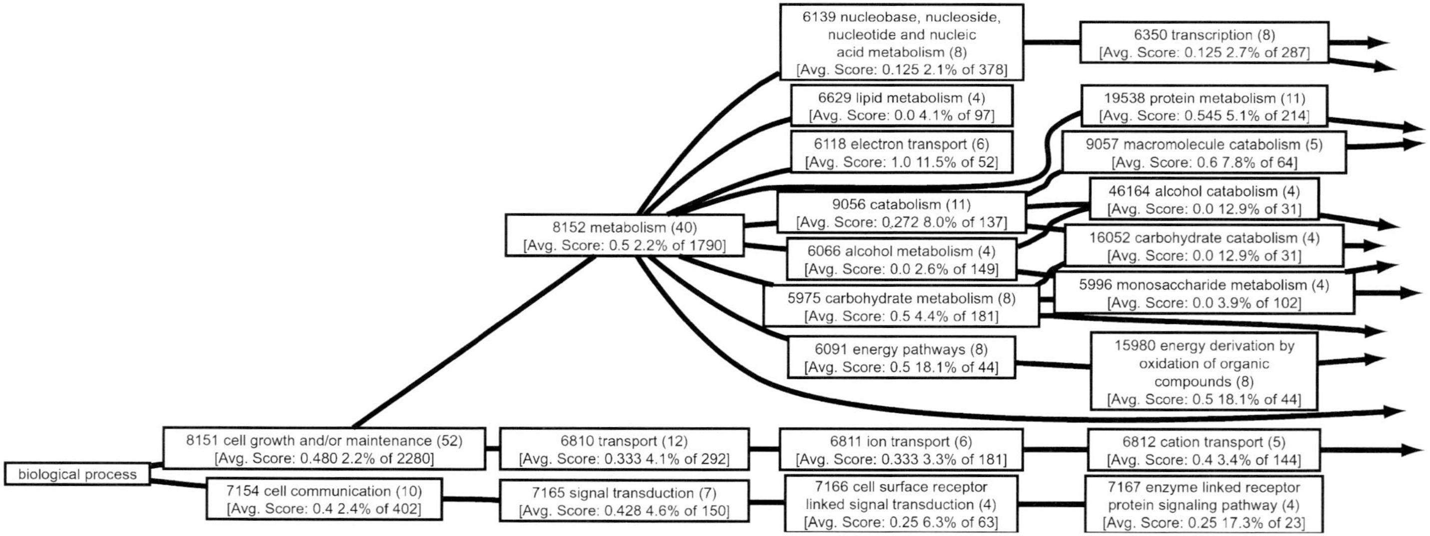

Fig. 3.7 Gene ontology figures are drawn from the most general category on the left to progressively more specific categories on the right. The quality and specificity of the results are reflected in the length of the branches. For example, a very general category represents many probesets. We expect a certain number of probes to match such a general category purely by chance. As we proceed to the right, the categories represent fewer probesets and are more specific. It is much less likely for a group of probesets to match such a small category by chance. This is reflected in the percentage value, which tends to increase to the right. The arrows pointing to the right indicate more specific categories that are not shown.

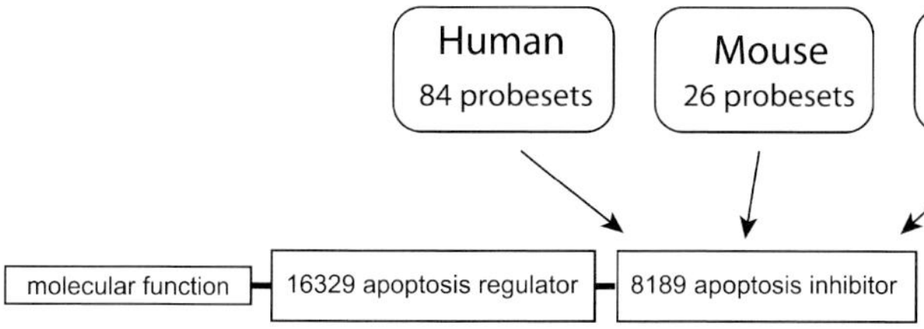

Fig. 3.8 Functional annotations facilitate biological interpretation across models. In this example, the molecular function 'apoptosis inhibitor' can be seen regardless of the animal model in use. This strategy avoids the difficulties of mapping probe sequences between models.

3. Knowledge of biological functions is transferable between biological models. It is very difficult to relate expression patterns to a different animal strain or even to a different animal genus without functional knowledge. Sequence-level mapping between models, such as human and mouse, is provided in NetAffx™. Such low-level mapping is very useful when conserved biological pathways are compared between animal models. When the biological pathways are divergent between the animal models, sequence-level comparison is often not possible. A high-level functional annotation can be helpful, because biological function tends to be conserved even when sequences are not (Figure 3.8) (Pearson 1996; Retief et al. 1999).
4. Not all the transcripts represented on an array have known functional annotations. Conversely, many genes are represented by more than one probeset. These conditions create a technical bias in the GO trees.
5. An ontology, like any literature search, is based on current knowledge and therefore subject to current biases. Fortunately, gene ontologies externalize biases. That is, unlike a personal bias, which cannot be easily measured or corrected, GO provides a structure in which the bias can be easily recognized (Kim and Falkow 2003). In a literature search it is natural to focus on the one or two functional categories that are of interest. The converse is more problematic: ignoring transcripts that are unexplained. Unexplained changes in expression are rarely reported, yet may indicate an unexpected toxic response. Gene ontologies help broaden our focus by displaying an overview of the significant functional categories that may otherwise be ignored.
6. Gene ontologies provide context. For example, if a given gene description is not recognized by itself, it may be recognized in the context of the GO hierarchy.
7. Xenobiotic functions are not explicitly mapped. Pathological responses to toxins are often recruited from normal biological processes. Since the normal biological process is mapped, it remains for the operator to judge when a response is pathological. For example, the well known cytochrome P450 phase 1 toxicological response genes are mapped under the biological function of electron transport.

Improving GO Interpretation with Statistics

Biological interpretation is often subjective but can be made more objective by incorporating statistical methods. Statistics tests examine specific hypotheses and summarize the significance with a *p* value. These *p* values guide the interpretation of analytical results. Several statistical methods can be used to test the significance of a GO node or function.

Implications

1. Concordance tests between a list of probesets and the list of genes within a node are very flexible. Typically, a concordance test either uses a chi-square approximation to the *p* value or a finds an exact probability through a computationally intensive procedure (Zeeberg et al. 2003). These approaches take into account the possibility that this event may occur purely by chance, which is difficult to assess without statistical guidance.

2. Some methods incorporate probeset scores (–log (*p* value)) derived from an experiment. For example, they may sum the probeset scores of all probesets associated with a GO node. The significance of this sum can then be evaluated by meta-analytic methods such as Fisher's method.

3. Bootstrap or permutation methods are another flexible means of evaluating the significance of scores. These methods allow the evaluation of any reasonable node score against the null hypothesis that this score occurred simply by chance. These methods indicate the relative significance of all nodes within the tree. This practical approach allows us to focus on the appropriate level of detail.

4. Statistical tests are valid if their assumptions fit the data. For example, many statistical tests assume that transcript profiles are independent. In reality, transcripts are frequently coregulated. Statistical tests are sensitive and powerful tools for detecting deviations from 'chance' assumptions, but judgment is still required to evaluate these results in a biological context.

5. The use of annotations in conjunction with expression profiles allow us to build more sophisticated statistical models. For example, if we know that two transcripts are functionally related, that knowledge can become *a priori* in a Bayesian model, because the coregulation is more significant than the regulation of one transcript by itself.

Peptide Information

Proteins are the functional manifestation of the genes represented on the array. When possible, the sequences of the proteins associated with the transcripts are provided in NetAffx™. Standard PFAM and BLOCKS motif annotations and BLASTp (Altschul et al. 1997) similarity searches are also included within NetAffx™. These standard-motif–based recognition systems annotate only approximately 51% of the human proteome (Lander et al. 2001). To provide more extensive information the

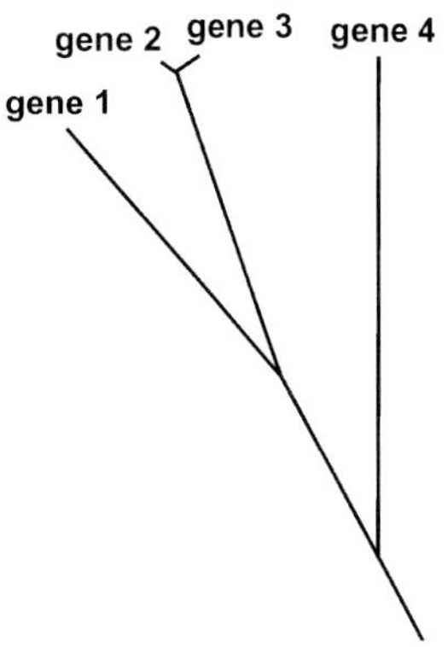

Fig. 3.9 Phylogenetic distances between genes having similar expression profiles. In this example, four transcripts with similar expression patterns were identified by clustering and examined for functional relationships. The protein sequences associated with the transcripts were aligned with ClustalX, and phylogenetic distances were measured with PHYLIP at http://evolution.genetics.washington.edu/phylip.html (Retief 2000). Genes 2 and 3 are more closely related than genes 1 and 4. It is assumed that these distances reflect the similarities in protein function. Such an assumption can form the basis for further testing.

high-level Structural Classification of Proteins (SCOP) is included, which represents domains in the Protein Databank (PDB) based on a hierarchical structure of evolutionary relatedness (Murzin et al. 1995). The SCOP classifications are created at Affymetrix and described in detail at http://www.affymetrix.com/support/technical/whitepapers/scop_whitepaper.pdf. The goal is to provide protein family-level annotations that allow classification of probesets based on protein structure and function.

Implications

1. Peptides provide information on previously uncharacterized genes. By comparing protein sequences we can establish the relationships among gene family members or among closely related genes (Figure 3.9). Since proteins with similar sequences often have similar structures and hence functions, we can use this strategy to characterize new genes (Pearson 1996; Wood and Pearson 1999).
2. Functional elements can be found directly. Protein functional elements from databases such as PFAM, BLOCKS, and EC and many others can be searched directly. For example, it may be possible to find a functional element in common with co-expressed genes.
3. Enzyme Commission (EC) numbers classify enzymes based on the type of reaction catalyzed, substrate, and reagents/cofactors. Apart from the functional information, these numbers provide a controlled vocabulary to link the array information to other platforms and technologies. For example, EC numbers can be used to relate microarray results to data obtained from two-dimensional proteomic gels.

3.1.4 Conclusions

Microarray design involves a series of choices to capture the breadth of the genome while maintaining transcript specificity and reproducibility. The unique characteristics of Affymetrix GeneChip® probeset design and probeset selection have implications that influence data analysis and experimental design. Using this information along with a careful experimental design provides more interpretable information from the biological model. When correctly applied, microarrays provide more information from *in vitro* systems early in the drug development process, before expensive drug synthesis scale-up. More information from rat experiments allows better decisions to be made before committing to expensive dog or primate studies. These are the promises of toxicogenomics.

3.1.5
Introduction to GeneChip® DNA Mapping Microarrays

It has long been known that individuals respond differently to drugs and toxins. One of the most frequently asked questions to physicians is "Why me, Doc?" (Calabrese 1986; Calabrese 1996; Olden and Guthrie 2001). These individual differences in drug response are one of the greatest challenges in moving a drug successfully into the clinic (Lazarou et al. 1998; Park and Pirmohamed 2001). The interactions between genetic susceptibility and environmental toxins also complicate accurate risk assessment in environmental toxicology (Au 2001; Marchant 2003 a; Marchant 2003 b). The study of inherited response to drugs or toxins is commonly referred to as pharmacogenetics or toxicogenetics. Idiosyncratic toxin responses may also have a genetic component, but they are usually considered in a class of their own due to their rarity, severity, and lack of dose dependence (Ulrich et al. 2001).

The change in RNA expression as measured by various toxicogenomic techniques can be regarded as a phenotype. This phenotype is a combination of genotypic, environmental, and other effects that can be difficult to distinguish from one another. If we want to study inherited risk we should study the genotype directly. Until recently the techniques to measure genetic variation, such as micro satellites and sequencing were cumbersome and expensive. However it is possible to adapt the same microarray technology used for RNA abundance measurements to detect DNA polymorphisms fast and efficiently.

Implications

1. DNA microarrays provide a direct measure of the genotype. The inherited component is therefore much easier to interpret than indirect, phenotypic measurements.
2. Genomic DNA microarrays measure DNA, which is more stable and easy to transport than RNA.
3. Inherited, germline mutations can be determined in any accessible tissue such as blood.
4. The application of single nucleotide polymorphism (SNP) detection arrays and resequencing arrays are complimentary. SNP detection arrays map the complete

genome and are useful when the polymorphic region is not known. Once a polymorphic region has been identified resequencing arrays can determine the exact mutations involved.

3.1.6 GeneChip® DNA Mapping Microarray Technology

In this section the term DNA microarrays refers to microarrays that are designed to measure DNA polymorphisms, as opposed to expression arrays that are designed to measure RNA abundance. The premise of all DNA microarray designs is that a 25 base nucleotide probe can be destabilized by a single nucleotide change at the center of the probe. This destabilization is used in the expression arrays to create mismatch (MM) probes (see Section 3.1.2.2). Arrays can be designed either to detect single nucleotide polymorphisms (SNPs), or to resequence entire DNA regions.

3.1.6.1 DNA Resequencing Arrays

A single GeneChip® microarray reaction can resequence 30kb of double stranded DNA and future designs will undoubtedly cover larger regions. This ability allows researchers to focus on a number of genes of interest or known polymorphic regions. It is well known that polymorphisms in specific genes or regulatory regions can lead to adverse drug responses. For example, the P450 enzyme gene family is responsible for a range of adverse reactions (Guengerich et al. 1987; Ingelman-Sundberg et al. 1994; Oscarson 2001; Pirmohamed and Park 2003). Of the 40 human cytochrome P450 enzymes identified so far, about 8 have been found to be responsible for the oxidation of most drugs and Industrial chemicals. Phase II enzymes are also highly polymorphic between different ethnic and racial populations and can lead to different drug responses in different populations (Bell et al. 1993; Landi 2000). Phase I and II enzyme families have therefore been the candidates of choice for detailed study.

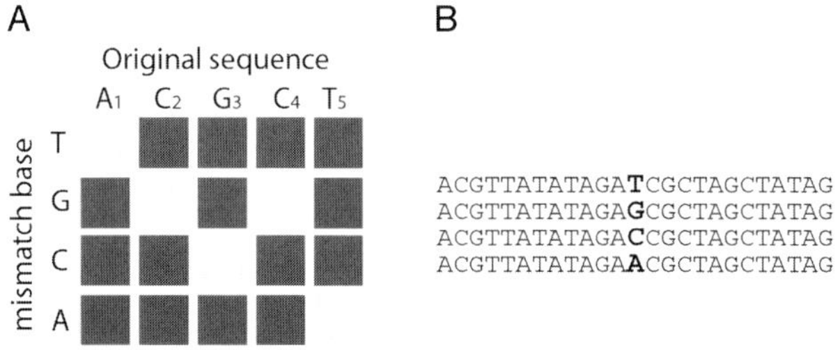

Fig. 3.10 Illustration of a GeneChip® resequencing array. (A) The squares represent cells on the array. For each base of the genomic sequence (positions 1, 2, 3 and 5 in the horizontal row) there are 4 corresponding probes in the vertical columns. The 4 probes each contain one of the 4 possible nucleotides in the center position. The center position corresponds to the mismatch (MM) position on expression arrays. (B) Sequences of the 4 probes that have their center bases corresponding to the base in position A_1. The bold characters indicate bases at the center position. If the center base matches the genomic sequence the cell will have high image intensity. If the center position does not match, the probes will not hybridize and the cells will be dark. The sequence can be read directly form the array.

Implications

1. The information gained by resequencing may provide insight into the biological consequence of polymorphisms.
2. By focusing on a small region of the genome, or a family of enzymes, confounding polymorphisms in other areas of the genome may be missed. This may be one of the reasons why studies of P450 enzyme families are sometimes inconclusive or contradictory (Garte 2001). Enzymes function in the context of a pathway or in concert with other enzymes. If any of the other enzymes involved in the pathway are affected by a polymorphism, it will influence the outcome of the experiment. This risk may be mitigated by increasing the size of the study or by running the study in conjunction with genome mapping (SNP) arrays (see below).
3. The major impact to date of polymorphic P450 expression has been on pre-clinical drug development. Up to now the direct clinical impact of P450 polymorphisms on prediction of ADRs has been limited, mainly due to the small size of the studies and the cost (Pirmohamed and Park 2003).
4. The data produced by a resequencing array is the same as standard sequencing reactions. However there are technical differences:
   a) The sequences produced from a resequencing array do not have to be trimmed, aligned, or concatenated.
   b) Data analysis is minimal.
   c) Both strands are sequenced in the same reaction.
   d) Base stacking in GC-rich areas is eliminated.
   e) The confidence measure of each base is high, so each array is equivalent to several standard sequencing runs.

3.1.6.2 DNA Mapping (SNP) Arrays

Due to the high frequency of polymorphisms in drug susceptibility genes, it is likely that more than one gene will be involved in most instances of inherited adverse drug reactions (Garte 2001). Whole genome single nucleotide polymorphism (SNP) profiling is an unbiased method of determining genetic predisposing factors for adverse drug responses (Pirmohamed and Park 2001). Once a polymorphic region is found, resequencing arrays can determine the exact sequences in that region. Until now these studies have been limited due to the high cost and time involved.

Implications

1. Screening for SNPs does not require prior knowledge of the genes involved. This technique, given that the experiment is designed appropriately, can determine associations between polymorphisms of many genes.

2. Microarrays measure all the targeted SNPs of an individual in a single reaction. As an increasing number of individuals in a population are screened, the data accumulates and can be analyzed before the study is completed. In this way gross indicators can be determined early and the information can be used to expand or redirect the study to find more subtle effects.
3. Some GeneChip® arrays can screen as many as 100,000 SNPs in a single reaction. This high SNP density may reduce the size of some studies and determine polymorphic regions more precisely.
4. Only 250ng of genomic DNA is required for a SNP assay (www.affymetrix.com). This makes testing viable on small blood or other tissue samples.

3.1.7 Conclusion

Toxicogenomics and the study of RNA expression profiles are providing valuable insights into mechanisms of toxic responses. The power of microarrays is not that they do anything new: they just bring an extreme efficiency to RNA abundance measures. It is this efficiency, and the massive amount of data that it produce, that is advancing our knowledge of cellular drugs responses and the field of toxicology as a whole. Toxicogenetics, the application of microarrays to detect inherited drug responses, is the next logical step. The speed and efficiency with which microarrays can map polymorphisms promise to produce an equally profound change in our knowledge of how individuals and populations respond to drugs and environmental toxins. The answer to "Why me, Doc?" may be at hand.

3.2 Experimental Design and Data Analysis

3.2.1 Introduction

The vast amount of data produced in a microarray experiment is both exciting and daunting to a biologist new to the field. To a statistician, microarray analysis is both appealing and technically challenging, given the low number of replicates compared with the large number of transcripts. Both the biological and statistical issues are addressed in the experimental design and data analysis process. The first steps are setting goals, running a pilot study to determine the optimum number of replicates, and designing a full scale experiment. Next, we apply data quality assessment, normalization, statistical modelling, and biological interpretation to bring us to our goal. In toxicogenomics the goal may be may be identifying off-target effects or identifying a mechanism of toxicity. In this section we focus on Affymetrix GeneChip® technology from the experimental design through to the data interpretation.

3.2.2
Experimental Design

In the typical toxicology laboratory relatively few experimental designs are used, and those are usually well established, based on sound statistics and many years of experience. Toxicogenomic experiments are no different. However, the sensitivity of the technique and the volume of data produced can be a challenge. In this section we discuss how to focus the experiment to get to the desired result most efficiently.

3.2.2.1 Setting Goals

Explicitly stating a goal before starting an experiment may seem pedantic to most scientists. However, once committed to an experiment, few things can save as much money, time, and effort as a keeping a clear goal in mind. In toxicology the main goal is usually to determine the toxic effects of drugs. Or more formally stated: the goal is to test the hypothesis that the drugs are not toxic. This may include investigating the mechanism of toxicity, toxic response, or critical dose. Additional goals may include the control of biological factors that influence results, control of technical errors, and the control of costs. Microarrays produce an extraordinary abundance of information, and the temptation to follow every interesting lead, new hypothesis, or new analysis method can be irresistible. An important part of experimental design and analysis is knowing when to stop.

Implications

1. When secondary goals are added to an experiment there is a risk of over-specification. In other words, we ask too many questions from too few replicates. When an experiment is over-specified the assumptions of the statistical models can be compromised. For example, if we ask whether expression increases over time, a simple linear model may be sufficient, because there is an assumption of an approximately linear response. However, if we change the question to ask whether there is a change in expression, there is no longer an assumption of linearity. In this case an ANOVA would be appropriate, because it can detect transient changes in expression. Importantly, ANOVA analysis requires more time points and does not tell us if expression increased over time. Ideally, there should be enough time and concentration sampling points to account for all real responses. In practice, the number of samples that can be processed in an experiment is limited, and the experimental design is of necessity a compromise. The experimenter should keep the compromises in the experimental design in mind when interpreting the results.
2. "If you torture the data long enough it will confess." This adage, attributed to John Freund, points to an important yet frequently neglected part of experimental design: defining the end of data analysis. Defining the end of the analysis is distinguished from goal setting by the recognition that a given study may not satisfy

the experimenter's expectations. The natural temptation is to reanalyze the data, often with different methods, until the sought-after answer is evident. This *post hoc* approach can be very misleading. Statistical tests run serially do not have the same authentic probability of success as one test run in isolation. That is, if test after test is run until one test is 'significant' the value of that significance is suspect. Eventually, if a sufficient number of *t* tests are performed on random data, the probability of getting a *t* test of 95% confidence approaches 100%. More specifically, if 100 tests are made, the chances of getting at least one false positive for which the *p* value is 0.05 or lower is 99.4% (Cobb 1997). Serial analysis without multiple comparison correction is therefore inherently suspect. This effect is recognized and is addressed by multiple comparison correction techniques such as Bonferroni. With microarray data this problem is greatly magnified, due to the large number of transcripts and the comparatively small number of samples. Always remember that measuring 10 transcripts of five rats or 20 000 transcripts of five rats has only the statistical power of five. If your analysis of five rats does not definitively answer your key question, test more animals or use the information you gained to redesign the experiment. There is far more value in replicating the biology than manipulating the data.

3. Experimental design should be guided by the analysis you plan to apply. For example, a statistical model that assumes a continuous response such as linear regression fails if the response is not linear. But if there are too few time points, there is no indication that the model has failed and real results, such as rapid fluctuations in gene expression, may be missed.

4. The experimental design should match the technology employed. In two-colour microarray experiments all measurements are relative. To avoid forced pairing of samples and controls, it is common practice to use a pooled control on all arrays to facilitate relative measurements. In single-colour experiments, such as GeneChip® arrays, controls should not be pooled. Pooling controls reduces the power of the statistical analysis significantly. The optimal experimental design, in which there is an equal number of control and treated samples, is balanced. The decision to treat samples and controls as paired or not can be taken later at the analysis stage.

5. A hypothesis is usually tested by a statistical test. For any statistical test, sufficient replication is required to guarantee sufficient statistical power and confidence. By replication, we are referring to biological replicates such as rats. A simple approach to estimating the number of replicates required in an experiment is discussed in detail later.

6. Unexpected variables may become apparent. For example, in typical toxicological experiments the time of day when the animals are sacrificed is not important. However, it is well known that many genes are regulated by circadian rhythms and that the abundance of some transcripts varies widely during the course of a day (Ueda et al. 2002), so in microarray experiments time of day is a variable that needs to be controlled. With *in vitro* experiments, changes in culture conditions can be expected to induce expression of a large number of genes. In Figure 3.11,

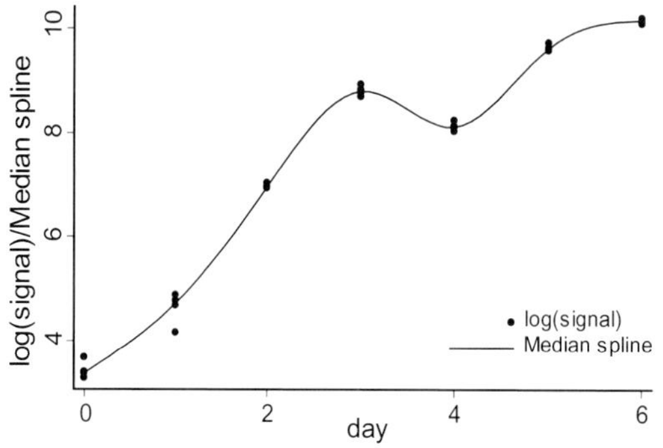

Fig. 3.11 An unexpected event during a time series. In this example, gene expression from four replicates of a chemically treated cell line was perturbed when the medium was replaced on the third day. The expression pattern, although still linear enough to be observed, has a greatly reduced quality of linear fit. This begs the question of how many other almost-linear responses were missed due to the environmental event.

the change in expression on day 4 was traced to changing the culture media on the previous day. True biological replication and controlled techniques serve to minimize these effects. When control is not possible, the only viable substitute is randomization and sufficient replication.

7. The cost of a microarray experiment has many components, such as labour, financial, and ethical when human donors or animal experiments are used. When increasing the number of replicates, these costs must be traded off against the increased power and sensitivity of the test. Clearly, these tradeoffs are very laboratory-dependent and also depend on the experimental system used. However, it is universally true that it is better to answer a single question well than to ask many poorly.

8. The cost of data analysis and data interpretation is usually underestimated. To reduce the number of arrays used, it is tempting to develop complex experimental designs in which many variables are measured simultaneously. However, increasing the design complexity increases the difficulty of sample treatment and data analysis. The complexity of biological interpretation also increases. These complex answers may require subsequent clarifying experimentation, which increases the overall cost of achieving the experimental goal. A better approach is to break a large experiment into more manageable smaller experiments. A pilot study is useful in this regard, because the experimenter can try to interpret the simplified experiment and potential issues can be addressed before committing to a large experiment.

3.2.2.2 **Statistical Approaches**

Each microarray measures several thousand transcripts. In a typical experiment we expect the abundance of some transcripts to change due to the experimental parameters we are testing while other transcripts change purely by chance. To extract authentically changed transcripts from changes that occurred by chance, statistical issues must be addressed: the choice of test, the determination of significance, and the interpretation of results. In this section we focus on selecting an appropriate statistical test and confidence threshold to extract authentically changed transcripts from those changes that occurred by chance.

Implications

1. Statistical tests do not eliminate the possibility that running more replicates, time points, or concentration points would uncover a previously undetected response. In other words, the tests described here identify a significant toxic response in the context of the experimental design. If no response is found this does not mean that no response exists, but only that no response was measurable with the number of arrays employed.
2. Samples are usually independent. In a typical experiment a set of animals are randomly divided into control and treatment. After the experiment the animals are sacrificed and samples taken. When several samples are obtained serially from the same individual, for example, blood samples on days 0, 1, 2, and 3, different statistical models are appropriate, because these measurements are not independent (Box et al. 1978). In the following discussion we assume that all samples are from different animals and are therefore independent.

Parametric vs. Nonparametric Tests

The choice of statistical tests for a typical toxicogenomics experiment can be divided into two classes: parametric and nonparametric. Nonparametric tests determine change in rank order and ignore the magnitude of expression changes. The advantage of this approach is that it does not require the data to be normally distributed. Nonparametric tests include the Wilcoxon Signed Rank test or the Mann–Whitney test for comparisons when there are two variables and the Kruskal–Wallis test for multivariate analysis. Parametric tests include the *t* test for comparisons when there are two variables and ANOVA for multivariate tests. Parametric tests assume that the data are normally distributed. If that assumption is indeed true, parametric tests are the most powerful and accurate tests we can apply. If the data are not normally distributed, we have to use less powerful nonparametric tests. Data are rarely perfectly normally distributed, so the choice of using parametric or nonparametric approaches is not clear and is often debated.

Implications

1. When they are valid, parametric tests are more statistically powerful than nonparametric tests. This means that more probesets should pass a threshold based on *p* values from ANOVA than would pass if the *p* values were based on a nonparametric test of the same data.
2. Log-transformed microarray data approximate a normal distribution. Even though it is not perfectly normal, it is close enough to allow the use of parametric tests. To confirm the accuracy of parametric tests, such as *t* tests and ANOVA, on log-transformed signal data we can use the residuals. Residuals are the measurement errors, in this case the differences between each observed value and the mean of all observations. If parametric tests are valid, the residuals should be normally distrib-

uted. At first glance, the residuals for all genes are not normally distributed (Figure 3.12 A). Observe that low signal values are more variable than moderate-to-high signal values. This means that the variance is unstable across intensity and therefore the residuals are unstable. A standardized measure is the difference between each observation and the mean divided by the standard deviation of the measurements. A standardized residual therefore removes the effect of the differing variances on the measurement. The standardized residuals are nearly perfectly normal (Figure 3.12 B and Table 3.1). The instability of the variance over intensity fully explains the non-normality in the distribution of residuals. As a result, we can predict when parametric tests will be the most accurate. The practical implication is that in the rare instances in which a signal level changes over several orders of magnitude, the

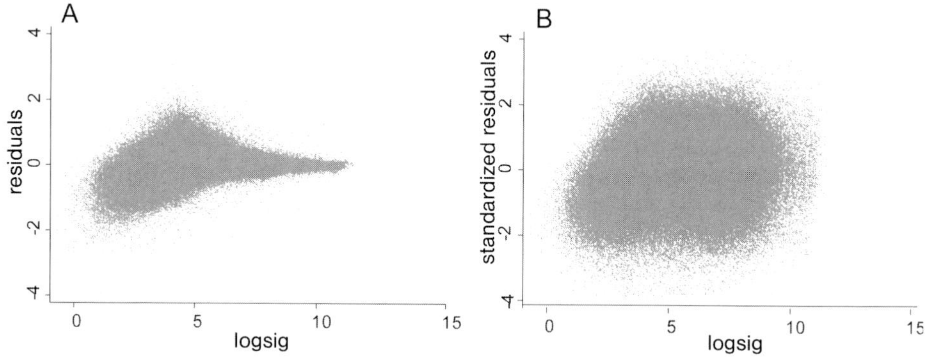

Fig. 3.12 Residuals of ANOVA for each probeset over a time series. The *x* axis represents the log-transformed signal values. (A) Pattern of residuals over signal intensity. Such a non-normal pattern may influence the accuracy of *p* values produced by a parametric test. (B) The standardized residuals have a random scatter consistent with the assumptions of parametric tests. The practical result of this observation is the *p* values derived from ANOVA of the log signal are reasonably accurate for the majority of probesets. For those rare probesets that change dramatically and therefore have dramatically changed variance, the *p* values are less accurate. As a rule, variance-stabilizing methods minimize these effects, allowing us to get accurate *p* values from parametric tests.

Tab. 3.1 Summary data for residuals. These distributions demonstrate that divergence of residuals from normal is an effect of the instability of variance across intensity and that, for most genes that do not change, this instability does not affect the *p* value, as the standardized residuals are nearly perfectly normal. We expect therefore that only those rare probesets that change dramatically in magnitude will have inaccurate *p* values.

	Residuals	*Standardized residuals*	*Ideally normal residuals*
Mean	–2.31e–11	–7.20e–11	0
Standard deviation	0.3995765	1.000002	1
Variance	0.1596614	1.000004	1
Skewness	–0.2025563	–0.1261272	0
Kurtosis	6.9743	2.9944	3

p value estimate is less accurate. For typical, small changes in signal, the difference in variance is small and the *p* values is accurate.

3. The *p* values provided by a multiclass nonparametric test such as the Kruskal–Wallis test is more significant (lower *p* value) for linear responses than for a non-linear response (Figure 3.13). A nonparametric test is based on rank order. For example, in a linear time response, there are changes in rank order at every time point, but a spiking pattern may only have changes in rank order for a single time point. This is not necessarily true for a nonparametric test when the magnitude of change is also taken into effect. This is an example of the principle that the mechanics of a statistical test may crucially influence which probesets are selected by *p* value and therefore the interpretation of the results.

4. Each time or dose point may have a different biological significance. By contrast, statistical tests treat each time point in a concentration series identically. If the bio-

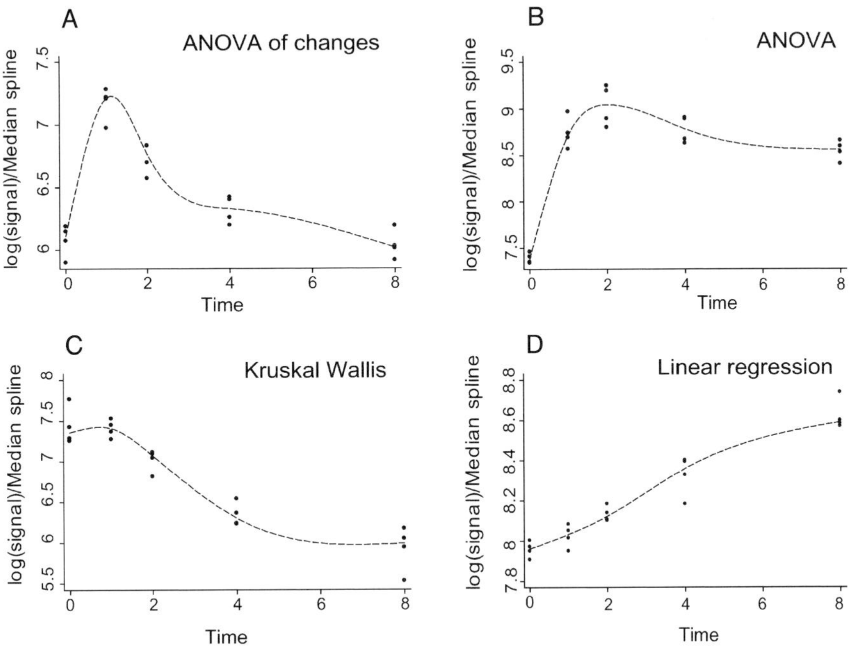

Fig. 3.13 Gene expression responses to time (log(signal) as a function of time in hours) from four different probe sets with the lowest (best) *p* values produced by four analytical methods. Each of panel represents four replicates of the same probeset. (A) ANOVA of changes. Time and the differences between time points were tested by a categorical ANOVA. This is a good technique for finding transient spikes. (B) ANOVA model with time treated as a categorical variable. (C) Kruskal–Wallis test. This signal response is nearly linear, because a linear change with time appears to have the most significant rank order changes. Patterns such as those in (B) are much less likely to be discovered by the Kruskal–Wallis test than those in (A), because in (B) the gene is relatively stable in ranking over most of the time course. (D) Linear regression of log-transformed data with time. This method cannot detect the patterns in (A) or (B), as the divergence from linearity is penalized.

logical significance of a time point changes, it should be reflected in the statistical model. For example, toxicology experiments may split time into two classes that correspond to acute and chronic responses. The decision to treat time and dose as a continuous variables or as class variables should be explicitly made, based on the biology. The gene expression pattern in Figure 3.13 A is not readily captured by models in which time is continuous. Furthermore, in the context of a toxicological response the rapid change in the transcript in Figure 13 B in the 0 to 1 h time interval is much more interesting than the same response at any other time point.

5. Vehicle and naïve controls are commonly used in toxicology. Toxins are usually dissolved in a solvent or 'vehicle' when applied to a system. The vehicle by itself may have a significant response that needs to be controlled. Usually this is done by comparison to a 'naïve' control that has not been exposed to the vehicle or the toxin. The responses for these two types of controls can be classed together in an ANOVA, because neither response is related to the toxin. However, modelling the naïve and vehicle controls in a split-plot design more accurately reflects the experiment (Cobb 1997, Chapter 8, Section 3).
6. Matching the logic of the statistical test to the biological interpretation is very important. Do not use an experimental design without first verifying that valid interpretation of the statistical results addresses the questions of biological interest.

Setting Thresholds: Multiple Comparison Correction

In a typical microarray experiment *p* values form a continuous population from very significant (near zero) to insignificant (near one) response. This allows us to rank probesets by significance of response. It is easy to judge significance at the extremes of the population, but exactly where to draw the line between significant and not significant is not so clear. If we select a threshold that is too relaxed, we risk including probesets that have not authentically changed – false positives (type 1 errors). On the other hand, if we make the threshold too stringent, we risk excluding authentically changed probesets – false negatives (type 2 errors). If a single probeset is tested, then a *p* value of 0.05 or lower denotes a significant change or, more formally stated, a rejection of the null hypothesis. This allows one false positive for every 20 tests (5 for every 100 tests). In microarray experiments in which thousands of probesets are tested simultaneously, this low threshold captures nearly all true positives but also a vast number of false positives. For applications in which false positives are costly, we must devise more stringent selection methods.

Implications

1. Generally, there is no clear break in the distribution of *p* values that can reasonably be used as a basis for setting a threshold. In an ideal dataset for which all assumptions are met, *p* values are a statement of probability. However, based on observed distributions of residuals, microarray experiments may not always give accurate *p* values. The degree of inaccuracy varies with data quality and the amount

of change. Given this fact, we can protect against overly optimistic *p* values by applying very stringent multiple comparison methods. The simplest multi-test correction method is the Bonferroni correction, which is optimized for a small number of tests. For microarray experiments in which thousands of genes are tested simultaneously, the correction is extraordinarily strict. The Bonferroni threshold can be considered to be the upper bound, in that no genes that pass this threshold are expected to be false positives. Despite the stringency of the Bonferroni correction, this approach has been successful in microarray experiments (Cheng et al. 2002; Wayne and McIntyre 2002; Wittwer et al. 2002; Bennett et al. 2003; Dow 2003). Several more complex corrections have been developed but are not widely employed because of their computational complexity (Efron and Tibshirani 2002; Westfall et al. 2002; Reiner et al. 2003).

2. If only one or two probesets pass the Bonferroni threshold when many changes are expected, then the experiment was statistically under-powered. If further replication or variance reduction is impractical, then use the *p* values as a ranking method. Once the probesets are ranked, the most significantly changed probesets can be selected from the top of the list. Although this approach does not address the multiple comparison problem or provide an analytical threshold, it does order the probesets by relevance. In such situations no statement of statistical confidence is possible.

3. The population of *p* values that pass a threshold is not normally distributed. The majority of values are close to the threshold, which exacerbates the effect of changing the threshold on the population that pass (Figure 3.14). Thus, the probesets that pass the threshold have relatively high *p* values and are very sensitive to the test used and the number of replicates. The range of *p* values and the distance from the threshold of a given gene are much more informative.

4. We recommend transforming *p* values to scores ($-\log_{10}(p \text{ value})$) so that they can be viewed more intuitively. Higher scores reflect higher significance and the differences between 0.1 and 0.001 can readily be seen.

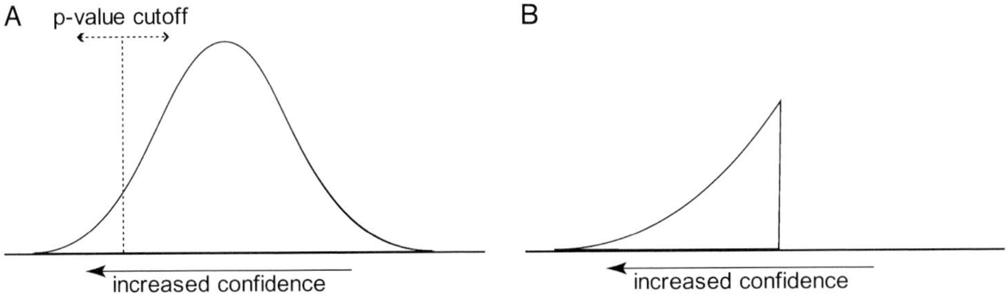

Fig. 3.14 Values that pass a threshold are not normally distributed. (A) Histogram of a normally distributed population to which we apply a threshold. (B) The population that passes the threshold. The newly created list has a majority of probesets having relatively low confidence; that is, most of the probesets are close to the threshold.

3.2.2.3 Clustering and Classification

Clustering methods have gained wide acceptance in toxicogenomics. Although not rigorous statistically, they do have value in ordering and exploring data. Clustering is extensively reviewed elsewhere (Wang et al. 1999; Retief 2000; Everitt et al. 2001). This section is intended as a guide to using clustering as an exploratory method in conjunction with statistical tests. The clustering techniques described here are unguided and can be divided into two types: hierarchical and not hierarchical. 'Not hierarchical' refers to a range of techniques including self-organizing maps, *k* means, and correlation methods. During clustering a second level of normalization is applied. In the MAS5.0 software the arrays are normalized. In the clustering techniques the probesets are normalized.

Implications

1. Clustering is sensitive and may reveal associations that are otherwise obscured.
2. The validity of clustering results can be difficult to assess.
3. Clustering techniques can be improved if used in conjunction with statistical techniques. For example, use a statistical filter before clustering to remove transcripts that have not significantly changed.
4. If transcripts are classed together as signatures, that knowledge can be built into a statistical model. In this way we test whether each biologically relevant signature is influenced by a drug instead of testing each transcript. The advantage of this classification is that we test a modest number of hypotheses instead of a hypothesis for each transcript. As a result, our multiple testing problem is reduced and the Bonferroni multiple comparison correction method is more appropriate. Signature classes are best defined through empirical testing. However, clustering methods can be used to define signatures, especially if the number of clusters is rigorously defined by a GAP statistic (Tibshirani et al. 2000; Kerr and Churchill 2001; Dudoit and Fridlyand 2002, 2003)

Hierarchical Clustering

Hierarchical clustering techniques can be divisive or agglomerative. In each case the data are progressively divided or combined until all possible nodes are accounted for.

Implications

1. Hierarchical clustering is best applied to small datasets such as chips, samples, experiments, or individuals.
2. Only one tree is produced, regardless of how many trees may be equally likely.
3. In each clustering step a decision is made as to how to group the data. This decision is propagated into the next step. When a large number of decisions are

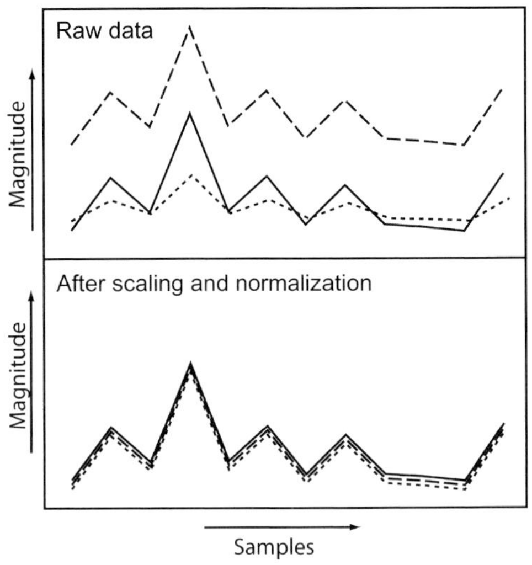

Fig. 3.15 Scaling and normalization simplifies the data, but some information is lost. The traces each represent a transcript in the form of a probeset. Clustering the raw data produces clusters based on the magnitude as well as the shape of the expression pattern. After scaling and normalization, the data are greatly simplified and it is clear all three probesets have the same expression pattern. The information that one of the probesets was expressed at much higher levels than the others is lost.

made, such as when clustering probesets, many errors are possible and the results are generally not reliable.

4. An indication of the confidence in the clustering can be obtained by using bootstrapping techniques. Bootstrapping is very computationally intensive but significantly improves the quality of the interpretation (Efron et al. 1996 a, b).
5. Some hierarchical clustering methods use tree building algorithms in which the lengths of branches reflect the distance or difference between nodes. Those methods are easy to identify, because the trees they produce have different branch lengths. These branch lengths are very helpful in estimating relative distances between branches. However, this is not as useful as bootstrapping.
6. Normalization, as the term is applied in the clustering context, changes the question asked and the interpretation. For example, after normalization the level of expression is no longer taken into account, because that information is lost (Figure 3.15). In other words, after normalization, clustering is performed on the pattern of expression changes, not on the level of those changes. Normalization simplifies the data and may elucidate patterns that may otherwise be hidden.

Self-organizing Maps, *k* Means, and Correlation Coefficient Methods

Nonhierarchical clustering methods use various strategies to calculate the distance between all data points in multidimensional space. The results are then grouped in a number of user-defined clusters (Tamayo et al. 1999).

Implications

1. Self organizing maps, *k* means, and correlation coefficient methods are best applied to large datasets such as probesets. Errors do not propagate as in hierarchical clustering, and the calculations are fast.
2. The user needs to define the number of nodes. This implies that the results are somewhat user-dependent and not totally objective. The gap statistic can be employed to provide a principled basis for selecting the number of nodes (Tibshirani et al. 2000).
3. Some techniques, such as self-organizing maps, use a random number generator to determine the order of the distance calculations. Different analysis runs on the same dataset may give slightly different answers. This reflects the true uncertainty in the dataset but can be disconcerting. This uncertainty or lack of robustness is corrected in more recent clustering methods (Bickel 2003).

Principal Component Analysis

Principal component analysis (PCA) and related techniques such as singular value decomposition (SVD) are usefully grouped with these exploratory techniques. In brief, PCA describes the variability of the data based on a series of components. Ideally, the first three components should capture the bulk of the variability in the dataset. This is an excellent exploratory technique and should be one of the first to be applied to a dataset. The results can usually act as a guide for further statistical testing.

Implications

1. PCA detects patterns in the data without supervision and is therefore a very good exploratory technique.
2. PCA assumes linearity and is therefore is best applied to log-transformed signal values.
3. If the majority of the variation is captured in more than two dimensions, the plot should be checked in three dimensions to make sure the best possible view of the data is obtained.
4. The results can be difficult to interpret, because no *p* value is reported and the key dimension may not relate to any known variable.

3.2.2.4 Toxicology Variables

Time and dose are the two variables of most interest to toxicologists. Although these variables can be handled the same in a statistical model, there are some special considerations.

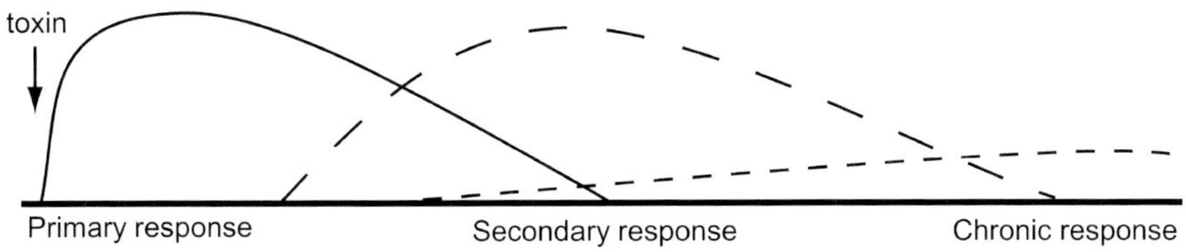

Fig. 3.16 The analysis and experimental design may depend on the time point chosen.

Time

In toxicogenomics the considerations for selecting a time point are the same as for a typical toxicology experiment. For example, in a multi-timepoint toxicology study we usually expect an immediate response, often by the phase I and phase II enzymes, followed by intermediate and long-term responses (Figure 3.16). Transcript-level responses are some of the earliest biological responses to an insult, so often changes in transcription can be detected before typical toxicology end-points (Waring et al. 2001). Time points should usually be shortened to detect informative early responses. Pilot studies are very helpful for determining the optimal time points for an experiment. In a genome-wide array we can observe both transient and continuous changes, so more than one statistical model may be appropriate. The final choice of statistical model depends on the question asked.

Implications

1. Changes in transcript levels can be detected very sensitively and usually precede changes in protein levels or histology (Waring et al. 2001). For this reason, time points used in microarray experiments may need to be shorter than for standard toxicological end points.
2. Although clinical assays may define genes of interest, the patterns of enzymatic response may not be indicative of genetic expression patterns. For example, if a toxin increases troponin T levels in the bloodstream, this does not mean that it will be particularly informative to focus on the expression profiles of genes in the troponin T pathway. Therefore, when a statistical model of expression is chosen, we recommend using one that detects the broadest range of patterns possible.
3. The number of time points measured in a toxicology experiment is usually limited, so the statistical model to apply is not always obvious. For example, a strong reaction that occurs at only a single timepoint may be as interesting as a linear increase. If we assume a continuous change, as in a linear or polynomial fit, we may miss transient changes. When the purpose is to identify patterns without *a priori* assumptions about their form, ANOVA, unlike Kruskal–Wallis or linear fits, is most likely to capture all responses (Figure 3.13).

4. Although there are many specialized statistical methods for time courses (Peña et al. 2000), in general, microarray time courses have too few time points for one to apply such methods properly. As a result, novel methods have been developed (Ghosh 2002; Xu et al. 2002; Peddada et al. 2003).

5. In time course experiments designed to study chronic exposure, small doses of a toxin are usually applied over a period of time. In such experiments, transient changes in the expression patterns are much less likely to occur, and measures of continuous change, such as linear or polynomial fitting, are more appropriate.

Dose

The same statistical models that apply to time can also be applied to dose. The type of experiment affects the appropriate model to use.

Implications

1. In an acute study, we expect a rapid, transient response, and methods such as ANOVA or *t* tests are commonly used.

2. In a chronic study, in which small doses are supplied over a period of time, spikes in the gene expression profiles are much less likely.

3. Regardless of the experimental design, treating the arrays as discrete measurements with ANOVA models is a useful quality measure. Such an analysis provides an indication of whether an array is an outlier due to an unforeseen effect.

3.2.2.5 Pilot Study

We strongly recommend performing pilot studies. Pilot studies are simple experiments that focus on a single variable. When we refer to a pilot study this includes a pilot analysis and biological interpretation. Refining methods after a small scale study is faster, cheaper, and more effective than developing complex mathematical fixes well after the fact. Pilot studies have great practical value and save time and money in the long run.

Implications

1. In any complex multistep process such as microarray analysis it is reasonable to expect that some difficulties will not be foreseen. Pilot studies allow the experimenter to recognize potential problems and address them before committing to the full-scale experiment.

2. If the biological goal is not well defined, a pilot experiment helps to focus the question.

3. Pilot studies provide an estimate of the variance that can be used to determine how many replicates are needed to answer the key question. Pilot studies gener-

ate standard deviations for each gene. These standard deviations are can be used as good first estimates for the number of replicates required for a parametric test (nonparametric requirements are higher). These methods of replicate estimation are best for two-way comparisons that use a *t* test and are more difficult for complex ANOVA designs that use the F test but are still possible.

4. Data gathered from the pilot experiment are not lost but can be incorporated into the complete experiment. This is another example of a multiple-comparison problem, and some adjustment in the *p* value may be required (see section on setting thresholds: multiple comparison correction in Section 3.2.2.2).

3.2.2.6 Replication

Replicates in a statistical context should effectively reproduce the entire question of interest. Thus, when we refer to replicates in the context of toxicology microarray experiments, we mean biological replicates in which each replicate is a treated or control animal. Multiple arrays from the same tissue, RNA extract, or other partial product are often called technical replicates but are more accurately called repeated measures or pseudo replicates.

Implications

1. Error estimates and sample size calculations derived from pseudo replicates underestimate the number required, because variation in expression derived from pseudo replicates is lower than that from true replicates.
2. Repeated measures do have some value. For example, the mean of three pseudo replicates should be more accurate and robust than a single measure. One should remember that signal values are based on a set of probe pairs that are in themselves a set of 11 or more pseudo replicates. Adding additional arrays as pseudo replicates to an experiment increases the expense without addressing biological variation, which is usually greater than technical variation.
3. True replicates and pseudo replicates have two sources of error: the measurements from true replicates are independent, whereas those from pseudo replicates are dependent. Mixing true replicates and pseudo replicates together in one experiment greatly complicates data analysis. The problem is tractable but should not be ignored, as it can influence interpretation.
4. Changes in transcript levels between pseudo replicates do not reflect a biological response.

Estimating the Number of Replicates

In this section we provide a simplified method that provides a rough estimate of the number of replicates required for a parametric test, such as ANOVA or *t* test (van Belle 2002). The assumptions and limitations of the method are discussed. A spreadsheet program is sufficient for these calculations.

To estimate the number of replicates in a microarray study we must define the following:

- the desired magnitude of change in expression level,
- the expected variance of signal for the probeset of interest,
- the statistical test. In this section we focus on parametric tests.

Step 1: Decide on the proportional change (PC) in expression between controls and treatment that you want to measure. A signal log ratio of at least 2 (a 100% change) can serve as a starting point. Keep in mind that many reproducible changes in gene expression are small and may fall below this cutoff. A better approach is to use a pilot study to determine a PC that will capture 25% to 50% of all changes.

$$\mathrm{PC} = \frac{\text{mean of treated } \log(\text{signals}_{\text{experiment}}) - \text{mean of treated } \log(\text{signals}_{\text{controls}})}{\text{mean of treated } \log(\text{signals}_{\text{controls}})}$$

As we are interested only in the magnitude of change, we take the absolute value of the PC. Next we rank the |PC| and take percentiles. From these percentiles we can say that a PC of 25% or better should select 40% of all genes at a given variance (Table 3.2).

Step 2: Estimate the variability of the signal measurements by calculating the coefficient of variance (CV). For this estimate we combine the signal values for control and treated samples:

$$\mathrm{CV} = \text{standard deviation of } \log(\text{signal}) / \text{mean of } \log(\text{signal})$$

As the CVs differ for each transcript, we cannot treat them identically. A practical approach is to divide the transcripts into quartiles based on their CV. To do this, calculate the CVs for all transcripts and rank them from lowest to highest. The list can then be divided into four equal parts. The highest CV in each quartile represents the range of variability. These numbers are then entered into the sample size estimation formula:

$$N = \frac{8\,\mathrm{CV}^2}{\mathrm{PC}^2}\left[1 + (1 - \mathrm{PC})^2\right]$$

By applying this formula four times, we get four sample-size numbers N, one for each quartile. The N we select for our full-scale experiment determines the number of transcripts we expect to test well. If we select the N for the first quartile, where CV is lowest, we expect reasonable answers for 25% of the transcripts in our final experiment (Table 3.2).

In Table 3.2, a 10% change in the top 25% most stably changed probesets would require four replicates.

Tab. 3.2 Sample size calculation. See text for explanation.

Percentile	*CV*	*Property change*	*Replicates*[a]
25	0.053	0.50	0[b]
		0.25	1[b]
		0.10	4
		0.05	17
50	0.124	0.50	1[b]
		0.25	3
		0.10	22
		0.05	94
75	0.205	0.50	2[b]
		0.25	8
		0.10	61
		0.05	256
99	0.488	0.50	10
		0.25	48
		0.10	345
		0.05	1451

a) Values are rounded to the nearest integer.
b) Three replicates are the minimum for statistical tests, so for these estimates use three replicates.

Implications

1. The ideal number of replicates is different for each transcript.
2. Variance may not be the same before and after treatment. If a transcript is rare in a control state but highly expressed after treatment, we would overestimate the number of replicates or transcripts that are increased by treatment and underestimate the number of replicates need for a transcript that decreases due to treatment. To address this difference, we combine both control and treated signals in our calculation of CV.
3. The appropriate PC cutoff depends on the PC for transcripts of interest. For example, if we observe in the pilot study that an important transcript has a PC of 10% (0.1) and a CV ranked in the lowest 50%, then we use these values in our formula to find N. For the sample data used to generate Table 3.2 we would require 22 replicates.
4. If very few or no genes are significantly changed by the treatment, you may need to lower the PC or adapt the experimental conditions to yield a higher PC.
5. The calculated numbers of replicates are rough estimates. These calculations depend on the quality and relevance of the pilot data. These calculations also depend on the assumptions shared by parametric tests, i.e., normality and equality of variance. This method does not address the multiple comparison problem (Section 3.3.2.2).

6. As noted, the number of replicates required is based on the variance. Any technique that stabilizes the variance affects the number of replicates required according to these calculations (Section 3.2.3.2).

The Effect of Variance Stabilization on Replicate Estimation

The estimate for the number of replicates can be improved if we stabilize variance. In Table 3.3 we consistently see that using corrected values requires fewer replicates. This mathematical correction is detailed below in Section 3.2.3.2 on data correction. This demonstrates the benefits of designing the full-scale experiment with the analysis method in mind.

Tab. 3.3 Sample size calculation after variance stabilization.

Percentile	*CV*		*Property*	*Number of replicates*	
	Original	*Corrected*	*change*	*Original*	*Corrected*
25	0.053	0.038	0.5	0 [a]	0 [a]
25	0.053	0.038	0.25	1 [a]	0 [a]
25	0.053	0.038	0.1	4	2 [a]
25	0.053	0.038	0.05	17	9
50	0.124	0.056	0.5	1 [a]	0 [a]
50	0.124	0.056	0.25	3	1 [a]
50	0.124	0.056	0.1	22	4
50	0.124	0.056	0.05	94	19
75	0.205	0.072	0.5	2 [a]	0 [a]
75	0.205	0.072	0.25	8	1 [a]
75	0.205	0.072	0.1	61	7
75	0.205	0.072	0.05	256	31
99	0.488	0.125	0.5	10	1 [a]
99	0.488	0.125	0.25	48	3
99	0.488	0.125	0.1	345	23
99	0.488	0.125	0.05	1451	95

a) Three replicates are the minimum for statistical tests, so for these estimates use three replicates. In this table 'corrected' means data that was variance-stabilized.

3.2.2.7 **Pooling**

Pooling samples reduces the complexity of an experiment and its analysis. Pooling also results in irretrievable loss of information. Balancing the gains and loss of pooling is a design decision having many implications.

Implications

1. Once RNA samples are mixed, it is impossible to identify outliers or misclassification events.

2. Unlike standard toxicological endpoints, which provide a single measure per animal, microarrays provide thousands of measures. As a result, subtle environmental effects may generate more outlier transcripts. If you pool you do not observe these outliers, which may confound your results.

3. Pooling reduces variance as long as multiple pools are created for control and treatment conditions. That is, the variability of data from three pools of three mice should be lower than the variability obtained from nine mice. With inbred animals this advantage is small.

4. Pooling introduces bias, as a mixed sample is equivalent to an arithmetic average. An arithmetic error is assumed to be a random constant *added* to the signal. In reality, the predominant error in microarray experiments is a random constant by which the signal is *multiplied*. By taking the log signal we make the factor additive, so that the mean is a representative measure of the group. After pooling this kind of transformation is not possible. In pooled data any outlier disproportionately affects the signal. Pooled signals are often higher than the mean of the log signal of individual measurements due to this bias (Figure 3.17).

5. Pooling limits statistical power. The most problematic use of pooling is when no replicate pools are produced and only a single control array is compared to a single treatment. This approach has all the disadvantages of pooling without the key benefit of variance reduction. When all animals are combined into a single pool, the user is forced to select genes on the basis of magnitude alone (Figure 3.18). This approach is sensitive to outliers and precludes statistical testing.

6. Pooling limits the ability to select significantly changed transcripts. It is clear from Figure 3.18 that the genes selected by the different methods are very different. The labels in the figure define the interpretation of those genes if the pooling method was applied. Probable false positives indicate the many genes that have extreme signal log ratios pooled between experiments and controls but are not consistently measured. These false positives are termed 'probably' false, because they were not bench-validated. The cost savings realized by pooling would likely be lost by validating many of these transcripts that are highly changed in trans-

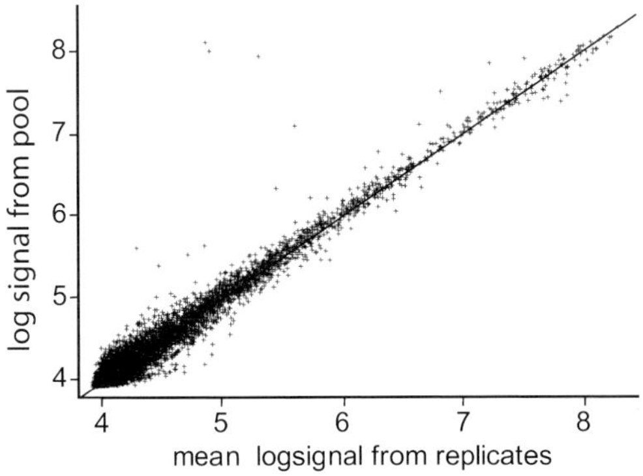

Fig. 3.17 The difference between the log signal from pooled samples and the signal from the mean of the log signals. Note that most differences are on one side of the diagonal. This bias is introduced by the pooling.

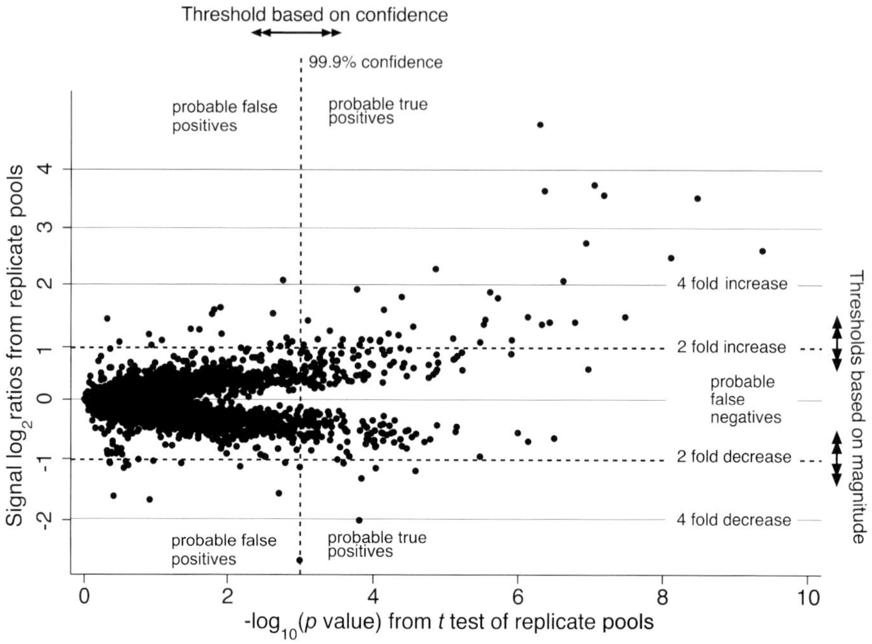

Fig. 3.18 Information lost by pooling. The y axis is the signal $\log_2$ ratio between one pool of controls and one pool of treated samples. The horizontal lines represent two-fold and four-fold cutoff values (the log ratio is base 2). If only two pools are available these horizontal lines would be the only method available for finding differentially expressed genes. The x axis is the statistical significance. Here, 'statistical significance' is the p value calculated by a t test of the replicates. By taking the $-\log_{10}$ (p value), the scale becomes equivalent to orders of magnitude. This means that 3 represents a 99.9% confidence level. If replicates exist, this test can be performed and genes are selected by the use of the vertical line representing 99% confidence. This dataset contains many significant but small changes that would be missed by pooling.

cript abundance. By contrast, the probable false negatives are very consistent, reproducible differences between treatment and control that do not meet the two- or four-fold requirement. Changes in transcription of these genes are the more subtle changes that are reliable and potentially meaningful but which are missed by pooling.

3.2.3
Data Assessment and Correction

A crucial part of the analytical process is the assessment of data quality. By capturing and evaluating array-wide and probeset-specific quality metrics, you can often diagnose the cause of low-quality data. After detecting quality issues, you must decide whether to remove the data or to attempt a correction.

Implications

1. Complete failures are easy to recognize by using standard guidelines. However, these guidelines do not reveal gradual erosions in data quality. To flag gradual changes early, more sensitive quality parameters are needed. Comparable historical data can be used to create guidelines.
2. Capture as much information about the experimental conditions as possible. For example, where more than one technician works on an experiment, that variable needs to be captured. Should a problem arise, these parameters can be used to diagnose the cause. A list of quality measures we find useful is provided (Table 3.4).
3. Some irreplaceable samples, such as muscle biopsies or post mortem tissues, may not yield good quality RNA. In such situations it is reasonable to relax the quality measures to test critical questions. When quality metrics are relaxed, subtle changes are lost. This lowered quality should be kept in mind when the data are interpreted.
4. Once suspect data are uncovered and discarded, care must be taken in interpreting the data. For example, *p* values generated from censored data do not represent true probabilities. Diagnostic tools, such as the examination of residuals and outliers, should be used only before data censoring.

3.2.3.1 **Quality Control**

Quality control should take place at every step of the experimental process and only arrays that pass all quality criteria should go on to the analysis process. The following is a review of the quality metrics commonly used with GeneChip arrays (Figure 3.19).

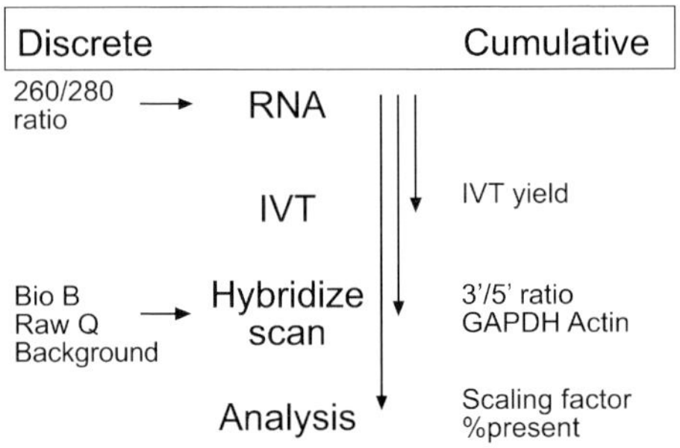

Fig. 3.19 Quality metrics. Discrete measures give an indication of the progress of one step in the process. For example, Bio B reports the efficiency of the labelling and hybridization, but does not tell us anything about the RNA quality. Cumulative measures report the success of all previous steps in the process. For example, a percent-present measure in the normal range indicates the success of all previous steps in the process: the RNA was of good quality, the hybridization and labelling worked well, and the software was applied properly. Divisions between quality measures are seldom this clear. For example, background primarily reports the hybridization reaction, but it is often influenced by sample quality (see Table 3.2 for descriptions of terms).

Tab. 3.4 Key quality-control measures.

Variable	***Description***
260/280 ratio (upon isolation) 260/280 ratio (upon processing)	The absorbance of the RNA should be measured at 260 and 280 nm to determine sample concentration and purity. The A260/A280 ratio should be close to 2.0 for pure RNA (ratios between 1.9 and 2.1 are acceptable).
Scale factor	When the two arrays are globally scaled to the same Target Intensity, the scaling factor for a poorly hybridized sample will be much higher than for a properly hybridized sample.
RawQ	A measure of the pixel-to-pixel variation of probe cells on a GeneChip® array.
Background average	A measurement of signal intensity caused by auto-fluorescence of the array surface and non-specific binding.
Percent present	The number of probe sets called "Present" by the software relative to the total number of probe sets on the array.
Actin 3′ 5′ ratio GAPDH 3′ 5′ ratio	Signal values of the 3′ probe sets for actin and GAPDH are compared to the Signal values of the corresponding 5′ probe sets. The ratio of the 3′ probe set to the 5′ probe set is generally no more than 3 for the 1-cycle assay.
BioB	BioB represents a gene in the biotin synthesis pathway of E. coli. This transcript is added to the hybridization mixture as a control.
IVT yield (micrograms cRNA)	The yield produced by the *in vitro* transcription (IVT) reaction.

Quality Metrics for Each Array

Global metrics are those quality measures that are reported as a single value per array (Figure 3.19). These global metrics are detailed in the GeneChip® Expression Analysis Technical Manual at http://www.affymetrix.com/support/technical/manual/expression_manual.affx and in the GeneChip Expression Analysis Data Analysis Fundamentals at https://www.affymetrix.com/support/downloads/manuals/data_analysis_ fundamentals_manual.pdf. Table 3.4 serves as a reminder of quality measures we find useful.

Collectively, these metrics monitor system performance and sample quality.

Implications

1. Global metrics are intended to reflect the quality of the entire array and are insensitive to local effects that affect only a small number of probesets.
2. Global measures track laboratory mistakes, as bench processing errors are generated on an array-by-array basis.

3. Global quality metrics do not address array comparisons. If two arrays are at opposite extremes of the acceptable range, inaccuracy may be observed only when the arrays are compared.

4. The experiment may influence quality measures. For example, if a treatment introduces severe necrosis, the RNA quality can be expected to be lower. In such instances, i. e., when quality metrics track with biological factors, then vast numbers of transcripts may be reported as falsely changed. A pilot study may detect this problem.

3.2.3.2 Data Correction: Normalization and Transformation

Once low-quality data are identified, there are two analytical options: remove or correct the data. Since removing data may require repeating an experiment to replace the data, there is a strong incentive to attempt correction. Unfortunately, data that are made to look good via transforms are not the same as data that are authentically good. To maintain data integrity, any correction method should be recorded, transparent, and reversible.

Implications

1. Some correction methods are based on models that compensate for well understood sources of error. These methods include the normalization or scaling methods, which are intended to correct for scanner or spatial defects (Yang et al. 2002). These normalization methods, based on physical properties, are easily justified.

2. Some normalization methods are designed to correct perceived flaws in the structure of the data. For example, the log transformation of signal measures has an additive error with a roughly normal distribution. As mentioned below in the section on variance stabilization this transformation helps the data fit the assumptions of parametric tests.

3. Quantile normalization, lowess normalization (Dudoit et al. 2000), and variance stabilization methods (Durbin et al. 2002; Huber et al. 2002; Rocke and Durbin 2003) alter the data to fit a preconceived data structure. The physical cause of the unsatisfactory data structure may not be accounted for or even understood. These methods are difficult to justify.

4. Data integrity must be maintained. For many correction methods, for example lowess, it very difficult to record the degree of correction and to revert to the original data. For these methods it is imperative that the original data be retained.

5. A measure of the severity of the correction should be recorded to aid the biological interpretation. If a correction is severe for a given array, this may indicate poor data quality.

6. Correction methods often negate quality control parameters. This may give the experimenter undue confidence in the data and lead to incorrect interpretation of the results. For example, lowess methods eliminate saturation effects so that detecting saturation after lowess normalization is difficult.

7. Transforming the data may remove authentic biological changes (Finkelstein et al. 2002; Quackenbush 2002).

8. Interpretations based on transformed data do not directly reflect biological measurements. For example, a prediction based on the log transformed signal is not as intuitive as a more direct measure of transcript abundance.

Carefully applied, data correction methods have demonstrated real value in improving the tractability of data analysis. However, biologists need to be aware that complex methods that do not report the degree of correction or allow for easy reversibility of the data may over-correct. Data correction is not a substitute for quality control.

Variance Stabilization

Low-level transcripts are more variable than high-level transcripts, which imply that the variance is not the same for all transcripts. This violates the assumption of normality for ANOVA. If the data are not corrected, we have to use nonparametric tests that are much less powerful. The following is a simple, practical strategy to remove bias. More complex and exact methods for variance stabilization are also available and have been applied to microarrays (Huber et al. 2002; Rocke and Durbin 2003).

In the first step we add a correction factor to the signal prior to log-transformation. The factor we use is based on the average background produced by the MAS software. At the time of writing, the average background for GeneChip® microarray experiments is roughly 100, with a standard deviation of approximately 25. If we add 50 (two standard deviations of background), we can be confident that our correction is in proportion to the noise. In practice, this addition stabilizes the CV across signal values (Figure 3.20). The value can be adjusted to suit specific experimental conditions or arrays. The second step is to transform the signal values into log values, usually natural logs. This change normalizes the error so that parametric tests function as expected. This rescaling greatly inflates the importance of signal values that are near zero. These low values are close to the background and are usually attributable to noise.

Implications

1. This method is effective, simple, and reversible.

2. Any correction such as this should be recorded, especially if the data are stored in a database.

3. This correction reduces the number of replicates required (see Section 3.2.2.6).

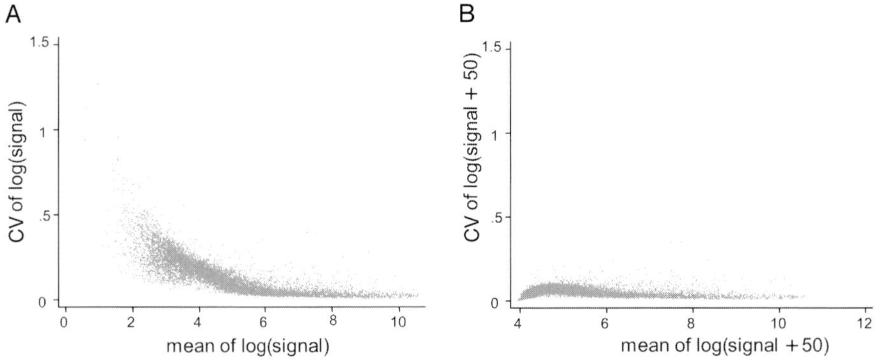

Fig. 3.20 Variance stabilization. (A) Coefficients of variance (CV) of log signal for each gene (*y* axis) against the mean of log-transformed signals produced by MAS 5.0 (*x* axis). (B) The CV of ln(signal + 50) for each gene against the mean of ln(signal + 50). Adding 50 prior to log transformation stabilizes the variance seen in A. The result of this simple invertible transformation is that parametric tests such an ANOVA perform more effectively.

4. This transform produces data that more closely fit the assumptions that underlie ANOVA models.

3.2.4
Comparing Results

The output of a microarray experiment is usually a list of probesets, ranked according to *p* values. To compare results between experiments or even between laboratories, we must compare lists. Intuitively we expect microarray experiments run under identical conditions to provide identical, or near-identical, lists of significant genes. Due to the nature of statistics, this expectation is rarely if ever met. To make effective list comparisons we need to understand how the expected variability in our signal measurements alters *p* values.

3.2.4.1 **Venn Diagrams**

Venn diagrams are the most common method used to display intersects between lists (Figure 3.21). The display is attractive and easily read, but oversimplifies the un-

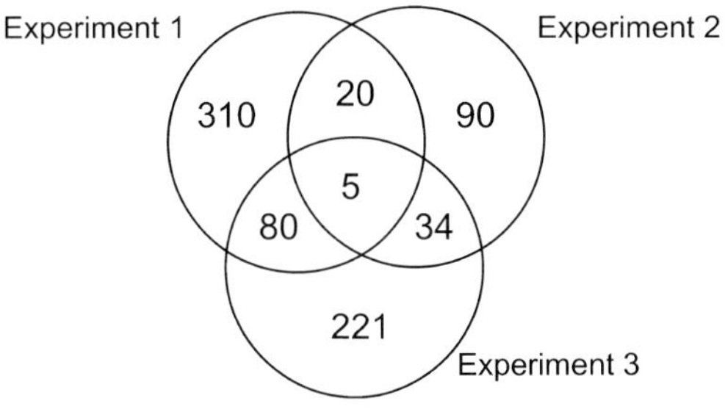

Fig. 3.21 A Venn diagram showing intersects between lists. This approach represents the intersection between data sets at only one *p* value, thereby oversimplifying the relationships between groups.

derlying data model. One simplification is that Venn diagrams treat all transcripts as equivalent, whereas microarrays result in a continuum of response and statistical significance.

Implications

1. An experiment represents a partial view of the complete biological response. The completeness of the view depends on the scope of the experimental design and the statistical power of the test. The practical result is that Venn diagrams, which are based on strict thresholds, underestimate the number of probesets in common between lists (Figure 3.22).
2. In a microarray experiment, we aim to separate the small number of authentic changes in expression from random changes in expression (Figure 3.23). To do this we usually apply a strict statistical threshold. We expect such a strict cutoff to exclude many authentic changes (false negatives) and yet include some false changes (false positives). Every time we create a list, false negative and false positive errors are created (Figure 3.24). During list comparisons the accumulation of false negatives is especially severe. A false negative is an authentic change in transcript abundance that does not pass the threshold and is excluded from the list. When we compare several lists, each containing such false negatives and false positives, we progressively lose real results until, if we compare enough lists, no agreement whatsoever remains. This effect is not unique to microarrays but is a

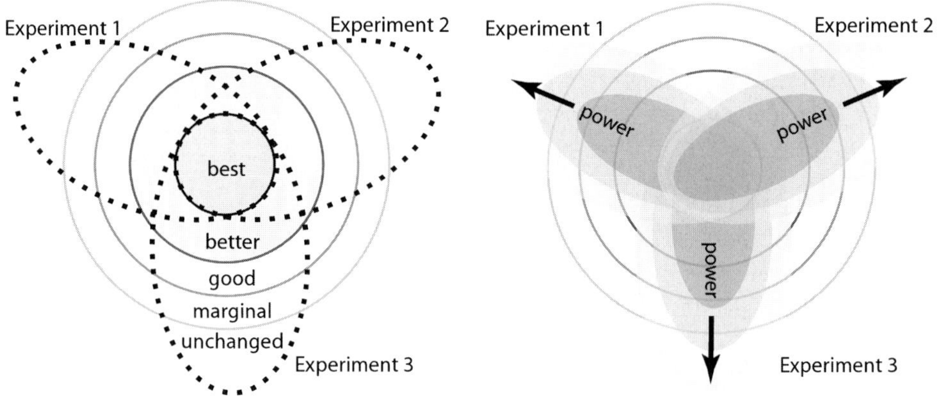

Fig. 3.22 Overlap between lists. An experiment represents a partial view of the biological response. The circles represent the biological reality, in which there is a smooth gradation from the 'best' responding transcripts to those that are 'unchanged'. In any single experiment, represented by a dashed ellipse, we are likely to measure the 'best' responders, and increasingly less likely to measure poorer responses. The result is that when we compare experiments, only the very best responders are consistent, but we under-represent poorer responses. In experiments with limited power, typically due to too few replicates, we may not be able to measure anything beyond 'good' responses, and the consequent correlation between lists is poor or non-existent.

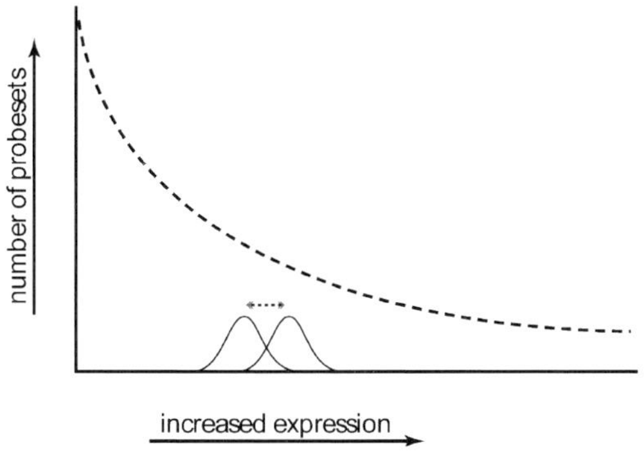

Fig. 3.23 In a typical microarray experiment, the vast majority of transcripts do not change. We are only interested in looking at the changes in a small subpopulation of transcripts that change in response to our experimental variables.

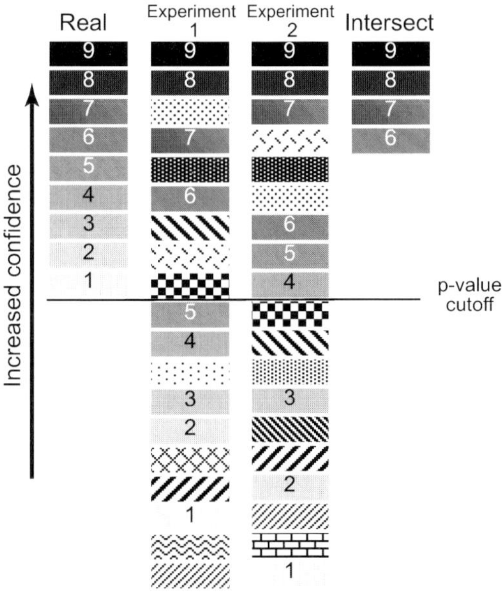

Fig. 3.24 The effect of false changes when comparing lists. Exp1 and Exp2 represent the lists, and each box represents a probeset. The probesets are arranged according to confidence, with highest confidence (lowest *p* value) at the top. 'Real' represent the authentic, real changes occurring in the cell. In the lists produced in Exp1 and Exp2 the real changes are interspersed with false positives, and false negatives fall below the *p* value threshold. The intersect shows probesets common to Exp1 and Exp2 that pass the *p* value threshold. The intersect is a significant under-representation of the 'Real' list.

known statistical effect produced by any measurement that includes some error. The model in Figure 3.25 illustrates the effect of false positives and negatives on list comparisons.

3. Venn diagrams represent an arbitrary slice through the data, treating all probesets as equivalent. This does not suit the data model, because *p* values fall along a continuum in which some probesets have a very good *p* value while others have a very poor *p* value.

3.2.4.2 Rank Correlations between Lists

Rank correlations between probeset lists generated from different experiments overcome many of the problems associated with Venn diagrams. Rank correlations are

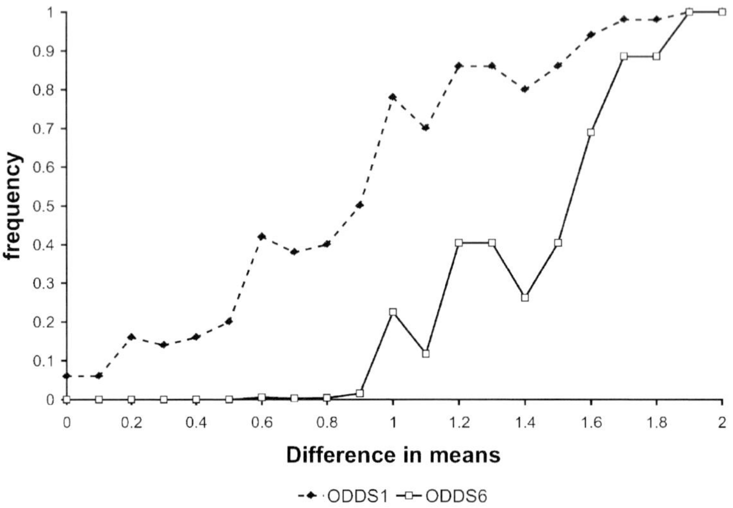

Fig. 3.25 An in silico simulated gene expression experiment. We simulated an experiment run six times. Each experiment simulated array data for approximately 5000 probesets. To do this, the number and quantity of differences between control and treatment were fixed and a known random error was added. With this approach the number and magnitude of all expression changes are known. All of these artificial changes in expression were identical for each user and the random error was of the same magnitude. A *t* test was then used to create a list of statistically significant differences between control and treatment for each experiment. This list of detected changes, i. e., those that pass the threshold, was then compared to the actual changes for every experiment. The dashed line represents the observations for one user. The *x* axis represents differences in means between control and treatment for all six experiments. Note that as the difference increases the chance of detecting statistically significant changes steadily increases. The solid line represents the proportion of changes detected by all six experimenters. The difference in means must be at least 100% (1) to detect any actual differences. Only more replicates or a greater degree of change improves the chance of agreement. This demonstrates that list agreement is low due to an inherent characteristic of statistical tests and is independent of the technology used.

based on the following model: a biological response typically affects a number of transcripts, each to a different extent. In other words, when a group of genes are activated, the degree of change in expression of each gene is falls along a range of values: the expression of some genes are highly changed, while others are moderately changed. Nonspecific changes that affect all transcripts should not affect the relative expression changes of the activated genes. Consistency of ranking can therefore be used to distinguish specific from nonspecific changes (Figure 3.26).

If authentically changed transcripts are ranked, it is possible to empirically estimate the p value threshold between specifically and nonspecifically changed genes with the following model (Figure 3.27):

Step 1: Select a series of lists of probesets that pass an increasingly stringent p value threshold. For practical reasons we use $-\ln(p \text{ value})$, so a threshold of 1 generates a list in which all probe sets have an $-\ln(p \text{ value}) > 1$. The benefit of log-transforming

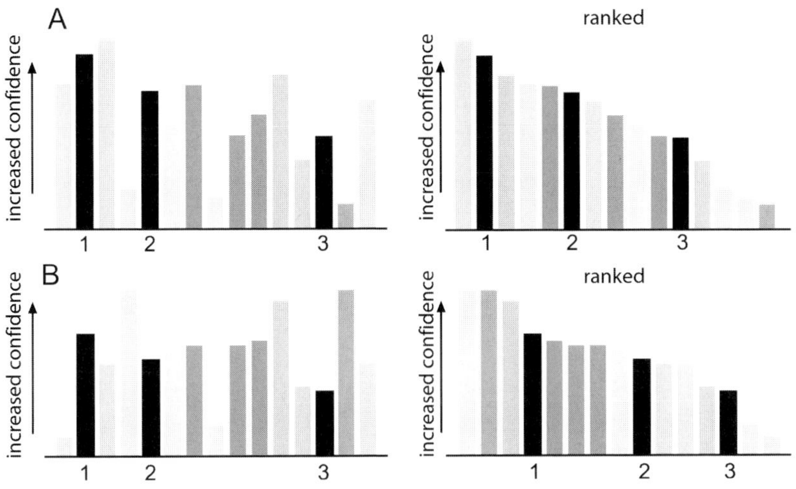

Fig. 3.26 A ranking strategy to determine specifically changed transcripts. In this hypothetical model, each bar represents the confidence level that a specific transcript had changed. The black bars each represent a specific transcript that has changed its expression level in response to a stimulus. (A) Left: the initial results; right: the same results after they were ranked according to increasing level of confidence. (B) A second experiment measuring response to the same stimulus. The rankings of the black bars, which represent the specific responders, remain constant, but the rankings of all the grey, nonspecific bars are different.

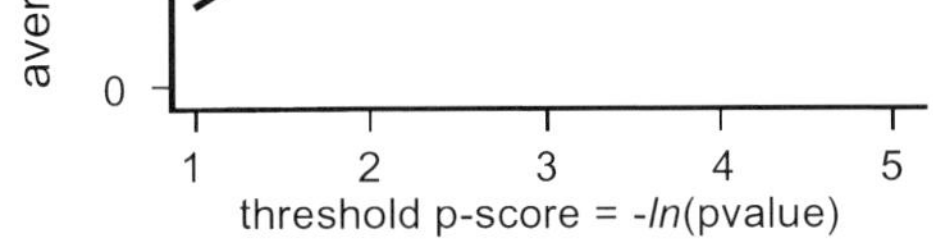

Fig. 3.27 Spearman's rank correlation at increasing stringency. A threshold of 1 indicates that all probesets for which $-\ln(p) > 1$ are selected. The first data point represents the average of five Spearman's rank correlations (values) calculated between the ranked baseline list A that passes threshold 1 and the ranked lists from all other experiments in Fig. 3.26. Data point 2 is the averaged values of the ranked list passing threshold 2, and the ranked lists from all other experiments A through E. This process is repeated for thresholds 3, 4, and 5. If the order of probesets between the lists is equivalent, then the correlation is high (ρ near 1).

the p values is that this change in scale makes the differences between very significantly changed transcripts (those having very low p values) visible.

Step 2: Calculate a Spearman's rank correlation, (rho) between a list of –log (p values) derived from experiment A and each subsequent list derived from experiments A through E.

Step 3: Average all the values to reduce the influence of single comparisons.

Implications

1. Comparing the two ranked lists where one list passes a threshold allows us to look past that threshold into the second list. This means that in the second list some new probesets appear that are not found in the first list. To capture and assess this effect, count the number of probesets in the second list and divide by the number found in the first list. Rank correlations represent only the probesets that are common to both lists.
2. As the threshold is increased we expect the lists to grow shorter, as fewer significantly changed transcripts are progressively excluded. Correspondingly, agreement in the ranks between the lists (based on average ρ) should increase until the optimum number of authentically changed probesets is included in the list. If we extend the threshold even further, the correlations reaches a plateau or may even decrease, due in part to the ever-shrinking number of genes examined. The optimum threshold (3.5 in Figure 3.27), provides a guide for selecting a p-value cutoff. The maximum average rank correlation also provides a relative measure of the number of consistently changed transcripts among all experiments.
3. If the average ρ does not improve as the threshold increases. The experiments may not involve equivalent biological effects and should not be compared.

3.2.4.3 Correlating Biological Functions Between Lists

Correlation of biological functions, such as gene ontology (GO) functions, can be used to compare lists. (GO annotations are discussed in detail, Section 3.1.3.1). The usual purpose of an experiment is to elucidate a biological function. If experiments that should yield the same biological response are compared at the functional level, this approach avoids many of the list-comparison problems. Although not statistically rigorous, this strategy can be of great practical value.

Implications

1. This approach is robust against false negatives. Each biological function is usually represented by several probesets. For example, if 11 probesets represent a biological function and five of them are captured by the list, the biological function is

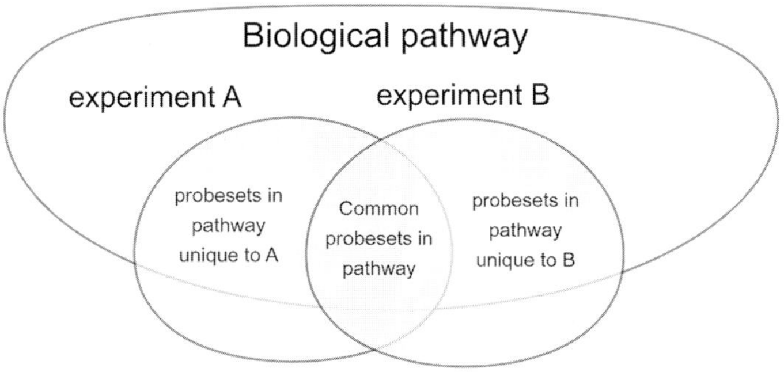

Fig. 3.28 Biological pathways may agree between lists, even if the actual probesets vary.

still indicated. If the second list captures six probesets the function is still indicated even if none of these probesets are common between the lists (Figure 3.28).

2. This approach is robust against false positives. The GO viewer (discussed elsewhere) allows the operator to set a minimum number of probesets that must be mapped to a function before the function is displayed. Random false positives are expected to be scattered among random functions so that this minimum requirement is not met and the false positives are not displayed.

3.2.5 Conclusions

Microarray experiment results are the outcome of a number of factors such as the array design, the experimental design, the data analysis, and the biological interpretation. Each step in the process should be carried out with an eye fixed firmly on the goal – the biological answer to a specific hypothesis. Ideally, the first step should be a pilot experiment to gain experience and to define the parameters, such as time, dose, and number of replicates to use in the full-scale experiment. Throughout the process, the integrity of the data should be maintained by careful quality control and practical data analysis. Good experimental design, which includes a plan for data analysis, maintains the integrity of the analysis. It is much better to run additional replicates or to repeat part of the experiment than to resurrect bad data with ingenious methods. Ultimately, the goal of the process is to link statistically validated result with a cogent biological interpretation. Ideally, this interpretation should produce a mechanism of action for observed toxic effects. The mechanism of action can then form a context for standard toxicological end-points. Through such principled, goal-orientated experiments, toxicogenomics will ultimately deliver on the promise of faster, more effective, and safer drugs.

References

Aardema M.J. and MacGregor J.T. Toxicology and genetic toxicology in the new era of 'toxicogenomics': impact of '-omics' technologies. *Mutat Res* 2002 **499**, 13–25.

Altschul S.F., Madden T.L., Schaffer A.A., Zhang J., Zhang Z., Miller W. and Lipman D.J. Gapped BLASTand PSI-BLAST: a new generation of protein database search programs. *Nucleic Acids Res* 1997 **25**, 3389–3402.

Ashburner M., Ball C.A., Blake J.A., Botstein D., Butler H., Cherry J.M., Davis A.P., Dolinski K., Dwight S.S., Eppig J.T., et al. Gene ontology: tool for the unification of biology. The Gene Ontology Consortium. *Nat Genet* 2000 **25**, 25–29.

Au W.W. Life style factors and acquired susceptibility to environmental disease. *Int J Hyg Environ Health* 2001 **204**, 17–22.

Bell D.A., Taylor J.A., Paulson D.F., Robertson C.N., Mohler J.L. and Lucier G.W. Genetic risk and carcinogen exposure: a common inherited defect of the carcinogen-metabolism gene glutathione S-transferase M1 (GSTM1) that increases susceptibility to bladder cancer. *J Natl Cancer Inst* 1993 **85**, 1159–1164.

Bennett L., Palucka A.K., Arce E., Cantrell V., Borvak J., Banchereau J. and Pascual V. Interferon and granulopoiesis signatures in systemic lupus erythematosus blood. *J Exp Med* 2003 **197**, 711–723.

Bickel D.R. Robust cluster analysis of microarray gene expression data with the number of clusters determined biologically. *Bioinformatics* 2003 **19**, 818–824.

Box G.E.P., Hunter W.G. and Hunter J.S. (1978) *Statistics for Experimenters: An Introduction to Design, Data Analysis, and Model Building*. Wiley, New York.

Burczynski M.E., McMillian M., Ciervo J., Li L., Parker J.B., Dunn R.T., Hicken S., Farr S. and Johnson M.D. Toxicogenomics-based discrimination of toxic mechanism in HepG2 human hepatoma cells. *Toxicol Sci* 2000 **58**, 399–415.

Calabrese E.J. Ecogenetics: historical foundation and current status. *J Occup Med* 1986 **28**, 1096–1102.

Calabrese E.J. Biochemical individuality: the next generation. *Regul Toxicol Pharmacol* 1996 **24**, S58–67.

Cheng R.Y., Alvord W.G., Powell D., Kasprzak K.S. and Anderson L.M. Microarray analysis of altered gene expression in the TM4 Sertoli-like cell line exposed to chromium(III) chloride. *Reprod Toxicol* 2002 **16**, 223–236.

Cobb G.W. (1997) *Introduction to Design and Analysis of Experiments*, pp. 454–455. Springer-Verlag, New York.

Dahlquist K.D., Salomonis N.,Vranizan K., Lawlor S.C. and Conklin B.R. GenMAPP, a new tool for viewing and analyzing microarray data on biological pathways. *Nat Genet* 2002 **31**, 19–20.

Doniger S.W., Salomonis N., Dahlquist K.D., Vranizan K., Lawlor S.C. and Conklin B.R. MAPPFinder: using gene ontology and GenMAPP to create a global gene-expression profile from microarray data. *Genome Biol* 2003 **4**, R7.

Dow G.S. Effect of sample size and *p*-value filtering techniques on the detection of transcriptional changes induced in rat neuroblastoma (NG108) cells by mefloquine. *Malar J* 2003 **2**, 4.

Dudoit S. and Fridlyand J. A prediction-based resampling method for estimating the number of clusters in a dataset. *Genome Biol* 2002 **3**, RESEARCH0036.

Dudoit S. and Fridlyand J. Bagging to improve the accuracy of a clustering procedure. *Bioinformatics* 2003 **19**, 1090–1099.

Dudoit S.,Yang Y.H., Callow M.J. and Speed T.P. Statistical methods for identifying differentially expressed genes in replicated cDNA microarray experiments. *Stats, UC Berkeley, Tech Rep* 2000 **578**.

Dunn R.T. II and Kolaja K.L. Gene expression profile databases in toxicity testing. In: M.E. Burczynski (ed.): *An Introduction to Toxicogenomics*, CRC Press, Boca Raton, FL, 2003, pp. 213–224.

Durbin B.P., Hardin J.S., Hawkins D.M. and Rocke D.M. A variance-stabilizing transformation for gene-expression microarray data. *Bioinformatics* 2002 **18 Suppl 1**, S105–110.

Efron B. and Tibshirani R. Empirical Bayes methods and false discovery rates for microarrays. *Genet Epidemiol* 2002 **23**, 70–86.

Efron B., Halloran E. and Holmes S. Bootstrap confidence levels for phylogenetic trees. *Proc Natl Acad Sci U S A* 1996 a **93**, 7085–7090.

Efron B., Halloran E. and Holmes S. Bootstrap confidence levels for phylogenetic trees. *Proc Natl Acad Sci U S A* 1996 b **93**, 13429–13434.

Everitt B.S., Landau S. and Leese M. (2001) *Cluster Analysis*. 4 edn. Edward Arnold, London.

Finkelstein D., Ewing R., Golub J. and Sterky F. Microarray data quality analysis: lessons from the AFGC project. *Plant Mole. Biol* 2002 **48**, 119–131.

Fodor S.P., Read J.L., Pirrung M.C., Stryer L., Lu A.T. and Solas D. Light-directed, spatially addressable parallel chemical synthesis. *Science* 1991 **251**, 767–773.

Fodor S.P., Rava R.P., Huang X.C., Pease A.C., Holmes C.P. and Adams C.L. Multiplexed biochemical assays with biological chips. *Nature* 1993 **364**, 555–556.

Garte S. Metabolic susceptibility genes as cancer risk factors: time for a reassessment? *Cancer Epidemiol Biomarkers Prev* 2001 **10**, 1233–1237.

GeneChip® Expression Analysis Technical Manual http://www.affymetrix.com/support/technical/manual/expression_manual.affx

GeneChip® Expression Analysis Technical Manual http://www.affymetrix.com/support/technical/manual/expression_manual.affx

Gerhold D., Lu M., Xu J., Austin C., Caskey C.T. and Rushmore T. Monitoring expression of genes involved in drug metabolism and toxicology using DNA microarrays. *Physiol Genomics* 2001 **5**, 161–170.

Ghosh D. Resampling methods for variance estimation of singular value decomposition analyses from microarray experiments. *Funct Integr Genomics* 2002 **2**, 92–97.

Guengerich F.P., Beaune P.H., Umbenhauer D.R., Churchill P.F., Bork R.W., Dannan G.A., Knodell R.G., Lloyd R.S. and Martin M.V. Cytochrome P-450 enzymes involved in genetic polymorphism of drug oxidation in humans. *Biochem Soc Trans* 1987 **15**, 576–578.

Huber W.,Von Heydebreck A., Sultmann H., Poustka A. and Vingron M. Variance stabilization applied to microarray data calibration and to the quantification of differential expression. *Bioinformatics* 2002 **18 Suppl 1**, S96–S104.

Ingelman-Sundberg M., Johansson I., Persson I., Oscarson M., Hu Y., Bertilsson L., Dahl M.L. and Sjoqvist F. Genetic polymorphism of cytochrome P450. Functional consequences and possible relationship to disease and alcohol toxicity. *Exs* 1994 **71**, 197–207.

Irizarry R.A., Bolstad B.M., Collin F., Cope L.M., Hobbs B. and Speed T.P. Summaries of Affymetrix GeneChip probe level data. *Nucleic Acids Res* 2003 **31**, e15.

Kanehisa M. The KEGG database. *Novartis Found Symp* 2002 **247**, 91–101; discussion 101–103, 119–128, 244–152.

Kanehisa M. and Goto S. KEGG: Kyoto encyclopedia of genes and genomes. *Nucleic Acids Res* 2000 **28**, 27–30.

Kanehisa M., Goto S., Kawashima S. and Nakaya A. The KEGG databases at GenomeNet. *Nucleic Acids Res* 2002 **30**, 42–46.

Kerr M.K. and Churchill G.A. Bootstrapping cluster analysis: assessing the reliability of conclusions from microarray experiments. *Proc Natl Acad Sci USA* 2001 **98**, 8961–8965.

Kim C.C. and Falkow S. Significance analysis of lexical bias in microarray data. *BMC Bioinformatics* 2003 **4**, 12.

Lander E.S., Linton L.M., Birren B., Nusbaum C., Zody M.C., Baldwin J., Devon K., Dewar K., Doyle M., FitzHugh W., et al. Initial sequencing and analysis of the human genome. *Nature* 2001 **409**, 860–921.

Landi S. Mammalian class theta GSTand differential susceptibility to carcinogens: a review. *Mutat Res* 2000 **463**, 247–283.

Lazarou J., Pomeranz B.H. and Corey P.N. Incidence of adverse drug reactions in hospitalized patients: a meta-analysis of prospective studies. *Jama* 1998 **279**, 1200–1205.

Li J. and Johnson J.A. Comparative studies using cDNA vs. oligonucleotide arrays. In: M.E. Burczynski (ed.): *An Introduction to Toxicogenomics*, CRC Press, Boca Raton, FL, 2003, pp. 17– 27.

Liu G., Loraine A.E., Shigeta R., Cline M., Cheng J.,Valmeekam V., Sun S., Kulp D. and Siani-Rose M.A. NetAffx: Affymetrix probesets and annotations. *Nucleic Acids Res* 2003 **31**, 82–86.

Marchant G. Genomics and toxic substances: part II–Genetic susceptibility to environmental agents. *ELR* 2003 a **33**, 10641–10667.

Marchant G. Genomics and toxic substances: part I–Toxicogenomics. *ELR* 2003 b **33**, 10071–10093.

Martinez M.J., Aragon A.D., Rodriguez A.L., Weber J.M., Timlin J.A., Sinclair M.B., Haaland D.M. and Werner-Washburne M. Identification and removal of contaminating fluorescence from commercial and in-house printed DNA microarrays. *Nucleic Acids Res* 2003 **31**, e18.

Murzin A.G., Brenner S.E., Hubbard T. and Chothia C. SCOP: a structural classification of proteins database for the investigation of sequences and structures. *J Mol Biol* 1995 **247**, 536–540.

Nakao M., Bono H., Kawashima S., Kamiya T., Sato K., Goto S. and Kanehisa M. Genome-scale gene expression analysis and pathway reconstruction in KEGG. *Genome Inform Ser Workshop Genome Inform* 1999 **10**, 94–103.

Nuwaysir E.F., Bittner M., Trent J., Barrett J.C. and Afshari C.A. Microarrays and toxicology: the advent of toxicogenomics. *Mol Carcinog* 1999 **24**, 153–159.

Ogata H., Goto S., Fujibuchi W. and Kanehisa M. Computation with the KEGG pathway database. *Biosystems* 1998 **47**, 119–128.

Ogata H., Goto S., Sato K., Fujibuchi W., Bono H. and Kanehisa M. KEGG: Kyoto encyclopedia of genes and genomes. *Nucleic Acids Res* 1999 **27**, 29–34.

Olden K. and Guthrie J. Genomics: implications for toxicology. *Mutat Res* 2001 **473**, 3–10.

Oscarson M. Genetic polymorphisms in the cytochrome P450 2A6 (CYP2A6) gene: implications for interindividual differences in nicotine metabolism. *Drug Metab Dispos* 2001 **29**, 91–95.

Park B.K. and Pirmohamed M. Toxicogenetics in drug development. *Toxicol Lett* 2001 **120**, 281–291.

Pearson W.R. Effective protein sequence comparison. *Methods Enzymol* 1996 **266**, 227–258.

Peddada S.D., Lobenhofer E.K., Li L., Afshari C.A., Weinberg C.R. and Umbach D.M. Gene selection and clustering for time-course and dose–response microarray experiments using order-restricted inference. *Bioinformatics* 2003 **19**, 834–841.

Peña D., Tiao G. and Tsay R. *A Course in Time Series Analysis.* Wiley, New York, 2000.

Pirmohamed M. and Park B.K. Genetic susceptibility to adverse drug reactions. *Trends Pharmacol Sci* 2001 **22**, 298–305.

Pirmohamed M. and Park B.K. Cytochrome P450 enzyme polymorphisms and adverse drug reactions. *Toxicology* 2003 **192**, 23–32.

Quackenbush J. Microarray data normalization and transformation. *Nat Genet* 2002 **32** (Suppl), 496–501.

Reiner A., Yekutieli D. and Benjamini Y. Identifying differentially expressed genes using false discovery rate controlling procedures. *Bioinformatics* 2003 **19**, 368–375.

Retief J.D. Phylogenetic analysis using PHYLIP. *Methods Mol Biol* 2000 **132**, 243–258.

Retief J.D., Lynch K.R. and Pearson W.R. Panning for genes: a visual strategy for identifying novel gene orthologs and paralogs. *Genome Res* 1999 **9**, 373–382.

Retief J.D. Phylogenetic analysis using PHYLIP. *Methods Mol Biol* 2000 **132**, 243–258.

Rocke D.M. and Durbin B. Approximate variance-stabilizing transformations for gene-expression microarray data. *Bioinformatics* 2003 **19**, 966–972.

Scheel J., von Brevern M.C. and Storch T. Transcriptional profiling in toxicology. In: M.E. Burczynski (ed.): *An Introduction to Toxicogenomics,* CRC Press, Boca Raton, FL, 2003, pp. 81–98.

Tamayo P., Slonim D., Mesirov J., Zhu Q., Kitareewan S., Dmitrovsky E., Lander E.S. and Golub T.R. Interpreting patterns of gene expression with self-organizing maps: methods and application to hematopoietic differentiation 17. *Proc Natl Acad Sci USA* 1999 **96**, 2907–2912.

Tibshirani R., Walther G. and Hastie T. Estimating the number of clusters in a dataset via the gap statistic. *JRSSB* 2000 **63**, 411–423.

Ueda H.R., Chen W., Adachi A., Wakamatsu H., Hayashi S., Takasugi T., Nagano M., Nakahama K., Suzuki Y., Sugano S., et al. A transcription factor response element for gene expression during circadian night. *Nature* 2002 **418**, 534–539.

Ulrich R. and Friend S.H. Toxicogenomics and drug discovery: will new technologies help us produce better drugs? *Nat Rev Drug Discov* 2002 **1**, 84–88.

ULRICH R.G., BACON J.A., BRASS E.P., CRAMER C.T., PETRELLA D.K. and SUN E.L. Metabolic, idiosyncratic toxicity of drugs: overview of the hepatic toxicity induced by the anxiolytic, panadiplon. *Chem Biol Interact* 2001 **134**, 251–270.

VAN BELLE G. *Statistical Rules of Thumb*. Wiley, New York, 2002.

WANG J.T.L., SHAPIRO B.A. and SHASHA D.E. (1999) *Pattern Discovery in Biomolecular Data: Tools, Techniques, and Applications*. Oxford University Press.

WARING J.F., JOLLY R.A., CIURLIONIS R., LUM P.Y., PRAESTGAARD J.T., MORFITT D.C., BURATTO B., ROBERTS C., SCHADT E. and ULRICH R.G. Clustering of hepatotoxins based on mechanism of toxicity using gene expression profiles. *Toxicol Appl Pharmacol* 2001 **175**, 28–42.

WAYNE M.L. and MCINTYRE L.M. Combining mapping and arraying: an approach to candidate gene identification. *Proc Natl Acad Sci USA* 2002 **99**, 14903–14906.

WESTFALL P.H., ZAYKIN D.V. and YOUNG S.S. Multiple tests for genetic effects in association studies. *Methods Mol Biol* 2002 **184**, 143–168.

WITTWER M., FLUCK M., HOPPELER H., MULLER S., DESPLANCHES D. and BILLETER R. Prolonged unloading of rat soleus muscle causes distinct adaptations of the gene profile. *FASEB J* 2002 **16**, 884–886.

WOOD T.C. and PEARSON W.R. Evolution of protein sequences and structures. *J Mol Biol* 1999 **291**, 977–995.

XU X.L., OLSON J.M. and ZHAO L.P. A regression-based method to identify differentially expressed genes in microarray time course studies and its application in an inducible Huntington's disease transgenic model. *Hum Mol Genet* 2002 **11**, 1977–1985.

YANG Y.H., DUDOIT S., LUU P., LIN D.M., PENG V., NGAI J. and SPEED T.P. Normalization for cDNA microarray data: a robust composite method addressing single and multiple slide systematic variation. *Nucleic Acids Res* 2002 **30**, e15.

ZEEBERG B.R., FENG W., WANG G., WANG M.D., FOJO A.T., SUNSHINE M., NARASIMHAN S., KANE D.W., REINHOLD W.C., LABABIDI S., et al. GoMiner: a resource for biological interpretation of genomic and proteomic data. *Genome Biol* 2003 **4**, R28.

4
Toxicogenomics Applications of Open-platform High Density DNA Microarrays

Mark McCormick and Emile F. Nuwaysir

4.1
Introduction

Toxicogenomics is based on the principle that changes in gene expression can be used as predictors of toxicity and perhaps to discern the mode of action of a particular compound. Under this paradigm, transcription profiles are generated from as many genes as possible, preferably the entire genome of the organism, when exposed to a given model toxicant. This transcriptome data can then serve as a training set to develop a more predictive and robust assay based on the expression profiles of a smaller number of genes, perhaps hundreds.

In the last several years, pilot studies have validated this approach in simple model systems using classical toxicants as test compounds. Some of these studies have suggested that differential expression of a very small number of genes, from 10 to 300, may be sufficient to serve as markers for toxicity [1–6].

Thus, the ideal tool to carry out toxicogenomics testing would be a microarray platform that can perform whole-genome analyses to identify the signature gene list, as well as run smaller focused arrays in extremely high throughput. The ability to run both genome-scale and focused arrays on the identical technology platform is critical to avoiding errors associated with inter-platform data comparison.

The standard method for high-density oligonucleotide microarray manufacture [7–9] takes advantage of three simple tools: (1) DNA phosphoramidite synthesis chemistry, (2) photolithography, and (3) photochemistry. This method has been used to synthesize hundreds of thousands of 25-mer oligonucleotides in parallel on solid supports.

Although the method is extremely powerful, the synthesis chemistry employed to date is relatively inefficient, and the required photolithographic masks are relatively expensive. These two characteristics make long-oligo microarrays (e.g. 60-mers) difficult and expensive to produce. Also, the photolithographic masks are inherently inflexible (changing a single probe requires the manufacture of an entire new set of masks), thus making the tool impractical for the design and redesign of smaller focused arrays for toxicogenomics.

Handbook of Toxicogenomics: Strategies and Applications. Edited by Jürgen Borlak

ISBN: 3-527-30342-1

A more recent technology developed by NimbleGen Systems employs photolithography to manufacture microarrays but obviates the need for photolithographic masks to pattern light [10–13]. The method instead utilizes the Digital Micromirror Device (DMD) developed by Texas Instruments [14, 15] to pattern light using only digital input.

This DMD-based approach to microarray manufacture has all the fundamental advantages of conventional photolithographic manufacturing techniques, including high density, high information content, parallel chemical synthesis, and manufacturing scalability. However, using the DMD, photolithographic masks are not required. This eliminates the fundamental cost and time barriers associated with the manufacture of custom high-density microarrays. Also, since the synthesis cycle for a given array is relatively short (approximately three hours) and the design process is digital (and therefore very low cost), an iterative approach to array design can be employed, in which experimental results can be used to improve the design of subsequent experiments.

The DMD is an array of 786 432 aluminium mirrors contained within a 17.4×13.1 mm area; each mirror is 16 μm square and arranged on a 17 μm centre-to-centre spacing [14, 15]. Figure 4.1 shows an external view of a DMD device, as well as micrographs of a section of the mirror array and the individual mirror substructure. Higher-density micromirror arrays are available from Texas Instruments, which offer 1.3×10^6 individual mirrors or more. Each mirror is mounted on a torsion hinge and can be deflected 10° in the positive or negative direction from the neutral state in a voltage-dependent manner. Mirrors tilted in the $+10^\circ$ orientation deflect light into the light path and onto the flow cell, while mirrors deflected in the -10° orientation deflect light out of the light path and onto an absorber. Using this method, sharply focused spatially resolved, digitally generated light patterns can be created.

Using these patterns of light in combination with photochemistry, DNA arrays can be manufactured. Figure 4.2 shows an overview of this synthesis process using

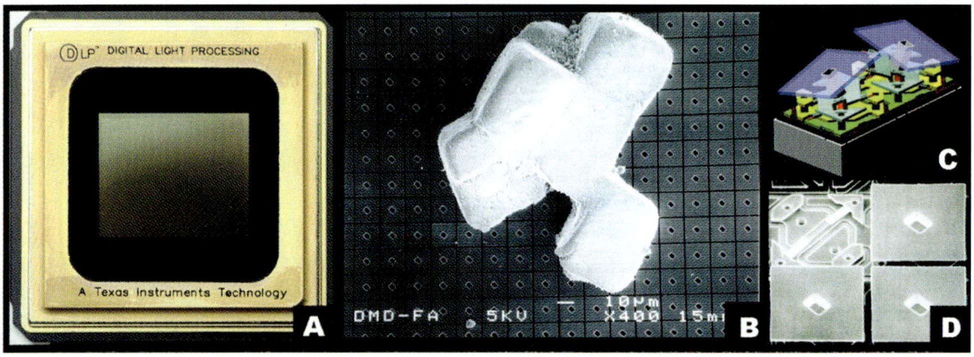

Fig. 4.1 DMD structure. (A) Texas Instruments Digital Micromirror Device. (B) Photomicrograph of a section of the micromirror array, with a grain of table salt shown for comparison. Each mirror is 16 μm square, on a 17 μm pitch. (C) Diagram of two micromirrors, with one mirror in the 'off' position and one mirror in the 'on' position. (D) high-resolution photomicrograph of four micromirror structures, with one micromirror removed to show the underlying microelectromechanical architecture. (Images courtesy of Texas Instruments Inc.).

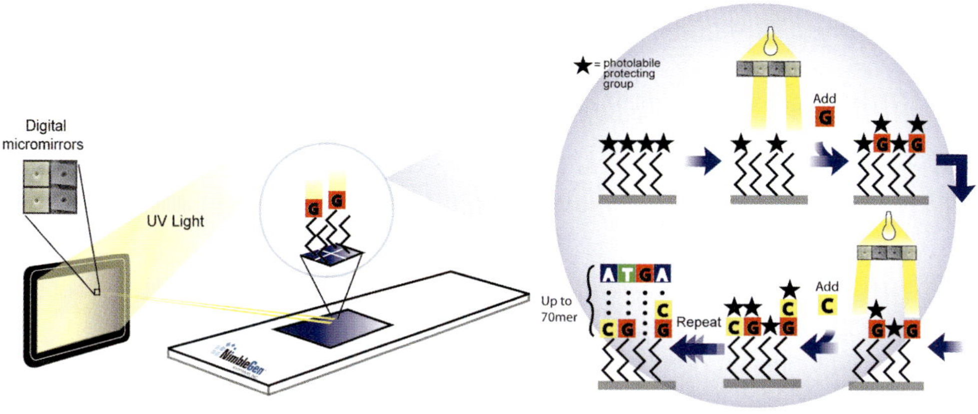

Fig. 4.2 Method for manufacture of microarrays using the NimbleGen Maskless Array Synthesizer. The UV light source is projected by the mirror array onto locations where photodeprotection is required. To the right is a graphical depiction of the sequential spatially addressed addition of nucleotides to the growing array.

the DMD. In the first step, two out of four of the possible synthesis sites are illuminated, resulting in deprotection of the surface-bound nucleotide and allowing for the subsequent coupling of the G nucleotide. In the next step, two different positions on the array are illuminated, resulting in coupling of the C nucleotide at those specific locations. By repeating this process, the desired oligonucleotide polymers can be synthesized in parallel.

Figure 4.3 shows the interior architecture of the NimbleGen Maskless Array Synthesizer (MAS). As shown in the figure, the fundamental components of the NimbleGen MAS instrument are the Texas Instruments DMD, an optical subassembly for illumination of the DMD, an imaging subassembly for refocusing the light projected from the DMD onto the activated substrate, a flow cell, and DNA synthesis chemistry including monomers with photolabile protecting groups. Not shown in this figure is the MAS fluidics delivery system, which is an Expedite DNA synthesizer from Applied Biosystems. With the exception of the fluidics station, a small optical shutter, and the micromirrors, there are no moving parts within the MAS unit. This results in a stable and robust instrument design that is amenable to desktop microarray manufacture in the average laboratory.

The digital nature of the light patterns created by the DMD, combined with the fact that each mirror is independently addressable, allows for spots of varying sizes or centre-to-centre distances (pitch) to be synthesized. Virtually any pattern based on the 16 μm mirror size can be created. Figure 4.4 is a hybridization image in which the same oligonucleotide probes have been synthesized in four different formats on the same array. In Figure 4.4 A, each probe was synthesized using four mirrors in a 2×2 block that were functionally grouped during synthesis. This results in a spot that is 33 μm square (16 μm mirror + 1 μm space + 16 μm mirror) on a 51 μm pitch. As shown in the figure, a border of inactive mirrors surrounds each block of four

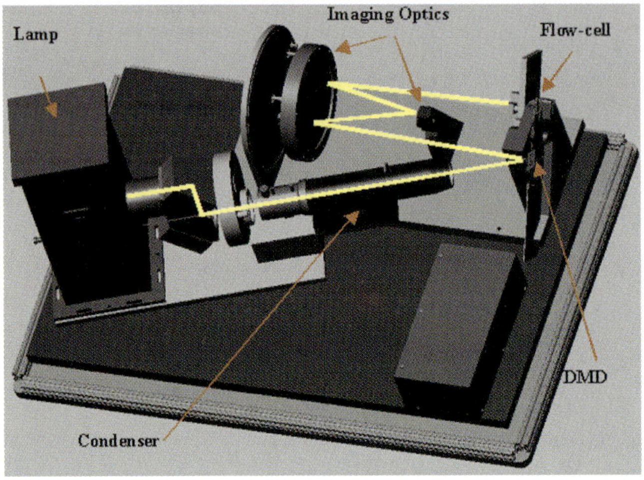

Fig. 4.3 NimbleGen maskless array synthesizer. Depicted is a cutaway view of the MAS in which the thick white line illustrates the light path from its origin at the lamp, through the optics, to the flow cell. The digital micromirror device (DMD) reflects the required light patterns through the optical pathway to project a 1 : 1 image on the flow cell. The system can produce very high-contrast images, allowing the synthesis of arrays of oligonucleotides with lengths of up to 80 nucleotides.

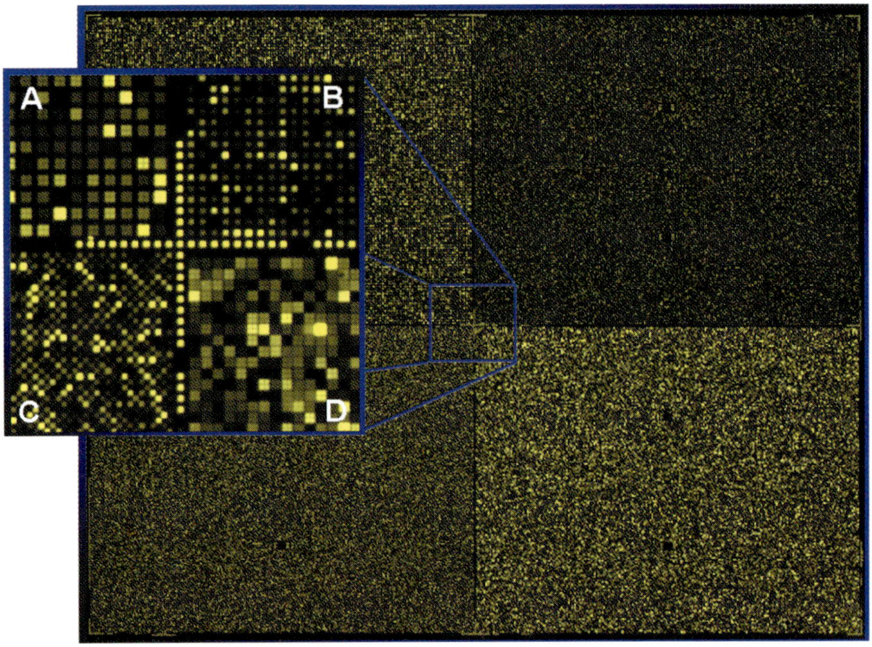

Fig. 4.4. Feature density options of NimbleGen arrays. A variety of feature sizes and densities are available on NimbleGen arrays. In this experiment, identical probes specific for a subset of mouse genes were arrayed in four different probe formats on a single array and hybridized with cRNA derived from mouse liver total RNA.

Tab. 4.1 Array designs available with the NimbleGen gene expression platform.

Array format	*Total probes*	*Feature size*	*Pitch*	*Illustration*
1_2	393 216	16 μm	34 μm [1)]	Figure 4.4 C
1_4	196 608	16 μm	34 μm	Figure 4.4 B
4_4	196 608	33 μm	34 μm	Figure 4.4 D
4_9	87 296	33 μm	51 μm	Figure 4.4 A

1) 24 μm centre-to-centre spacing on the diagonal.

active mirrors, resulting in four active mirrors in a total group of nine used to synthesize a single spot; thus, this format is referred to as 4_9. By varying the number of grouped mirrors and the proportion of dormant mirrors used as spacers, microarrays with a large number of possible spot sizes and pitches can be created, such as the 1_4, 1_2, and 4_4 formats shown in Figure 4.4 B–D, respectively.

Table 4.1 details the standard array formats offered by NimbleGen. As many as 393 216 features (probes) can be synthesized on a single custom array in the highest density 1_2 format. In any of these formats, the oligonucleotides can vary in length from 1-mers up to a maximum of 80-mers. Since all spots are synthesized in parallel, spot size, pitch, and feature quantity do not affect manufacturing costs.

On a typical array, probes are placed within a defined layout of control elements. These control elements are designed to control for possible variations in the synthesis and/or hybridization of the array. Figure 4.5 demonstrates the layout and number of these control probes. As shown in the figure, the 'A' probes are used to test overall uniformity of the array synthesis, and the corner probes also serve as fiducial marks for automated image analysis (image location, grid alignment, and feature intensity extraction). More than 600 'A' probe replicates are distributed throughout the entire array. 'B' probes are base-specific synthesis controls, represented 112 times on the array. 'C' probes are a six-point spike-in standard curve that demonstrates the limit of detection (sensitivity) and linear range of the array. These sets are replicated 56 times throughout the array. 'D' probes are a 10-point photometric standard curve used to assess synthesis efficiency with varying light dosage and are replicated 12 times on the array. In total more than 1200 quality-control probes are incorporated into every array.

4.2
Genome-scale Expression Profiling

Using the full complement of 393 216 available features, an entire genome can be represented on a NimbleGen microarray. This allows a researcher to study the expression of all the genes in an organism simultaneously. This capability is a critical element for the first step of the toxicogenomics paradigm – the identification of gene expression signatures. Figure 4.6 shows an example dataset from large-scale gene expression profiling using custom NimbleGen arrays in *Saccharomyces cerevisiae*. Fig-

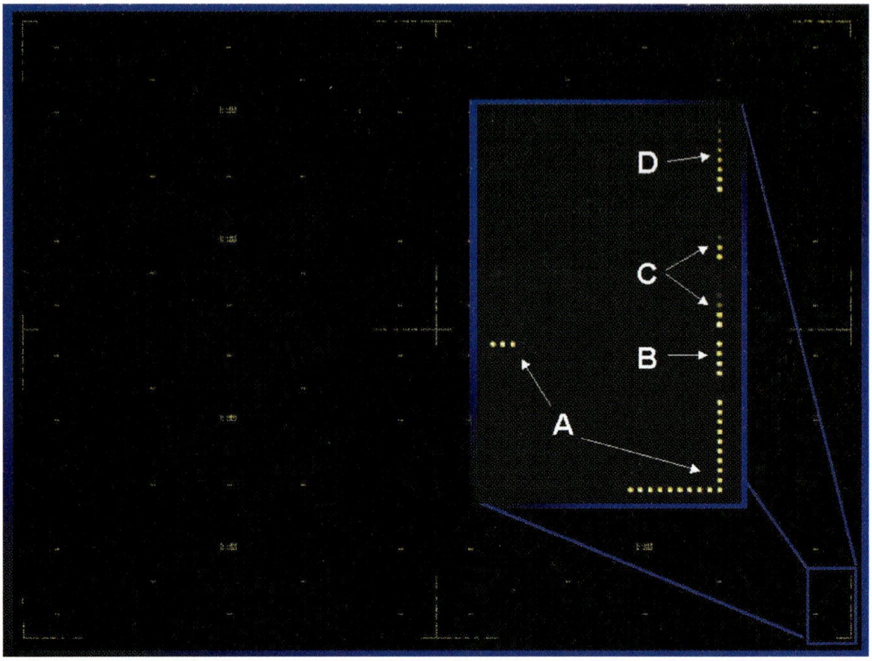

Fig. 4.5 Quality-control features. Standard NimbleGen array designs include a minimum of 1200 different control features. Customer-specified controls can also be included. The array in this figure was hybridized to a cocktail of Cy-3 labelled spike-in controls to illuminate their positions on the array.

ure 4.6 (left) shows data from a replicate hybridization of the same sample on two independent arrays, for which the R^2 correlation is approximately 0.998. The average gene expression value for each of the 6200 genes in the organism is plotted. In Figure 4.6 (right), the x axis represents data acquired from yeast grown on glucose medium, while the y axis shows data from yeast grown on galactose medium.

4.3 Multiplex Array Hybridization with NimbleScreen 12

NimbleGen arrays provide an unprecedented feature density for custom, user-defined, in situ–synthesized arrays. However, the available capacity of 393 216 probes often exceeds the number of probes required for some assays. Screening of a relatively small set of signature genes in a toxicogenomics assay is an archetypal example of such an array application, in which a relatively small set of optimized probes (e.g., 5000) is preferable to a larger set of genome-scale probes (e.g., 400 000). With sufficient replicates of training set data and linkage of observed differential gene expression in signature genes to histopathology-based observations, the required pro-

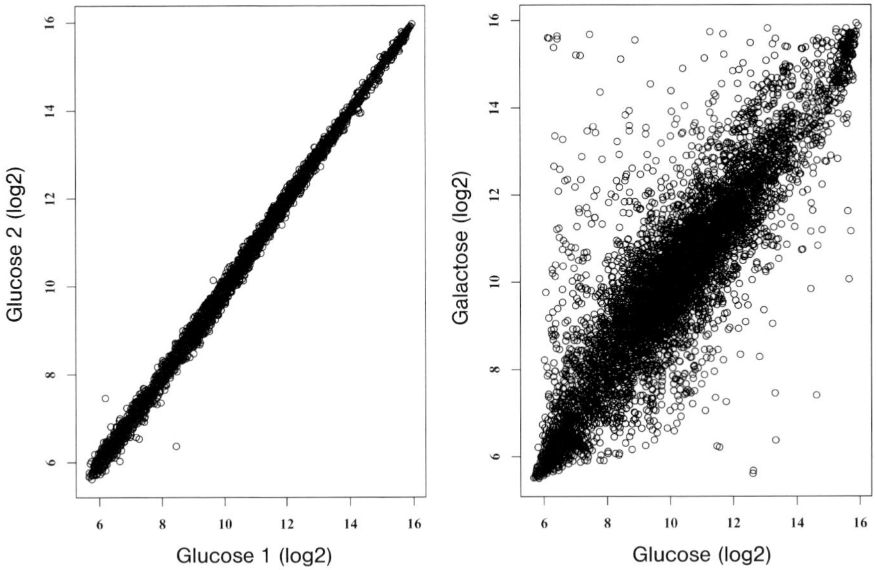

Fig. 4.6 Gene expression. Left: Data from replicate hybridizations of the same labelled yeast RNA to two independent arrays. Right: Differential gene expression depending on whether yeast is grown on glucose (*x* axis) or galactose (*y* axis) medium.

spective screening set may be fully contained in an array of a few thousand probes. With these reduced probe set requirements, the NimbleGen array capacity can be more efficiently used by dividing the array into a grid of individual subarrays and processing multiple samples in parallel.

Multiplex processing of replicate subarrays provides a cost-effective means to perform time- or dose-dependent studies of differential gene expression. Dose dependency studies of differential gene expression are a critical method, because they help resolve therapeutic and toxic dose levels and establish the therapeutic index of a candidate drug. Temporal studies are useful in distinguishing circadian expression patterns from those attributable to toxicity, particularly when compared to untreated controls. The ability to conduct twelve independent microarray experiments within a single custom high-density DNA microarray has the potential to greatly accelerate the development and application of toxicogenomics for routine screening of a wide variety of chemical entities.

We have developed a multiplex DNA microarray technology, termed NimbleScreen 12, which permits the processing of 12 samples in parallel on a single array. The individual subarrays are arranged in a 3×4 grid of circular 'wells'. Each well contains up to 13 500 independent features. Probe sets are synthesized, in situ, within the wells using the previously described synthesis method. The area surrounding the wells is made hydrophobic by a proprietary process. The result is a surface that contains 12 regions of higher hydrophilicity, as shown in Figure 4.7. The

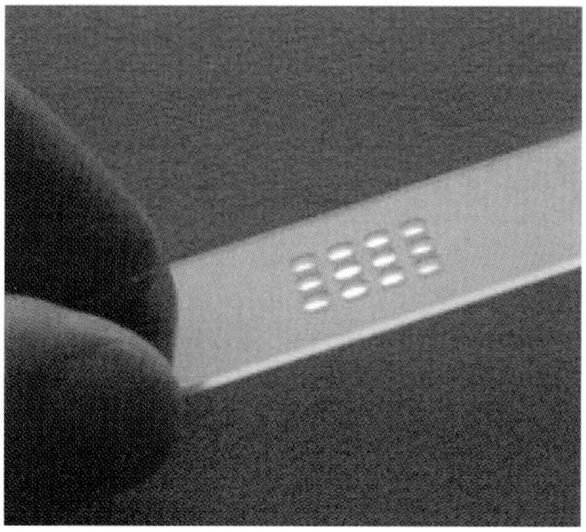

Fig. 4.7 Water droplets on a hydrophobic grid. The hydrophobic layer of NimbleScreen 12 causes individual water droplets to remain bound with high contact angles within the array areas while sheeting off the surrounding areas.

location of the grid of wells is precisely aligned with a sample containment fixture, engineered to maintain sample alignment with array areas and stable hydration for long-duration hybridizations.

The optimal sample volume in the current configuration is 6 μL. The chamber formed by the containment fixture is bound by O-ring seals to prevent sample evaporation. An auxiliary reservoir within the chamber acts as a hydration donor to saturate the enclosed chamber volume. The fixture has been extensively tested under a variety of hybridization conditions and temperatures and has proven to be a reliable method for sequestering multiple samples on an array surface.

By contrast, other methods for parallel processing of samples on a single array typically involve the placement of an adhesive-backed barrier on the array surface to segregate samples. The use of physical barriers can pose a higher risk of experimental failure due to misalignment of the barrier relative to the array location, inadequate hydration of the entire array area leading to severe nonuniformity, or barrier failure leading to sample cross-contamination. In addition, depending on the width of the barriers employed, a significant percentage of the slide area may be occupied by the barriers and unavailable for probe synthesis or hybridization. These risks and drawbacks are largely eliminated with the design of NimbleScreen 12.

4.4
NimbleScreen 4

For the routine screening of larger probe sets, an intermediate level of multiplex sample hybridization has been developed, termed NimbleScreen 4. In this format, the available array is divided into a 2 × 2 grid of subarrays within which up to 55 000 user-defined probes can be synthesized. The working sample volume is 10–30 μL, and the method of sample containment is analogous to that in NimbleScreen 12. A template for four-well array design is available as an option for array layouts. The sample fixture described above is employed for four-well hybridizations, but the in-

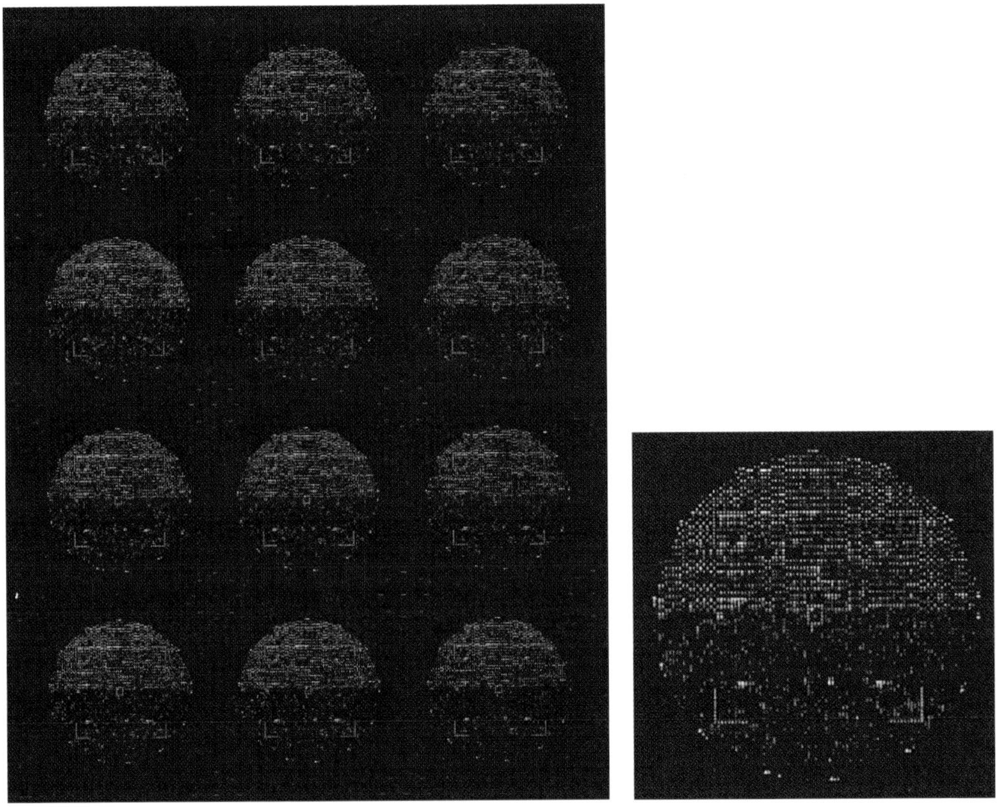

Fig. 4-8 Nimble Screen 12 gene expression profiling. The image schown is a NimbleScreen 12 hybridization of mouse liver cRNA to a mouse liver/spleen design. Genes empirically selected for high-level expression in mouse liver were placed in the upper half of each well and genes highly expressed in spleen were placed in the lower half. The inset shows a close up view of one of the wells. The interwell r^2 values for the extracted data sets had an average of 0.9972.

terchangeable sample insert is replaced with one designed to align and contain four samples, rather than 12. The sample volume is optimized to incorporate a small bubble during sample loading. The bubble facilitates sample mixing as the fixture is rotated during hybridization, providing hybridization uniformity. The higher probe capacity of the four-well system may be well suited to the evaluation of smaller toxicogenomic training sets in which a larger number of samples is desired, for example, when working with smaller genomes or applying a training set with a reduced number of genes. With a capacity of up to 55 000, it is possible to query expression levels of 10 000 genes with a representation of five probes per gene in each of the four wells of NimbleScreen 4.

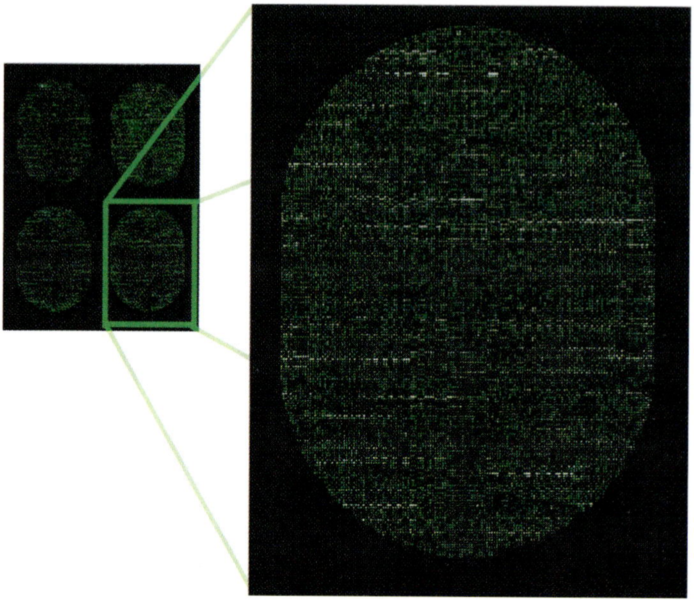

Fig. 4-9 Nimble Screen 12 gene expression profiling. The array shown incorporates probes sets derived from genes previously determined to be highly expressed in mouse liver and spleen (an expanded set analogous to Figure 4-7) tiled and interleaved. Each well was hybridized with mouse liver cRNA. Each well contains 55,000 features and includes a mismatch control for each perfect match probe.

4.5
Software for Open-platform Array Design

Because the NimbleGen array technology is essentially an 'open source' platform, users may use their own probe sets and design arrays according to their experimental requirements. To facilitate the design of NimbleGen arrays, software was developed to provide a graphical interface for array layout. A graphical representation of the array surface and drag-and-drop functionality greatly facilitate the incorporation of probe sets into array designs. The software has default templates for the design of 1-plex, 4-plex, and 12-plex arrays. The only limitation placed on 12-well array design is the capacity of each well. Individual wells in NimbleScreen 12 have probe capacities that are layout-dependent. Probe layouts in the 1_4 pattern can accommodate 6789 probes per well. Similarly, 4_4 layouts can hold 6606 probes, and 1_2 layouts can hold 13 747. A free version of the software is available for download [19]. The probe sets can be imported from tab-delimited text files, and users may design 12 identical subarrays or a unique set of probes for each array, as desired. The probes can be arranged in either a random or nonrandom manner within each well, and the software has additional features that facilitate the array design process.

4.6 Multiplex Array Control Elements

The NimbleScreen 12 template incorporates a set of several hundred standard control probes that are used during array manufacture to monitor array quality. Each individual well contains multiple replicates of a set of 12 unique probes that are present around the circumference of the well and represented in a grid in the centre of the well. The circumferential probes provide a functional confirmation that the subarray and sample are in proper alignment and adequately hydrated during hybridization. If the sample is misaligned or the sample volume inadequate, these probes reveal measurable nonuniformity in signal intensity. When samples are prepared for hybridization, a unique control oligonucleotide, complimentary to one of the grid of 12 control probes is added, at saturating concentration, to monitor for cross-contamination. In this way, any cross-contamination between samples results in detectable signal in more than one control probe in any affected wells.

One additional advantage of NimbleScreen 12 is the reduced sample requirement relative to the full array format. For typical differential gene expression work, a total of 10 µg of labelled cRNA is required for full-array hybridizations. By contrast, only 250 ng of cRNA is required for an individual well in NimbleScreen 12. This reduction in sample results in a proportionate reduction in sample labelling costs. The decreased sample may also make possible the screening of smaller cell or tissue samples, which may be very important when testing precious drug candidates of limited availability.

4.7 Multiplex Array Consistency

One requirement for prospective toxicogenomics screening is that the array results observed for the training set be consistent with those observed for the screening set. In addition, any array-based screening method required that arrays demonstrate a high degree of intra- and inter-array signal consistency. Although global shifts in intensity can, to a certain extent, be adjusted by dataset normalization, the best array results are obtained from the most consistently manufactured arrays.

The reproducibility of 12-well hybridizations has been tested by comparison of inter-well correlations of replicate hybridizations. Table 4.2 is an example comparison of mouse liver cRNA hybridized to a set of genes selected from mouse liver and spleen. The average difference values for every gene in the set were compared between each well and the remainder of the wells in the array by a least-squares fit linear correlation. As can be seen in the table, the data were highly reproducibly from well to well with an average R^2 value of 0.997. The same level of reproducibility is achieved when comparing 1-plex and 12-plex data for comparable probe sets. The fact that the results are highly consistent in the transition from the full array to the 12-well format provides good assurance that the results observed during training set development will hold during routine screening set deployment.

Tabl. 4.2 Well-to-well dataset reproducibility. Twelve replicates of a mouse liver probe set containing 6789 features were synthesized in a 12-plex array and hybridized with 12 aliquots from the same sample. The data were extracted and average difference values for each gene were calculated. The datasets for each well were compared by least-squares fit linear correlation, and the inter-well R^2 values are shown in the table. The average R^2 value for the set was 0.9972.

	Well 1	Well 2	Well 3	Well 4	Well 5	Well 6	Well 7	Well 8	Well 9	Well 10	Well 11	Well 12
Well 1	1.000	0.998	0.997	0.997	0.997	0.996	0.996	0.998	0.996	0.995	0.994	0.996
Well 2	–	1.000	0.998	0.998	0.998	0.998	0.998	0.999	0.998	0.996	0.996	0.998
Well 3	–	–	1.000	0.997	0.998	0.999	0.997	0.998	0.998	0.996	0.997	0.998
Well 4	–	–	–	1.000	0.999	0.997	0.998	0.998	0.997	0.996	0.997	0.997
Well 5	–	–	–	–	1.000	0.998	0.998	0.998	0.998	0.996	0.998	0.997
Well 6	–	–	–	–	–	1.000	0.998	0.998	0.999	0.997	0.998	0.997
Well 7	–	–	–	–	–	–	1.000	0.999	0.998	0.997	0.998	0.997
Well 8	–	–	–	–	–	–	–	1.000	0.999	0.997	0.997	0.997
Well 9	–	–	–	–	–	–	–	–	1.000	0.996	0.998	0.996
Well 10	–	–	–	–	–	–	–	–	–	1.000	0.998	0.997
Well 11	–	–	–	–	–	–	–	–	–	–	1.000	0.997
Well 12	–	–	–	–	–	–	–	–	–	–	–	1.000

4.8 Conclusions

The principal paradigm of toxicogenomics requires a broad transcriptome survey to identify target genes whose shifts in expression can be linked to toxicity response. Once identified, this working set of transcriptome targets can be used in the routine screening of a larger number of samples in a higher-throughput mode. Ideally, the same DNA microarray technology can be applied to both survey and screening modes to allow direct comparison of datasets through the assay development process. The high-density, open-platform, microarray technology described here is well positioned to support the transition from toxicity target identification through optimization to routine sample screening in a facile, flexible way.

References

1. Bulera SJ, Eddy SM, Ferguson E, Jatkoe TA, Reindel JF, Bleavins MR, De La Iglesia FA (**2001**) RNA expression in the early characterization of hepatotoxicants in Wistar rats by high-density DNA microarrays. *Hepatology 33*: 1239–1258.
2. Hamadeh HK, Bushel PR, Jayadev S, Martin K, DiSorbo O, Sieber S, Bennett L, Tennant R, Stoll R, Barrett JC, Blanchard K, Paules RS, Afshari CA (**2002**) Gene expression analysis reveals chemical-specific profiles. *Toxicol Sci 67*: 219–231.
3. Hamadeh HK, Bushel PR, Jayadev S, DiSorbo O, Bennett L, Li L, Tennant R, Stoll R, Barrett JC, Paules RS, Blanchard K, Afshari CA (**2002**) Prediction of compound signature using high density gene expression profiling. *Toxicol Sci 67*: 232–340.
4. Thomas RS, Rank DR, Penn SG, Zastrow GM, Hayes KR, Pande K, Glover E, Silander T, Craven MW, Reddy JK, Jovanovich SB, Bradfield CA (**2001**) Identification of toxicologically

predictive gene sets using cDNA microarrays. *Mol Pharmacol 60*: 1189–1194.

5. Waring JF, Jolly RA, Ciurlionis R, Lum PY, Praestgaard JT, Morfitt DC, Buratto B, Roberts C, Schadt E, Ulrich RG (**2001**) Clustering of hepatotoxins based on mechanism of toxicity using gene expression profiles. *Toxicol Appl Pharmacol 175*: 28–42.
6. Waring JF, Ciurlionis R, Jolly RA, Heindel M, Ulrich RG (**2001**) Microarray analysis of hepatotoxins *in vitro* reveals a correlation between gene expression profiles and mechanisms of toxicity. *Toxicol Lett 120*: 359–368.
7. Bushel PR, Hamadeh HK, Bennett L, Green J, Ableson A, Misener S, Afshari CA, Paules RS (**2002**) Computational selection of distinct class- and subclass-specific gene expression signatures. *J Biomed Inform 35*: 160–170.
8. Fodor SP, Read JL, Pirrung MC, Stryer L, Lu AT, Solas D (**1991**) Light-directed, spatially addressable parallel chemical synthesis. *Science 251*: 767–773.
9. Pease AC, Solas D, Sullivan EJ, Cronin MT, Holmes CP, Fodor SA (**1994**) Light-generated oligonucleotide arrays for rapid DNA sequence analysis. *Proc Natl Acad Sci USA 91*: 5022–5026.
10. Lockhart DJ, Solas D, Sullivan EJ, Cronin MT, Holmes CP, Fodor SA (**1996**) Expression monitoring by hybridization to high-density oligonucleotide arrays. *Nat Biotechnol 14*: 1676–1680.
11. Singh-Gasson S, Green RD, Yue Y, Nelson C, Blattner F, Sussman M, Cerrina F (**1999**) Maskless fabrication of light-directed oligonucleotide microarrays using a digital micromirror array. *Nat Biotechnol 17*: 974–978.
12. Nuwaysir EF, Huang W, Albert TJ, Pitas A, Nuwaysir AK, Singh J, Richmond T, Gorski T, Berg JP, Ballin J, McCormick M, Norton J, Pollock T, Sumwalt T, Butcher L, Porter D, Molla M, Hall C, Blattner F, Sussman MR, Wallace RL, Cerrina F, Green RD (**2002**) Gene expression analysis using oligonucleotide arrays produced by maskless photolithography. *Genome Research 12*: 1749–1755.
13. Albert TJ, Norton J, Ott M, Richmond T, Nuwaysir AK, Nuwaysir EF, Stengele K, Green RD (**2003**) Light-directed 5′–3′ synthesis of complex oligonucleotide microarrays for large-scale genotyping. *Nucleic Acids Research 31*: e35, 1–9.
14. NimbleGen Systems Inc. website: http://www.nimblegen.com/
15. Van Kessel PF, Hornbeck LJ, Meier RE, Douglass MR (**1998**) A MEMS-based projection display. *Proc IEEE, 86*: 1687–1704.
16. Sampsell JB. (**1994**) Digital micromirror device and its application to projection displays. *J Vac Sci B12*: 3242–3246.
17. Paules R (**2003**) Phenotypic anchoring: linking cause and effect, *Environ Health Perspect 111*: A338–339.

5
Mass Spectrometry and Proteomics: Principles and Applications

Uwe Rapp

5.1
Introduction

Since the invention of the term 'proteomics' the meaning has been adjusted several times, e.g., by adding words for specific characterization. As of today, three specific categories have been identified and are in use: expression proteomics, interaction proteomics, and structural proteomics [1]. In toxicoproteomics one would mainly apply the expression 'proteomics methodology' as discussed later.

This chapter focuses on methodologies involving mass spectrometry (MS). However, related techniques that are essential for the success of MS are discussed as well. The pros and cons of the various approaches are discussed, although in proteomics the methods that are optimal are heavily influenced by the analytical goal behind a biochemical or biological question. A short view of informatics closes the chapter, but the focus is mainly on the workflow and software modules, because they make the analytical techniques used practical and comprehensible.

The main application areas in which MS is used as key technology [2] are:

- Identification of proteins in large-scale projects resulting in libraries for different tissues, body fluids, or organisms. An example is the human brain protein project [3], which is now under way, for which a consortium of laboratories is trying to identify all human brain proteins as completely as possible. Many other projects are in progress for protein mapping of different species.
- Determination of changes in the proteome pattern under various influences, such as stress, toxic substances, changes in environmental conditions. Here, the up- and down-regulation, or more precisely the protein abundance, is monitored. This means that quantification of the amounts of protein is the essential point. Several techniques are in use; some are based on detection of fluorescence introduced by chemical labels prior to two-dimensional (2D) gel separation. Others are based on MS, such as the ICAT (isotope-coded affinity tag) technology [4] and related techniques [5], in which isotopically labelled quantification markers are, for example in ICAT, covalently bound to cysteine. In principle, all cysteine-containing proteins

Handbook of Toxicogenomics: Strategies and Applications. Edited by Jürgen Borlak

ISBN: 3-527-30342-1

can be quantified; however, all groups reactive to the derivatization protocol are modified as well.

- In-depth analysis of individual proteins that can be separated by gel electrophoresis or chromatographic techniques. Modifications, especially post-translational modifications, but also mutations of the DNA reflected in the protein sequence, are to be determined. Here, very recently the top–down approach, analysing intact proteins, has had an impact [6].
- Use of the protein pattern for global screening in clinical proteomics. For example, the protein mixture obtained from diseased tissue is analyzed after specific fractionation, and bioinformatics tools are used to classify protein patterns based on pattern-recognition methods [7]. Mass spectrometry is essential for these applications and becomes even more important for the identification of biomarkers, which in turn are closely related to the in-depth analysis mentioned above.

5.2 Analysis Tools in Proteomics

Techniques are basically applied in three steps in proteomics projects:

- Separation and fractionation of proteins, including enrichment if required.
- Mass spectrometric analysis.
- Data evaluation resulting in identification or quantification or PTM (post translational modification) detection.

5.2.1 Separation Techniques

Why are separation techniques required? Could the mass spectrometer not deal with the sample in total? This is known as the shotgun approach. In general, one can say that any reduction of the complexity of the sample at the front end significantly pays off later on, in the performance of MS and in easier evaluation of datasets. The shotgun approach is successful only if the sample complexity is reduced or if a certain compartment or protein complex of limited complexity is under investigation.

- Gel-based systems, either 1D or 2D, are widely used; 2D gels especially have a resolution that is unmatched until now and can separate several thousand protein spots [8]. A special feature of 2D gels, in addition to information on the pI and molecular mass, is the separation of isoforms that cannot be separated by chromatography [9]. Zoom gels covering smaller pH ranges are very attractive when only a fraction is of interest. In general, there is a trend to use 1D gels, since they are easier and faster to run and often yield sufficient resolution [2]. The presence of several proteins in one spot or in a gel band can be accepted, because the mass spectrometer used in the next analysis step is, to a certain extent, a mixture analysis system, provided the complexity is limited to only a few proteins.

- In recent years liquid chromatography systems have been becoming competitive with the gel-based techniques. A requirement is a flow rate in the nanoflow range, to achieve the sensitivity required – the low femtomol to attomol range. The introduction of commercial systems for nanoflows at 50 to 500 nL min^{-1} together with columns of, e.g., 75 μm i.d. have made this technology very attractive. The separation power is sufficient for moderately complex protein mixtures – usually, enzymatic digestion mixtures. A chromatographic run requires about 60 min total analysis time. A new development is the use of monolithic columns [10], for which the total run times are as low as 10–15 min. However, the requirements respecting the scan speeds of the mass spectrometer then are very stringent, and instruments a few years old cannot cope with these demands. In the meantime, chromatographic systems with microflows (several μL min^{-1}) are being used as well. However, they cannot achieve the same sensitivity as the nanoflow systems.
- 2D liquid chromatography (2D nanoHPLC) is being developed but is still in its infancy [11]. Typically, as the first dimension a stepwise-increased salt gradient eluting, for example, a strong anion-exchange column is followed by a standard reversed-phase separation as the second dimension. The separation power is high; however, the runs require many hours or even a whole day, depending on the tuning of the salt gradients. Huge datasets are acquired when these systems are coupled to ESI–MS systems running in an automatic alternating mode of MS and MS/MS spectra acquisition. It seems that redundancy may create problems during evaluation, because a large portion of the MS/MS spectra is not used, not required, or not interpretable.
- Multidimensional chromatography approaches (MudPIT) [12] are now under development and have yet to prove their possible superiority to 2D gel-based systems.
- Capillary electrophoresis (CE) seems to be very useful, although it is not used much. The analysis times are very short, and in one run proteins and peptides can be separated. In addition, 2D–LC–CE couplings are possible. Sensitivities are comparable to those achieved with a straight 2D nanoLC experiment [13].
- Other techniques, such as free-flow electrophoresis (FFE), have been well known for years [14]; however, they have not attracted much attention in practice [15].

5.2.2 Mass Spectrometric Techniques

Two ionisation technologies for mass spectrometers have, since their invention and commercialisation, revolutionized measurements in the protein analysis area:

- Matrix-assisted laser desorption/ionisation (MALDI).
- Electrospray ionisation (ESI).

These two ionisation techniques are coupled to different types of mass analysers, such as time-of-flight (TOF), ion traps (IT), quadrupole (Q), and several hybrid configurations, such as triple quadrupole (QqQ), Q–q–TOF, Q–q–Fourier transform (FT)

MS, Trap–TOF, TOF/TOF, and others. The hybrid mass spectrometers are called tandem mass spectrometers.

It is commonly accepted that MALDI–TOF instruments are ideal for very rapid, accurate determinations of peptide mass fingerprint (PMF) spectra resulting from 2D gel–separated and digested proteins. In principle, several thousand spectra per day can be measured [16]. Automation is available that uses fuzzy-logic methods for intelligent acquisition of spectra in MS and MS/MS modes of operation [17]. The entire workflow from the 2D gel via picking, digestion, MS measurement in MS and MS/MS mode, to database search for identification of proteins is today under complete software control when commercial equipment is used [18].

ESI-coupled instruments are operated as MS/MS instruments and therefore give more structurally related information, although being significantly slower for a single sample, due to the separation technologies usually coupled up-front. The classical nanospray arrangement is no longer a preferred system because of suppression effects with complex mixtures and insufficient sensitivity.

The main characteristics of the above-mentioned mass spectrometers are the determination of molecular masses of intact or enzymatically digested proteins. This is a first dimension of information, which is often sufficient to identify a protein: in sequenced genomes such as those of *Escherichia coli*, yeast, or humans, typically 60%–80% of the samples can be identified this way. However, for the remaining samples the MS/MS mode has to be used, where, as a second dimension of information, the structural aspect is determined. The molecular ion species are fragmented and sequence-specific fragments are generated which can in turn give a highly specific identification of a protein. Typically, sequence tags of varying length are used to identify the proteins via database searches. The MS/MS techniques are ideally suited for complete de novo sequencing, especially when redundant data, for example, from a MALDI–TOF/TOF and an ESI–IT, are available [19].

MALDI [20] and ESI [21] are well documented as methods, as are the characteristics of the above mentioned mass spectrometers, and are not discussed here.

5.3 Application

The separation of proteins from a cell line using 2D gel processing is presented below. This example should serve as a model system for the total workflow during a proteomics investigation and illustrates how well the identification of proteins by PMF works and when MS/MS spectra have to be added for successful identification, using the MALDI–TOF/TOF technology or the ESI–IT technology to generate MS/MS spectra.

5.3.1 Experimental Details

Proteins from a human cell lysate, separated by 2D gel electrophoresis followed by colloidal Coomassie Blue staining, were provided by Dr. Hanno Langen (Roche,

Basle, Switzerland). The Coomassie-stained spots were excised by using a spot-picking robot and then trypsin-digested with a digestion/preparation robot using a commercially available chemical kit (kit and robots were from Bruker Daltonik). Thirty percent of the digestion solution was applied by the thin-layer method to 600 μm MALDI AnchorChip targets (Bruker Daltonik); the remaining 70% was used for ESI analysis without any further purification.

MALDI–TOF MS and MS/MS

Spectra were acquired on a MALDI–TOF/TOF mass spectrometer (ultraflex from Bruker Daltonik) in the MS and MS/MS mode of operation. The instrument was equipped with a 2-GHz digitizer, delayed-extraction ion source, LIFT cell, gridless double stage reflectron, and timed ion selector for precursor ion selection. Up to 10 MS/MS spectra were acquired from an individual spot on the target.

LC–MS/MS

The LC–MS/MS spectra were acquired on an Esquire HCT ion-trap instrument (Bruker Daltonik) connected to an Ultimate nano HPLC system (Dionex/LC Packings) equipped with a 75 μm i.d. PepMap column 15 cm long and of 5-μm particle size.

In the experiment discussed here the workflow chosen for analysing all samples with all three MS techniques was (1) MALDI–TOF for PMF spectra, (2) MALDI–MS/MS (TOF/TOF), and (3) nanoHPLC–ESI–MS/MS for generation of fragment spectra.

Overall, 86 spots were selected from the gel and automatically digested, MS analysed, and processed by using Mascot as a database search engine.

5.3.2 Results

From the 2D gel (Figure 5.1), 86 spots were identified and analysed using different parameter settings for the database search. The influence of the settings on the time needed for the total analysis and the quality of identification were studied to find an optimal approach for larger proteome studies. Table 5.1 summarizes the proteins identified. The overall success rate after the whole automatic process was 97%.

Figure 5.2 shows the effect of different stringency criteria for identification of a protein. For the 'relaxed' scoring, a PMF Mascot scoring of >100 was accepted as sufficient for identification. Hits <100 had to be remeasured in MALDI–MS/MS mode. However, the majority of the 66 spots could be identified by using PMF alone. The remaining 20 were identified via TOF/TOF (6) or nanoHPLC–ESI–MS/MS (14). Overall, the analysis time was about 14 h. The PMF measurements of 66 spots required 33 min in all, the 6 spots identified by MALDI–MS/MS needed 30 min, and the other 14 spots for which nanoHPLC–MS/MS was used required 13 h. The time values include the instrument running times and the evaluation procedures.

The 'stringent' mode allowed for identifications at Mascot scores >300. Here, the easy and fast PMF was sufficient for identification of only 25 spots. The majority of spots (61) had to be measured in MS/MS mode: 17 of them received good scores by the use of MALDI–TOF/TOF and the rest of the 44 spots had to be measured by na-

Tab. 5.1 List of proteins from the 2D gel identified on the basis of MALDI-TOF and TOF/TOF as well as LC-ESI MS/MS spectra.

Spot	*Identified protein*
1	(P16949) Stathmin (phosphoprotein p19)
2	(P16949) Stathmin (phosphoprotein p19)
3	(P15531) Nucleoside diphosphate kinase A (EC 2.7.4.6)
4	(P32119) Peroxiredoxin 2 (EC 1.11.1.-)
5	(P32119) Peroxiredoxin 2 (EC 1.11.1.-)
6	(P09211) Glutathione S-transferase P (EC 2.5.1.18)
7	(P09936) Ubiquitin carboxyl-terminal hydrolase isozyme L1
8	(P43487) Ran-specific GTPase-activating protein
9	(A25530) Tropomyosin alpha 3 chain
10	?
11	?
12	(P28066) Proteasome subunit alpha type 5 (EC 3.4.25.1)
13	(P28066) Proteasome subunit alpha type 5 (EC 3.4.25.1)
14	(P12004) Proliferating cell nuclear antigen
15	(P12004) Proliferating cell nuclear antigen
16	(P06748) Nucleophosmin (NPM)
17	(Q15181) Inorganic pyrophosphatase (EC 3.6.1.1)
18	(P06748) Nucleophosmin + tetratricopeptide repeat protein 1
19	(P07195) L-lactate dehydrogenase B chain (EC 1.1.1.27)
20	(P05388) 60S acidic ribosomal protein P0
21	(P12277) Creatine kinase, B chain (EC 2.7.3.2)
22	(P02570) Actin, cytoplasmic 1
23	(P50502) Hsc70-interacting protein (Hip)
24	(P34932) Heat shock 70-kDa protein 4
25	(P05218) Tubulin beta-5 chain
26	(P05209) Tubulin alpha-1 chain
27	(P05209) Tubulin alpha-1 chain + (A25074) vimentin
30	(P08107) Heat shock 70-kDa protein 1
31	(P07900) Heat shock protein HSP 90-alpha
32	(P55072) Transitional endoplasmic reticulum ATPase
33	(P08107) Heat shock 70-kDa protein 1
34	(P48643) T-complex protein 1, epsilon subunit
35	(Q02790) FK506-binding protein 4 (EC 5.2.1.8)
36	(P07237) Protein disulfide isomerase precursor
37	(P78371) T-complex protein 1, beta subunit
38	(P17987) T-complex protein 1, alpha subunit
39	(P49368) T-complex protein 1, gamma subunit
40	(P40227) T-complex protein 1, zeta subunit
41	(P06733) Alpha enolase (EC 4.2.1.11)
42	(O43175) D-3-phosphoglycerate dehydrogenase (EC 1.1.1.95)
43	(P31948) Stress-induced-phosphoprotein 1
44	(P12268) Inosine-5′-monophosphate dehydrogenase 2
45	(P06733) Alpha enolase (EC 4.2.1.11)
46	(Q99832) T-complex protein 1, eta subunit

Tab. 5.1 (continued)

Spot	Identified protein	Spot	Identified protein
47	(P04075) Fructose bisphosphate aldolase A (EC 4.1.2.13)	67	(P47756) F-actin capping protein beta subunit
48	(P78417) Glutathione transferase omega 1 (EC 2.5.1.18)	68	(Q99426) Tubulin-specific chaperone B
49	(P25786) Proteasome subunit alpha type 1 (EC 3.4.25.1)	69	(P25788) Proteasome subunit alpha type 3 (EC 3.4.25.1)
50	(P05217) Tubulin beta-2 chain	70	(P28072) Proteasome subunit beta type 6 precursor
51	(P00938) Triosephosphate isomerase (EC 5.3.1.1)	71	(O75832) 26S proteasome non-ATPase regulatory subunit 10
52	(P18669) Phosphoglycerate mutase 1 (EC 5.4.2.1) (EC 5.4.2.4)	72	(Q99436) Proteasome subunit beta type 7 precursor
53	(P09329) Ribose-phosphate pyrophosphokinase I (EC 2.7.6.1)	73	(L76416) Similar to SMT3
54	(P05217) Tubulin beta-2 chain	74	(O75347) Tubulin-specific chaperone A
55	(P09429) High mobility group protein 1	75	(P05387) 60S acidic ribosomal protein P2
56	(P05092) Peptidyl-prolyl cis-trans isomerase A (EC 5.2.1.8)	76	(A60167) Acidic ribosomal protein P2
57	(P23528) Cofilin, non-muscle isoform	77	(P02593) Calmodulin
58	(Q06830) Peroxiredoxin 1 (EC 1.11.1.-)	78	(A49798) Nucleoside diphosphate kinase
59	(Q9UQ80) Proliferation-associated protein 2G4	79	(Q15185) Telomerase-binding protein p23
60	(O35753) TATA-binding protein-interacting protein 49	80	(P52565) Rho GDP-dissociation inhibitor 1
61	(O43175) D-3-phosphoglycerate dehydrogenase (EC 1.1.1.95)	81	(P39687) Potent heat-stable protein phosphatase 2A inhibitor
62	(P30101) Protein disulfide isomerase A3 precursor	82	(S43309) Probable HLA class II-associated protein PHAPI, human
63	(P31943) Heterogeneous nuclear ribonucleoprotein H	83	(P42655) 14-3-3 protein epsilon
64	(Q13347) Eukaryotic translation initiation factor 3 subunit	84	(O00299) Chloride intracellular channel protein 1
65	(Q9Y3F4) UNR-interacting protein	85	(P08865) 40S ribosomal protein SA
66	(P06733) Alpha enolase (EC 4.2.1.11)	86	(P19338) Nucleolin
		87	(P14625) Endoplasmin precursor
		88	(Q07244) Heterogeneous nuclear ribonucleoprotein K

Fig. 5.1 2D gel of lysed HEK293 cells (335 μg), with the identified spots numbered. Spots discussed in more detail in this chapter are circled.

noHPLC–MS/MS. The total analysis time for this stringent procedure was 44 h. This was due to the high percentage of MS/MS measurements that required nanoHPLC–ESI as methodology, because each spot with a certain number of peptides requires a complete LC run, which takes about 40–60 min. The measuring times for these analyses could be shortened significantly, to 10–15 min per run or spot, if a monolithic column had been used, which have recently become commercially available. However, the scan speed of the mass spectrometer has to cope with the very narrow peaks, which is not possible for many instruments for which the scan speeds are in the range of several seconds per full scan. Ion traps are very suitable for this task, since their scan speeds exceed 25 000 u s^{-1}.

„Relaxed“: Score below 100 -> must be further analyzed

Spot #	MALDI MS	MS/MS	LC-MS/MS
32	506		
38	474		
37	452		
33	447		
30	427		
24	426		
47	416		
26	411		
51	397		
46	394		
45	391		
43	359		
25	355		
36	354		
87	347		
40	335		
53	334		
39	329		
34	322		
50	319		
65	314		
59	310		
44	309		
84	309		
27	299		
21	296		
17	292		
41	288		
31	281		
52	275		
35	272		
14	269		
58	265		
19	263		
1	260		
22	254		
49	248		
63	244		
66	237		
81	234		
88	234		
20	229		
64	223		
68	222		
86	222		
4	220		
42	218		
23	217		
83	213		
62	208		
69	206		
48	199		
7	194		
61	193		
3	178		
71	178		
57	175		
12	172		
85	156		
67	149		
74	145		
56	142		
75	135		
18	130		
79	111		
72	104		
8	86	171	
76	77	155	
80	79	132	
70	96	126	
16	58	124	
55	98	106	
60	0	0	865
9	0	0	490
6	41	65	489
78	0	0	388
77	0	0	208
82	0	0	193
15	0	0	170
5	0	0	125
73	0	0	125
54	0	0	114
13	0	0	96
2	0	0	44

„Stringent“: Score below 300 -> must be further analyzed

Spot #	MALDI MS	MS/MS	LC-MS/MS
32	506		
38	474		
37	452		
33	447		
30	427		
24	426		
47	416		
26	411		
51	397		
46	394		
45	391		
43	359		
25	355		
36	354		
87	347		
40	335		
53	334		
39	329		
34	322		
50	319		
65	314		
59	310		
44	309		
84	309		
21	296	622	
22	254	606	
52	275	557	
41	288	522	
58	265	520	
4	220	520	
14	269	506	
20	229	506	
17	292	474	
42	218	460	
3	178	452	
63	244	369	
27	299	362	
66	237	356	
35	272	348	
49	248	341	
31	281	326	
64	223	306	
61	193	240	977
60	0	0	865
62	208	208	821
19	263	287	806
86	222	232	768
23	217	217	747
88	234	247	735
67	149	149	733
83	213	250	723
7	194	231	557
85	156	298	542
81	234	245	530
69	206	298	502
68	222	290	498
12	172	229	495
56	142	174	494
9	0	0	490
6	41	65	489
71	178	178	480
57	175	259	469
48	199	280	423
76	77	155	406
18	130	167	397
78	0	0	388
79	111	122	373
55	98	106	365
80	79	132	329
8	86	171	315
75	135	195	276
74	145	212	222
72	104	104	215
77	0	0	208
16	58	124	204
82	0	0	193
70	96	126	187
15	0	0	170
5	0	0	125
73	0	0	125
54	0	0	114
1	260	288	107
13	0	0	96
2	0	0	44

Fig. 5.2 Comparison of scoring values for all identified spots after using 'relaxed' or 'stringent' parameters for identification.

When we investigated some of the results in detail, we found the following:

The Mascot results for spot 25 (Figure 5.3) shows its clear identification from the PMF spectrum at a score of 355. The spectrum is rich in peptides that belong to the protein identified. The sequence coverage is 70% (28 peptides), with an intensity coverage of 69%

Looking at spot 68 (Figure 5.4), we find that MALDI MS/MS just confirms the PMF identification but gives no further insight, except that we have determined some additional peptide sequences. A 53% sequence coverage and 13 peptides were obtained. However, careful investigation of all the peptides under ESI–MS/MS conditions revealed a nice peptide fragment spectrum (Figure 5.4c) that could not be attributed to another protein. This finding makes it very likely that a protein of much lower abundance is present. One might be successful in identifying it by repeating the measurement with more sample.

Spot 27 (Figure 5.5) was well identified (as vimentin) with a score of 299 from the PMF spectrum. However, detailed analysis by MALDI–MS/MS, in addition to yielding an increase in the score for vimentin, indicated the presence of a second component of lower intensity, which turned out to be tubulin. Here, the limited resolution of the gel could be improved by the mixture analysis capabilities together with the sequencing tool of mass spectrometry. The values for the main component were 74% sequence coverage and 23 peptides.

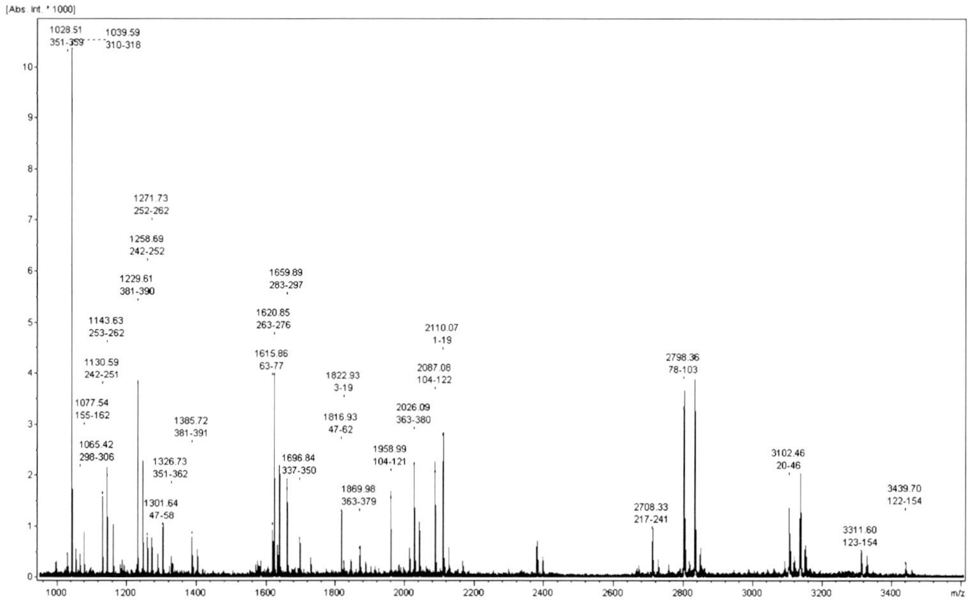

(A)

Fig. 5.3 (A) PMF spectrum of spot 25 from the gel in Figure 5.1. (B) Table showing matching peptides, accuracies of mass determination, and sequence annotations from the database. (C) Sequence coverage map based on the PMF spectrum.

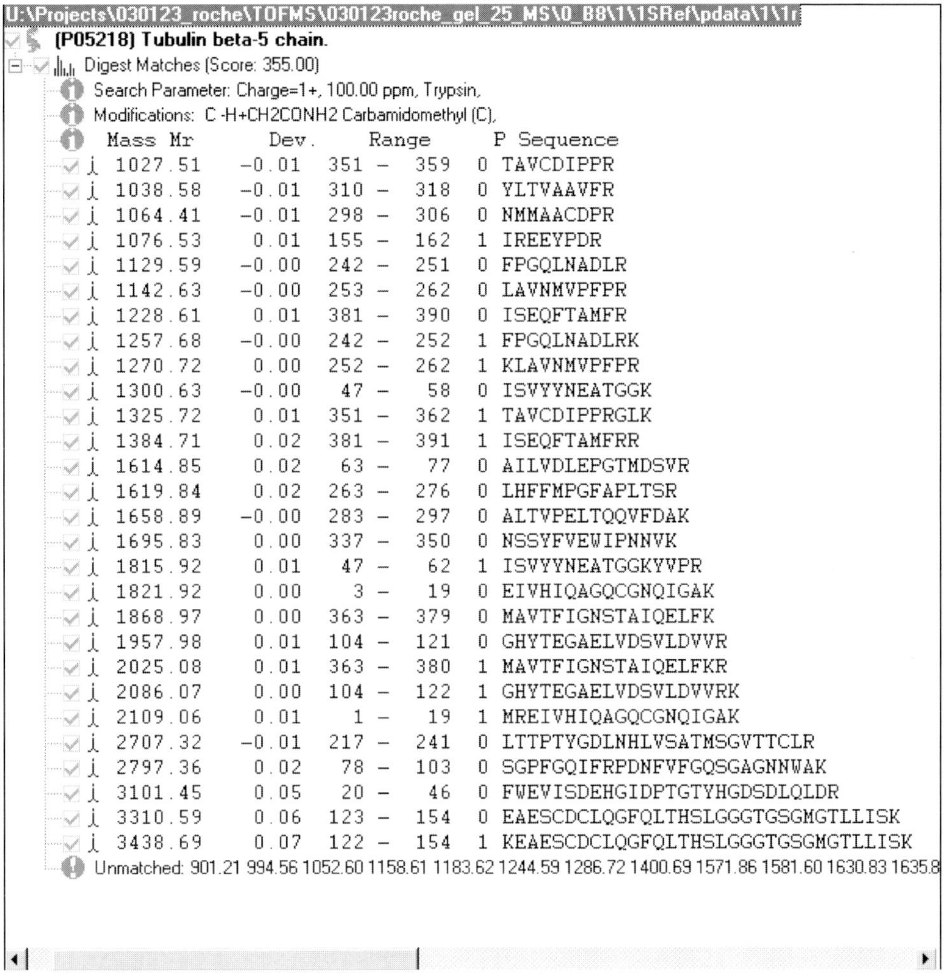

(B)

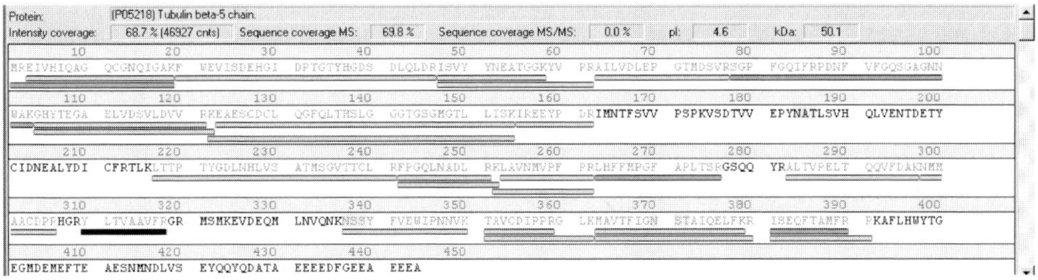

(C)

Fig. 5.3 (continued)

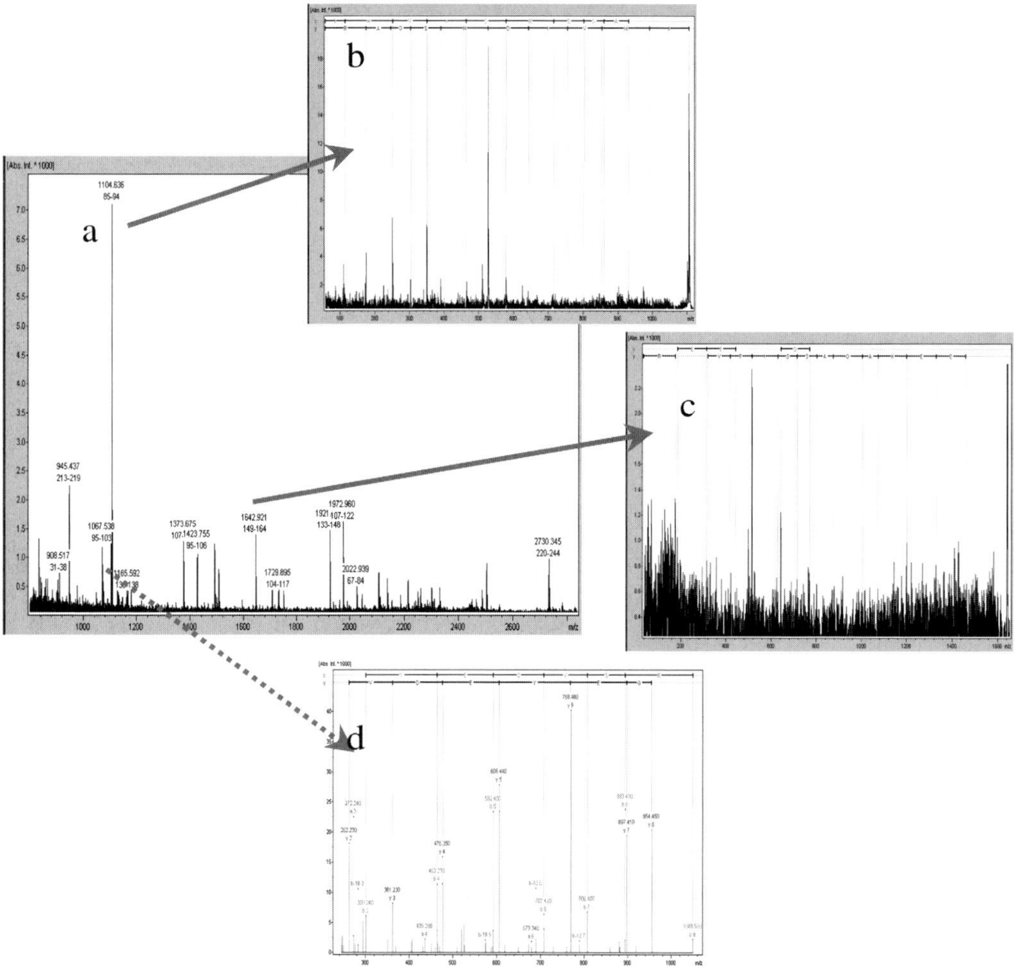

Fig. 5.4 (A) PMF spectrum of spot 68 from the gel in Figure 5.1. (B) MALDI–TOF MS/MS spectrum at *m/z* 1104.6 with sequence assignment (y and b series). (C) MALDI–TOF MS/MS spectrum at *m/z* 1642.9 with sequence assignment (y and b series). (D) LC–ESI–MS/MS spectrum at *m/z* 1067.5 using the doubly charged species with sequence assignment.

Finally, sometimes MALDI–TOF and MALDI–TOF/TOF data did not result in an identification. Consequently, a nanoHPLC–MS/MS run was the only possibility for identification. With the relaxed criterion for this set of proteins, 14 gel spots or 16% of the spots had to be investigated with the second instrument and methodology, whereas with the stringent criterion this was true for 44 gel spots (51%). The increased number of gel spots for ESI–MS/MS analysis is obviously responsible for the extended analysis time, since the nanoHPLC runs are very time-consuming.

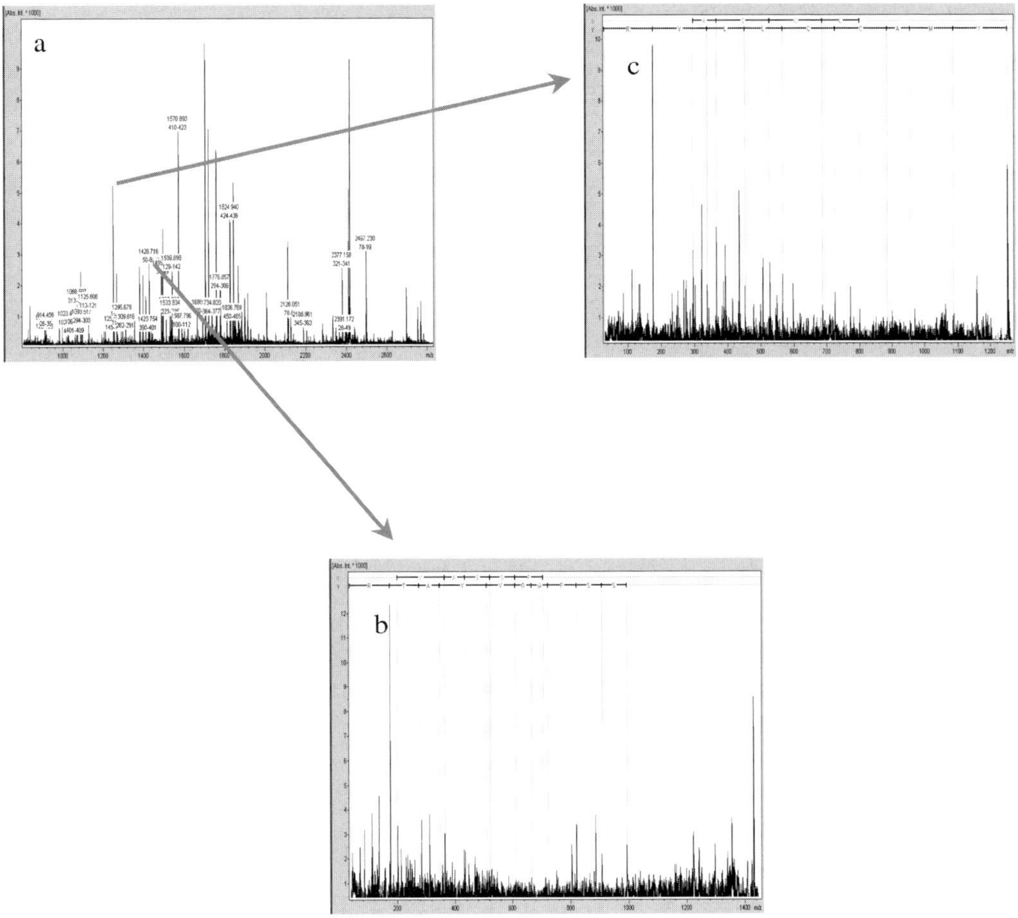

Fig. 5.5 (A) PMF spectrum of spot 27 from the gel in Figure 5.1. MALDI–TOF MS/MS spectra at (B) m/z 1428.7 and (C) m/z 1249.6.

The MALDI–PMF spectrum of spot 77 was insufficient for a successful database search, although it looks at a first glance to be rich in peptide masses (Figure 5.6A). However, ESI–MS/MS analysis resulted in very high scoring with good-quality spectra. For the final identification, six peptide fragment spectra could be used, only two of the parent ion masses (m/z 1754.9 and 1844.9) being present in the PMF spectrum. The other parent ions found in the ESI data were most likely suppressed in the MALDI spectrum. The remaining peaks could not be interpreted easily.

In summary, one can say that the protein identifications were possible by applying routine protocols and using automatic measurements and evaluation procedures. This is not always possible. If too many spots remain unidentified, the more tedious manual interpretation has to be chosen, in which various alternatives are tested by adjusting the evaluation parameters.

Besides the identification of large numbers of proteins for proteomic studies, it now appears that in-depth analysis of proteins is of increasing importance. This is also true when a larger number of spots from a gel cannot be identified by using the standard strategy, as mentioned earlier. For this task, the above techniques form the basis of the approach; however, they require even more sophisticated tools, especially with respect to software programs. Reasons for lack of identification are manifold, including the following:

- Low or very high protein molecular weight, resulting in too few tryptic peptides or too many ubiquitous peptides, respectively.
- Unfavourable enzymatic cleavage sites, resulting in very small or a low number of very large peptides.
- Post-translational modifications.
- Sequence errors caused by various reasons (e. g., wrong ORF).
- Protein sequence not contained in the database (SwissProt, NCBI, or others), no genome sequence available.

In most of these situations, manual evaluation of the MS/MS spectra using trial and error methods is required. Such procedures are time-consuming but yield a very

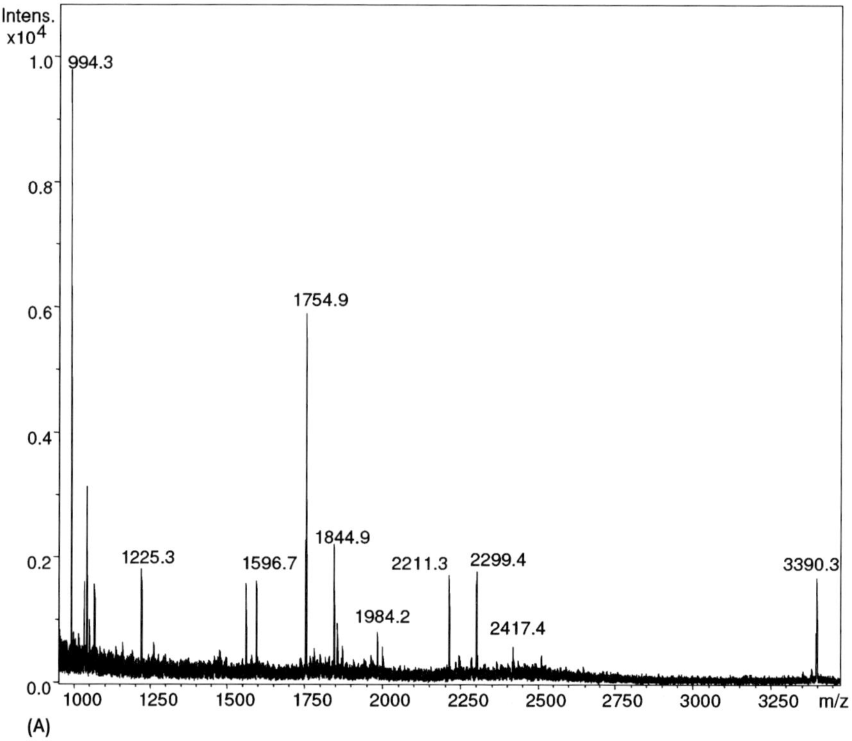

Fig. 5.6 (A) PMF spectrum of spot 77 from the gel in Figure 5.1. LC–ESI MS/MS spectra at (B) m/z 1754.9 and (C) m/z 1844.9.

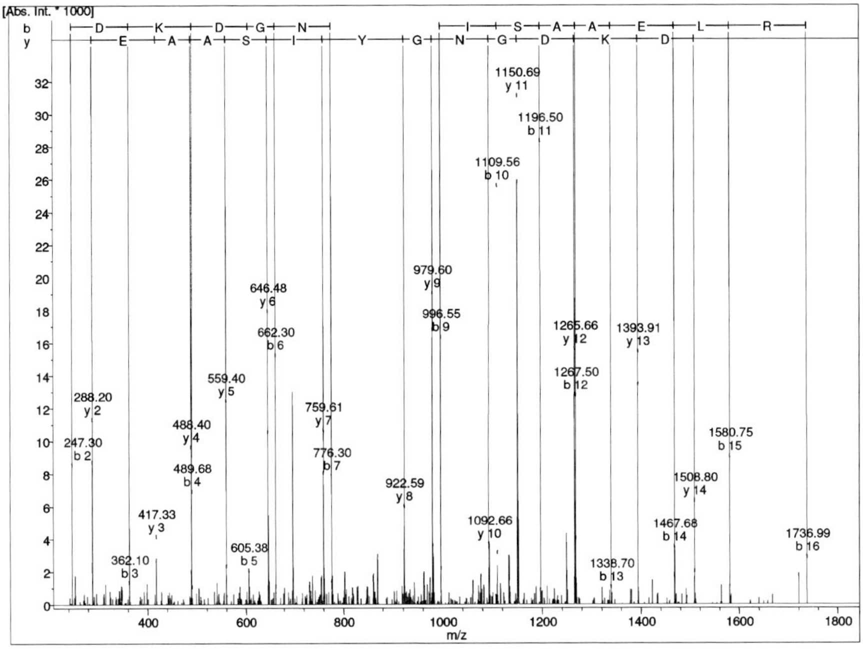

(B)

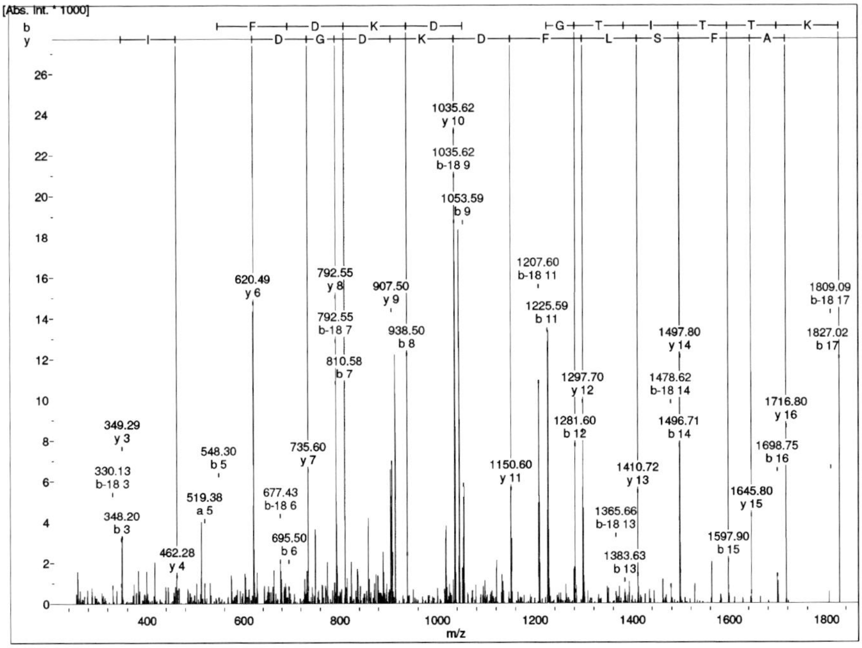

(C)

Fig. 5.6 (continued)

detailed knowledge of individual proteins, which for many studies may be essential. The principal techniques are to use software programs designed for the determination of modifications and mutations. In addition, de novo sequencing techniques are now available, which can be assisted by homology searches using MS BLAST.

The extent, size, and number of data files generated in proteomics projects is continually increasing. Several projects have to be managed and compared, and relations to other results using even different methods such as gene expression measurements are desired. For these purposes, relational databases based on Microsoft SQL or Oracle software are now on the market. The systems perform archival and retrieval of data and comparison of datasets; by using XML as a universal data exchange format, they can interface with databases outside the MS world.

5.3.3
Top–Down Analysis

The methodology discussed above can be called a bottom–up strategy, because from peptides (the bottom) having relatively low molecular weights, we reach conclusions regarding intact proteins with higher molecular weights (up). It is a type of puzzle-solving using the peptide molecular weights and sequence tags.

In contrast to this approach, the top–down methodology means that the structure or a verification procedure starts with the intact protein. Two technologies have recently been introduced for top–down proteomics:

- Fourier transform mass spectrometry (FT–MS), together with ES ionization and electron capture dissociation (ECD) for the generation of fragments, leading to sequencing. The outstanding performance of FT–MS in accuracy (in the 1 ppm range) for molecules as well as fragments makes this approach feasible.
- T3 sequencing [22] uses MALDI–TOF/TOF technology in which, first, an in-source decay (ISD) initiates fragmentation which typically includes the N and C termini; then, the ISD fragments are selected for MS/MS spectra, yielding the sequence and including the information about the terminus. This strategy seems to be extremely promising and effective for the analysis of recombinant proteins, for which the determination of the termini is crucial.

5.4
Summary and Outlook

This chapter gave an overview of the various techniques that are now available and in use in proteomics analysis, together with an example of an automatic measurement using MALDI–TOF and TOF/TOF and nanoHPLC–MS/MS techniques. The combination of them results in a clear identification of spots picked from 2D gels. The definition of when a scoring value identifies a protein was discussed by means of two criteria, relaxed and stringent. In this example all identifications could be performed using both settings, the stringent being more time consuming but yielding more sequence information. Depending on the analytical questions, the parameters can be adjusted for extremely detailed (stringent) or less strict, for example, when a large amount of information is already available and the identification is intended more as a confirmation. The experiments showed that with commercial equipment automatic measurements of gel-separated protein mixtures is possible with a high success rate. High-throughput proteomics is in my opinion a misleading term, because it does not say anything about the success of protein identification. In other words, the real task, which I tried to demonstrate with the example discussed here, is to perform proteomics analysis under high-throughput conditions and with high success.

In the future, in addition to high-throughput analyses, many questions will arise that require a very detailed analysis, for example, in the context of structure–function relationships. Here, the tools discussed in this chapter will have to be supplemented by techniques that are just now being developed, such as top–down approaches or targeted analysis for specific PTMs.

Acknowledgements

I thank Markus Macht, Detlev Suckau, Peter Hufnagel, and Ulrike Schweiger-Hufnagel for their assistance in supplying spectra and discussing the manuscript.

References

1. Blackstock, W.P. and Weir, M.P. *Trends Biotechnol.* **1999**, 17, 121–127.
2. Pandey, A. and Mann, M. *Nature* **2000**, 405, 837–846.
3. Human Proteome Organisation website: http://www.hupo.org/
4. Li, J., Steen, H. and Gygi, S.P. *Mol. Cell Proteomics* **2003**, 11, 1198–1204.
5. Chakraborty, A. et al. *J. Chromatogr.*, A **2002**, 949, 173–184.
6. Zabrouskov, V., Giacomelli, L., Van Wijk, K.J. and McLafferty, F.W. *Science* **1999**, 284, 1289–1290

6a. Sze, S.K., Je, Y., Oh, H.B., McLafferty, F.W. *Anal. Chem.* **2003**, 75, 1599–1603

6b. Suckau, D. and Resemann, A. *Anal. Chem.* **2003**, Web Release, DOI: 10, 1021/ac034362b.

7. Petricoin, E.F., Ardekani, A.M., Hitt, B.A., Levine, P.J., Fusaro, V.A., Steinberg, S.M., Mills, G.B., Simone, C., Fishman, D.A., Kohn, E.C., Liotta, L.A. *Lancet* **2002**, 359, 572–577.
8. Klose, J.; Nock, C., Herrmann, M., Stuhler, K., Marcus, K., Blueggel, M., Krause, E., Schalkwyk, L.C., Rastan, S., Brown, S.D., Bussow, K., Himmelbauer, H. Lehrach, H. *Nat. Genet.* **2002**, 4, 385–393.
9. Kalume, D.E., Kieffer, S., Rafn, K., Skou, L., Andersen, S.O., Roepstorff, P. *Biochim. Biophys. Acta* **2003**, 1645, 152–163.
10. Ishizuka, N. et al. J. *Chromatogr.*, A **2002**, 960, 85–96.
11. Peng, J., Elias, J.E., Thoreon, C.C., Licklider, L.J., Gygi, S.P. *J. Proteomics Res.* **2003**, 2, 43–50.
12. Washburn, M.P., Wolters, D., Yates, J.R. *Nat. Biotechnol.* **2001**, 19, 242–247.
13. Neusuess, C., Pelzing, M., Macht, M. *Electrophoresis* **2002**, 23, 3149–3159.
14. Zischka, H., Weber, G., Weber, P.J., Posch, A., Braun, R.J., Buhringer, D., Schneider, U., Nissum, M., Meitinger, T., Ueffing, M., Eckerskorn, C. *Proteomics* **2003**, 3, 906–916.

15. RIGHETTI, P.G., CASTAGNA, A., HERBERT, B., REYMOND, F., ROSSIER, J.S. *Proteomics* **2003**, 3, 1397–1407.
16. BERNDT, P., HOBOHM, U., LANGEN, H. *Electrophoresis* **1999**, 20, 3521–3526.
17. JENSEN, O.N., MORTENSEN, P., VORM, O., MANN, M. *Anal. Chem.* **1997**, 69, 1706–1714.
18. SUCKAU, D., RESEMANN, A., SCHUEREN-BERG, M., HUFNAGEL, P., FRANZEN, J., HOLLE, A. *Anal. Bioanal. Chem.* **2003**, 376, 952–965.
19. AEBERSOLD, R., GOODLETT, D.R. *Chem. Rev.* **2001**, 101, 269–295.
20. KARAS, M., HILLENKAMP, F. *Anal. Chem.* **1988**, 60, 2299–2301.
21. FENN, J.B., MANN, M., MENG, C.K., WONG, S.F., WHITEHOUSE C.M. *Science* **1989**, 246, 64–71.
22. SUCKAU, D., REZEMANN, A. *Anal Chem.* **2003**, 75, 5817–5824.

6
Covalent Protein Modification Analysis by Electrospray Tandem Mass Spectrometry

Wolf D. Lehmann

6.1
Introduction

The one gene – one protein hypothesis of the early days of molecular biology has long been replaced by a much more complex view, in which flexibility and complexity are the main characteristics of the cellular proteome. In humans, current data suggest that the number of proteins with individual structure is greater than the number of genes at least by a factor of between 3 and 10. This increase is created by covalent modifications, which confer to the cellular proteome a broad functional flexibility, e. g., for stress response, cell–cell interaction in multicellular organisms, differentiation, mitosis, or apoptosis. A modification may directly alter the functionality or location of a protein, or it may trigger a protein–protein or protein–ligand interaction that results in noncovalent protein complexes with particular functions. The linkage between covalent protein modification and noncovalent protein interaction results in the number of functionally different proteins by far exceeding the number of protein-encoding genes on the DNA level, as schematically presented in Figure 6.1.

Since covalent modifications are directly linked to the regulation of protein function, their determination is an important challenge in numerous current proteomics projects aiming at the understanding of physiological and pathophysiological mechanisms. Due to recent instrumental improvements in mass spectrometry, this technique is a highly versatile tool for modification analysis, since the majority of modifications are related to a change in mass. Although the technology for protein identification by mass spectrometry is highly developed and automated, methods for recognition of covalent protein modifications are as yet less perfectly developed. The particular differences between protein identification and covalent protein modification analysis is demonstrated in Figure 6.2, which displays the results obtained when a protein gel band was identified by mass spectrometry (data derived from nanoESI–MS/MS and the search engine Mascot [1], see below).

In the analysis shown (Figure 6.2), 8 tryptic peptides were recognized, leading to a reliable identification of the protein as human cytokeratin 1 (score 300, all hits with a score >70 were significant with $p > 0.05$ in this search). However, this reliable re-

Handbook of Toxicogenomics: Strategies and Applications. Edited by Jürgen Borlak

ISBN: 3-527-30342-1

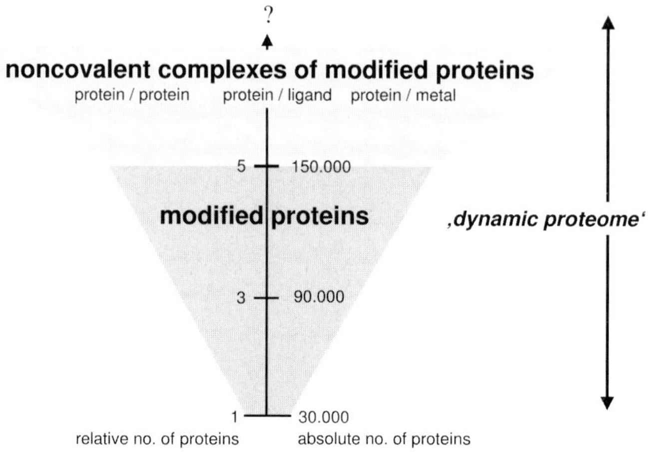

Fig. 6.1 The human proteome is much greater than the number of gene-encoded protein sequences, owing to covalent modification and noncovalent interactions of proteins. The (estimated) basic 30 000 genes are considered to be correlated to the (estimated) 30 000 human proteins. In reality, the complexity of a cellular proteome is strongly dependent on, for example, the differentiation and the functional state of a cell.

human keratin, type II
cytoskeletal 1 (Cytokeratin 1)

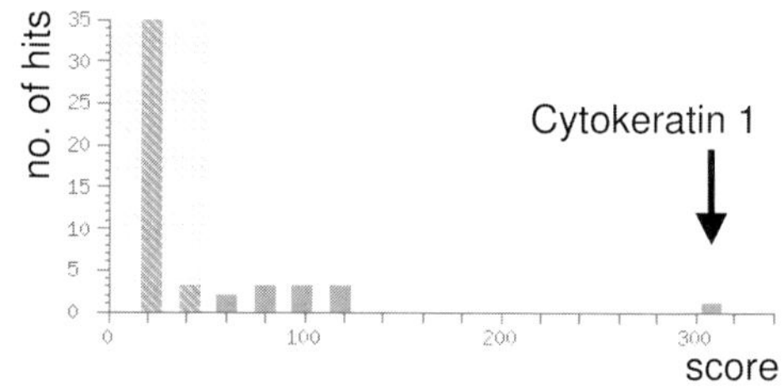

sequence coverage: 11 %

```
  1 MSRQFSSRSG YRSGGGFSSG SAGIINYQRR TTSSSTRRSG GGGGRFSSCG
 51 GGGGSFGAGG GFGSRSLVNL GGSKSISISV ARGGGRGSGF GGGYGGGGFG
101 GGGFGGGGFG GGGIGGGGFG GFGSGGGGFG GGGFGGGGYG GGYGPVCPPG
151 GIQEVTINQS LLQPLNVEID PEIQKVKSRE REQIKSLNNQ FASFIDKVRF
201 LEQQNQVLQT KWELLQQVDT STRTHNLEPY FESFINNLRR RVDQLKSDQS
251 RLDSELKNMQ DMVEDYRNKY EDEINKRTNA ENEFVTIKKD VDGAYMTKVD
301 LQAKLDNLQQ EIDFLTALYQ AELSQMQTQI SETNVILSMD NNRSLDLDSI
351 IAEVKAQYED IAQKSKAEAE SLYQSKYEEL QITAGRHGDS VRNSKIEISE
401 LNRVIQRLRS EIDNVKKQIS NLQQSISDAE QRGENALKDA KNKLNDLEDA
451 LQQAKEDLAR LLRDYQELMN TKLALDLEIA TYRTLLEGEE SRMSGECAPN
501 VSVSVSTSHT TISGGGSRGG GGGGYGSGGS SYGSGGGSYG SGGGGGGGRG
551 SYGSGGSSYG SGGGSYGSGG GGGGHGSYGS GSSSGGYRGG SGGGGGGSSG
601 GRGSGGGSSG GSIGGRGSSS GGVKSSGGSS SVRFVSTTYS GVTR
```

Fig. 6.2 Typical search results obtained in a protein identification analysis (by nanoESI–MS/MS, see below) performed with the search engine Mascot (www.matrixscience.com). These results contain no information on covalent modifications of this protein, including in the region covered by the identified peptides.

sult contains no information about covalent modifications of this protein. The identified tryptic peptides cover only 12% of the total sequence, so that for about 88% of the protein no information is obtained at all. Moreover, identification of the sequences (bold in Figure 6.2) in their unmodified form does not exclude the additional presence of a modified variant. In the following, the instrumental background of covalent protein modification analysis by electrospray ionisation (ESI) mass spectrometry (MS) is summarized, and corresponding analytical strategies and results are presented and discussed.

6.2 Electrospray Ionization

In the early 1980s an active period for development of new soft ionisation methods led to the creation of MALDI (matrix-assisted desorption/ionisation) and electrospray ionisation (ESI) [2, 3], which opened new avenues to the use of mass spectrometry in biochemical analysis. In ESI, ion formation is achieved by spraying the analyte solution (water/organic solvent mixtures or even only water) from a small tip that is at high potential, so that, depending on the polarity of the applied potential, small droplets with an excess positive or negative charge are formed. The spray is formed at ambient pressure near a small aperture of the mass spectrometer providing a connection to the mass analyser system, which is kept under high vacuum. The droplets are sucked into the mass analyser system and are desolvated by passing through the interface region (hot drying gas curtain or heated capillary), and ions are formed which are focussed into an ion beam. Experimental observations and theoretical calculations have led to the ion-evaporation model and the charged-residue model for electrospray ionisation, which have been comprehensively reviewed [4]. The original flow rates of ESI were in the range of several $\mu L\ min^{-1}$, and under these conditions the spray was supported by a concentric nebulisation gas. The subsequently developed nanoESI variant works with flow rates of 15–30 $nL\ min^{-1}$ [5, 6], and at these flow rates complete nebulisation is achieved without an additional stream of gas. The introduction of the nanoESI technique has had a great impact on the application of ESI–MS in the life sciences by drastically reducing the required sample amount. Together with its robust performance, this has led to a rapid acceptance of nanoESI in the bioanalytical field. Recently, a further reduction in flow rates (and thus sample consumption) by about one order of magnitude has been reported [7] showing that the technical possibilities of this approach are not yet fully exploited.

6.3 Tandem Mass Spectrometry

Tandem mass spectrometry (MS/MS), originally introduced to study physicochemical properties of small molecules [8], found its way into bioanalytics in combination with soft ionisation methods. MS/MS gives access to the structural characterization of analytes in mixtures by allowing the recording of compound-specific fragment ion spectra without the need for their isolation in a pure state. By mass analysis, a single analyte is isolated and fragmented by collision-induced dissociation (CID), and its fragment ions are analysed in a second stage of mass analysis. The first instrument type designed for tandem MS analysis in biochemistry was the triple quadrupole instrument [9], consisting of three quadrupole analysers. Q1 operates as the first mass analyser, Q2 is designed and operated as a collision cell, and Q3 performs the second stage of mass analysis. In the product ion scan mode, a precursor ion is selected with Q1 and fragmented in Q2, followed by fragment ion analysis in Q3. Moreover, this type of instrument can selectively detect all analytes in a mixture exhibiting a certain neutral loss (neutral loss scan) or all analytes forming a certain fragment ion (precursor ion scan mode). This mode of analysis is named 'tandem in space', since the single steps proceed in spatially separate units of the tandem MS system.

The 'tandem in time' systems are either 3D [10] or 2D (linear) [11] ion traps, schematically displayed in Figure 6.3.

In these ion trap systems, ions are trapped, selectively fragmented, and mass analysed by the use of a single device. The 3D ion trap consists of a ring electrode with electrically isolated end caps, through which the ions are introduced for trapping and ejected for mass analysis. The 2D (linear) ion trap is a compact arrangement of three electrically separated quadrupole analysers. The ions are introduced concentrically into the central quadrupole system, which performs both stages of mass analysis and the intermediate fragmentation step. The ions are ejected either axially or perpendicularly for detection. Ion traps have the unique ability to perform multistage MS/MS experiments (MS^n), in which the product ions of a fragmentation process are selected as precursor ions for the next fragmentation step. In spite of their extreme specificity, MS^n techniques have so far found only sporadic application in protein modification analysis. Ion traps can be operated at variable resolution (low to moderately high resolution) (see below); however, due to the low scan speed required for increased resolution, complete spectra are usually recorded at low to medium resolution.

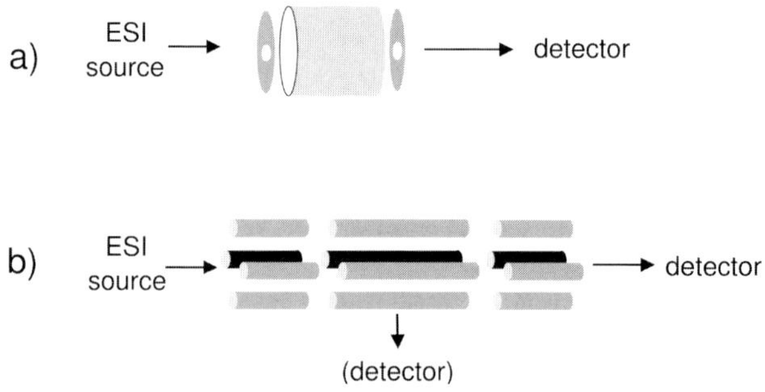

Fig. 6.3 Tandem in time MS systems implemented as (a) 3D ion trap or (b) 2D (linear) ion trap. In the central part of these analyzers, the ions are trapped, selectively fragmented, and mass-analyzed by dynamic electromagnetic fields in the presence of a mediator/collision gas (mostly He).

6.4
Q–TOF and Q–FT–ICR Systems

Q–TOF and Q–FT–ICR systems represent two high-resolution tandem in space MS/MS systems, in which different mass analysis principles for the two stages of mass analysis are employed (hybrid systems) [12, 13]. The second stage of mass analysis, which can also be active in the MS mode, is performed with a reflectron TOF (time-of-flight) or a FT–ICR (Fourier transform ion cyclotron resonance) analyser, which are both characterized by high mass resolution (TOF: 7000 to 25 000; FT–ICR: 50 000 to 10^6). The remarkable feature of these systems is that high resolution and high MS/MS sensitivity are achieved simultaneously. The arrangement of a Q–TOF system [13] is displayed schematically in Figure 6.4.

Whereas Q–TOF systems have already reached a relatively wide distribution in the field of bioanalytics, the implementation of Q–FT–ICR is still in its early stages. In these latter systems, the second mass analyser consists of an ICR cell positioned in the centre of a superconducting magnet, where the captured ions cycle with a frequency (cyclotron frequency) determined by their m/z ratio. By their movement, they induce an oscillating induction in the ICR cell walls, which by Fourier transform analysis is converted into a mass spectrum with m/z scale. The near future will see more applications of this high-end mass analysis technique in the biological sciences.

6.4.1
Resolution

In TOF–MS analyses the FWHM (full width at half maximum) definition of mass spectral resolution is commonly used. With this definition, the mass spectrometric resolution can be determined by analysing the peak shape of a single peak (Figure

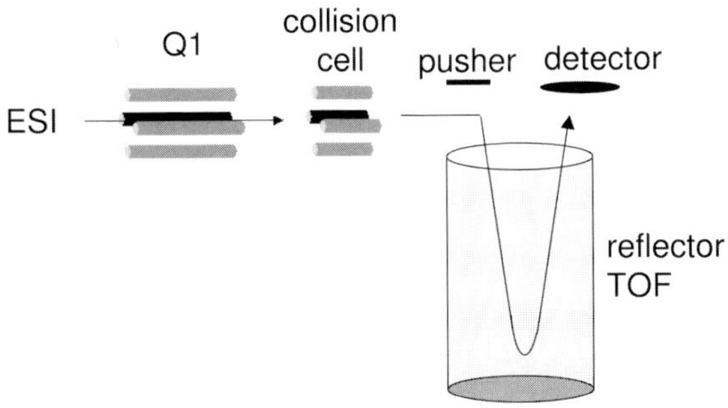

Fig. 6.4 Setup of a Q–TOF tandem MS system, representing a tandem in space instrument. In the MS/MS mode, Q1 selects the precursor ion, which is fragmented in the collision cell. The reflectron TOF analyser then allows the fragment ion mass spectrum to be recorded at high resolution. Single-stage MS spectra (survey spectra) can also be recorded at high resolution by operating Q1 as an ion transmission element only.

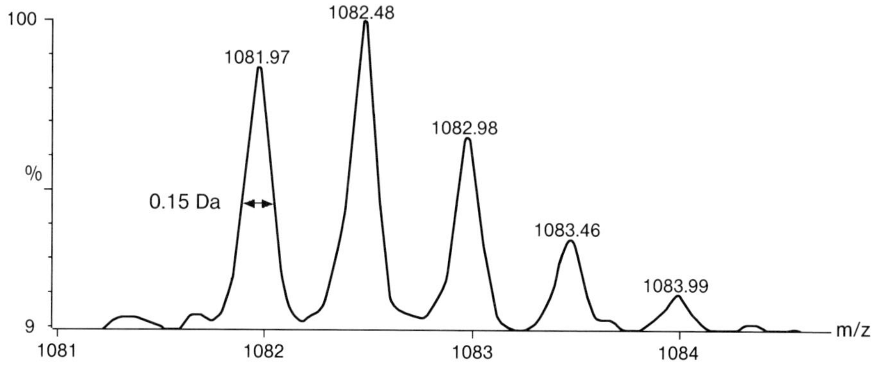

Fig. 6.5 Calculation of the mass spectral resolution from the (raw data) molecular ion signal of a peptide. The peak at *m/z* 1082 has a width of 0.16 Da at 50% of its height. According to the FWHM definition (full width at half maximum), the resolution is calculated as about 7000 (= 1082/0.15).

6.5). Dividing the *m/z* value of a peak by its width at 50% intensity yields the resolution. The molecular ion group of a peptide (Figure 6. 5) analysed in this way results in a mass spectrometric resolution of about 7000. This spectrum was acquired using a Q–TOF instrument.

6.4.2
Mass Accuracy

The key parameter determining the mass error is the resolution, although other parameters such as instrument calibration and stability also exert an influence on the accuracy of the mass determinations. The mass error is often measured as a relative property and given in units of ppm (parts per million). Mass values extracted from spectra recorded at low to medium resolution (500–5000) are usually in the range from about 100 to 1000 ppm, those extracted from spectra recorded at high resolution (>5000) cover the range from 2 to 100 ppm. In principle, each measured mass value should be accompanied by an error, so that its significance can be scored. For a realistic determination of this error, researchers should carefully determine this error on their instrument(s) in their own laboratories. Of course, the statistical nature of this error (SD of the mean, SD of a single value, 2 SD, 3 SD, etc) has to be specified so that a meaningful correlation to actual experimental data can be performed. In practice, numerous parameters can influence accurate mass data acquired at high resolution, including the absolute ion intensities, laboratory temperature, instrument warm-up during data analysis, etc., since the instruments are usually operated near the limit of their electronic and conceptual performance. Therefore, in analysing unknowns, the use of relaxed error limits is recommended to avoid false negative results due to erroneously underestimated error limits.

6.5 Peptide Sequencing by Electrospray Tandem Mass Spectrometry

Peptides and proteins are linear biopolymers consisting of amino acid building blocks connected by amide bonds (peptide bonds), which link a carboxy and an amino function of two vicinal amino acids. In this way, each peptide or protein has one amino terminus and one carboxy terminus. Peptides are conventionally displayed in one- or three-letter amino-acid codes from left to right, starting with the N terminus and ending with the C terminus. In collision-induced dissociation of protonated peptides [14–17], cleavage of the peptide bond is the predominant fragmentation reaction, whereas sidechain fragmentations are of minor importance (Figure 6.6).

Normally, the peptide bond is the strongest bond in the protein backbone, since it has a partial double bond character. However, in protonated peptides, the extra proton(s) have a certain probability of residing on the N atoms of the backbone. In this position, they weaken the peptide bond by destroying its partial double bond character (Figure 6.6 b). This leads to preferential fission of the peptide bond in CID of protonated peptides. The fragmentation behaviour results in two fragment ion series. The N-terminal ions are called b ions, and the b ions have a 5-ring oxazolone structure at their newly formed end [17, 18] (a ions are also N-terminal ions and have one CO unit less than the corresponding b ions). The C-terminal ions are called y ions and have a structure similar to that of a normal peptide ion. In accord with this explanation is the observation that MS/MS spectra of negative ions of peptides are much less informative with respect to sequence than are positive ion MS/MS spectra [19], since they lack the phenomenon of proton-induced backbone cleavage.

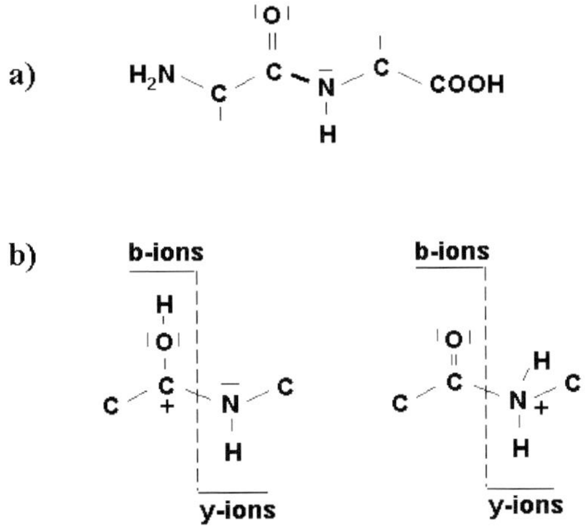

Fig. 6.6 Schematic display of the peptide bond and its fragmentation in protonated peptides following CID. (a) Structure of the peptide bond. (b) Protonation of the O or N atom of the peptide bond, as postulated to occur in protonated peptides. Fragment ions containing the N-terminal part are called b ions, those with the C-terminal part are y ions [17]. (See the text for further discussion).

6.6
Protein Modifications and Their MS/MS Reactions

So far, >100 covalent modifications of proteins have been described [e.g., 20–22]. The annotated protein database SwissProt [23] is a rich source of well established covalent protein modifications. Many covalent modifications are accompanied by an increase in molecular weight and an increase in acidity (lower pI value), including deamidation, phosphorylation, sulfation, N-acylation, and cysteic acid formation. A selection of covalent modifications is given in Table 6.1, together with information about signature fragmentation reactions after CID.

The stability of the covalent modifications under the CID conditions can vary considerably. As a demonstration, Figure 6.7 shows survey MS spectra of two peptides of identical sequence, which carry a phosphotyrosine or a sulfotyrosine residue at the third position from the C terminus. Although the phosphotyrosine peptide shows a stable molecular ion signal, the sulfotyrosine peptide exhibits strong loss of SO_3 from the sulphate ester group even under standard (usually nonfragmenting) conditions.

Following CID, the sulfotyrosine peptide exhibits a spectrum identical to that of the unmodified peptide, since loss of SO_3 results in the formation of a tyrosine residue. In contrast, the phosphotyrosine residue is so stable that a phosphotyrosine immonium ion is formed, which can be used as a marker ion – Figure 6.8 shows the low-mass region of the CID spectra of these two tyrosine-modified peptides. These MS/MS spectra, recorded under identical conditions, show the Y immonium ion at *m/z* 163 for the sulfated peptide and the pY immonium ion at *m/z* 216 for the phosphorylated peptide. Those fragment ions that do not contain the modified tyrosine residue are observed at identical *m/z* values for both peptides.

a)
b)
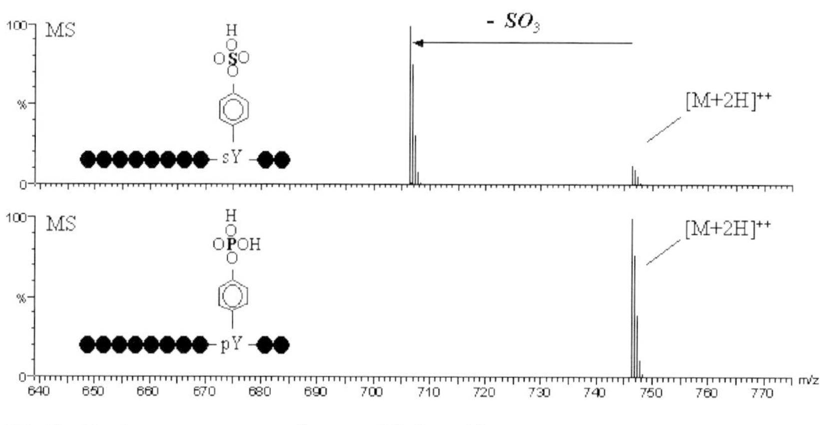

Fig. 6.7 Positive ion survey spectra of two modified peptides, carrying (a) a sulfotyrosine residue or (b) a phosphotyrosine residue. The phosphotyrosine peptide shows a stable molecular ion signal, whereas the sulfotyrosine peptide exhibits a strong loss of SO_3 even without the CID step.

Tab. 6.1 Selection of abundant covalent protein modifications and their signature reaction (if one occurs) in positive ion electrospray MS after collision-induced dissociation.

Protein modification	***Mass shift***	***CID signature ions or reactions (m/z values)***
N-terminal demethionylation	– 131 Da	none
Thiazole formation between Cys and Ser	– 20 Da	
Succinimide formation at Asn	– 18 Da	none
pyro-Glu formation from Glu	– 18 Da	
pyro-Glu formation from Gln	– 17 Da	none
Disulfide formation Cys-Cys	– 2 Da	doubled ^{18}O content after digestion in $H_2{}^{18}O$
Deamidation at Asn, Gln	+ 1 Da	none
Methylation at His	+ 14 Da	meHis immonium ion at 124
Methyl ester formation at the C terminus	+ 14 Da	none
Hydroxylation at proline	+ 16 Da	hydroxy-P immonium ion at 86
Oxidation at Met	+ 16 Da	loss of 64 = CH_3-SOH
Dimethylation at Arg	+ 28 Da	neutral loss of 45, 87 dimethylammonium ion at 46, dimethylcarbodiimidium ion at *m/z* 71
Formylation at Lys	+ 28 Da	formyl-b_1 ion for N-terminal formylation
Acetylation	+ 42 Da	acetyl-b_1 ion for N-terminal acetylation acetyl-Lys-(-NH_3) immonium ion at 126
Trimethylation at Lys	+ 42 Da	neutral loss of 59 me-Lys and dime-Lys immonium ions at 98, 112
Carbamoylation	+ 43 Da	carbamoyl-b_1 ions for N-terminal carbamoylation
Nitration at Tyr	+ 45 Da	nitroTyr immonium ion at 181
Oxidation of Cys to Cysteic Acid	+ 48 Da	none
Phosphorylation at Ser, Thr	+ 80 Da	loss of H_3PO_4 = 98 Da 69 Da or 83 Da distance in fragment ion series
Phosphorylation at Tyr	+ 80 Da	loss of HPO_3 = 80 Da, pY immonium ion at 216
Sulfation at Tyr	+ 80 Da	loss of SO_3 = 80 Da (strong)
Phosphorylation at hydroxyproline	+ 96 Da	dehydro-P immonium ion at 68
Iodination at Tyr	+ 126 Da	I-Tyr immonium ion at 262
N-terminal gluconoylation	+ 178 Da	
N-terminal myristoylation to myrG	+ 210 Da	b_0 at 211, a_1 at 240, b_1 at 268
O-GlcNAc addition at Ser, Thr	+ 203 Da	GlcNac-H_2O ion at 204
Palmitoylation at Cys	+ 238 Da	acyl ion at 239
Dioidination at Tyr	+ 252 Da	I_2-Tyr immonium ion at 388
N-terminal 6-phosphogluconoylation	+ 258 Da	
Glutathionylation	+ 305 Da	
ADP-ribosylation	+ 541 Da	
Glycosylation	+ >1 kDa	oxonium ions at 163, 204, 366
Ubiquitination	+ ca. 8 kDa	internal K-GG unit after tryptic digestion

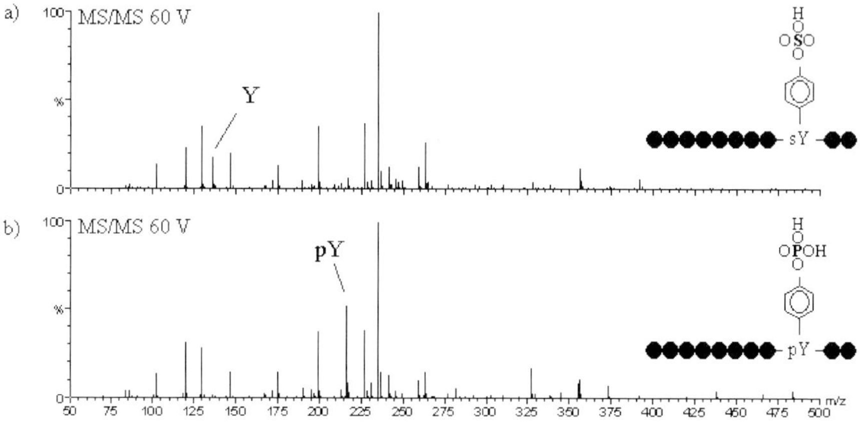

Fig. 6.8 Low-mass CID spectra of the two peptides shown in Figure 6.6. (a) The MS/MS spectrum of the sulfopeptide shows abundant Y immonium ion at *m/z* 136; (b) the corresponding spectrum of the phosphotyrosine peptide instead shows an abundant pY immonium ion at *m/z* 216.

Modifications lost as neutral entities can be specifically detected by neutral loss scanning. Those giving rise to specific marker ions can be detected by precursor ion scanning or by extraction of mass-specific ion traces from a pool of MS/MS spectra.

6.7 Detection of Protein Modifications by MS and MS/MS

In this section some aspects of protein modification analysis, i. e., characterization of isolated proteins, are discussed. Figure 6.9 provides a visual display of the MS and MS/MS dimensions of a protein digest analysis. In front, the survey MS spectrum of a protein digest is displayed. Orthogonal to this survey spectrum is the MS/MS dimension, with a single MS/MS spectrum given as example.

The sequence- and modification-specificity of the MS approach is located in the MS/MS dimension, since the MS/MS spectrum contains both molecular weight and structural specificity, whereas the survey MS mode is confined to molecular weight specificity. A particularly beneficial property of the MS/MS with respect to the MS mode is its improved sensitivity in spite of reduced ion currents, due to the drastically reduced nonspecific background. Thus, MS/MS analysis is simultaneously more specific and more sensitive than MS analysis. On this background, the final aim in all modification analyses is the acquisition of a high-quality MS/MS spectrum, which allows a trustworthy identification of the peptide sequence and of the modification and also pinpoints the modified site within the sequence. An MS/MS spectrum of a modified peptide may contain all this desired information even in a partially redundant form. The chance that the aim can be reached improves as the signal-to-noise (S/N) ratio of the acquired MS/MS spectrum improves. A simple

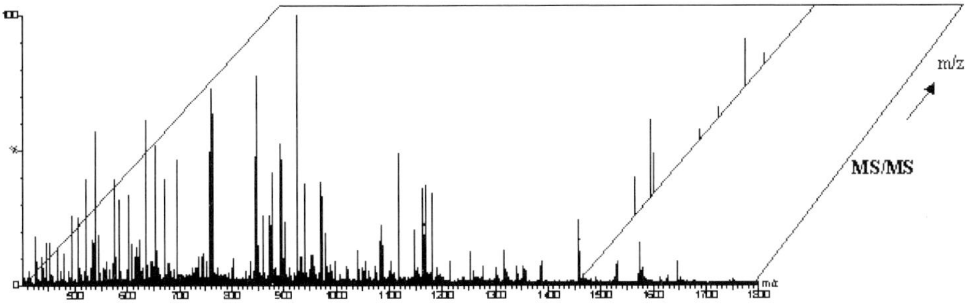

Fig. 6.9 Display of the analytical dimensions of MS and MS/MS analysis. The survey MS analysis shows molecular mass specificity only, whereas the MS/MS analysis has molecular mass and structural specificity.

measure to improve the S/N ratio is to increase the data acquisition time, since the S/N ratio improves in proportion to the square root of acquisition time. Figure 6.10 shows this basic principle with the example of an MS/MS spectrum that was acquired for different time intervals. For demonstration of the improvement achieved, the acquired raw MS/MS spectra data were used for protein database interrogation via the search engine Mascot.

As is evident from Figure 6.10, the score of the correct hit increases strongly as the acquisition time is increased from 6 to 30 s. In modification analysis, one would like to recognize the modifications on the level of the MS survey scan, since then one could direct the MS/MS product scan effectively to the ions of the modified peptide(s). Unfortunately, the MS spectrum of a protein digest yields much less information concerning protein modifications than does the MS/MS mode. This obvious dilemma has led to the development of a variety of strategies. One answer to this situation is the acquisition of all possible product ion spectra, e.g., in the nanoESI–MS to MS/MS switching mode, in the Q–TOF neutral loss/precursor ion scan mode (which also proceeds via product ion spectrum recording), or in the LC–MS/MS mode. In this way a group of modified peptides may be recognized by some generic property, such as loss of H_3PO_4 from phosphoserine peptides or formation of the pY immonium ion from phosphotyrosine peptides. Another answer is to try to recognize modified peptides candidates with methods other than ESI–MS analysis or to enrich subsets of modified peptides before MS/MS analysis to reduce the sample complexity. By all these approaches, analytical sensitivity is increased, which in turn improves the probability of successful identification and spotting of a covalent modification. These strategies are presented and discussed in the following sections for selected examples.

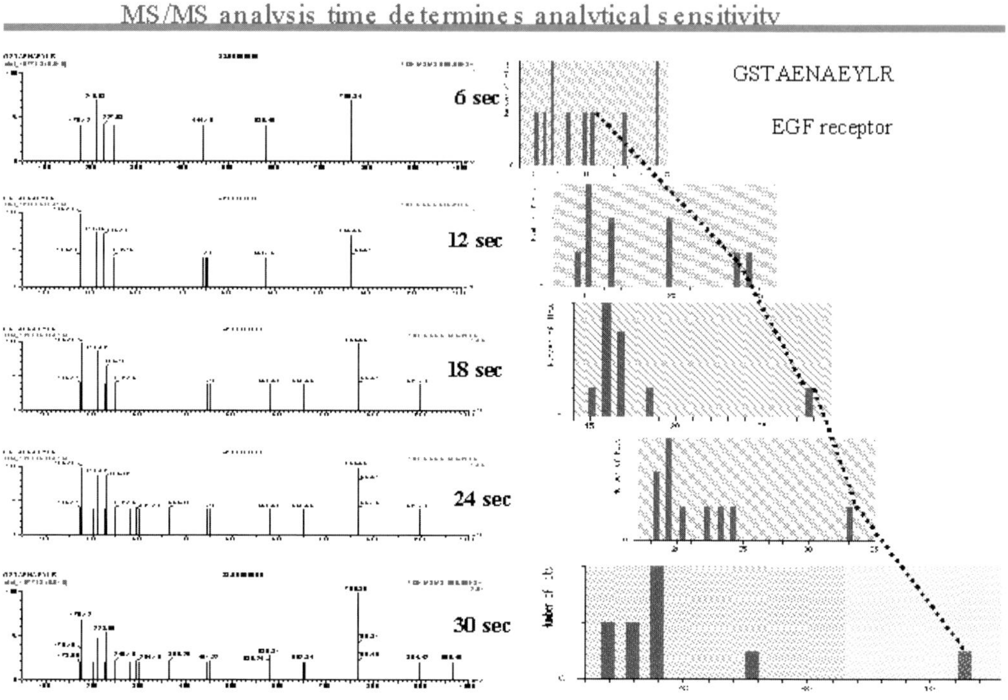

Fig. 6.10 A very dilute solution of a synthetic tryptic peptide (sequence from human EGF receptor) was subjected to nanoESI–MS/MS for the various acquisition times indicated. The raw MS/MS spectra data were used for database searching via Mascot, and the graphical search reports are shown with the correct hits connected by a dotted line. It is evident that the score of the correct hit increases with increasing acquisition time and approaches the significance threshold at a measurement period of about 30 s (significance threshold at the right border of the shaded area).

6.7.1
Phosphorylation

Reversible phosphorylation is a common and functionally highly important covalent protein modification involved in many vital cellular processes, including regulation of enzyme activities, protein localization, signal transduction events, mitosis, apoptosis, and carcinogenesis. The outstanding biological background and pharmaceutical interest in phosphorylation events have triggered an impressive number of studies on the molecular details of this covalent modification. In the last two decades roughly a thousand papers have appeared in this area, in which mass spectrometry was used as analytical tool in some form. As is exemplified below, most if not all mass spectrometric principles and procedural innovations in the field of covalent modification analysis can be found in the area of protein phosphorylation analysis.

Neutral Loss Scan

Most protein phosphorylation events occur at serine and threonine residues. Upon CID, serine and threonine phosphopeptides exhibit a characteristic loss of H_3PO_4 not observed for unmodified peptides [e. g., 24, 25].

This specific feature can be used to detect Ser- and Thr-phosphopeptides. Figure 6.11 shows the spectra obtained when a sample of protein kinase A was in-gel digested with elastase and subjected to nanoESI–MS analysis using scanning for neutral loss of 98 Da. In this way, specific detection of singly charged phosphopeptides is achieved [26]. Digestion with elastase instead of the usual trypsin was selected, because elastase generates peptides with a smaller molecular weight, and because the loss of H_3PO_4 was found to proceed most effectively for small phosphopeptides with molecular weights between 400 and 1000 Da. The phosphopeptide candidates spotted in this way in the digest mixture are then selected for product ion scanning for sequencing and for pinpointing the phosphorylation site.

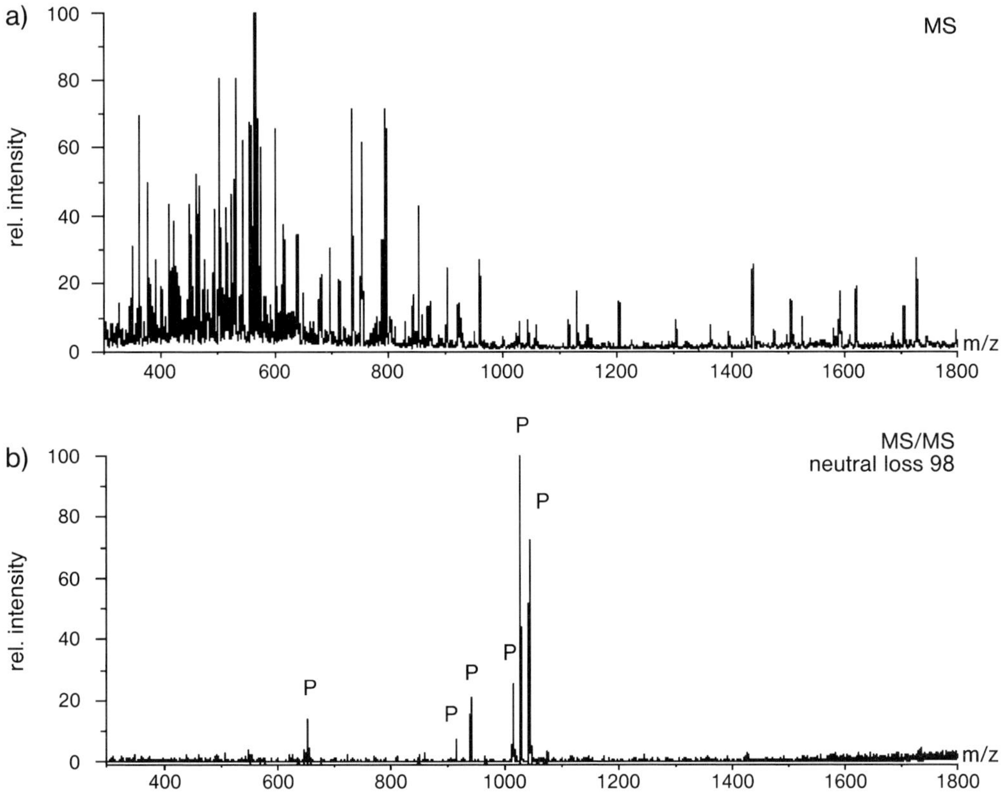

Fig. 6.11 NanoESI–MS analysis of an elastase digest of protein kinase A. (a) Survey MS; (b) neutral loss scan (98 Da) selectively showing the singly charged phosphopeptides present in the mixture (triple quadrupole analysis).

PO_3^- Marker Fragment

In negative ion mode CID, Ser-, Thr-, and Tyr-phosphopeptides generate a PO_3^- fragment at m/z 79, which can be used for recognition of the corresponding phosphopeptides in LC–MS by skimmer CID [27, 28] or by nanoESI–MS and precursor ion scanning [29]. Following their recognition in negative ion mode, the corresponding molecular ion signals are selected in positive ion mode for their characterization by MS/MS, since negative ion product ion spectra of have a poor sequence information content [19].

Enrichment of Phosphopeptides by IMAC

Phosphopeptides can be specifically enriched by immobilized metal affinity chromatography (IMAC), which utilizes the interaction of chelator-immobilized three-valent cations such as Fe^{3+} or Ga^{3+} with the phosphate group [30–32]. The efficiency of this approach is shown in Figure 6.12, which shows the results of nanoESI–MS analysis

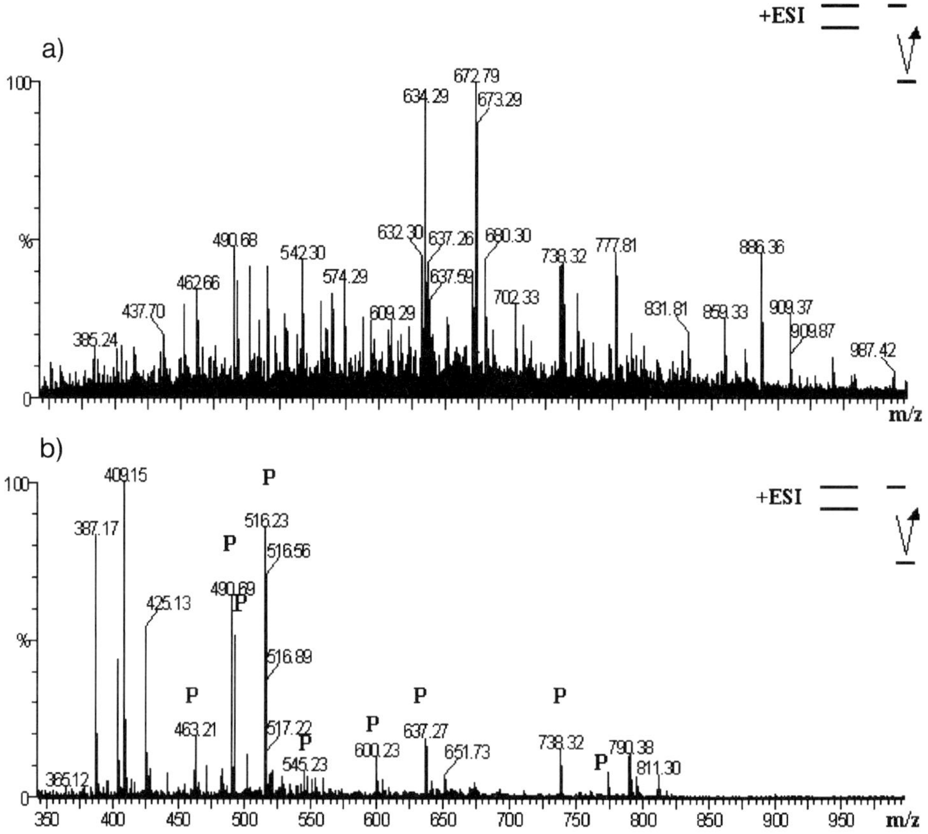

Fig. 6.12 Enrichment of phosphopeptides using IMAC. (a) NanoESI–MS survey spectrum of an elastase digest of protein kinase A. (b) The same sample and MS analysis as in (a) but after enrichment of phosphopeptides by IMAC. All signals labelled with 'P' were found to represent phosphopeptides upon subsequent product ion analysis. [33].

of an elastase digest of protein kinase A before and after enrichment of phosphopeptides by IMAC.

As can be seen by comparing Figure 6.12 a and b, the complexity of the peptide mixture is greatly reduced by the IMAC step, and most signals in the spectrum after IMAC (Fig. 5.12 b) were identified as phosphopeptides. The method also tends to enrich peptides having W or H residues or having (multiple) residues of D and E, since the sidechains of these amino acids also interact with free coordination sites of immobilized metal cations. Recently, methyl ester formation of free carboxyl groups was introduced to suppress the nonspecific interaction of D and E residues [34], and the efficiency of this measure was demonstrated in an application to the yeast proteome. Phosphopeptide enrichment by intermediate covalent binding to a solid support via a phosphoamide bond and subsequent release has also been demonstrated [35].

Enrichment of Ser- and Thr-Phosphopeptides

Phosphoserine and phosphothreonine peptides can be dephosphorylated by base treatment, resulting in dehydroalanine or dehydroaminobutric acid residues at the place of the former pS and pT residues, respectively. Thiol reagents can be coupled to these unique sites [36]; the utility of this procedure for the identification of phosphorylation sites by MS has been demonstrated [e. g., 37–39]. The exchange of phosphorylated sites (Ser, Thr) with a biotin tag and affinity-enrichment of the biotin-tagged peptides was demonstrated as an extension of this principle [40]. The replacement of phosphate groups at Ser and Thr by dimethylaminoethanethiol was demonstrated [41], since after oxidation this group generates a fragment ion at *m/z* 122 Da in positive ion mode CID, which then can be used as a specific marker ion in precursor ion scanning experiments in positive ion mode. Finally, addition of a radiolabeled tag after base-catalyzed dephosphorylation [42] resulted in the generation of radiolabeled phosphopeptide derivatives without the biological limitations of classical *in vitro* ^{32}P assays. These limitations originate mainly from the necessary incorporation of ^{32}P from either inorganic phosphate or ATP.

Enrichment of pTyr-Peptides by Anti-phosphotyrosine Affinity Methods

Phosphorylation at tyrosine is a relatively rare event (abundances of pSer, pThr, and pTyr are about 90 : 9:1), which nevertheless attracts high interest because of its involvement in many signal transduction cascades and its elevated occurrence in various diseases including cancer. Upon CID, phosphotyrosine residues are more stable than the corresponding pSer and pThr residues, because it results in the formation of a stable pTyr immonium marker ion [43]. The high specificity of anti-phosphotyrosine antibodies has been used successfully for specific enrichment of proteins phosphorylated at tyrosine. After digestion, the pTyr peptides were selectively recognized by precursor ion scanning for the pY immonium ion at *m/z* 216 and then sequenced by product ion scanning [44, 45]. Any CID-induced signature fragmentation reactions including the pY immonium ion formation are sequence-dependent [46]. Therefore, for pY detection in isolated proteins, a tyrosine-targeted product ion scanning strategy was proposed, which utilizes the known sequence of the protein under analysis [46] to achieve optimal sensitivity for detection of phosphotyrosine peptides (Figure 6.13).

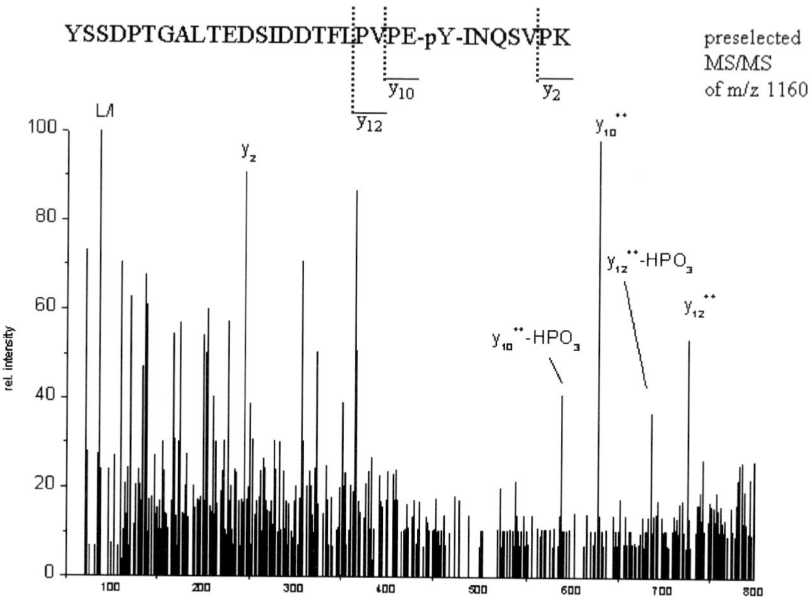

Fig. 6.13 NanoESI–MS/MS product ion spectrum recorded by tyrosine-targeted MS/MS analysis of a tryptic digest of human EGF receptor. The sample amount was less than one picomole, and the phosphopeptide was identified on the basis of the proline-directed fragments and the specific loss of HPO_3 typical of pTyr [46]. The pY marker ion was not detected.

Element Mass Spectrometry with ^{31}P Detection

The main limitation of using modification-specific fragmentation reactions for recognition of covalent modifications arises from their inherent dependence on the peptide sequence. In addition, molecular mass spectrometry methods as used in these approaches require particular measures for quantitative results to be obtained, such as individual isotopically labelled internal standards. The use of element mass spectrometry (ICP–MS, inductively coupled plasma) with ^{31}P detection overcomes these limitations, since this technique shows a generic sensitivity for the element selected. When applied to the task of protein phosphorylation analysis, this results in uniform sensitivity to all phosphopeptide species in a phosphoprotein digest. As an example, Figure 6.14 shows the LC–MS analysis of a tryptic digest of β-casein, which was coupled to ESI–MS and to ICP–MS [47]. The elution of a single monophosphorylated peptide is clearly recognizable in the ^{31}P trace.

As shown in Figure 6.14, ICP–MS achieves specific detection for the elution of phosphopeptides in LC eluates of phosphoprotein digests, since phosphorus in proteins occurs mostly in the form of phosphate esters. This new combination of element and electrospray mass spectrometry has been applied for the detection of phosphorylation sites in fibrinogen and fetuin [48] and has helped in the identification of so far unknown phosphorylation sites in recombinant and native polo kinases [49, 50]. Ele-

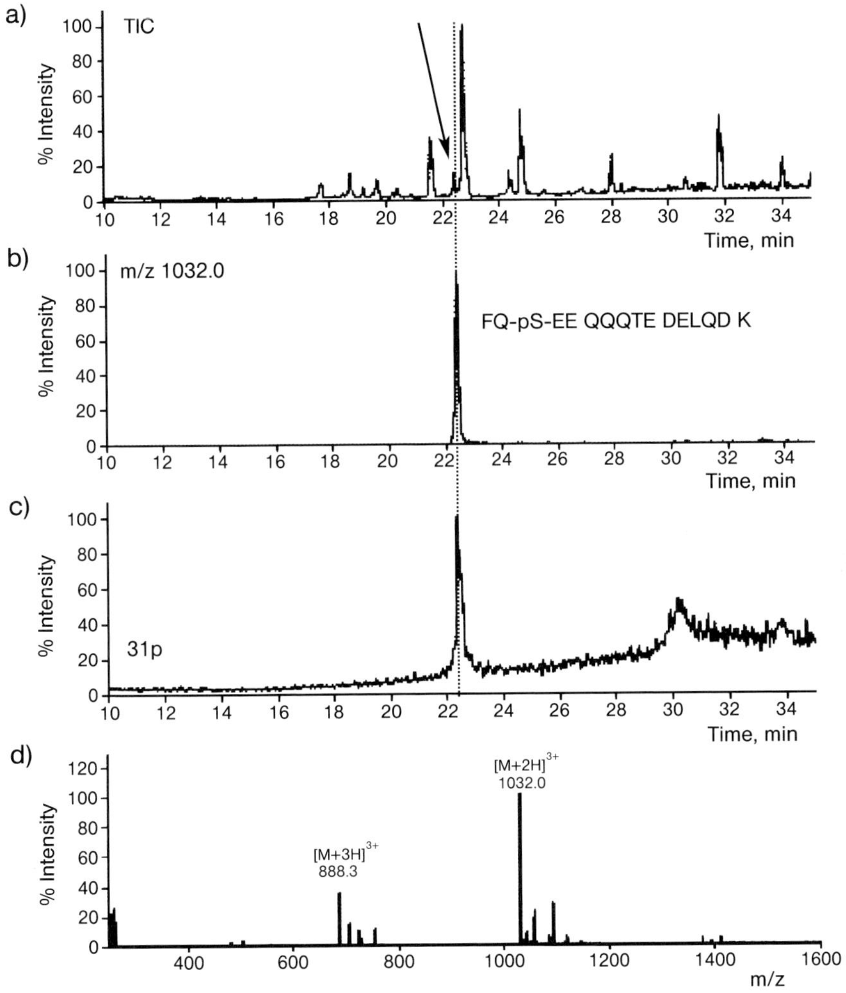

Fig. 6.14 Analysis of a tryptic digest of the phosphoprotein β-casein by LC coupled to element and electrospray MS. (a) Total ion current of the LC–ESI–MS analysis; (b) selected ion trace for *m/z* 1032, the $[M+2H]^{2+}$ ion of the indicated phosphopeptide; (c) ^{31}P trace determined by ICP–MS; (d) ESI mass spectrum at the top of the ^{31}P peak [47].

ment mass spectrometry also gives unique access to the degree of phosphorylation in phosphorproteins by simultaneous measurement of sulphur and phosphorus [51]. ICP–MS has also been used in combination with laser ablation for the detection of electrophoretically separated phosphoproteins [52]. The quantitative nature of the ICP signals provides valuable support for the (usually) nonquantitative results of the molecular MS techniques ESI and MALDI. For quantitative results to be achieved by these techniques, techniques based on stable isotope dilution have to be utilized [53–55].

6.7.2 Tyrosine Sulfation

Although sulfation at tyrosine is relatively frequent [56], only a few studies have been published on the use of mass spectrometry for analysis of protein tyrosine sulfation. One difficulty that may be responsible for this situation is that, in positive ion MS, sulfotyrosine effectively fragments by loss of SO_3 (Figure 6.7), resulting in a peptide or protein containing unmodified tyrosine as the end product. Nevertheless, detection of sulfotyrosine by MS has been reported, e.g., in coagulation factor VIII [57] and in some conotoxins [58].

6.7.3 Redox-related Modifications

Redox-related modifications include processes such as disulfide formation and glutathionylation [59]. Whereas disulfide-bridged peptides are difficult to sequence because they contain two N and two C termini, this feature is what can be used for their recognition after digestion in ^{18}O-labelled water [60]. The proteolytic incorporation of ^{18}O into the C termini means that disulfide-bridged peptides contain twice as much ^{18}O as do normal, linear peptides, allowing them to be discriminated [61].

Glutathionylation of cellular proteins has been observed to increase under oxidative stress [62]. Nitration at tyrosine is also an indicator of oxidative stress and of aging [63], since peroxinitrite attacks the meta positions of tyrosine and forms a stable nitrotyrosine. The formation of an L-nitrotyrosine residue at a certain position was monitored quantitatively by selected reaction monitoring using the 'native reference peptide' method [64]. Under CID conditions, the nitrotyrosine residue is stable and leads to the occurrence of a specific immonium ion at m/z 181.

6.7.4 Myristoylation

Acylation events preferentially occur at basic sites, such as the amino (N terminus, Lys) or guanidino (Arg) functions. Myristoylation usually occurs at the N terminus of proteins and is thought to support their localization at membranes [65]; for example, a variety G-proteins and kinases [66] are covalently modified at their N terminus, which then starts with a myrG unit. N-terminal acylation results in the formation of b_1 ions, which cannot normally be formed, since b ion formation proceeds mainly by a cyclic mechanism requiring a carbonyl function on the N-terminal side of the peptide bond to be cleaved. With an N-terminal myrG residue, the b_1 ion is found at m/z 268, and this characteristic ion is accompanied by two additional fragments at m/z 240 (a1) and m/z 211 (myristoyl acyl ion). By this characteristic triplet of marker ions, an N-terminal myrG structure can be reliably recognized, as shown in Figure 6.15 for the N-terminal peptide of a Golgi-associated protein [67].

Recording the MS/MS data at high resolution, as performed for the analysis shown in Figure 6.15, facilitates discrimination of the myrG-specific fragment ions

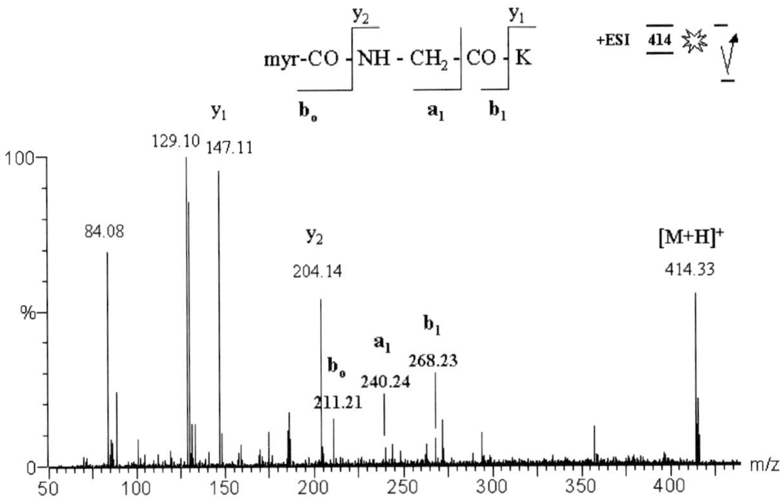

Fig. 6.15 NanoESI–MS/MS spectrum of the C-terminal peptide of a Golgi-associated protein. The myristoylation of this peptide is recognized according to the marker ion triplet at *m/z* 211, 240, and 268 [67].

from other peptide fragment ions in this mass region, since their accurate mass values show a significant high-mass shift due to the unusually high number of hydrogen atoms present.

6.7.5
Acetylation

N-terminal protein acetylation is a frequently observed phenomenon, which can occur with and without N-terminal demethionylation [68]. Addition of an acetyl group is assumed to play a role in regulating the proteolytic stability of a protein; it was observed that attachment of the acetyl group is influenced by the N-terminal sequence. As occurs for myristoylation, an N-terminal acetyl group triggers the formation of b_1 ions in CID of the corresponding N-terminally acetylated peptides. According to these *m/z* values (19 possible values), they can be recognized in a pool of MS/MS spectra. Such a pool of MS/MS spectra can be conveniently generated by, e.g., LC–MS/MS or nanoESI in combination with automated MS to MS/MS switching. In the latter method, the instrument automatically acquires MS/MS spectra from all peptide molecular signals present in the survey spectrum of a protein digest in an intensity-dependent order, starting with the most abundant signal. This pool of MS/MS spectra can be interrogated for the presence of ions with certain *m/z* values by extracting a selected ion chromatogram. Figure 6.16 shows such a data analysis performed on a pool of MS/MS spectra generated from a tryptic digest of dynamin A [69], which has the N-terminal sequence MDQL. Selected ion chromatograms were generated corresponding to the *m/z* values of the b_1, b_2, b_3, and b_4 ions in their acetylated form.

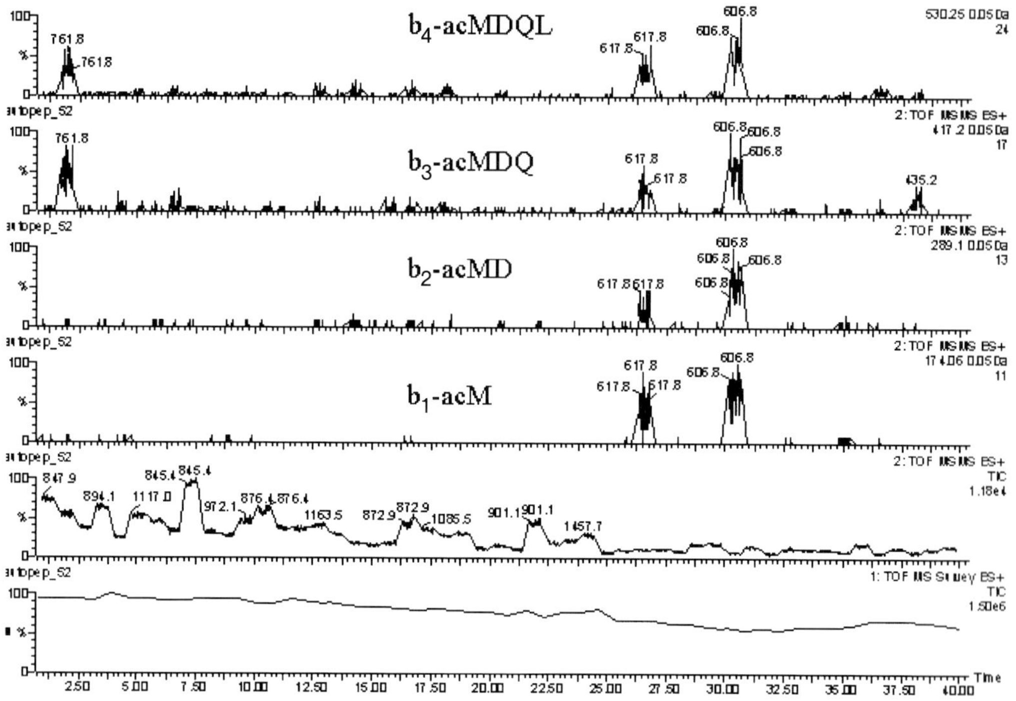

Fig. 6.16 Systematic search for the presence of N-terminal acetylation in dynamin A in a pool of MS/MS spectra acquired automatically by nanoESI–MS/MS from a total tryptic digest of this protein. For two precursor ion *m/z* values, hits are observed in all selected ion chromatograms; these correspond to the b_1 to b_4 ions in their acetylated form. These *m/z* values correspond to the doubly charged molecular ion of the acetylated N-terminal tryptic peptide and of its Na^+ adduct, respectively, which has the sequence acetyl-MDQLIPVINK. The broad peaks in the selected ion chromatograms arose because the program executes five MS/MS spectra at different collision offset values [69]. The two traces at the bottom represent the TIC traces for the MS/MS analyses and for the survey MS, respectively.

At two retention times, corresponding to the precursor ion values of *m/z* 606 and *m/z* 617, peaks occurred in all selected ion chromatograms. Inspection of the corresponding product ion spectra revealed the presence of the C-terminal peptide acetyl-MDQLIPVINK in its H^+/H^+ and in its mixed H^+/Na^+ forms. The two peaks in the upper left corner of Figure 6.16 correspond to an accidental isobaric overlap with some other fragment ions in the MS/MS data pool. Their absence from the b_1 and b_2 ion chromatograms shows that they are not significant.

Internal acetylation at Lys residues can also occur; they have, for instance, been detected by mass spectrometry in lens cristallins [70, 71] and in histones [72, 73]. MS/MS spectra of peptides with acetylated lysine residues exhibit marker ions at *m/z* 143 (immonium ion) and *m/z* 126 (immonium ion $-NH_3$); the latter was reported to show a higher specificity for acetyl-lysine [73].

6.7.6 Methylation

Methylation of proteins has been observed at Lys, Arg, and His residues. Histones represent a class of highly modified proteins that are methylated at numerous sites, as evident when intact histones were analysed by ESI MS analysis [74]. At Lys, mono-, di-, and trimethylation was observed. Trimethylation produces nearly the same mass shift as acetylation at Lys, but trimethylation and acetylation can be distinguished by high-resolution peptide molecular weight data and by specific fragment ions [73]. In MALDI MS/MS neutral loss of 59 was observed for peptides carrying an ε-trimethyl-Lys residue [75]; however, this may be a specific feature of singly charged peptide ions, as typically observed in MALDI MS. For arginine monomethylation dimethylation is observed [76, 77]. Specific detection of dimethylated arginine residues can be achieved by neutral loss of 45 and 87, and their isomeric forms can be discriminated on the basis of the dimethylammonium ion at *m/z* 46 and the *N,N*-dimethylcarbodiimidium ion at *m/z* 71.

6.7.7 Glycosylation

A substantial proportion of cellular proteins are glycosylated [78]. Glycosylation is, for instance, a typical feature of the extracellular domains of membrane proteins, for which the carbohydrate moiety can account for the major part of the total molecular weight of the glycoprotein. MS/MS spectra of N- or O-linked glycopeptides, at least when they contain a polymeric carbohydrate chain, are difficult to interpret. However, attractive methods for their detection in glycoprotein digests have been developed. For instance, pronase digestion of ribonuclease A generates a peptide digest mixture containing unmodified peptides in the low mass region, but in which all signals at *m/z* values >1000 are caused by glycopeptides [79], as demonstrated by MALDI MS analysis. Various ESI MS/MS studies have shown that marker ions originating from the carbohydrate part, such as oxonium ions at 163, 204, and 325, are highly selective for recognition of glycosylated peptides by precursor ion scanning [80–82]. Recently, this<<Q14>> has also been demonstrated for high-resolution MS/MS data [83]. Reversible modification of serine residues by glycosidic addition of *N*-acetylglucosamine has also been reported [84] at sites which may alternatively be phosphorylated [84]. Specific MS/MS detection of peptides modified by GlcNAc was successfully demonstrated on the basis of the corresponding oxonium ion at *m/z* 204 [85–87].

6.7.8 Ubiquitination

Ubiquitin is a small, highly conserved protein of about 8 kDa. It has a C-terminal sequence of Arg-Gly-Gly and becomes linked via its C terminus to Lys residues in other proteins via an isopeptide bond, a reaction that is known to initiate degradation of the ubiquitinated protein in the cell's proteasomes [88]. When a ubiquitinated protein is subjected to tryptic digestion, peptides with internal Lys-Gly-Gly branches are created as markers for the ubiquitinated sites, since the modified Lys residues are not cut by trypsin. This elegant principle has been used for mapping ubiquitination sites at the protein [89] and the proteome level [90]. Since the particular structure does not give rise to a specific fragment ion but rather to a molecular weight increase by +114 Da, the modified peptides were searched for by using software-supported interpretation of a pool of automatically acquired MS/MS spectra. In a proteomic study of ubiquitination [90], 110 lysines could be identified as ubiquitin target sites in the yeast proteome.

6.7.9
Isoaspartate Formation

The formation of isoaspartate and aspartate residues by spontaneous deamidation of specific Asn residues is a widely observed phenomenon in proteins [91] and is probably the most common type of nonenzymatic covalent modification. It proceeds via the β-aspartyl shift mechanism [91] via a succinimide intermediate and is accompanied by partial racemization of the newly formed aspartate and isoaspartate residues [92]. It is mainly considered to be a process correlated with protein ageing. Using electrospray tandem MS, significant differences in the product ion spectra of aspartate-containing peptides and their isoaspartate counterparts could be observed [93, 94]. LC–ESI–MS and nanoESI–MS/MS demonstrated the occurrence of isoAsp, D-Asp, and D-isoAsp in position 2 of the myristoylated N terminus of native bovine protein kinase A catalytic subunit [95].

6.8
Summary and Outlook

In the last years, massive progress has been achieved in the identification and characterization of covalent protein modifications at the molecular level. Synthetic modified peptides, modified reference proteins, recombinant proteins tailored for modification analysis, new analytical concepts, and instrumental innovations have all contributed synergistically to this impressive development. In contrast to genomic projects, which have a clearly defined end point, proteomic analyses are more open-ended tasks, owing to the complexity and dynamic nature of the proteome. In protein modification analysis, determination of the intact molecular weight of a modified protein is a kind of analytical end point; however, at a lower level, other modified forms besides the main form(s) may also be present, which may be overlooked, for example, when the dynamic range of the molecular weight determination method is insufficient for their detection. When a proteomic modification analysis end-point is desired, it is more difficult to define criteria to score the completeness of the analytical results. For this purpose, quantitative data describing the overall occurrence of a class of modifications would be helpful, followed by a quantitative summary of what has been detected. New methods for specific enrichment of modified subproteomes are also highly promising in this respect. On the instrumental side, the ongoing improvements in mass accuracy of MS/MS data will result in a greater proportion of successful modification analyses. The increased mass accuracy will also be essential for the discrimination between covalent modifications and allelic sequence modifications, if no signature fragmentations exist. Finally, the development of quantitative methods may lift the so far mostly qualitative protein modification analysis to a level of elevated biological impact.

References

1. D. N. Perkins, D. J. Pappin, D. M. Creasy, J. S. Cottrell. Probability-based protein identification by searching sequence databases using mass spectrometry data. *Electrophoresis* 1999, *20*, 3551–3567.
2. M. Yamashita, J. B. Fenn. Electrospray ion source: another variation of the free-jet theme. *J. Phys. Chem.* 1984, *88*, 4451–4459.
3. C. M. Whitehouse, R. N. Dreyer, M. Yamashita, J. B. Fenn. Electrospray interface for liquid chromatographs and mass spectrometers. *Anal. Chem.* 1985, *57*, 675–679.
4. P. Kebarle. A brief overview of the present status of the mechanisms involved in electrospray mass spectrometry. *J. Mass Spectrom.* 2000, *35*, 804–817.
5. M. Wilm, M. Mann. Electrospray and Taylor-cone theory, Dole's beam of macromolecules at last? *Int. J. Mass Spectrom. Ion Proc.* 1994, *136*, 167–180.
6. M. Wilm, M. Mann. Analytical properties of the nanoelectrospray ion source. *Anal. Chem.* 1996, *68*, 1–8.
7. S. Geromanos, G. Freckleton, P. Tempst. Tuning of an electrospray ion source for maximum peptide-ion transmission into a mass spectrometer. *Anal. Chem.* 2000, *72*, 777–790.
8. K. R. Jennings. The changing impact of the collision-induced decomposition of ions on mass spectrometry. *Int. J. Mass Spectrom.* 2000, *200*, 479–493.
9. R. A. Yost, G. C. Enke. Selected ion fragmentation with a tandem quadrupole mass spectrometer. *J. Am. Chem. Soc.* 1978, *100*, 2274–2275.
10. S. A. McLuckey, G. J. Van Berkel, D. E. Goeringer, G. L. Glish. Ion trap mass spectrometry using high-pressure ionization. *Anal. Chem.* 1994, *66*, 737A–743A.
11. J. C. Schwartz, M. W. Senko, J. E. P. Syka. A two-dimensional quadrupole ion trap mass spectrometer. *J. Am. Soc. Mass Spectrom.* 2002, *13*, 659–669.
12. R. A. Yost, R. K. Boyd. Tandem mass spectrometry: quadrupole and hybrid instruments. *Methods Enzymol.* 1990, *193*, 154–200.
13. H. R. Morris, T. Paxton, A. Dell, J. Langhorne, M. Berg, R. S. Bordoli, J. Hoyes, R. H. Bateman. High sensitivity collisionally-activated decomposition tandem mass spectrometry on a novel quadrupole/orthogonal-acceleration time-of-flight mass spectrometer. *Rapid Commun. Mass Spectrom.* 1996, *10*, 889–896.
14. D. F. Hunt, A. M. Buko, J. M. Ballard, J. Shabanowitz, A. B. Giordani. Sequence analysis of polypeptides by collision activated dissociation on a triple quadrupole mass spectrometer. *Biomed. Mass Spectrom.* 1981, *8*, 397–408.
15. M. Kinter and N. E. Sherman. *Protein Sequencing and Identification Using Tandem Mass Spectrometry.* Wiley Interscience, New York, 2000.
16. K. Biemann. Nomenclature for peptide fragment ions (positive ions). *Methods Enzymol.* 1990, *193*, 886–887.
17. D. Arnott, J. Shabanowitz, D. F. Hunt. Mass spectrometry of proteins and peptides: sensitive and accurate mass measurement and sequence analysis. *Clin. Chem.* 1993, *39*, 2005–2010.

18. A. Schlosser, W. D. Lehmann. Five-membered ring formation in unimolecular reactions of peptides: a key structural element controlling low-energy collision-induced dissociation of peptides. *J. Mass Spectrom.* 2000, *35*, 1382–1390.
19. J. H. Bowie, C. S. Brinkworth, S. Dua. Collision-induced fragmentations of the (M–H)-parent anions of underivatized peptides: an aid to structure determination and some unusual negative ion cleavages. *Mass Spectrom. Rev.* 2002, *21*, 87–107.
20. C. O'Donovan, R. Apweiler, A. Bairoch. The human proteomics initiative. *Trends Biotechnol.* 2001, *19*, 178.
21. UNIMOD protein modifications for mass spectrometry website at http://www.unimod.org/
22. Delta Mass Database of Protein Post Translational Modifications website at http://www.abrf.org/index.cfm/dm.home?AvgMass=all
23. ExPASy Proteomics Server website at http://www.expasy.ch
24. A. Tholey, J, Reed, W. D. Lehmann. Electrospray tandem mass spectrometric studies of phosphopeptides and phosphopeptide analogues. *J. Mass Spectrom.* 1999, *34*, 117–123.
25. J. P. DeGnore, J. Quin. Fragmentation of phosphopeptides in an ion trap mass spectrometer. *J. Am. Soc. Mass Spectrom.* 1998, *9*, 1175–1188.
26. A. Schlosser, R. Pipkorn, D. Bossemeyer, W. D. Lehmann. Analysis of protein phosphorylation by a combination of elastase digestion and neutral loss tandem mass spectrometry. *Anal Chem.* 2001, *73*, 170–176.
27. J. Ding, W. Burkhart, D. B. Kassel. Identification of phosphorylated peptides from complex mixtures using negative ion orifice-potential stepping and capillary liquid chromatography/electrospray ionisation mass spectrometry. *Rapid Commun. Mass Spectrom.* 1994, *8*, 94–98.
28. P. Jedrzejewski, W. D. Lehmann. Detection of modified peptides in enzymatic digests by capillary liquid chromatography/electrospray mass spectrometry and a programmable skimmer-CID acquisition routine. *Anal. Chem.* 1997, *69*, 294–301.
29. T. Kocher, G. Allmaier, M. Wilm M. Nanoelectrospray-based detection and sequencing of substoichiometric amounts of phosphopeptides in complex mixtures. *J. Mass Spectrom.* 2003, *38*, 131–137.
30. D. C. Neville, C. R. Rozanas, E. M. Price, D. B. Gruis, A. S. Verkman, R. R. Townsend. Evidence for phosphorylation of serine 753 in CFTR using a novel metal-ion affinity resin and matrix-assisted laser desorption mass spectrometry. *Protein Sci.* 1997, *6*, 2436–2445.
31. M. C. Posewitz, P. Tempst. Immobilized gallium(III) affinity chromatography of phosphopeptides. *Anal Chem.* 1999, *71*, 2883–2892.
32. P. Cao, J. T. Stults. Mapping the phosphorylation sites of proteins using on-line immobilized metal affinity chromatography/capillary electrophoresis/electrospray ionization multiple stage tandem mass spectrometry. *Rapid Commun. Mass Spectrom.* 2000, *14*, 1600–1606.
33. A. Schlosser, D. Bossemeyer, J. Bodem, I. Grummt, W. D. Lehmann. Identification of protein phosphorylation sites by a combination of elastase digestion, IMAC enrichment, and Q-TOF tandem mass spectrometry. *Proteomics* 2002, *2*, 911–918.
34. S. B. Ficarro, M. L. McCleland, P. T. Stukenberg, D. J. Burke, M. M. Ross, J. Shabanowitz, D. F. Hunt, F. M. White. *Phosphoproteome analysis by mass spectrometry and its application to Saccharomyces cerevisiae. Nat. Biotechnol.* 2002, *20*, 301–305.
35. H. Zhou, J. D. Watts, R. Aebersold. A systematic approach to the analysis of protein phosphorylation. *Nat. Biotechnol.* 2001, *19*, 375–378.
36. H. E. Meyer, E. Hoffmann-Posorske, H. Korte, L. M. Heilmeyer. Sequence analysis of phosphoserine-containing peptides: modification for picomolar sensitivity. *FEBS Lett.* 1986, *204*, 61–66.
37. K. A. Resing, R. S. Johnson, K. A. Walsh. Mass spectrometric analysis of 21 phosphorylation sites in the internal repeat of rat profilaggrin, precursor of an intermediate filament associated protein. *Biochemistry* 1995, *34*, 9477–9487.
38. H Jaffe, Veeranna, H. C. Pant. Characterization of serine and threonine phosphory-

lation sites in beta-elimination/ethanethiol addition-modified proteins by electrospray tandem mass spectrometry and database searching. *Biochemistry* 1998, *37*, 16211–16224.

39. A. J. Thompson, S. R. Hart, C. Franz, K. Barnouin, A. Ridley, R. Cramer. Characterization of protein phosphorylation by mass spectrometry using immobilized metal ion affinity chromatography with on-resin beta-elimination and Michael addition. *Anal. Chem.* 2003, *75*, 3232–3243.

40. Y. Oda, T. Nagasu, B. T. Chait. Enrichment analysis of phosphorylated proteins as a tool for probing the phosphoproteome. *Nat. Biotechnol.* 2001, *19*, 379–382.

41. H. Steen, M. Mann. A new derivatization strategy for the analysis of phosphopeptides by precursor ion scanning in positive ion mode. *J. Am. Soc. Mass Spectrom.* 2002, *13*, 996–1003.

42. E. Salih. Synthesis of a radioactive thiol reagent, I-*S*-[H-3]carboxymethyl-dithiothreitol: identification of the phosphorylation sites by N-terminal peptide sequencing and matrix-assisted laser desorption/ionization time-of-flight mass spectrometry. *Anal. Biochem.* 2003, *319*, 143–158.

43. H. Steen, B. Kuster, M. Mann. QTOF versus triple quadrupole MS for the determination of phosphopeptides by precursor ion scanning. *J. Mass Spectrom.* 2001, *36*, 782–790.

44. H. Steen, B. Kuster, M. Fernandez, A. Pandey, M. Mann. Tyrosine phosphorylation mapping of the epidermal growth factor receptor signaling pathway. *J. Biol. Chem.* 2002, *277*, 1031–1039.

45. A. Pandey, A. V. Podtelejnikov, B. Blagoev, X. R. Bustelo, M. Mann, H. F. Lodish. Analysis of receptor signaling pathways by mass spectrometry: identification of vav-2 as a substrate of the epidermal and platelet-derived growth factor receptors. *Proc. Natl. Acad. Sci. USA* 2000, *97*, 179–184.

46. M. Salek, A. Alonso, R. Pipkorn, W. D. Lehmann. Analysis of protein tyrosine phosphorylation by nanoelectrospray ionization high-resolution tandem mass spectrometry and tyrosine-targeted product ion scanning *Anal. Chem.* 2003, *75*, 2724–2729.

47. Wind, M.; Edler, M.; Jakubowski, N.; Linscheid, M.; Wesch, H.; Lehmann, W. D. Analysis of protein phosphorylation by capillary liquid chromatography coupled to element mass spectrometry with ^{31}P detection and to electrospray mass spectrometry. *Anal. Chem.* 2001, *73*, 29–35.

48. Wind, M.; Gosenca, D.; Kübler, D., Lehmann, W. D. Stable isotope phosphoprofiling of fibrinogen and fetuin subunits by element mass spectrometry coupled to capillary liquid chromatography. *Anal. Biochem.* 2003, *317*, 26–33.

49. Kelm, O.; Wind, M.; Lehmann, W. D.; Nigg, E. A. Cell-cycle–regulated phosphorylation of the *Xenopus* polo-like kinase Plx1. *J. Biol. Chem.* 2002, *277*, 25247–25256.

50. Wind, M.; Kelm, O.; Nigg, E.; Lehmann, W. D. Identification of phosphorylation sites in the polo-kinases Plx1 and Plk1 by a novel strategy based on element and electrospray high resolution mass spectrometry. *Proteomics* 2002, *2*, 1516–1523

51. Wind, M.; Wesch, H.; Lehmann, W.D. Protein phosphorylation degree: determination by capillary liquid chromatography and inductively coupled plasma mass spectrometry. *Anal. Chem.* 2001, *73*, 3006–3010.

52. Wind, M.; Feldmann, I.; Jakubowski, N.; Lehmann, W. D. Spotting and quantification of phosphoproteins purified by gel electrophoresis by laser ablation element mass spectrometry with phosphorus-31 detection. *Electrophoresis*, 2003, *24*, 1276–1280.

53. S. P. Gygi, B. Rist, S. A. Gerber, F. Turecek, M. H. Gelb, R. Aebersold. Quantitative analysis of complex protein mixtures using isotope-coded affinity tags. *Nat. Biotechnol.* 1999, *17*, 994–999.

54. S. A. Gerber, J. Rush, O. Stemman, M. W. Kirschner, S. P. Gygi. Absolute quantification of proteins and phosphoproteins from cell lysates by tandem MS. *Proc. Natl. Acad. Sci. USA* 2003, *100*, 6940–6945.

55. D. Bonenfant, T. Schmelzle, E. Jacinto, J. L. Crespo, T. Mini, M. N. Hall, P. Jenoe. Quantitation of changes in protein phosphorylation: a simple method based on stable isotope labeling and mass spectrometry. *Proc. Natl. Acad. Sci. USA* 2003, *100*, 880–885.

56. C. Niehrs, R. Beisswanger, W. B. Huttner. Protein tyrosine sulfation. *Chem. Biol. Interact.* 1994, *92*, 257–271.

57. J. C. Severs, M. Carnine, H. Eguizabakl, K. K. Mock. Characterization of tyrosine sulfate residues in anthemophilic recombinant factor VIII by LC ESI tandem MS and amino acid analysis. *Rapid Commun. Mass Spectrom.* 1999, *13*, 1016–1023.

58. J. L. Wolfender, F. Chu, H. Ball, F. Wolfender, M. Fainzilber, M. A. Baldwin, A. L. Burlingame. Identification of tyrosine sulfation in *Conus pennaceus* conotoxins a-PnIA and a-PNIB: further investigation of labile sulfo- and phosphopeptides by ESI, MALDI and API MALDI MS. *J. Mass Spectrom.* 1999, *34*, 447–454.

59. P. Ghezzi, V. Bonnetto. Redox proteomics: identification of oxidatively modified proteins. *Proteomics* 2003, *3*, 1145–1153.

60. M. Schnölzer, P. Jedrzejewski, W. D. Lehmann. Protease-catalyzed incorporation of ^{18}O into protein fragments and its application to protein sequencing. *Electrophoresis* 1996, *17*, 945–953.

61. J. J. Gorman, T. P. Wallis, J. J. Pitt. Protein disulfide bond determination by mass spectrometry. *Mass Spectrom. Rev.* 2002, *21*, 183–216.

62. M. Fratelli, H. Demol, M. Puype, S. Casagrande, I. Eberini, M. Salmona, V. Bonetto, M. Mengozzi, F. Duffieux, E. Miclet, A. Bachi, J. Vandekerckhove, E. Gianazza, P. Ghezzi. Identification by redox proteomics of glutathionylated proteins in oxidatively stressed human T lymphocytes. *Proc. Natl. Acad. Sci. USA*, 2002, *99*, 3505–3510.

63. Viner R.I., Ferrington D.A., Williams T.D., Bigelow D.J., Schoneich C. Protein modification during biological aging: selective tyrosine nitration of the SERCA2a isoform of the sarcoplasmic reticulum Ca^{2+}-ATPase in skeletal muscle. *Biochem. J.* 1999, *340*, 657–669.

64. B. B. Willard, C. I. Ruse, J. A. Keightley, M. Bond, M. Kinter. Site-specific quantitation of protein nitration using liquid chromatography/tandem mass spectrometry. *Anal. Chem.* 2003, *75*, 2370–2376.

65. M. Resh. Fatty acylation of proteins: new insights into membrane targeting of myristoylated and palmotoylated proteins. *Biochim. Biophys. Acta* 1999, *1451*, 1–16.

66. P. T. Jedrzejewski, A. Girod, A. Tholey, N. Konig, S. Thullner, V. Kinzel, D. Bossemeyer D. A conserved deamidation site at Asn 2 in the catalytic subunit of mammalian cAMP-dependent protein kinase detected by capillary LC–MS and tandem mass spectrometry. *Protein Sci.* 1998, *7*, 457–469.

67. H. B. Eberle, R. L. Serrano, J. Fullekrug, A. Schlosser, W. D. Lehmann, F. Lottspeich, D. Kaloyanova, F. T. Wieland, J. B. Helms. Identification and characterization of a novel human plant pathogenesis-related protein that localizes to lipid-enriched microdomains in the Golgi complex. *J. Cell Sci.* 2002, *115*, 827–838.

68. R. A. Bradshaw, W. W. Brickey, K. W. Walker. N-terminal processing: the methionine aminopeptidase and N-alpha-acetyl transferase families. *Trends Biochem. Sci.* 1998, *23*, 263–267.

69. A. Schlosser, B. Klockow, D. J. Manstein, W. D. Lehmann. Analysis of post-translational modification and characterization of the domain structure of dynamin A from *Dictyostelium discoideum*. *J. Mass Spectrom.* 2003, *38*, 277–282.

70. P. P. Lin, R. C. Barry, D. L. Smith, J. B. Smith. In vivo acetylation identified at lysine 10 of human lens aA-crystallin. *Prot. Sci.* 1998, *7*, 1451–1457.

71. V. N. Lapko, D. L. Smith, J. B. Smith. In vivo carbamoylation and acetylation of water soluble human lens aB-crystallin. *Prot. Sci.* 2001, *10*, 1130–1136.

72. J. Y. King, K. W. Kim, H. J. Kwon, D. W. Lee, J. S. Yoo. Probing lysine acetylation with a modification-specific marker ion using high-performance liquid chromatography/electrospray–mass spectrometry with collision-induced dissociation. *Anal Chem.* 2002, *74*, 5443–5449.

73. K. Zhang, H. Tang, L. Huang, J. W. Blankenship, P. R. Jones, F. Xiang, P. M. Yau, A. L. Burlingame. Identification of acetylation and methylation sites of histone H3 from chicken erythrocytes by high-accuracy matrix-assisted laser desorption ionization-time-of-flight, matrix-

assisted laser desorption ionization-post-source decay, and nanoelectrospray ionization tandem mass spectrometry. *Anal Biochem.* 2002, *306*, 259–269.

74. R. E. Schweppe, C. E. Haydon, T. S. Lewis, K. A. Resing, N. G. Ahn. The characterization of protein post-translational modifications by mass spectrometry. *Acc. Chem. Res.* 2003, *36*, 453–461.

75. J. Hirota, Y. Satomi, K. Yoshikawa, T. Takao. Epsilon-*N,N,N*-trimethyllysine–specific ions in matrix-assisted laser desorption/ionization–tandem mass spectrometry. *Rapid Commun. Mass Spectrom.* 2003, *17*, 371–376.

76. J. Yague, J, Vazquez, J. A. Lopez de Castro. A post-translational modification of nuclear proteins, NG, NG-dimethyl-Arg, found in a natural HLA class I peptide ligand. *Prot. Sci.* 2000, *9*, 2210–2217.

77. J. Rappsilber, W. J. Friesen, S. Paushkin, G. Dreyfuss, M. Mann. Detection of arginine dimethylated peptides by parallel precursor ion scanning mass spectrometry in positive ion mode. *Anal. Chem.* 2003, *75*, 3107–3114.

78. R. Apweiler, H. Hermjakob, N. Sharon. On the frequency of protein glycosylation as deduced from analysis of the SWISSPROT database. *Biochim. Biophys. Acta* 1999, *1473*, 4–8.

79. P. Juhasz, S. A. Martin. The use of non-specific proteases in the characterization of glycoproteins by high resolution TOF MS. *Int. J. Mass Spectrom. Ion Processes* 1997, *169–170*, 217–230.

80. M. J. Huddleston, M. F. Bean, S. A. Carr. Collisional fragmentation of glycopeptides by ESI LC/MS and LC/MS/MS: methods for selective detection of glycopeptides in protein digests. *Anal. Chem.* 1993, *65*, 877–884.

81. S. Carr, M. Huddleston, M. Bean, Selective identification and differentiation of N- and O-linked oligosaccharides in glycoproteins by LC–MS. *Prot. Sci.* 1993, *2*, 183–196.

82. M. A. Ritchie, A. C. Gill, M. Deery, K. Lilley, Precursor ion scanning for detection of and structural characterization of heterogenous glycopeptide mixtures. *J. Am. Soc. Mass Spectrom.* 2002, *13*, 1065–1077.

83. J. Jebanathirajah, H. Steen, P. Roepstorff. Using optimised collision energies and high resolution high accuracy fragment ion selection to improve glycopeptide detection by precursor ion scanning. *J. Am. Soc. Mass Spectrom.* 2003, *14*, 777–784.

84. Wells L., Whalen S. A., Hart G. W. L. Wells, S. A. Whalen, G. W. Hart. O-GlcNAc: a regulatory post-translational modification. *Biochem. Biophys. Res. Commun.* 2003, *14*, 435–441.

85. K. D. Greis, B. K. Hayes, F. I. Comer, M. Kirk, S. Barnes, T. L. Lowary, G. W. Hart. Selective detection and site-analysis of O-GlcNAc–modified glycopeptides by beta-elimination and tandem electrospray mass spectrometry. *Anal. Biochem.* 1996, *234*, 38–49.

86. P. A. Haynes, R. Aebersold. Simultaneous detection and identification of O-GlcNAc–modified glycoproteins using liquid chromatography–tandem mass spectrometry. *Anal Chem.* 2000, *72*, 5402–5410.

87. R. J. Chalkley, A. L. Burlingame. Identification of novel sites of *O-N*-acetylglucosamine modification of serum response factor using quadrupole time-of-flight mass spectrometry. *Mol. Cell Proteomics* 2003, *2*, 182–190.

88. A. M. Weissman. Themes and variations on ubiquitylation. *Nat. Rev. Mol. Cell. Biol.* 2001, *2*, 169–178.

89. L. A. Marotti, R. Newitt, Y. Wang, R. Aebersold, H. G. Dohlman. Direct identification of a G protein ubiquitination site by mass spectrometry. *Biochemistry* 2002, *41*, 5067–5074.

90. J. Peng, D. Schwartz, J. E. Elias, C. C. Thoreen, D. Cheng, G. Marsischky, J. Roelofs, D. Finley, S. P. Gygi. A proteomics approach to understanding protein ubiquitination. *Nat. Biotechnol.* 2003, *21*, 921–926.

91. D. W. Aswad, M. V. Paranandi, B. T. Schurter. Isoaspartate in peptides and proteins: formation, significance, and analysis. *J. Pharm. Biomed. Anal.* 2000, *21*, 1129–1136.

92. S. Ritz-Timme, M. J. Collins. Racemization of aspartic acid in human proteins. *Ageing Res. Rev.* 2002, *1*, 43–59.

93. W. D. Lehmann, A. Schlosser, G. Erben, R. Pipkorn, D. Bossemeyer, V. Kinzel. Analysis of isoaspartate in peptides by electrospray tandem mass spectrometry. *Prot. Sci.* 2000, *9*, 2260–2268.

94. L. J. Gonzalez, T. Shimizu, Y. Satomi, L. Betancourt, V. Besada, G. Padron, R. Orlando, T. Shirasawa, Y. Shimonishi, T. Takao. Differentiating alpha- and beta-aspartic acids by electrospray ionization and low-energy tandem mass spectrometry. *Rapid Commun. Mass Spectrom.* 2000, *14*, 2092–2102.

95. V. Kinzel, N. Konig, R. Pipkorn, D. Bossemeyer, W. D. Lehmann. The amino terminus of PKA catalytic subunit: a site for introduction of posttranslational heterogeneities by deamidation: D-Asp2 and D-isoAsp2 containing isozymes. *Prot. Sci.* 2000, *9*, 2269–2277.

7
Chromatin Immunoprecipitation-based Identification of Gene Regulatory Networks

Monika Niehof and Jürgen Borlak

7.1
Introduction

7.1.1
Importance of Identifying Transcriptional Regulatory Networks in Toxicogenomics

Administered in critical doses, drugs and chemicals can damage organs and tissues by turning numerous genes on or off. Changes in the expression patterns of target genes indicate toxic action and are manifested as multiple toxicological endpoints detectable by transcriptome analysis. Microarray technology allows measuring transcriptional modulation of thousands of genes after exposure to xenobiotics. Induction or repression of genes is mediated by an altered protein–DNA binding pattern of nuclear transcription factors (TFs). TFs are regulatory proteins that bind to the promoters or enhancers of their respective target genes and thereby affect gene expression and potentially lead to dysfunction of target organs. Approximately 2000 TFs [1, 2] are responsible for controlling the entire gene expression from development and differentiation to metabolic functions. A major challenge in genomic research today involves identifying more of their respective target genes.

Regulation of gene transcription is a multifactorial process. TFs bind to a specific DNA sequence in the control region of a gene and interact with so-called general basal factors to recruit RNA polymerase II to the transcription start site of a gene. These proteins together form a multiprotein complex that permits regulated mRNA synthesis [3]. Initiation of transcription is frequently the result of binding of many different TFs to cognate DNA binding sites, which enables combinatorial control of gene expression. An additional level of complexity is provided by protein–protein interactions between TFs and cofactors and between synergistically acting TFs [4]. The activation of a gene requires accessibility of TFs, cofactors, and basal factors to the regulatory region. Chromatin remodelling complexes change chromatin structure by altering DNA–histone contacts within a nucleosome and make regions of the genome accessible to target transcription factor binding [5]. Several transcriptional coactivators contribute to chromatin remodelling [6].

Handbook of Toxicogenomics: Strategies and Applications. Edited by Jürgen Borlak

ISBN: 3-527-30342-1

Involvement of different kinds of TFs and cofactors in specific target gene regulation allows the integration of several signalling pathways. Identifying the target genes for specific TFs as well as discovering the crosstalk mechanism involved will lead to understanding the transcriptional network.

The liver is the first organ that encounters toxins that have been absorbed through the intestines. One of the major roles of the liver is detoxification and metabolism of xenobiotics [7]. Particularly with regard to predicting the toxic action of xenobiotic compounds, identification of all targets of liver-specific TFs (for review see Schrem et al. [8, 9]) would constitute great progress in toxicogenomics. Substances could be grouped mechanistically by targeting the same TF pattern, and prediction of toxic action would then be possible through analyses of changes in TF binding prior to observable damage to the tissue.

7.1.2
Chromatin Immunoprecipitation to Analyze Target Genes

One of the most useful techniques for studying the complex process of gene regulation is the chromatin immunoprecipitation (ChIP) procedure. ChIP enables the specific association of a given TF with DNA within living cells to be examined. In the standard ChIP assay, proteins are crosslinked to DNA at their actual binding sites, and specific protein–DNA complexes are isolated by immunoprecipitation. After reversal of crosslinking and purification of DNA specifically associated with the protein of interest, specific DNA sequences can be examined by PCR with gene-specific primers [10–12]. A positive result confirms that a TF is bound *in vivo* to a gene previously described by other means. In the past few years, an increasing number of potential TF targets have been proved or revised by using the ChIP assay (examples are given in [13–17]). A modified ChIP protocol with subsequent cloning steps is used to examine DNA sequences specifically precipitated by antibodies against given TFs, with no prior knowledge of the targets. This method therefore allows the immunoselection of novel *in vivo* target genes [18]. It is an elaborate, but immensely worthwhile, multistep method carried out in only a few laboratories [19–26].

7.2
Description of Methods

A schematic outline of the method is presented in Figure 7.1 (for reviews see [10–12, 18]). In this section we describe the important steps in detail, point out some of the problems, and discuss diverse strategies.

7.2.1
Crosslinking Applications

The initial step is crosslinking of living cells. Formaldehyde is particularly useful for this purpose and is the most frequently used reagent. The chemical targets for

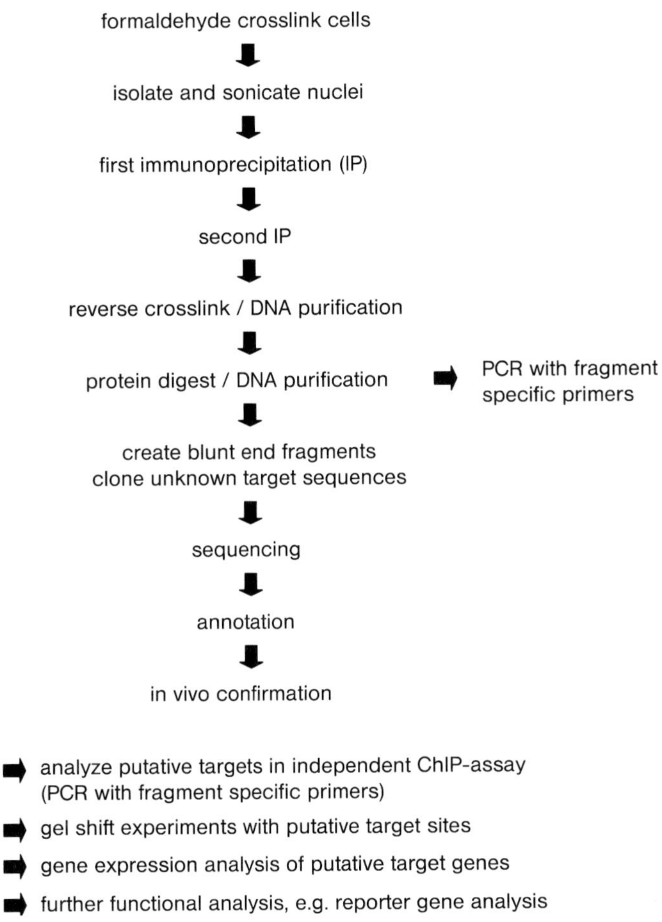

Fig. 7.1 Flow chart of chromatin immunoprecipitation assay (ChIP assay) for cloning procedure and target gene analysis.

formaldehyde are primary amino groups (lysines, arginines, histidines) and the adenine, guanine, and cytosine bases. Crosslinking leads to both protein–protein and protein–DNA crosslinks, bridging distances of about 2 Å [27, 28]. Both types of crosslinks can be reversed selectively, so that DNA and proteins can be further analyzed separately. Extended incubation at 65 °C breaks protein–DNA bonds, and reversing protein–protein crosslinks requires temperatures close to boiling [29, 30]. Formaldehyde is active over a wide range of buffer conditions and temperatures and penetrates biological membranes; thus, crosslinking can be done with intact cells. Nucleosomal proteins are usually analyzed after a crosslinking time of about 10 min at a final concentration of 1% formaldehyde. The extent of crosslinking is an important parameter. Longer exposure to formaldehyde leads to loss of immunoprecipitated material, and overfixed cells are refractory to sonication [12]. Formaldehyde is a moderate denaturant to proteins and interferes with protein secondary structure, resulting in unfolding of proteins. Therefore, excessive crosslinking can result in reduced antigen availability. During immunoprecipitation, polyclonal antibodies are preferred to monoclonals to avoid potential epitope masking problems in crosslinked material. It is important to test the ability of the antibody to recognize its antigen in fixed material.

Ultraviolet (UV)-induced crosslinking has been successfully applied to study *in vitro* protein–DNA interactions [31, 32]. UV laser-induced protein–DNA crosslinking occurs in two distinct steps. In the first step, the bases of DNA are excited by light absorption. This excitement rapidly gives rise to radical cations of nucleic bases, resulting in chemical crosslinking and macromolecular damage, mainly to DNA. Completion of the crosslinking reaction occurs in less than a microsecond [32]. The chemical reaction of laser-induced protein–DNA crosslinking is poorly understood [31]. Nanosecond or picosecond UV laser irradiation prevents artifactual rearrangement during crosslinking. Some laboratories use conventional UV sources, but prolonged irradiation is required with conventional UV light, which allows redistribution of proteins [31]. Laser-induced reactions, as opposed to those generated by conventional UV sources, lead to higher crosslinking efficiency [32]. UV lasers for crosslinking applications have often been custom-modified, and the critical parameters – the combination of intensity and pulse length – have to be carefully checked for each new application [33]. Furthermore, different proteins and different DNA sequences might require different irradiation parameters [33, 34].

In contrast to formaldehyde fixation, UV laser irradiation does not cause protein–protein crosslinks [35] but does induce lesions in DNA [31, 32, 36], with possible consequences for subsequent PCR or cloning procedures. These lesions can be easily detected by treatment with chemical reagents; therefore, UV crosslinking is mainly used in footprinting assays to analyze protein–DNA interactions *in vitro* or in isolated nuclei. Nevertheless, UV illumination (especially for *Drosophila* embryos), as well as UV laser crosslinking coupled with ChIP assays, are carried out in a few laboratories [26, 37–39].

However, in combination with immunoprecipitation of targets, formaldehyde is the most commonly used method for *in vivo* protein–DNA crosslinking. A key advantage of formaldehyde, especially in subsequent target cloning, is the fully reversible crosslinking [12, 18].

7.2.2
Chromatin Fragmentation

After crosslinking, nuclei are isolated and then nuclear extracts are prepared. Formaldehyde-fixed cells are highly resistant to restriction enzyme digestion or DNase I treatment. Therefore, soluble chromatin can be produced efficiently only by mechanical shearing [10, 11]. Sonication is a rapid and simple way to shear chromatin fragments and to generate rather uniformly sized pieces of DNA with well defined lengths. The addition of glass microbeads prior to sonication improves the shearing efficiency [18]. The conditions for sonication with a particular sonicator have to be

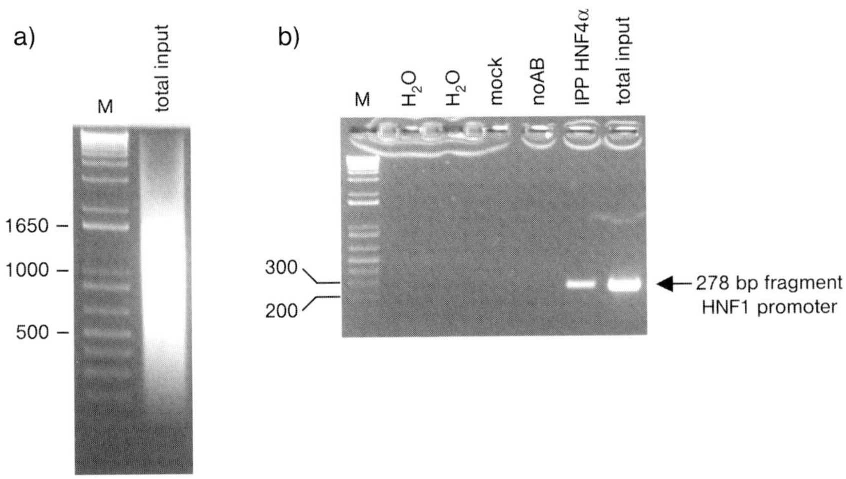

Fig. 7.2 Examples of preliminary setup experiments before ChIP cloning. (a) Effect of sonication conditions. DNA fragments, the majority of which were between 500 and 1600 bp long, were generated with four 20-s pulses from a W-250-classic sonicator (Branson) equipped with a microtip and operated at setting cycle 50%, output control 5. Between each pulse the samples were allowed to cool for 20 s in an ice bath. DNA was purified and analyzed by agarose gel electrophoresis and ethidium bromide staining. (b) HNF4α ChIP experiment in Caco2 cells for HNF1α as positive target. A ChIP experiment was performed in Caco2 cells with an antibody against HNF4α (IPP HNF4α) or no antibody (noAB). After DNA purification, samples were subjected to PCR with primers designed for the HNF1α promoter as the HNF4α-positive target. A mock probe and a portion of the total input sample were also examined by PCR.

tested beforehand, because the sonication time and number of pulses required vary, depending on the sonicator, cell type, and extent of crosslinking. Therefore, DNA is isolated after fragmentation and analyzed by agarose gel electrophoresis and ethidium bromide staining to determine how many cycles of sonication are needed to shear the chromatin to a certain size range. An example of such an experiment for the human epithelial cell line Caco2 is shown in Figure 7.2a.

7.2.3 Immunoprecipitation of Proteins

After preparation of nuclear extracts and chromatin fragmentation, specific TFs, together with crosslinked DNA, are recovered from cell lysates by addition of specific antibodies and adsorption onto protein A–Sepharose beads. The immunoprecipitation step requires stringent conditions. The composition of buffers used for cell lysis, immunoprecipitation, and washing determines the stringency of analyses. Varying the type and concentration of denaturing and nondenaturing detergents (Triton X-100, sodium deoxycholate, and sodium dodecylsulphate) and salts in lysis and wash buffers may be helpful in adapting the procedure to a particular application. The outcome of the experiment depends on the quality of antibodies used. They should possess high affinity for the antigen and should cross-react minimally with other proteins. Using affinity-purified antibodies is highly recommended. To prevent recovering unspecific DNA during immunoprecipitation, chromatin should first be precleared with blocked protein A–Sepharose. Even though the goal of these experiments is to characterize the immunoprecipitated DNA, it is absolutely necessary to control the efficiency of precipitation by analyzing the protein content in the precipitate. For this purpose an aliquot is heated to 95 °C in conventional SDS–polyacrylamide gel electrophoresis gel-loading buffer in the presence of 0.5 M 2-mercaptoethanol for 30 min to 1 hour to reverse protein–protein crosslinks, prior to SDS–PAGE [29, 30].

7.2.4 DNA Isolation and PCR Analyses

For identification of *in vivo* targets of a given protein, after immunoprecipitation of crosslinked chromatin the DNA is purified and analyzed by a PCR reaction in which the immunoprecipitated material is used as a template for amplification with gene-specific primers ('target gene analysis'). Such analysis requires the removal of all proteins from the immunopurified chromatin fraction. The DNA is isolated from samples after reversal of crosslinking by heat treatment, extensive digestion with proteinase K, and purification [18]. Bound and unbound sequences are represented equally in the genome and are amplified accordingly from the total input sample. Only sequences specifically isolated by the factor of interest give rise to PCR products from the immunoprecipitated material. In parallel, a control immunoprecipitation with no antibody should be carried out to monitor nonspecific binding of DNA. A mock sample, which contains buffer without chromatin, should also be carried through the entire immunoprecipitation procedure and DNA isolation, to control for DNA contamination of buffer and wash solutions. Figure 7.2B represents a successful ChIP experiment in Caco2 cells with an HNF4α antibody and subsequent PCR analysis with primers designed for the HNF1α promoter as an HNF4α-positive target.

7.2.5 Cloning Strategies

By subcloning and sequencing the immunoprecipitated DNA, it is possible to modify the ChIP procedure for identifying unknown interaction sites. Therefore, changes to the standard protocol are required, especially to eliminate as much of the nonspecific DNA as possible [18]. Two sequential immunoprecipitations with aliquots of the same TF-specific antibody decrease the amount of nonspecific DNA. It is important to confirm that the second immunoprecipitation was successful before proceeding to the cloning procedure. Some antibodies cannot efficiently recognize protein complexes after elution, possibly because some proteins do not renature appropriately for antibody recognition. Therefore, this step must be closely monitored before cloning.

If sequencing of small fragments (200–300 bp) results in a majority of highly repetitive DNA fragments, then shearing of chromatin to larger fragments during preparation is advised, and only cloned DNA fragments of at least 500 bp should be analyzed [18]. Nevertheless, small fragments can result in positive targets [25], possibly because of differences in kind of beads, mode of blocking reaction, or preclearance of probes.

The amount of DNA after the second immunoprecipitation step is very small, resulting in two different cloning strategies: direct cloning [18] and cloning including PCR amplification steps [40]. The disadvantage of the linker-mediated PCR amplification procedure lies in the difficulties of amplifying sequences with high GC content, and a significant percentage of mammalian promoter regions are GC-rich. The PCR amplification step may preferentially amplify AT-rich, nonpromoter sequences, creating a false abundance of these sequences in the cloning pool. To compensate for the low DNA yield after the second immunoprecipitation step, direct cloning requires running several identical immunoprecipitation reactions in parallel, the products of which are pooled after the DNA purification step. A schematic outline of the cloning procedure is presented in Figure 7.3. T4 DNA polymerase is used to create blunt-ended immunoprecipitated fragments, which can be directly cloned into a blunt vector. Increasing the molar ratio of ChIP DNA to vector in the ligation reaction increases the probability of cloning larger fragments, but increasing the DNA concentration also decreases the overall ligation efficiency. Testing various insert-to-vector ratios is therefore recommended, as well as monitoring the transformation efficiency. Blunt-end ChIP DNA processed with an A-addition kit can subsequently be cloned in a T/A vector, which can improve transformation efficiency. Positive clones are screened by restriction enzyme analysis, sequenced, and then analyzed.

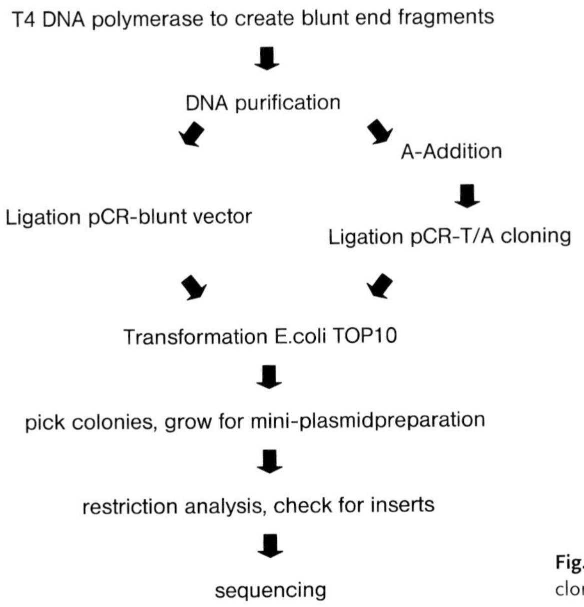

Fig. 7.3 Schematic outline of cloning procedure.

7.2.6
Target Validation

Although a large fraction of nonspecific DNA is removed in the second immunoprecipitation step, it is very difficult to completely eliminate it [18]. Therefore, it is extremely important to validate each clone obtained by the ChIP cloning method. The first step in confirming the clones is to perform independent standard ChIP experiments with subsequent PCR analyses using clone-specific primers. These analyses eliminate false positives, which can occur by random chance or be acquired by nonspecific precipitation. It is impossible to completely eliminate all nonspecific DNA, so some false positives are unavoidable [18]. Examples of true- and false-positive clones of HNF4α targets obtained with the ChIP cloning assay are shown in Figure 7.4. Work on identi-

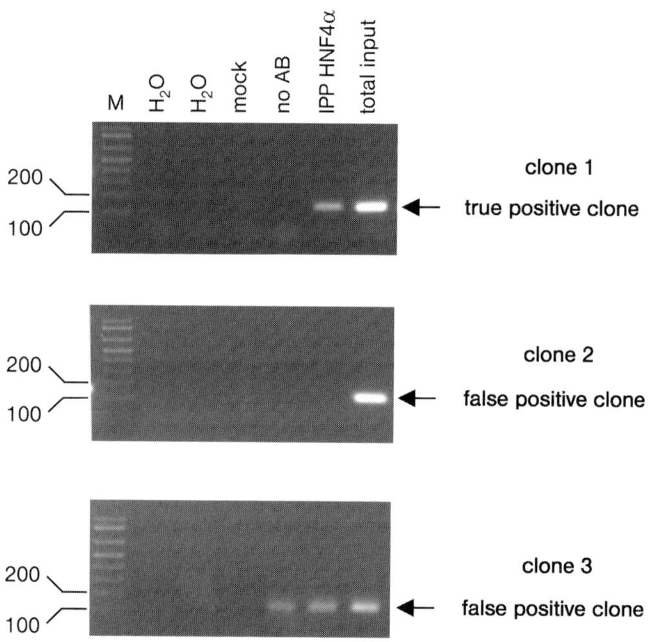

Fig. 7.4 Examples of true- and false-positive clones obtained with the ChIP cloning assay for HNF4α targets in Caco2 cells. A ChIP experiment (performed separately from the ChIP experiment for cloning) was performed in Caco2 cells with an antibody against HNF4α (IPP HNF4α) or no antibody (noAB). After DNA purification, samples were subjected to PCR with primers designed for the potential target clones (clone 1 = primers for a fragment of 147 bp, clone 2 = primers for a fragment of 124 bp, clone 3 = primers for a fragment of 126 bp). A mock probe and a portion of the total input sample were also examined by PCR. *Top:* Example of a true-positive clone. PCR fragments were generated in the IPP HNF4α sample, but not in the no-antibody control (clone 1). *Middle:* Example of a false-positive clone isolated due to random chance without confirmation in the subsequent experiment. PCR fragments were not generated in either the IPP HNF4α sample or the no-antibody control (clone 2). *Bottom:* Example of a false-positive clone due to nonspecific isolation without confirmation in the subsequent experiment. PCR fragments were generated in the IPP HNF4α sample as well as in the no-antibody control (clone 3).

fying and characterizing new HNF4α targets by the ChIP cloning procedure is still in progress and will be reported later [41, 42].

The confirmed genomic fragments are annotated in the human genome database, and potential regulatory regions are further characterized for factor binding sites. Inspection of cloned fragments with bioinformatics-generated matrices for TF binding sites [43–48] enables implementation of specific electrophoretic mobility-shift assays (EMSA). It is likely to identify clones with and without consensus binding sites for the factor [19]. Recruitment of a TF to DNA is possible in consequence of interaction with other DNA binding proteins. Formaldehyde induces protein–protein crosslinks [12] and thus has the potential to connect proteins to DNAs that they do not contact directly. It is also possible that the promoter context may greatly influence TF binding efficiency within the cellular environment [19]. Synergy of some TFs is mediated in part by cooperative DNA binding *in vivo*. Others have previously shown that site-specific DNA binding proteins can regulate transcription through sequence elements that diverge from the consensus [49, 50].

In addition to characterizing factor binding sites, it is essential to monitor the functional relevance of the identified targets. These additional studies can include analyzing the expression profiles of target genes by RT–PCR as well as analyzing the functional relevance of the characterized binding sites in reporter gene assays. Ultimately, expression of potential target genes has to be down-regulated in the knockout mouse for the corresponding TF.

7.3 Successfully Reported ChIP Cloning for New Target Identification

The first demonstration that formaldehyde crosslinking combined with the modified chromatin immunoprecipitation assay can be used to clone promoters that are direct *in vivo* targets of a mammalian TF was published by Weinmann et al. in 2001 [19]. They cloned, confirmed, and described three novel E2F target genes. So far, subsequent studies have described new targets for E2A [23], Egr1 [24], EWS/ATF-1 [25], *Drosophila* TF engrailed [26], RUNX1 [20], BARX2 [21], Smad4 [22]. These studies are summarized in Table 7.1. Solana et al. [26] were the only group to use UV light instead of formaldehyde for crosslinking *Drosophila* embryos before isolating genomic targets. Some studies varied the conventional cloning after immunoprecipitation. For example, Jishage et al. [25] used the transcriptional activity of the fragments for detection (see Section 7.4.2), and DeBelle et al. [24] used a multiplex PCR step for target identification. The literature summary shows that some confirmed targets failed to contain consensus binding sites [19, 26] (for discussion see Sections 7.2.6 and 7.4.1). Unfortunately, only a few of the predicted consensus sites have been tested by EMSA. The ratio of confirmed targets to total reported clones varied among the studies but nevertheless show that the ChIP cloning strategy was normally limited to the identification of a small number of target genes. Multiple targets are localized (if actual information is available) in intronic regions [21, 23, 26]. Greenbaum et al. [23] were able to confirm immunoprecipitation of the putative promoter region

Tab. 7.1 Summary of reports of successful ChIP cloning for new target identification with subsequent validation.

Reference	*Crosslink*	*TF*	*Species*	*Total clone number reported*	*Number of confirmed targets*	*Localization*	*With consensus site*	*EMSA* [a]	*Reporter gene assay*	*Gene expression monitoring*
19	FA [b]	E2F	human	28	9	3 promoter 6 no information	1 out of 3 analyzed	2 out of 2 analyzed	2 out of 2 analyzed	3 out of 3 analyzed
23	FA	E2A	mouse	13	8	1 intronic sequence 7 no information	8	no	no	1 out of 1 analyzed
24	FA	Egr1	human	1	1	no information	no information	1 out of 1 analyzed	1 out of 1 analyzed	1 out of 1 analyzed
25	FA	EWS/ATF-1	human	62	6 out of 16 clones with consensus site	3 clones in the vicinity or inside of genes 3 clones far away from transcription initiation site	6	1 out of 1 analyzed	6 out of 6 analyzed	6 out of 6 analyzed
26	UV light	engrailed	*Drosophila*	542	no ChIP confirmation, 203 further analyzed	47% intronic 53% intergenic	49 out of 107	4 out of 4 analyzed	1 out of 1 analyzed	12 out of 14 analyzed
20	FA	RUNX1	human	1	1	promoter	1	1 out of 1 analyzed	1 out of 1 analyzed	1 out of 1 analyzed
21	FA	BARX2	human	60	21	25% intronic 35% within 50 kb up or down of annotated genes 30% greater than 50 kb from a gene	13 sites reported	9 out of 13 analyzed	14 out of 19 analyzed	8 out of 11 reduced by RNAi
22	FA	Smad4	mouse	60	1	promoter	yes	no	1 out of 4 analyzed	1 out of 1 analyzed

a) Electrophoretic mobility shift assay.
b) Formaldehyde.

of a newly identified intronic E2A target clone, suggesting multiple binding sites for the factor. Intronic enhancers have become well known in recent years [51] and are located predominantly in intron 1 and intron 2. For example, intron enhancers have been described for three HNF4α targets (aldolase B [52, 53], apolipoprotein B [54], and adenosine deaminase [55]).

Some publications have reported similar or modified approaches to isolating genomic fragments, but those studies did not use follow-up experiments to confirm *in vivo* binding of the factor of interest to the isolated DNA [38, 56–63]. One of these studies used a UV laser instead of formaldehyde for crosslinking [38]. But, due to the lack of *in vivo* confirmation, it is difficult to be sure if any of the clones in these studies corresponded to real *in vivo* targets [18].

7.4 Problems and Potential Strategies

7.4.1 Elimination of Nonspecific DNA and Protein–Protein Crosslinking

As discussed in Section 7.2.5, elimination of nonspecific DNA, by carefully adapting the protocol, greatly improves the yield of real target clones. In summary, the important criteria are monitoring the fragment length, chromatin preclearance with blocked protein A–Sepharose, use of affinity-purified antibodies, stringent conditions during immunoprecipitation and in the wash buffers, and using two sequential immunoprecipitations. Because it is very difficult to completely eliminate nonspecific DNA, confirmation of target sequences in separate ChIP experiments is extremely important [18].

Some reported clones failed to contain consensus binding sites and showed no protein binding under *in vitro* assay conditions [19, 26]. However, they are summarized under confirmed targets because they have been verified in separate immunoprecipitation experiments. During initiation of transcription, a specific TF interacts with several coactivators and basal TFs. Binding of different TFs as part of a multiprotein complex leads to combinatorial control of gene expression. Formaldehyde causes not only protein–DNA but also protein–protein crosslinks [12]. Thus, a 3-dimensional, higher-order structure is crosslinked, and an immunoprecipitated fragment would not necessarily represent a direct DNA partner of a protein. Instead, it could reveal a distant site that was in contact through the multimeric protein interactions of the chromatin structure. The identified site might recruit the analyzed TF through cooperative binding with synergized TFs [64].

7.4.2 Enrichment of Target Promoters and High-throughput Screening

The described ChIP cloning strategy is applicable only to identification of a limited number of target genes, because of the difficulties encountered in the entire procedure. Enrichment of promoter sequences in screening procedures would be preferable. Various attempts have been made with this aim.

Jishage et al. [25] described the DIGR approach (DNA–protein crosslinking, immunopurification, and GFP reporter assay) for identifying EWS/ATF-1 targets. The distinguishing feature of DIGR is the combination of ChIP and GFP reporter gene assays. Immunoprecipitated DNA fragments were subcloned in a GFP reporter vector and cotransfected with the EWS/ATF-1 expression vector. The screening procedure resulted in identification of 62 clones, out of 15 000 from a library, that showed increased green fluorescence intensity and therefore contained potential responsive elements. Sequence analysis revealed that 16 clones contained the consensus binding site; of these, 6 clones were confirmed by separate ChIP experiments. The remaining 46 clones with no potential common sites were not checked further. Isolated fragments were located not only in the promoter region but also far upstream or downstream of the coding region of genes. In contrast to conventional cloning after chromatin immunoprecipitation, the DIGR method uses transcriptional activity as the detection approach. The DIGR method has the potential to isolate any responsive elements functioning at regions other than promoters. However, it is time-consuming and does not necessarily give higher yields of confirmed clones (Table 7.1).

The most promising high-throughput screening method is a microarray-based approach. First, a DNA microarray-based technique that identifies genomic sites bound directly to DNA-binding factors was developed for living yeast cells [40, 65–68]. Genome-wide location analysis, named 'ChIP on a chip', was achieved by combining the ChIP procedure (formaldehyde crosslinking) with DNA microarray technology. Briefly, immunoprecipitated DNA was amplified and labelled with a fluorescent dye, and a sample of control DNA with a different fluorophore. Both pools of labelled DNA were hybridized to a single DNA microarray containing all yeast intergenic sequences. The ability to combine chromatin immunoprecipitation with microarray analysis is a promising means of increasing the number of targets isolated.

However, similar analysis of mammalian cells is more difficult, because of the lack of a comparable genomic microarray representing a major portion of the intergenic regions, due to the vastly greater size of the mammalian genome. Therefore, Ren et al. [69] developed a DNA microarray that contained PCR products spanning the proximal promoters of 1200 human cell cycle–regulated genes and focussed their studies on E2F. Weinmann et al. [18, 70] used a DNA microarray containing human genomic fragments that were isolated on the basis of their high CpG content, because approximately 50% of mammalian gene promoters are associated with CpG islands [71, 72]. They probed a CpG island microarray with immunoprecipitated chromatin and no-antibody–precipitated DNAs labelled with different fluorescence dyes to provide a high-throughput method for identification of E2F *in vivo* target promoters. Recently, CpG island microarrays were also used to identify targets that are bound *in vivo* by Rb [73] and by c-myc [74]. CpG island microarrays are mainly suited to analyzing housekeeping genes, because genes showing tissue-specific expression are usually not associated with CpG islands [72, 75].

Martone et al. [76] used a whole chromosome genomic microarray (human chromosome 22, PCR-products with a mean size of 700 bp) to search for TF target-genes.

They identified unexpected intronic binding of p65/NF-kappaB (1. intron 12%, other introns 28%), whereas 9% binding of transcription factor was detected 1 kb upstream and 18% 5 kb upstream of transcription start site. Consensus and nonconsensus sequence binding sites were found at equal frequency, which points to the possibility of the immunoprecipitation of targets through protein-protein interactions as seen by us in ChIP-cloning experiments. Cawley et al. [77] mapped an unexpectedly large number of in vivo binding sites for SP1, cMyc and p53 using high-density oligonucleotide arrays (25-nucleotide oligomers) within human chromosome 21 and 22. Only 22% of these regions are located at the 5′ terminus of protein-coding genes while 36% lie within or 3′ to well-characterized genes and are significantly correlated with noncoding RNAs with today unknown function, which were detected by RNA transcription analysis using the same chips [77]. Though 'ChIP on a chip experiments' revealed a large number of potential targets, they were only, in part, verified by immunoprecipitation. Martone et al. [76] chose 75 sites out of 209 and confirmed thereof 59 (20% false positive). Odom et al. [78] constructed a DNA microarray containing promoter regions (PCR-products spanning 700 bp upstream and 200 bp downstream of transcription start sites) of 13000 human genes on the basis of NCBI annotation for TF target-gene identification. In the case of HNF4α the number of targeted genes was unexpected high and corresponded to half of the actively transcribed genes, identified by RNA polymerase II immunoprecipitation. A 16% frequency of false positives was reported and only 48 of 1575 potential HNF4α target genes (corresponding to 3%) were verified in separate gene-specific ChIP-experiments. 'ChIP on a chip experiments' will therefore be invaluable, but there is the need for thorough evaluation of findings.

7.5 Challenges for the Future

Future development of mammalian DNA microarrays representing a major portion of intergenic regions would be a great advancement in the genome-wide location analysis of potential targets by 'ChIP on a chip'. Researchers have looked for various types of signals around the transcriptional start site to improve promoter prediction [75]. The RNA polymerase II core promoters can be classified into two main classes, one associated with CpG islands and the other not. The first class corresponds to the so-called housekeeping genes. The second class of promoters, typically corresponding to genes showing tissue-specific expression, constitute a bottleneck in trying to obtain accurate promoter predictions. Hannenhalli et al. [75] explored the possibility of improving promoter prediction by combining several biologically relevant features. However, computational prediction of promoters for genes with no associated CpG islands, by looking only in the immediate neighbourhood of the transcription start site, may not even be possible. This is because the majority of regulatory DNA in vertebrate genomes is found in islands of highly structured chromatin, and it is likely that the genes of the second class may have their 'basal' transcription level controlled by non-core TF binding far from the start site of transcription.

Currently, the best-accepted promoter prediction tool is PromoterInsepctor (based on libraries of IUPAC words extracted from training sequences), presented by Scherf et al. [79], which has achieved ca. 40% sensitivity and specificity on large genomic sequences. Overall, generation of mammalian DNA microarrays that represent a total of promoter regions is not foreseeable today, but development of specific DNA microarrays with preselected targets is suited to carrying out 'ChIP on a chip' experiments, as shown by Ren et al. for E2F [69].

Recently, various computer algorithms have been developed for searching genomic databases for potential TF binding sites. They have been used successfully for the TFs E2F [80], p53 [81–83], HNF1α [84, 85], HNF4α [86], and c-myc [87]. Incorporation of the modular organization of regulatory regions into promoter models is essential for development of an in-silico approach [47, 48]. The most basic form of regulatory modules are composite elements consisting of pairs of functional TF binding sites that act synergistically [43–46]. These were successfully used for database searches that were independent of direct sequence similarity [46]. Computer-predicted binding sites could be confirmed or rejected by subsequent chromatin immunoprecipitation assays for E2F [80], c-myc [87], and p53 [82]. Experimentally verified motifs from ChIP experiments enable improved computer algorithms to be developed [88]. Therefore, linkage of bioinformatics tools for searching potential TF binding sites with ChIP assays for validation will be a promising tool for identification of unknown targets.

Coupling TF overexpression with cDNA microarray analysis is a possible way to gain insight into a network of genes that are regulated by a given factor. But the genes identified in a cDNA microarray are not necessarily direct targets of the TF, because it is possible that the deregulated gene expression is due to indirect effects resulting from changes in signal-transduction cascades. Recently, information resulting from coupling TF overexpression or loss of expression with cDNA microarray analyses was used to identify new targets with conventional ChIP experiments. The ChIP assay was used to confirm or reject selected potential E2F [89], Egr1 [90], and p53 [91] targets.

In the future, identification of genes regulated by specific TFs in the humane genome may be achieved by the integration of human genomic sequence information, genome-wide gene-expression analysis, bioinformatics in-silico approaches considering composite modules, and confirmation of target gene expression. In particular, feedback coupling between computer analyses and ChIP experiments as a tool for validation of bioinformatics-based identification of target genes, with the goal of creating improved training sequences (necessarily with regard to interacting factors), is the most promising approach to enabling analysis of global gene-regulatory networks.

References

1. Tupler R, Perini G, Green MR: Expressing the human genome. *Nature* 2001, 409:832–833.
2. Venter JC, Adams MD, Myers EW, Li PW, Mural RJ, Sutton GG, Smith HO, Yandell M, Evans CA, Holt RA, et al.: The sequence of the human genome. *Science* 2001, 291:1304–1351.
3. Wolberger C: Multiprotein–DNA complexes in transcriptional regulation. *Annu Rev Biophys Biomol. Struct.* 1999, 28:29–56.
4. Reese JC: Basal transcription factors. *Curr Opin Genet Dev* 2003, 13:114–118.
5. Martens JA, Winston F: Recent advances in understanding chromatin remodeling by Swi/Snf complexes. *Curr Opin Genet Dev* 2003, 13:136–142.
6. Grunstein M: Histone acetylation in chromatin structure and transcription. *Nature* 1997, 389:349–352.
7. Duncan SA: Transcriptional regulation of liver development. *Dev Dyn* 2000, 219:131–142.
8. Schrem H, Klempnauer J, Borlak J: Liver-enriched transcription factors in liver function and development. I. The hepatocyte nuclear factor network and liver-specific gene expression. *Pharmacol Rev* 2002, 54:129–158.
9. Schrem H, Klempnauer J, Borlak J: Liver-enriched transcription factors in liver function and development. Part II: the C/EBPs and D site-binding protein in cell cycle control, carcinogenesis, circadian gene regulation, liver regeneration, apoptosis, and liver-specific gene regulation. *Pharmacol Rev* 2004, 56: 291–330.
10. Orlando V, Strutt H, Paro R: Analysis of chromatin structure by *in vivo* formaldehyde cross-linking. *Methods* 1997, 11:205–214.
11. Hecht A, Grunstein M: Mapping DNA interaction sites of chromosomal proteins using immunoprecipitation and polymerase chain reaction. *Methods Enzymol* 1999, 304:399–414.
12. Orlando V: Mapping chromosomal proteins *in vivo* by formaldehyde-crosslinked chromatin immunoprecipitation. *Trends Biochem Sci* 2000, 25:99–104.
13. Strutt H, Paro R: The polycomb group protein complex of *Drosophila melanogaster* has different compositions at different target genes. *Mol Cell Biol* 1997, 17:6773–6783.
14. Boyd KE, Wells J, Gutman J, Bartley SM, Farnham PJ: c-Myc target gene specificity is determined by a post-DNA binding mechanism. *Proc Natl Acad Sci USA* 1998, 95:13887–13892.
15. Hake SB, Masternak K, Kammerbauer C, Janzen C, Reith W, Steimle V: CIITA leucine-rich repeats control nuclear localization, *in vivo* recruitment to the major histocompatibility complex (MHC) class II enhanceosome, and MHC class II gene transactivation. *Mol Cell Biol* 2000, 20:7716–7725.
16. Schepers A, Ritzi M, Bousset K, Kremmer E, Yates JL, Harwood J, Diffley JF, Hammerschmidt W: Human origin recognition complex binds to the region of the latent origin of DNA replication of Epstein–Barr virus. *EMBO J* 2001, 20:4588–4602.
17. Sasaki Y, Ishida S, Morimoto I, Yamashita T, Kojima T, Kihara C, Tanaka T, Imai K, Nakamura Y, Tokino T: The p53 family member genes are involved in the Notch signal pathway. *J Biol Chem* 2002, 277:719–724.
18. Weinmann AS, Farnham PJ: Identification of unknown target genes of human transcription factors using chromatin immunoprecipitation. *Methods* 2002, 26:37–47.
19. Weinmann AS, Bartley SM, Zhang T, Zhang MQ, Farnham PJ: Use of chromatin immunoprecipitation to clone novel E2F target promoters. *Mol Cell Biol* 2001, 21:6820–6832.
20. Hug BA, Ahmed N, Robbins JA, Lazar MA: A chromatin immunoprecipitation screen reveals protein kinase Cbeta as a direct RUNX1 target gene. *J Biol Chem* 2004, 279: 825–830.
21. Stevens TA, Iacovoni JS, Edelman DB, Meech R: Identification of novel binding elements and gene targets for the homeodomain protein BARX2. *J Biol Chem* 2004, 279: 14520–14530.

22. SEKI K, HATA A: Indian hedgehog gene is a target of the bone morphogenetic protein signaling pathway. *J Biol Chem* 2004, 279: 18544–18549.

23. GREENBAUM S, ZHUANG Y: Identification of E2A target genes in B lymphocyte development by using a gene tagging-based chromatin immunoprecipitation system. *Proc Natl Acad Sci USA* 2002, 99:15030–15035.

24. DEBELLE I, WU JX, SPERANDIO S, MERCOLA D, ADAMSON ED: In vivo cloning and characterization of a new growth suppressor protein TOE1 as a direct target gene of Egr1. *J Biol Chem* 2003, 278:14306–14312.

25. JISHAGE M, FUJINO T, YAMAZAKI Y, KURODA H, NAKAMURA T: Identification of target genes for EWS/ATF-1 chimeric transcription factor. *Oncogene* 2003, 22:41–49.

26. SOLANO PJ, MUGAT B, MARTIN D, GIRARD F, HUIBANT JM, FERRAZ C, JACQ B, DEMAILLE J, MASCHAT F: Genome-wide identification of *in vivo Drosophila* Engrailed-binding DNA fragments and related target genes. *Development* 2003, 130:1243–1254.

27. MCGHEE JD, VON HIPPEL PH: Formaldehyde as a probe of DNA structure. I. Reaction with exocyclic amino groups of DNA bases. *Biochemistry* 1975, 14: 1281–1296.

28. MCGHEE JD, VON HIPPEL PH: Formaldehyde as a probe of DNA structure. II. Reaction with endocyclic imino groups of DNA bases. *Biochemistry* 1975, 14: 1297–1303.

29. JACKSON V: Studies on histone organization in the nucleosome using formaldehyde as a reversible cross-linking agent. *Cell* 1978, 15:945–954.

30. SOLOMON MJ, VARSHAVSKY A: Formaldehyde-mediated DNA–protein crosslinking: a probe for *in vivo* chromatin structures. *Proc Natl Acad Sci USA* 1985, 82:6470–6474.

21. ANGELOV D, KHOCHBIN S, DIMITROV S: UV laser footprinting and protein–DNA crosslinking: application to chromatin. *Methods Mol Biol* 1999, 119:481–495.

32. DIMITROV SI, MOSS T: UV laser-induced protein–DNA crosslinking. *Methods Mol Biol* 2001, 148:395–402.

33. RUSSMANN C, TRUSS M, FIX A, NAUMER C, HERRMANN T, SCHMITT J, STOLLHOF J, BEIGANG R, BEATO M: Crosslinking of progesterone receptor to DNA using tuneable nanosecond, picosecond and femtosecond UV laser pulses. *Nucleic Acids Res* 1997, 25:2478–2484.

34. LEJNINE S, DURFEE G, MURNANE M, KAPTEYN HC, MAKAROV VL, LANGMORE JP: Crosslinking of proteins to DNA in human nuclei using a 60 femtosecond 266 nm laser. *Nucleic Acids Res* 1999, 27:3676–3684.

35. HOCKENSMITH JW, KUBASEK WL, VORACHEK WR, VON HIPPEL PH: Laser cross-linking of nucleic acids to proteins: methodology and first applications to the phage T4 DNA replication system. *J Biol Chem* 1986, 261:3512–3518.

36. RUSSMANN C, STOLLHOF J, WEISS C, BEIGANG R, BEATO M: Two wavelength femtosecond laser induced DNA–protein crosslinking. *Nucleic Acids Res* 1998, 26:3967–3970.

37. CARR A, BIGGIN MD: A comparison of *in vivo* and *in vitro* DNA-binding specificities suggests a new model for homeoprotein DNA binding in *Drosophila* embryos. *EMBO J* 1999, 18:1598–1608.

38. SANTORO R, WOLFL S, SALUZ HP: UV-laser induced protein/DNA crosslinking reveals sequence variations of DNA elements bound by c-Jun *in vivo*. *Biochem Biophys Res Commun* 1999, 256:68–74.

39. TOTH J, BIGGIN MD: The specificity of protein–DNA crosslinking by formaldehyde *in vitro* and in *Drosophila* embryos. *Nucleic Acids Res* 2000, 28:e4.

40. REN B, ROBERT F, WYRICK JJ, APARICIO O, JENNINGS EG, SIMON I, ZEITLINGER J, SCHREIBER J, HANNETT N, KANIN E, VOLKERT TL, WILSON CJ, BELL SP, YOUNG RA: Genome-wide location and function of DNA binding proteins. *Science* 2000, 290:2306–2309.

41. NIEHOF M, ZEMLIN, R, BORLAK J: *In vivo* ChlP-cloning of novel HNF4alpha gene targets. *In preparation.*

42. NIEHOF M, BORLAK, J: HNF4alpha targets novel kinases in diabetic rat kidney and brain. *Submitted 2004.*

43. KEL OV, ROMASCHENKO AG, KEL AE, WINGENDER E, KOLCHANOV NA: A compilation of composite regulatory elements affecting gene transcription in vertebrates. *Nucleic Acids Res* 1995, 23: 4097–4103.

44. Lavorgna G, Boncinelli E, Wagner A, Werner T: Detection of potential target genes in silico? *Trends Genet* 1998, 14:375–376.

45. Kel A, Kel-Margoulis O, Babenko V, Wingender E: Recognition of NFATp/AP-1 composite elements within genes induced upon the activation of immune cells. *J Mol Biol* 1999, 288:353–376.

46. Klingenhoff A, Frech K, Quandt K, Werner T: Functional promoter modules can be detected by formal models independent of overall nucleotide sequence similarity. *Bioinformatics.* 1999, 15: 180–186.

47. Werner T: Models for prediction and recognition of eukaryotic promoters. *Mamm Genome* 1999, 10:168–175.

48. Gailus-Durner V, Scherf M, Werner T: Experimental data of a single promoter can be used for in silico detection of genes with related regulation in the absence of sequence similarity. *Mamm Genome* 2001, 12:67–72.

49. Halle JP, Haus-Seuffert P, Woltering C, Stelzer G, Meisterernst M: A conserved tissue-specific structure at a human T-cell receptor beta-chain core promoter. *Mol Cell Biol* 1997, 17: 4220–4229.

50. Hines WA, Thorburn J, Thorburn A: A low-affinity serum response element allows other transcription factors to activate inducible gene expression in cardiac myocytes. *Mol Cell Biol* 1999, 19: 1841–1852.

51. Le Hir H, Nott A, Moore MJ: How introns influence and enhance eukaryotic gene expression. *Trends Biochem Sci* 2003, 28:215–220.

52. Gregori C, Porteu A, Lopez S, Kahn A, Pichard AL: Characterization of the aldolase B intronic enhancer. *J Biol Chem* 1998, 273:25237–25243.

53. Gregori C, Porteu A, Mitchell C, Kahn A, Pichard AL: In vivo functional characterization of the aldolase B gene enhancer. *J Biol Chem* 2002, 277:28618–28623.

54. Antes TJ, Goodart SA, Chen W, Levy-Wilson B: Human apolipoprotein B gene intestinal control region. *Biochemistry* 2001, 40:6720–6730.

55. Dusing MR, Brickner AG, Lowe SY, Cohen MB, Wiginton DA: A duodenum-specific enhancer regulates expression along three axes in the small intestine. *Am J Physiol Gastrointest Liver Physiol* 2000, 279:G1080–G1093.

56. Tomotsune D, Shoji H, Wakamatsu Y, Kondoh H, Takahashi N: A mouse homologue of the *Drosophila* tumour-suppressor gene l(2)gl controlled by Hox-C8 *in vivo*. *Nature* 1993, 365:69–72.

57. Strutt DI, White RA: Characterisation of T48, a target of homeotic gene regulation in *Drosophila* embryogenesis. *Mech Dev* 1994, 46:27–39.

58. Grandori C, Mac J, Siebelt F, Ayer DE, Eisenman RN: Myc–Max heterodimers activate a DEAD box gene and interact with multiple E box-related sites *in vivo*. *EMBO J* 1996, 15:4344–4357.

59. Phelps DE, Dressler GR: Identification of novel Pax-2 binding sites by chromatin precipitation. *J Biol Chem* 1996, 271:7978–7985.

60. Robinson L, Panayiotakis A, Papas TS, Kola I, Seth A: ETS target genes: identification of egr1 as a target by RNA differential display and whole genome PCR techniques. *Proc Natl Acad Sci USA* 1997, 94:7170–7175.

61. Cohen-Kaminsky S, Maouche-Chretien L, Vitelli L, Vinit MA, Blanchard I, Yamamoto M, Peschle C, Romeo PH: Chromatin immunoselection defines a TAL-1 target gene. *EMBO J* 1998, 17:5151–5160.

62. Kim JH, Hui P, Yue D, Aycock J, Leclerc C, Bjoring AR, Perkins AS: Identification of candidate target genes for EVI-1, a zinc finger oncoprotein, using a novel selection strategy. *Oncogene* 1998, 17:1527–1538.

63. DeBelle I, Mercola D, Adamson ED: Method for cloning *in vivo* targets of the Egr-1 transcription factor. *BioTechniques* 2000, 29:162–169.

64. Wells J, Farnham PJ: Characterizing transcription factor binding sites using formaldehyde crosslinking and immunoprecipitation. *Methods* 2002, 26:48–56.

65. Iyer VR, Horak CE, Scafe CS, Botstein D, Snyder M, Brown PO:

Genomic binding sites of the yeast cell-cycle transcription factors SBF and MBF. *Nature* 2001, 409:533–538.
66. Lieb JD, Liu X, Botstein D, Brown PO: Promoter-specific binding of Rap1 revealed by genome-wide maps of protein-DNA association. *Nat Genet* 2001, 28: 327–334.
67. Simon I, Barnett J, Hannett N, Harbison CT, Rinaldi NJ, Volkert TL, Wyrick JJ, Zeitlinger J, Gifford DK, Jaakkola TS, Young RA: Serial regulation of transcriptional regulators in the yeast cell cycle. *Cell* 2001, 106:697–708.
68. Biggin MD: To bind or not to bind. *Nat Genet* 2001, 28:303–304.
69. Ren B, Cam H, Takahashi Y, Volkert T, Terragni J, Young RA, Dynlacht BD: E2F integrates cell cycle progression with DNA repair, replication, and G(2)/M checkpoints. *Genes Dev* 2002, 16: 245–256.
70. Weinmann AS, Yan PS, Oberley MJ, Huang TH, Farnham PJ: Isolating human transcription factor targets by coupling chromatin immunoprecipitation and CpG island microarray analysis. *Genes Dev* 2002, 16:235–244.
71. Antequera F, Bird A: Number of CpG islands and genes in human and mouse. *Proc Natl Acad Sci USA* 1993, 90: 11995–11999.
72. Ioshikhes IP, Zhang MQ: Large-scale human promoter mapping using CpG islands. *Nat Genet* 2000, 26:61–63.
73. Wells J, Yan PS, Cechvala M, Huang T, Farnham PJ: Identification of novel pRb binding sites using CpG microarrays suggests that E2F recruits pRb to specific genomic sites during S phase. *Oncogene* 2003, 22:1445–1460.
74. Mao DY, Watson JD, Yan PS, Barsyte-Lovejoy D, Khosravi F, Wong WW, Farnham PJ, Huang TH, Penn LZ: Analysis of Myc bound loci identified by CpG island arrays shows that Max Is essential for Myc-dependent repression. *Curr Biol* 2003, 13:882–886.
75. Hannenhalli S, Levy S: Promoter prediction in the human genome. *Bioinformatics* 2001, 17 Suppl 1:S90–S96.
76. Martone R, Euskirchen G, Bertone P, Hartman S, Royce TE, Luscombe NM, Rinn JL, Nelson FK, Miller P, Gerstein M, Weissman S, Snyder M: Distribution of NF-{kappa}B-binding sites across human chromosome 22. *PNAS* 2003, 100: 12247–12252.
77. Cawley S, Bekiranov S, Ng HH, Kapranov P, Sekinger EA, Kampa D, Piccolboni A, Sementchenko V, Cheng J, Williams AJ, Wheeler R, Wong B, Drenkow J, Yamanaka M, Patel S, Brubaker S, Tammana H, Helt G, Struhl K, Gingeras TR: Unbiased mapping of transcription factor binding sites along human chromosomes 21 and 22 points to widespread regulation of noncoding RNAs. *Cell* 2004, 116: 499–509.
78. Odom DT, Zizlsperger N, Gordon DB, Bell GW, Rinaldi NJ, Murray HL, Volkert TL, Schreiber J, Rolfe PA, Gifford DK, Fraenkel E, Bell GI, Young RA: Control of Pancreas and Liver Gene Expression by HNF Transcription Factors. *Science* 2004, 303: 1378–1381.
79. Scherf M, Klingenhoff A, Werner T: Highly specific localization of promoter regions in large genomic sequences by PromoterInspector: a novel context analysis approach. *J Mol Biol* 2000, 297: 599–606.
80. Kel AE, Kel-Margoulis OV, Farnham PJ, Bartley SM, Wingender E, Zhang MQ: Computer-assisted identification of cell cycle-related genes: new targets for E2F transcription factors. *J Mol Biol* 2001, 309:99–120.
81. Kannan K, Amariglio N, Rechavi G, Jakob-Hirsch J, Kela I, Kaminski N, Getz G, Domany E, Givol D: DNA microarrays identification of primary and secondary target genes regulated by p53. *Oncogene* 2001, 20:2225–2234.
82. Wang L, Wu Q, Qiu P, Mirza A, McGuirk M, Kirschmeier P, Greene JR, Wang Y, Pickett CB, Liu S: Analyses of p53 target genes in the human genome by bioinformatic and microarray approaches. *J Biol Chem* 2001, 276:43604–43610.
83. Hoh J, Jin S, Parrado T, Edington J, Levine AJ, Ott J: The p53MH algorithm and its application in detecting p53-responsive genes. *Proc Natl Acad Sci USA* 2002, 99:8467–8472.

84. Lockwood CR, Frayling TM: Combining genome and mouse knockout expression data to highlight binding sites for the transcription factor HNF1alpha. *In Silico Biol* 2002, 3: 6.

85. Lockwood CR, Bingham C, Frayling TM: In silico searching of human and mouse genome data identifies known and unknown HNF1 binding sites upstream of beta-cell genes. *Mol Genet Metab* 2003, 78: 145–151.

86. Ellrott K, Yang C, Sladek FM, Jiang T: Identifying transcription factor binding sites through Markov chain optimization. *Bioinformatics* 2002, 18 Suppl 2: S100–S109.

87. Fernandez PC, Frank SR, Wang L, Schroeder M, Liu S, Greene J, Cocito A, Amati B: Genomic targets of the human c-Myc protein. *Genes Dev* 2003, 17: 1115–1129.

88. Liu XS, Brutlag DL, Liu JS: An algorithm for finding protein–DNA binding sites with applications to chromatin-immunoprecipitation microarray experiments. *Nat Biotechnol* 2002, 20: 835–839.

89. Wells J, Graveel CR, Bartley SM, Madore SJ, Farnham PJ: The identification of E2F1-specific target genes. *Proc Natl Acad Sci USA* 2002, 99: 3890–3895.

90. Virolle T, Krones-Herzig A, Baron V, De Gregorio G, Adamson ED, Mercola D: Egr1 promotes growth and survival of prostate cancer cells. Identification of novel Egr1 target genes. *J Biol Chem* 2003, 278: 11802–11810.

91. Mirza A, Wu Q, Wang L, McClanahan T, Bishop WR, Gheyas F, Ding W, Hutchins B, Hockenberry T, Kirschmeier P, Greene JR, Liu S: Global transcriptional program of p53 target genes during the process of apoptosis and cell cycle progression. *Oncogene* 2003, 22: 3645–3654.

8
NMR Spectroscopy as a Versatile Analytical Platform for Toxicology Research

Olivia Corcoran

8.1
A Role for NMR in Toxicogenomics

In this post-genomic age, a prerequisite for establishing a predictive model for human toxicity remains a profound knowledge of the underlying mechanisms of molecular toxicity [1–3]. Over the next decade, the powerful and rapidly evolving technologies of toxicogenomics may greatly illuminate the molecular basis of toxicology towards this goal. However, a key challenge is to chronicle dose-related toxicity across complex and often interdependent levels of biomolecular organization with respect to mechanistic events that occur over time [2, 3]. Likewise, a central question of functional genomics is how to simply relate gene expression to pathophysiological endpoints in health and disease so that human toxicity is predictable [4]. A further problem is how to quantify the inherent genetic and metabolic variability in biological systems amongst individuals and across species. Solving these fundamental problems typically requires multivariate datasets and chemometrics to extract predictive value. It has been suggested that metabolic profiling by nuclear magnetic resonance spectroscopy (NMR) aims to measure the real outcome of potential changes suggested by genomics and proteomics [5]. Thus, it is likely that the future of toxicogenomics will rely on the integration of the genomic, proteomic, and metabolic sciences.

Compared to microarrays, differential display technology, and 2-dimensional (2D) gel electrophoresis–mass spectrometry [4], NMR has been established over the last two decades as a valuable tool for researching the molecular basis of toxicity. The exploratory nature of the technique has led to success in relating certain pathologies to underlying mechanisms of disease, including inborn errors of metabolism and coronary heart disease [6–8]. The increasing use of NMR in clinical settings is thus envisaged in the coming years. With this evolution comes the possibility of investigating toxicological pathologies directly in a hospital environment. Wide-ranging applications of NMR in toxicology already include the clinical diagnostics described above, evaluating suitable animal models for biomarkers of toxicity [9,10], detecting silent phenotypes in genetic models [11, 12], and assessing environmental toxicity [13–15].

Handbook of Toxicogenomics: Strategies and Applications. Edited by Jürgen Borlak

ISBN: 3-527-30342-1

This chapter aims to review the key role of NMR as a mature analytical platform used to chronicle the temporal and spatial alterations in the basal biochemical pathways as a result of molecular toxicity. The newly emerging field of metabonomics [2, 3], is defined as the measuring and mapping of the low molecular weight metabolites of an entire biological system, typically by NMR and pattern recognition. Here the focus is on the profiling and biomarker applications for which NMR has already become routine. The influence of NMR on the development and direction of toxicogenomics is considered afterwards.

8.2
Evolution of NMR Technologies in Toxicology Research

Before the 1970s NMR was predominantly used by chemists for determining the structures and purity of synthetic compounds. The application to biological fluids was discounted by many because proton NMR spectra of urine and plasma appeared too complicated to interpret. Technical obstacles also included the lack of efficient solvent suppression methods, analogue electronics, and poor sensitivity. As a rule, urine and plasma had to be freeze-dried and reconstituted in deuterated water to provide enough sensitivity for the available 60–200-MHz NMR instruments. The first paper to demonstrate NMR spectra of endogenous molecules in erythrocytes appeared in 1977, showing the conversion of glucose to lactate [16]. Tests for cancer based on lactate as a biomarker in NMR spectra of plasma appeared soon after and generated much excitement. However, the claims of sensitivity and selectivity were never proved, and an interesting discussion on this topic is provided in the literature [17].

Publications relating urinary composition to pathological states followed in the early 1980s. One of the first studies reported differences after fasting between normal and diabetic subjects [18]. Around the same time, one of the first examples of NMR applied to the study of toxicity reported the investigation of acetaminophen and metabolites on a 300-MHz system [19]. As the major urinary and plasma components were gradually assigned via systematic studies using standards and 2D spectra, the key advantages of NMR as an analytical platform for toxicology became apparent (Table 8.1).

In these early studies samples were analyzed by conventional NMR (using glass NMR tubes). Throughout the 1990s the development of flow-injection NMR (tubeless NMR), combined with 96-well plate formats, greatly accelerated the screening of biofluids and tissue extracts. Likewise, the advent of commercial probes for magic angle spinning NMR (MAS–NMR) enabled profiling of intact kidney, liver, and brain tissues. High-performance liquid chromatography coupled to NMR and mass spectrometry (LC–NMR–MS) quickly became routine in many pharmaceutical laboratories worldwide to identify biomarkers or potentially toxic metabolites within complex biofluids.

Tab. 8.1 Unique features of NMR as a research tool in toxicology.

1. Uniquely rich structural content includes chemical shifts, multiplicity, integrals, and intramolecular relationships.
2. Because NMR is a non-destructive detector, samples can be recovered for subsequent analysis by destructive techniques such as MS.
3. NMR is nonselective for most proton-containing analytes, which means that unexpected or novel biomarkers can often be detected.
4. Endogenous and xenobiotic metabolites can be monitored simultaneously in complex biofluids, which avoids the need to develop batches of assays.
5. Qualitative and, often, quantitative data are acquired.
6. A wide range of dynamic processes can be measured, including molecular motions in solution, chemical exchange, and ligand binding.
7. Minimal sample preparation, with requirements for as little as 5 μL, are needed when the latest microcoil probes are used.
8. High automation and relatively high-throughput are achieved, thanks to recent advances in NMR sensitivity.

8.2.1 Conventional NMR Spectroscopy

Solution state NMR spectroscopy is the study of molecules by recording the interaction of radiofrequency electromagnetic radiation with the nuclei of molecules in solution when placed in a strong magnetic field. The circulation of electrons around nuclei in different electronic environments creates local magnetic environments. These local magnetic fields give rise to characteristic chemical shifts suitable for functional group identification. Moreover, the presence of coupling between pairs of nuclei extending over 1–3 bonds establishes the connectivity between atoms and provides a powerful tool for structural elucidation including stereochemical information. However, the quantum basis of NMR, first described in 1946 by Bloch and Purcell (awarded a Nobel prize in 1952), is beyond the scope of this review. The interested reader is referred to several excellent textbooks on the principles of NMR [20, 21]. Here, the pivotal features that pertain to toxicology are presented in Table 8.1. Some milestones in NMR and the most important experiments routinely used for the assignment of metabolites in biofluid spectra are outlined in Table 8.2.

In brief, the goal is to elucidate the molecular structure by interpreting the relationships of NMR-active nuclei, typically protons (^{1}H) or carbon (^{13}C). Compared to protons, the relative sensitivity of carbon is only 0.16%, which imposes time restrictions on NMR experiments to determine carbon data. For drug discovery programmes where fluorine is present in the drug, the fluorine nucleus (with a high relative sensitivity of 83% relative to the proton) provides exquisite selectivity for drug-related material in urine and plasma, due to the lack of endogenous fluorine present in mammalian biofluids. To measure an NMR spectrum the biofluid (commonly

Tab. 8.2 Some significant dates in the evolution of NMR and toxicology.

Date	*Associated development*
1946	The detection of proton NMR signals is reported independently by Bloch in California and Purcell at Harvard.
1952	Nobel Prize for Physics is jointly awarded to Bloch and Purcell.
Mid 1950s	^{13}C NMR signals are first observed.
1950s–1970s	NMR is mostly the domain of organic synthetic chemists and NMR physicists.
1970s	Fourier transform (greater sensitivity) and 2D NMR (higher resolution) are introduced.
1977	Conversion of glucose to lactate is observed in erythrocytes by Brown et al.
1984	Nicholson and coworkers report urinalysis of normal and fasting diabetics by proton NMR and continue to develop this field over the next 20 years.
1985	Bales et al. report analysis of acetyl aminophen metabolites from urine, and the first applications of NMR in toxicology start to appear in the literature.
Late 1980s	First reports of LC–NMR although, due to technical limitations, the technique does not become routine until the mid 1990s.
1991	Nobel Prize for Chemistry to Ernst for pioneering work in 2D NMR.
1994	HRMAS is introduced for the analysis of tissues. Anthony et al. report NMR pattern-recognition techniques that provide new insights into predictive models of toxicity.
1997	Spraul and coworkers develop flow-injection NMR, which greatly facilitates screening of biofluids.
1999	In the post-genomic age, Nicholson, Lindon, and Holmes propose metabonomics.
2002	The first cryoflow probe is announced and applied to the analysis of APAP metabolites in urine (the gold standard for testing new hyphenated NMR methods). Online solid-phase extraction provides for greatly enhanced sensitivity.

100–500 μL of sample) is placed in a 5-mm glass tube and inserted into the bore of a superconducting magnet at field strengths ranging from 9.4 to 18.7 T. These are commonly referred to as 400–800-MHz NMR systems on the basis of the proton resonance frequency. The relaxation of nuclei following a train of RF pulses is then measured and translated into chemical shifts, coupling constants, and integration data. The resulting signals are presented typically as a 1-dimensional (1D) proton NMR spectrum (Figure 8.1). The term 1D refers to one dimension of *frequency*, as the *y* axis is the signal intensity. The spectrum is representative of a urine sample from a healthy volunteer; the most common urinary and plasma metabolites are catalogued elsewhere [17, 22]. The presence of a metabolite tends to be confirmed by spiking available standards into the biofluid sample. Thus, the main signals are often readily assigned. However, overlapping signals and multiplicity patterns tend to complicate assignments in 1D spectra. When abnormal and disease states differ

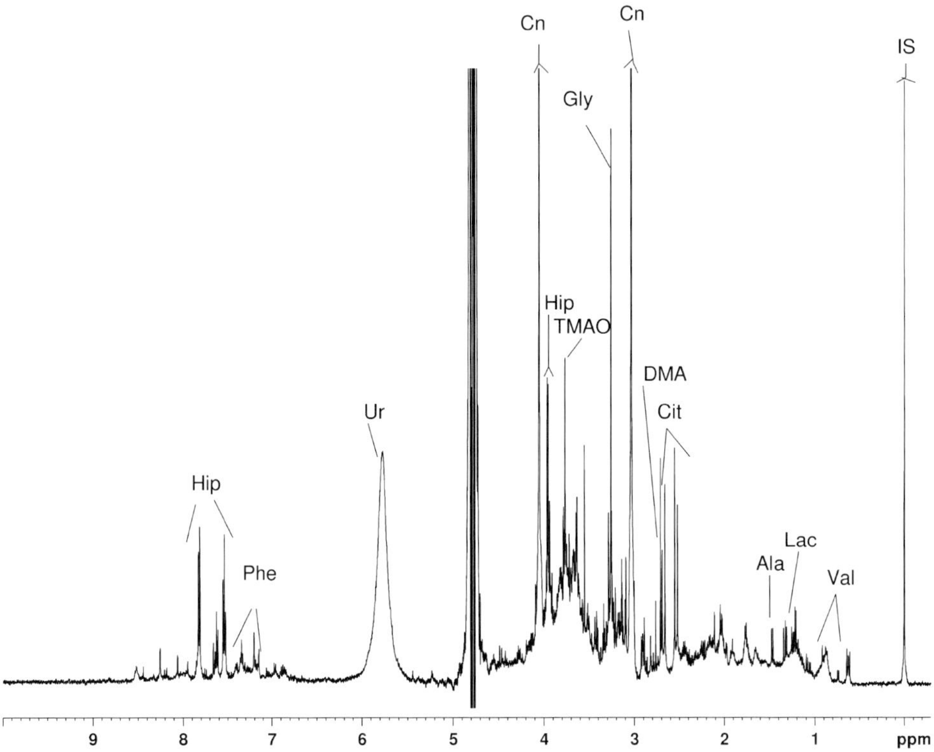

Fig. 8.1 A representative 500-MHz ^{1}H NMR spectrum of normal human urine, showing some assigned resonances.
Abbreviations: Ala, alanine; Cit, citrate; Cn, creatinine; DMA, dimethylamine; Gly, glycine; Hip, hippurate; IS, internal standard (TSP); Lac, lactate; Phe, phenylalanine; TMAO, trimethylamine-*N*-oxide; Ur, urea; Val, valine.

in metabolite composition, spiking of standards may aid assignment. However, it is often necessary to identify metabolites not encountered previously. In these instances 2D NMR experiments may enable deconvolution of latent information.

Throughout the 1960s and 1970s the introduction of Fourier transform to NMR and higher-dimensional NMR spectroscopy provided further incentives to use the technique for complex mixture analysis. The second Nobel Prize associated with the field of NMR was awarded to Richard Ernst in 1991 for his development of 2D NMR. The term refers to *two dimensions of frequency*, with the intensity of the NMR signals as the third dimension. Higher dimensionality can often simplify spectra and aid signal assignment. However, even with higher dimensionality, when signal overlap remains or concentrations of metabolites are below the detection limit (depending on the strength of magnet used, but at 800 MHz detectable concentrations tend to be >100 nM), the information in 2D NMR is often insufficient. Spectral editing can be used to simplify spectra; this comprises methods based on spin-echo, quantum coherence filters, and molecular differences in relaxation times and diffusion rates [17]. However, when 2D and spectral-edited experiments fail to solve the structure of an analyte present in a complex mixture, a sample purification step is often required. This typically includes solvent extraction, solid-phase chromatographic extraction (SPE), or freeze-drying. Alternatively, a chromatographic step followed by off-line NMR is commonly used.

8.2.2
Flow NMR Methods

The term flow NMR spectroscopy encompasses any platform that transfers samples or analytes from an autosampler or HPLC system to the NMR magnet using polyether ether ketone (PEEK) capillaries of 1–1.5 m length and internal diameter 0.1–0.25 mm. The term currently includes flow injection (FI–NMR) and direct injection (DI–NMR) for screening whole samples. It also covers the chromatography-based LC–NMR–MS for identifying analytes purified from a complex mixture.

8.2.2.1 Hyphenated LC–NMR–MS

As an alternative to off-line NMR after fractionating peaks from a HPLC chromatogram, so-called hyphenated NMR techniques have been commercially available from the early 1990s. Following the successful coupling of LC with MS, the direct coupling of LC to NMR and MS (LC–NMR–MS) permits more efficient identification of chromatographic peaks from complex mixtures. A 95%/5% post-column split to the NMR and MS instruments allows parallel measurement of NMR and MS data. The working modes include onflow, stop-flow, and loop-storage modes. Onflow mode involves acquisition of NMR spectra on the chromatographic mobile phase in real time and is thus limited by sensitivity. In stop-flow mode the flow is halted as soon as the LC peak is in the NMR probe. Thus, it is possible to accumulate NMR spectra over longer time periods to achieve greater NMR signal intensities, as shown in Figure 8.2. Loop-storage mode detects LC peaks by UV or MS for storage in online loops for NMR analysis later.

Full structural elucidation of novel drug metabolites is often possible using an ensemble of 1D ^{1}H NMR and MS^n data, especially when neither NMR nor MS alone can provide the unequivocal structure. This can occur due to NMR-silent functional moieties including heteroatoms, phenolic, nitro, amino, *N*-oxide, and sulphate groups. It can also occur due to the ambiguity of the position of a functional group on, for example, an aromatic ring, which cannot be solved by MS. The initial obstacles to the development of these hyphenated techniques were a lack of suitable interfaces, inefficient solvent suppression techniques, and lower magnetic field strengths, but these problems have since been solved. The evolution of LC–NMR and LC–NMR–MS has been reviewed [23, 24].

8.2.2.2 Flow–injection NMR

Following the successful development of LC–NMR–MS, the concept of flow-injection or so-called tubeless NMR was investigated by removing the HPLC column from the system [25]. Intact biofluid samples are transferred from an autosampler using

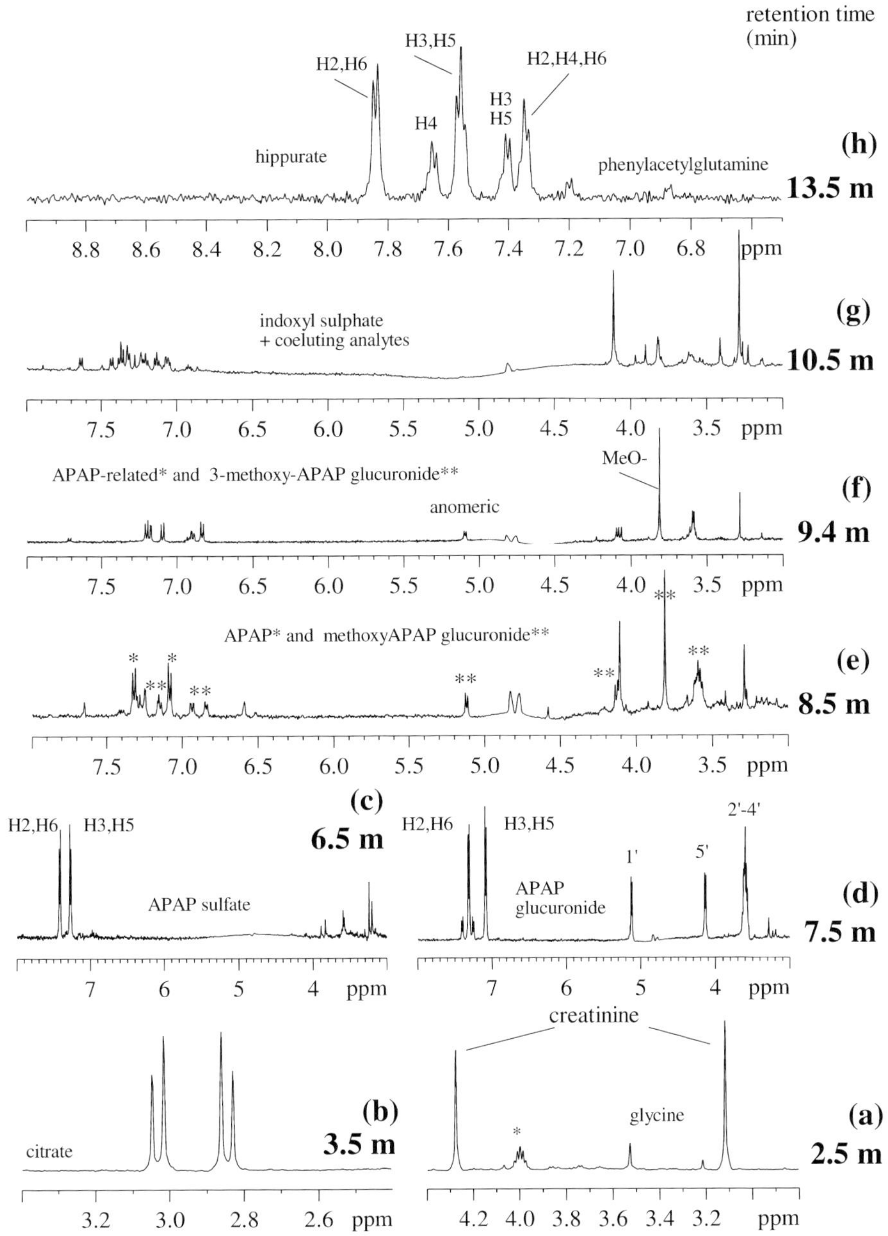

Fig. 8.2 500-MHz ^{1}H NMR spectra of acetaminophen (APAP) metabolites and endogenous urinary components acquired from LC–NMR–MS experiments. A cryoflow probe was used for enhanced sensitivity, and 100 μL of whole untreated urine was injected directly onto the LC column. (a, b, h) Data extracted from an onflow experiment, 16 accumulated scans. Stop-flow spectra: (c, d) 16 scans; (e) 128 scans; (f, g) 256 scans. (Reproduced with permission from reference [49], *Anal. Chem.* **2003**, *75*, 1536–1541. Copyright 2003 American Chemical Society).

96- or 384-well plates directly to the NMR magnet via a capillary. Important benefits of flow NMR are that fragile, expensive glass NMR tubes are not required, and the system is optimized for a minimum turnaround time to transfer, flush, and recover samples if necessary. Other aspects of conventional spectrometer operation, such as optimizing magnetic homogeneity for each sample, are also minimized due to the flow probe design. These combined advantages lead to typical turnaround times of less than a minute per 500 μL of urine sample on an optimized system at 600 MHz ^{1}H NMR observation frequency.

Flow-injection NMR has accelerated the screening of biofluid samples from vast numbers of animals needed to establish useful predictive models of toxicity. Inherent variability in dose–response and time-related urinary profiles exists even in a rodent population bred under strictly controlled conditions for research purposes. This variability arises from genetics, nutritional status, hormonal and diurnal variations, and sex differences [2, 3]. Unfortunately, in practice hundreds of animals may be required for statistical purposes to validate a model of toxicity. The implications of genetic variability are discussed in Chapter 21 of this volume.

8.2.3
HRMAS NMR of Tissues

A relative newcomer to the field of NMR in toxicology is high-resolution magic angle spinning (HRMAS) NMR spectroscopy. This provides spectra for intact semisolid tissues, which are of comparable resolution to conventional NMR spectra of tissue extracts. Tissue samples are spun in a rotor at speeds of typically 4–8 KHz at the magic angle of 54.7° so that dipolar coupling, bulk susceptibility, and chemical shift anisotropy effects are averaged to zero. This results in sharp spectral resonances, particularly for tissue samples that are heterogeneous in their bulk magnetic properties [26, 27]. The lower spin speeds do not disrupt tissue structure, and low-temperature experiments permit acquisition times of several hours before the tissue structure degrades. Compared with tissue extracts, which may require >0.25 g tissue, as little as 5 mg of sample tissue is needed for HRMAS – the technique is therefore appropriate for biopsy samples. HRMAS has been applied to kidney [14], liver [27], testes [13], and prostate tissue [28].

8.3
Metabolite Profiling by NMR

Identification of novel drug metabolites from complex mixtures has been a serious challenge for drug discovery scientists. In practice, metabolic profiling has two main objectives. The primary goal is profiling biofluids, tissues, and extracts thereof by conventional, flow, and HRMAS NMR to build predictive models of normal and abnormal (or toxicological) status. The secondary goal concerns the identification of drug metabolites and so-called biomarkers of underlying toxicity, which involves 2D NMR and, increasingly, LC–NMR–MS. Identifying the chemical structure of metabolites is especially important when studying the molecular basis of novel toxicities. This section aims to give the reader an appreciation of the role of these original NMR applications in clinical diagnosis, inborn errors of metabolism, and toxicology which preceded metabonomics as applied to the prediction of human toxicity.

The earliest NMR research relating urinary composition to physiological states reported differences between fasting normal and diabetic subjects [18]. Since that time NMR has been used to investigate interspecies differences [14, 17] and the urine of renal transplant patients [29]; and in a wide range of studies the exploratory power of NMR was used to investigate incidents of toxic drug doses [17]. Surprisingly few cases have been reported on the application of NMR to the study of clinical toxicological problems, probably due to the perceived lack of sensitivity, issues of validation, and the lack of routine access of clinical laboratories to NMR instrumentation. Recent advances in NMR technology (Section 8.5) should see an increase in these applications.

8.3.1 Inborn Errors of Metabolism

Rare inborn errors of metabolism (IEM) are often fatal in newborn infants if not quickly diagnosed and treated. Yet the diagnostics of hereditary metabolic diseases remains a challenge for clinical chemistry. This area has special relevance to the clinical domain of toxicogenomics: idiosyncratic reactions to drugs or an unusual urinary NMR profile might be explained by a silent metabolic phenotype. Often, the analysis of amino acids and organic acids alone cannot lead to a definitive diagnosis. Conventional methods include gas chromatography–MS (GC–MS) and specific enzyme assays. However, these are time-consuming, require considerable sample preparation, and are not general. NMR of biofluids has often been shown to be a powerful exploratory method, especially in light of the speed of analysis. Time is of crucial importance in the first hours of life for neonates exhibiting clinical symptoms of IEM.

The successful application of NMR in this field has been thoroughly documented [6, 17, 30–32]. A recent study by Wevers and colleagues [31] highlighted >20 metabolites present in over half the biofluid samples measured over a 10 year period that are not detected by routine metabolic screening techniques. These include ketoacids, glycerol, trimethylamine *N*-oxide, allantoin, and hippuric acid, amongst others. Over 55 inborn errors of metabolism have been catalogued using NMR, and a few key examples to illustrate the approach include phenylketonuria, 5-oxoprolinuria, alcaptonuria, maple syrup disease, and fish odour syndrome. Urinary biomarkers have already been catalogued for the most common IEMs [17, 31]. Although an invasive and potentially dangerous technique, several biomarkers from cerebrospinal fluid have also been reported [17, 31].

In addition, a prominent feature arising from these original IEM studies was the importance of sample preparation, which is relevant to all toxicogenomic studies by NMR. To avoid the problem of pH-dependent chemical shifts that arise from variable urinary pH, adjustment of the pH to either 2.5 or 7.4 has been discussed [17]. This adds to sample preparation time, can cause degradation of certain analytes, and may interfere with subtle intermolecular interactions of diagnostic value. These issues must be considered when constructing large databases of biofluid NMR spectra with the aim of building predictive models of toxicity.

Although NMR systems as low as 250 MHz can be used, research on IEMs is typically carried out at 500 MHz or higher. For now, NMR provides a complementary diagnosis to be confirmed, for example, by GC–MS analysis in the clinical chemistry laboratory, because of the greater sensitivity of GC–MS at lower concentrations of diagnostic metabolites. In time, research NMR laboratories using LC–NMR–MS will no doubt identify new diagnostic biomarkers of certain metabolic disorders. GC–MS assays of greater sensitivity could then be developed for routine use in the clinical chemistry laboratory. Indeed, the recent advances of flow-injection modes, coupled with the integrated chemical NMR analyzer (INCA) and cryoprobes for the highest sensitivity (section 8.5), should ensure an increasing use of NMR for large-scale screening for a variety of IEMs in the general population.

8.3.2
Reactive Metabolites

One of the major driving forces behind the use of NMR in toxicology has no doubt been the regulatory pressure on pharmaceutical companies to fully characterize metabolites of novel drug candidates in animal species as part of drug evaluation submissions. An internal motivation for these companies is also to identify reactive or toxic metabolites of novel drug candidates at the earliest stage possible so as to minimize attrition in later, more expensive, stages of the development pipeline. Hyphenated LC–NMR–MS has developed into a powerful technique for analyzing metabolites of novel drugs from complex mixtures, and its applications are reviewed elsewhere [23, 24].

A key illustrative example of the use of NMR for identifying reactive metabolites is the characterization of certain reactive and volatile metabolites, which is impossible by LC–MS and only feasible by LC–NMR [33]. Ester glucuronide metabolites of many acidic drugs are unstable in aqueous solutions at pH 7.4, due to the susceptibility of the acyl groups to internal and external nucleophilic attack. The chemical reactivity is well established and has been implicated in adverse drug reactions due to protein binding to bile transporter proteins [33]. In brief, the initial drug β-1-*O*-acyl glucuronide is formed enzymatically in the body as a polar conjugate that is readily excreted in the urine or bile (depending on the molecular weight). However, the drug moiety can then internally acyl-migrate around the glucuronide ring from positions 1 to 4 to produce positional isomers which also mutarotate. Analysis of reactive drug β-1-*O*-acyl glucuronides in urine requires collecting samples over ice and adjusting to acidic pH to stabilize the parent conjugate. LC–NMR was used to identify the highly reactive α-1-*O*-acyl isomer of naproxen glucuronide, which was previously discounted in drug metabolism and pharmacokinetic studies. Dynamic stopped-flow LC–NMR provided key kinetic data that confirmed that the highly reactive α-1-*O*-acyl isomer is part of the overall kinetic scheme. As this is a general chemical reaction of carbohydrates, observed also for zomepirac, tolmetin, and diflunisal acyl glucuronides, the presence of this isomer *in vivo* is therefore possible. This finding may have toxicological implications in the reactivity of these metabolites toward important cellular proteins. Similarly, LC–NMR–MS may be used to identify other reactive conjugates, including glutathione pathway metabolites and acyl coenzyme A thioester conjugates.

8.3.3
Animal Models of Toxicity

One of the most systematic programs of studies to date reporting the use of NMR to construct databases and metabolic models of drug toxicity has been the Consortium for Metabonomics Toxicology (COMET) [5, 34]. This project, of fundamental importance to the pharmaceutical industry, is constructing a database using 100 000 spectra (600-MHz ^{1}H NMR) of biofluids from 150 studies on laboratory rats treated with model toxic compounds of well defined modes and severity of toxicity. Chemometric methods are being used to characterize the time-related and dose-specific effects on the endogenous metabolic profiles to develop predictive models of toxicity for novel candidate drugs. Interlaboratory, intersite, and inter-instrument reproducibility in sample preparation and spectral acquisition have been investigated. In addition, a variety of new processing and chemometric methods have also been developed. The comparison of histopathology, clinical chemistry, and urine and serum measurements from six study centres suggested discernible interstudy differences, especially in the rate of progress and magnitude of response. Excellent reproducibility and robustness of metabonomics techniques are claimed to be highly competitive with the best proteomic analysis methods and are in significant contrast to genomic microarray platforms [34]. NMR-based metabonomics can also be used to characterize inter-animal variation, in direct contrast to current toxicogenomic protocols which often pool samples from individuals and suffer from poor interlaboratory reproducibility.

8.4
Biomarkers of Toxicity

For toxicogenomics it is important to be able to measure exposure to a toxin, to assess the severity or extent of response, and to predict likely responses. The response to a drug depends on the absorption, distribution, metabolism, and excretion (ADME) profile of that drug. The umbrella term 'biomarker' can refer to a single molecule or to a complex pattern of biochemical effects associated with a known pathological state (for example, enzyme induction or inhibition). Timbrell has further divided the term into biomarkers of exposure, response or effect, and susceptibility [35]. To provide useful results, any biomarker-based procedure must be quantitative, non-invasive, specific, easy to measure, related to biochemical mechanism, and sufficiently sensitive at realistic doses. Reactive drug metabolites, which bind to important cellular proteins and disrupt cellular function, can also provide biomarkers of toxicity. The formation of reactive metabolites is of toxicogenomic interest with respect to drug-metabolizing enzymes that exhibit polymorphisms in human populations, such as cytochrome P450 2D6 and 2C9 and the UGDT conjugation enzymes. Idiosyncratic reactions to certain drugs may therefore have a molecular basis that can be predicted based on an integrated genomic, proteomic, and metabolic profiling research strategy. Biomarkers in toxicology are reviewed elsewhere [35].

8.4.1 Organ Toxicity

Good biomarkers for organ toxicity are preferably obtained by non-invasive means; thus, urinalysis by NMR is arguably the most effective tool for cataloguing nephrotoxicity. Conventional clinical biomarkers are enzyme-based and thus relatively inexpensive for screening purposes. These typically include enzymes such as γ-GT, intermediates like ALA, and breakdown products in urine (5-hydroxymethyluracil). However, the disadvantage of serum enzymes is that changes tend to be transient and usually only indicate significant pathological damage. Because NMR is nonselective for most low molecular weight intermediates of metabolism, its advantage is in exploring biomarkers that may be detected by other methods only with great difficulty. Compared with bile and plasma, urine is relatively easy to analyze, as reflected by exhaustive reviews of urinalysis for model drug compounds and drugs in development, reported elsewhere [17]. Centrifugation and filtering are the minimal sample preparations required for urine and bile samples. Plasma samples also require a protein-precipitation step. The main problem is the identification of small amounts of metabolite in large dilute urine samples over the background of endogenous urinary components. Sample preparation is clearly an important step in this process if ^{1}H NMR is to provide useful structural data. Bile, however, is a more difficult matrix to analyze, as it contains high bile salt concentrations, micellar components, and detergent properties [17]. Other more exotic biofluids, albeit of less clinical importance, that can be probed for biomarkers of toxicity include amniotic fluid, milk, synovial fluid, aqueous and vitreous humour, saliva, and cyst fluid. These can provide useful windows into toxic mechanisms of specific organ and tissue damage in rodent models, but as yet few studies have been published.

The main organ toxicities studied by NMR have been hepatotoxicity [2, 3, 9, 10] and nephrotoxicity [2, 3, 10]. Early studies identified taurine as a biomarker for liver damage and creatine for testicular damage [35]. Nicholson and coworkers have argued that it is not any single biomarker but rather a combination of altered metabolites which are significantly changed over time that constitutes a more predictive model of toxicity [2, 3, 9, 10]. Building on the above studies, one of the most systematic programs to date using NMR to construct databases and metabolic models of drug toxicity has been the COMET program, as outlined in Section 8.3.3.

8.4.2
Forensic and Chemical Warfare Toxicology

NMR is not widely used in forensic toxicology, probably due to the perceived poor sensitivity and the lack of routine access to high-field (>500 MHz) NMR instrumentation. Some interesting historical examples using low-field magnets demonstrate the versatility of NMR for identifying biomarkers of poisoning. Cartigny and colleagues [36] reported on a 4-month-old girl who presented with agitation, fever, dehydration, and metabolic acidosis. Metabolites including *o*-hydroxyhippuric acid, 2,5-dihydroxyhippuric acid, and 2-hydroxybenzoic acid (salicylic acid) were observed in ^{1}H NMR spectra of freeze-dried urine, which indicated that she had been poisoned with aspirin. The pattern of unusual metabolites can provide a biomarker of aspirin poisoning. This result was remarkable in that an 80-MHz system was employed. NMR has also been used to monitor progressive liver failure following paracetamol-related overdose (10 g) [37]. In addition, the second-ever known instance of acute intentional tetrahydrofuran poisoning was also investigated by NMR of untreated urine and serum samples, and the results were confirmed by using GC–MS [38]. Poisonings with the herbicide paraquat were revealed by analyzing untreated urine samples using NMR [39]. The latter studies used 300-MHz NMR systems, which proves that useful evidence has been derived in poisoning cases even with routinely available instruments. However, for more subtle poisonings, higher field strengths would surely provide greater sensitivity and resolution. Another forensic investigation used a 200-MHz system to investigate the value of NMR in quantifying multiple components of saliva, including ethanol, as a direct measure of alcohol consumption [40].

An example from the drug-doping arena is a report on the use of ^{1}H NMR for measuring creatine in urine samples as a biomarker for the use of illegal dietary supplements by French athletes [41]. Creatine is not typically measured in clinical laboratories, and common methods such as LC–MS and capillary electrophoresis require much sample preparation. The detection limits by NMR were 1.31 mg L^{-1}, and the analysis of untreated urine samples took less than 10 min. Although forensic toxicology reports are scarce, it is evident that some forensic laboratories have access to conventional NMR systems.

In the field of warfare intelligence, preliminary results were recently reported from an integrated genomics, proteomics, and metabonomics approach to studying the toxicity of chemical warfare agents (CWAs) [42]. The toxicity of vesicant sulphur mustard (HD) in minipigs was investigated by Dillmann and colleagues with the goal of identifying exposure biomarkers, carrying out advanced drug development, validating models, and studying interspecies differences. Dose- and time-related urinary profiles were measured by NMR at 600 MHz, and thiodiglycol was identified as a metabolic marker of HD exposure. In addition, an *N*-acetylated cysteinyl sulphur mustard conjugate was also clearly observed. In these studies, it is clear that NMR provided valuable data with minimal sample preparation, without the need to preselect analytes for detection, and without the need to develop chromatographic techniques.

Application of newer NMR technologies in forensic toxicology has yet to be reported, but with the advancing NMR sensitivity described in Section 8.5 this is likely to change over the coming decade. Flow-injection NMR can be enabled on NMR systems of 300 MHz and higher. The INCA system (Section 8.5.2), which has minimal requirements for laboratory space and operator skill, will see increasing use in clinical laboratories. A conventional NMR system of 400 MHz and higher can also be upgraded by addition of an LC and MS system for analyzing drugs and metabolites in complex mixtures by LC–NMR–MS. Finally, the exploratory power of HRMAS for tissue analysis may be of value in autopsies and time-of-death studies.

8.4.3 Environmental Toxicity

Although most applications of NMR in environmental toxicity studies have been in the analysis of plants, terrestrial invertebrates, and rodent species, several important features with respect to biomarkers of toxicity are worth discussing briefly. Increasing regulatory demands for the formulation of objective measures of environmental pollution and damage have led to the study of biological systems that can qualitatively and quantitatively indicate exposure to pollutants. The identification of biomarkers is an important aspect in these developments. For example, tissue homogenates and coelomic fluids in the earthworm species *Eisenia andrei*, *Eisenia veneta*, and *Lumbricus rubellus* have been well documented by conventional NMR [43, 44]. These species are well known to accumulate metals above ambient concentrations. The biochemical response of worms subjected for 110 days to 40–160 mg Cu(II) kg^{-1} dry weight of soil revealed an elevation in whole-body free histidine correlated with increasing Cu(II) exposure, so this response was proposed as a novel molecular biomarker for Cu(II) exposure. Similar approaches to measuring environmental stressors have since been applied to the analysis of cadmium exposure in plant cell cultures [45] and may have widespread significance in the study of metal tolerance and toxicity in plant species.

Nicholson and collaborators are also building databases of dose- and time-related toxic responses of earthworms to small organic molecules including fluoroanilines and fluorobiphenyls. This approach particularly exploits the sensitivity and selectivity of ^{19}F NMR for toxin-related materials so as to elucidate metabolic pathways [46, 47]. The endogenous response is measured by 1D and 2D ^{1}H NMR combined with pattern-recognition techniques [44]. Potential novel markers in the earthworm for fluoroaniline toxicity were identified by HPLC–Fourier transform mass spectrometry and off-line ^{1}H and ^{13}C NMR. These included decreased 2-hexyl-5-ethyl-3-furansulfonate and increased inosine monophosphate [15]. This strategy illustrates the power of the combined technologies: using conventional NMR and pattern-recognition methods to profile extracts of the samples according to dose and time, followed by 2D NMR and LC–NMR/MS to characterize the individual analytes as biomarkers or patterns of response. Ultimately these patterns may provide data on the underlying biochemical mechanisms of toxicity.

In addition to dose- and time-related toxic responses, interspecies differences can complicate the choice of the best animal model for toxicity in man. A recent study in the environmental arena [14] reported the use of HR–MAS of kidney and conventional ^{1}H NMR of urine samples to conduct metabolic profiling of common wild mammals in the UK. These included the bank vole, wood mouse, white-toothed shrew, and the laboratory rat. Striking interspecies differences were measured in the concentrations and compositions of aromatic acids and lipids. The researchers concluded that metabolic data acquired from laboratory animals cannot be extended to wild species. Several recent papers have also emphasized the value of NMR in exploring interspecies differences in toxic response [2, 3], which will remain an important challenge in the emerging field of toxicogenomics.

8.5 Improvements in NMR Technology

8.5.1 Sensitivity and Throughput

The major criticism of NMR as a spectroscopic technique is often its inherent insensitivity. The sensitivity of NMR depends on the type of NMR experiment, the strength of the magnet, the multiplicity and number of protons in a signal of interest, and whether the signal is in a more or less crowded region of the spectrum. With poor sensitivity, there is low throughput, as long acquisition times are needed to obtain sufficient spectral information. It has been argued that NMR studies should be performed at the highest field available, for maximal sensitivity and greater spectral resolution. Currently, the highest field is 900 MHz, but such systems are expensive, so most biofluid analysis is carried out at 600 MHz. As field strengths increase, more NMR signals are resolved and an increasing number of metabolites must be assigned. For most diagnostic purposes, a 400-MHz system is adequate, but the spectra should always be interpreted with caution, as metabolites may be missed that might be observed with a higher-field system. In addition, typical sample preparation includes freeze-drying and solvent extraction, so care must be taken when interpreting the resulting profiles, as volatile and reactive metabolites tend to be lost from the sample. This is especially important when analyzing toxic and possibly reactive metabolites in drug toxicity screening programs.

NMR detection limits have advanced significantly with the recent introduction of so-called cryoprobes. The electronic components in these probes are cryogenically cooled to around 20 K. Operating at these temperatures, while the sample remains at ambient temperature, greatly decreases the electronic noise [48, 49]. As a result, the signal-to-noise ratio for cryoprobes is increased, on average, to four times that of conventional probes. This increase in signal-to-noise ratio has considerable implications for the NMR measurements; a 4-fold increase in sensitivity enables a 4-fold lower detection limit (for a given experiment time); and, for a given amount of sample, the experiment time is 1/16 that with a conventional probe. The first application of a cryogenic probe to the analysis of ^{13}C spectra of rat urine for metabolic profiling was reported by Nicholson and coworkers [48]. As these probes are also compatible with flow-injection NMR [49], it is envisaged that screening for toxicity will be greatly accelerated by cryoprobe technology.

LC–NMR–MS has also seen recent innovations for improving the sensitivity of routine 400–600-MHz instruments [24]. These include capillary-scale LC–NMR, online solid-phase extraction (LC–SPE–NMR), and cryogenic flow probes. Fully automated capillary-scale LC–NMR at 600 MHz was applied to the stop-flow analysis of 5–25 ng (on-column) of components in an extract of urine 4 h after a 1-g dose of acetaminophen [50]. This application employed a microcoil flow probe with an active volume of 1.5 μL. Another advance is online sample preparation to concentrate samples for NMR. Solid-phase extraction (SPE) is commonly used to clean up complex mixtures or to concentrate samples prior to LC analysis. In a new development termed LC–SPE–NMR, the SPE is used after the chromatographic separation to trap analytes in-line on mini-SPE cartridges (of dimensions 10 mm length × 1–3 mm i.d). Discrete analytes are detected by UV or MS and, with the aid of post-column addition of water, are diluted in-line and adsorbed on the SPE cartridges. Chromatographic solvents are nondeuterated, which reduces costs. Nondeuterated solvents also simplify the MS data by avoiding deuterium exchange with –OH, –NH, and $-NH_2$ groups. After multiple trappings of analytes from sequential injections of sample, each cartridge is dried with nitrogen to remove all residual protonated solvent. Pure deuterated solvent is used to then flush the peak into the NMR flow probe for analysis. Triple trapping a simple aromatic molecule gave a 6.8-fold increase in the signal-to-noise ratio with LC–SPE–NMR compared to a loop-storage experiment [50].

Finally, Spraul et al. [49] recently reported the introduction of the first cryoflow probe and applied it to the analysis of untreated urine taken 4 h post dosage of 500 mg acetaminophen. Besides the known glucuronide and sulphate metabolites, other minor novel metabolites hitherto unreported at 500 MHz were found. This strategy is generally applicable for samples containing mass-limited analytes, such as those from drug metabolism studies, biomarker analyses, and toxicity profiling.

8.5.2 Integrated NMR Chemical Analyzer

Even with the vast improvements in sensitivity and throughput, some major hurdles prevent NMR becoming a routine method in the clinical laboratory for toxicological analysis. Two main issues tend to be the siting of the NMR magnet and the perceived operator skill. Instruments are now available from 300–500 MHz with UltraShield™ superconducting magnets, so that the magnetic field is contained within the enclosure. These require only 2 m^2 of space and are readily installed in most laboratories. The system is termed the integrated NMR chemical analyzer (INCA) system [51]. It can also be equipped with a flow-injection instrument and a cryoprobe for greater sensitivity. The INCA system was designed for use by non-NMR spectroscopists who need the analytical power of modern FT–NMR but do not have the facility for a traditional NMR spectroscopy laboratory. Automation and user-friendly software requires a minimum of NMR knowledge, and the system can thus be used as a routine turnkey system by clinical analysts. As the use of NMR becomes more widespread in hospital environments and as biofluid NMR is taught as electives in clinical chemistry courses and continuing professional development programs, the role of NMR in toxicological research will be ensured by the necessity for in-house databases in the clinical research areas of interest.

8.5.3
Metabolic and Genetic Profiling

Publications on metabolic markers relating to genetic strain differences and disorders in rodents have been reported [11, 52], and these applications will increase rapidly in the next decade, particularly with the integration of genomic, proteomic, and metabonomics techniques. ^1H NMR and pattern recognition was used to examine the *mdx* mouse as a model of the muscle-wasting disease Duchenne muscular dystrophy (DMD) in which the muscle protein dystrophin is not expressed. Dystrophic mouse brain and cardiac tissue extracts showed distinct metabolic profiles with altered ratios of creatine, taurine, and choline-containing metabolites. It was suggested that these ratios could be used to correlate cerebral deficits with metabolic abnormalities in DMD sufferers by using NMR *in vivo* [52].

Scott and collaborators at Imperial College London have also been concerned with gene discovery using both animal and human models of the metabolic syndrome, which is the constellation of disorders related to insulin resistance and includes obesity, dyslipidaemia, diabetes mellitus, hypertension, and increased risk of atherosclerosis. A biological atlas of insulin resistance (BAIR) is currently under development using genetically engineered and environmental models of insulin resistance along with multimodality phenotyping [53]. This approach aims to integrate transcriptomics, phospho- and glycoproteomics, metabonomics, and structural biology to advance new hypothesis-driven research toward better understanding and treatment of metabolic syndrome.

Another clinically focused metabolic project that relies heavily on flow-injection NMR is the metabonomics and genomics in coronary artery disease (MAGICAD) project [5]. In a pilot study involving the ^1H NMR–PR analysis of serum samples from 80 patients, half of whom had severe coronary artery disease (CAD), >90% of the subjects with severe CAD were correctly diagnosed by the NMR–PR approach [8]. The BAIR and MAGICAD projects are amongst the first clinical projects to attempt to integrate the genomic, proteomic, and metabolic-profiling technologies, and these approaches may be extended to diagnostics in toxicogenomics.

8.6
Conclusions

NMR spectroscopy in toxicology research has evolved from the conventional NMR methods of the 1980s into a mature and versatile toolkit for studying the molecular bases of biochemical toxicology. The dual role of higher-throughput NMR profiling coupled with chemometrics, and the subsequent identification of biomarkers, is becoming well established as an analytical strategy. Continuing advances in magnet and cryoprobe technology, along with automated sample handling, ensure ever-greater sensitivity and throughput. Indeed, the establishment of expert systems for predicting toxicity based on metabolic profiling relies heavily on NMR as the central analytical platform.

The molecular basis of toxicity spanning several levels of biomolecular organization has already been well documented for chronic hepatotoxicity and nephrotoxicity in rodents, and certain biomarkers of organ-specific toxicity have been proposed. A key future challenge in toxicogenomics will, however, be to relate the gene–protein–metabolic endpoint relationship for subtle toxic pathologies. In addition, the classical toxicology parameters of dose- and time-responses, variability, and genetic susceptibility must all be factored into interspecies studies *in vitro*. Ultimately, the question remains as to the best *in vivo* model species for man for a given toxicity. NMR is certainly an important general method for measuring alterations in the low molecular weight metabolites that comprise a diagnostic metabolic signature for many clinical diseases and toxicities. Confirmation with data from the highly sensitive MS-based analytical techniques will provide further validation. In conclusion, the future of NMR in toxicology research is relatively assured, and it will be interesting to monitor the role of NMR in toxicogenomics as the molecular basis of genomic, proteomic, and metabolic science is explored.

Acknowledgements

The author thanks Dr Laurence Bugeon for helpful discussions. OC is a Maplethorpe Fellow at the University of London.

References

1. Timbrell, J. *Principles of Biochemical Toxicology*, Taylor & Francis, London, 2000.
2. Nicholson, J. K., Lindon, J. C. and Holmes, E.: „Metabonomics“: understanding the metabolic responses of living systems to pathophysiological stimuli via multivariate statistical analysis of biological NMR spectroscopic data. *Xenobiotica* 1999, **29**, 1181–1189.
3. Nicholson, J. K., Connelly, J., Lindon, J. C. and Holmes, E.: Metabonomics: a platform for studying drug toxicity and gene function. *Nat. Rev. Drug Discov.* 2002, **1**, 153–161.
4. Castle, A. L., Carver, M. P. and Mendrick, D. L.: Toxicogenomics: a new revolution in drug safety. *Drug Discovery Today*, 2002, **7**, 728–736.
5. Henry, C. M. New 'ome' in town. *Chem. Eng. News* 2002, **80**, 66–70.
6. Moolenaar, S. H., Engelke, U. F. H., Wevers, R.A.: Proton nuclear magnetic resonance spectroscopy of body fluids in the field of inborn errors of metabolism. *Ann. Clin. Biochem.* 2003, **40**, 16–24.
7. Otvos, J., Jeyarajah, E. and Bennett, D.: A spectroscopic approach to lipoprotein subclass analysis. *J. Clin. Ligand Assay* 1996, **19**, 184–189.
8. Brindle, J. T., Antti, H., Holmes, E., Tranter, G., Nicholson, J. K., Bethell, H. W. L., Clarke, S., Schofield, P. M., Mckilligin, E., Mosedale, D. E., Granger, D. J.: Rapid and noninvasive diagnosis of the presence and severity of coronary heart disease using ^{1}H NMR-based metabonomics. *Nat. Med.* 2002, **8**, 1439–1444.
9. Beckwith-Hall, B. M., Nicholson, J. K., Nicholls, A., Foxall, P. J. D., Lindon,

J. C., Connor, S. C., Abdi, M., Connelly, J. and Holmes, E.: Nuclear magnetic resonance spectroscopic and principal components analysis investigations into biochemical effects of three model hepatotoxins. *Chem. Res. Toxicol.* 1998, **11**, 260–272.

10. Holmes, E., Nicholls, A. W., Lindon, J. C., Ramos, S., Spraul, M., Neidig, P., Connor, S. C., Connelly, J., Damment, S. J. P., Hasleden, J. N. and Nicholson, J. K.: Development of a model for classification of toxin-induced lesions using ^{1}H-NMR spectroscopy of urine combined with pattern recognition. *NMR in Biomedicine,* 1998, **11**, 1–10.

11. Gavaghan, C. L., Holmes, E., Lenz, E., Wilson, I. D. and Nicholson, J. K.: An NMR-based metabonomic approach to investigate the biochemical consequences of genetic strain differences: application to the C57BL10J and Alpk:ApfCD mouse. *FEBS Lett.* 2000, **484**, 169–174.

12. Raamsdonk, L. M., Teusink, B., Broadhurst, D., Zhang, N., Hayes, A., Walsh, M. C., Berden, J. A., Brindle, K. M., Kell, D. B., Rowland, J. J., Westerhoff, H. V., van Dam, K., Oliver, S. G.: A functional genomics strategy that uses metabolome data to reveal the phenotype of silent mutations. *Nat. Biotech.* 2001, **19**, 45–50.

13. Griffin. J. L., Troke, J., Walker, L. A., Shore, R. F., Lindon, J. C. and Nicholson, J. K.: The biochemical profile or rat testicular tissue as measured by magic angle spinning ^{1}H NMR spectroscopy. *FEBS Lett.* 2000, **486**, 225–229.

14. Griffin, J. L., Walker, L. A., Garrod, S., Holmes, E., Shore, R. F., Nicholson, J. K.: NMR spectroscopy based metabonomic studies on the comparative biochemistry of the kidney and urine of the bank vole (*Clethrionomys glareolus*), wood mouse (*Apodemus sylvaticus*), white toothed shrew (*Crocidura suaveolens*) and the laboratory rat. *Comp. Biochem. Physiol.,* B 2000, **127**, 357–367.

15. Bundy, J. G., Lenz, E. M., Bailey, N. J., Gavaghan, C. L., Svendsen, C., Spurgeon, D., Hankard, P. K., Osborn, D., Weeks, J. A. and Trauger, S. A.: Metabonomic assessment of toxicity of 4-fluoroaniline, 3,5-difluoroaniline and 2-fluoro-4-methylaniline to the earthworm *Eisenia veneta* (Rosa): identification of new endogenous biomarkers. *Environ. Toxicol. Chem.* 2002, **21**, 1966–1972.

16. Brown, F. F., Campbell, I. D., Kuchel, P. W. and Rabenstien, D. L.: Human erythrocyte metabolism studied by ^{1}H spin echo NMR. *FEBS Lett.* 1977, **82**, 12–16.

17. Lindon, J. C., Nicholson, J. K. and Everett, J. R.: NMR spectroscopy of biofluids. *Annu. Rep. NMR Spectrosc.* 1999, **38**, 1–88.

18. Nicholson, J. K., O'Flynn, M. P., Sadler, P. J., Macleod, A. F., Juul, S. M. and Sonksen, P. H.: Proton-nuclear-magnetic-resonance studies of serum, plasma and urine from fasting and normal diabetic subjects. *Biochem. J.* 1984, **217**, 365–375.

19. Bales, J. R., Hingham, D. P., Howe, I., Nicholson, J. K. and Sadler, P. J.: Use of high resolution proton nuclear magnetic resonance spectroscopy for rapid multi-component analysis of urine. *Clin. Chem.* 1984, **30**, 426–432.

20. Derome, A. E. *Modern NMR Techniques for Chemistry.* Pergamon, Oxford. 1987.

21. Levitt, M. H. *Spin dynamics: basics of nuclear magnetic resonance.* Wiley, New York, 2001.

22. Fan, W. M.T.: Metabolite profiling by one- and two-dimensional NMR analysis of complex mixtures *Prog. Nucl. Magn. Reson. Spectrosc.* 1996. **28**, 161–219.

23. Albert, K. *On-line LC–NMR and Related Techniques,* Wiley, New York, 2002.

24. Corcoran, O. and Spraul, M.: LC–NMR–MS in drug discovery. *Drug Disc. Today* 2003, **8**, 624–631.

25. Spraul, M., Hofmann, M., Ackermann, M., Nicholls, A. W., Damment, S. J. P., Hasleden, J. N., Shockcor, J. P., Nicholson, J. K. and Lindon, J. C.: Flow injection nuclear magnetic resonance spectroscopy combined with pattern recognition methods: implications for rapid structural studies and high throughput biochemical screening. *Anal. Commun.* 1997, **34**, 339–341.

26. Moka, D., Vorreuther, R., Schicha, H., Spraul, M., Humpfer, E., Lipinski, M., Foxall, P. J. D., Nicholson, J. K. and Lindon, J. C.: Magic angle spinning proton nuclear magnetic resonance spectros-

copic analysis of intact kidney tissue samples. *Anal. Commun.* 1997, **34**, 107–109.
27. Waters, N. J., Holmes, E., Waterfield, C. J., Farrant, R. D. and Nicholson, J. K.: NMR and pattern recognition studies on liver extracts and intact livers from rats treated with α-napthylisothiocyanate. *Biochem. Pharmacol.* 2002, **64**, 67–77.
28. Tomlins, A. M., Foxall. P. J. D., Lindon, J. C., Lynch, M. J., Spraul, M., Everett, J. R. and Nicholson, J. K.: High resolution magic angle spinning ^{1}H nuclear magnetic resonance analysis of intact prostatic hyperplasic and tumor tissues. *Anal. Commun.* 1998, **35**, 113–115.
29. Foxall, P. J. D., Mellotte, G. J., Bending, M. R., Lindon, J. C. and Nicholson, J. K.: NMR spectroscopy as a novel approach to the monitoring of renal transplant function. *Kidney Int.* 1993, **43**, 234–245.
30. Iles, R., Hind. A. J. and Chalmers, R. A.: Use of proton nuclear magnetic resonance spectroscopy in detection and study of organic acidurias. *Clin. Chem.* 1985, **31**, 1795–1801.
31. Moolenaar, S. H., Engelke, U. F. H., Hoenderop, S. M. G. C., Sewell, A. C., Wagner, L. and Wevers, R. A.: Handbook of ^{1}H-NMR spectroscopy in inborn errors of metabolism. Heilbronn: SPS publications, 2002.
32. Lehnert, W. and Hunkler, D.: Possibilities of selective screening for inborn errors of metabolism using high-resolution ^{1}H-FT–NMR spectrometry. *Eur. J. Pediatr.* 1986, **145**, 260–266.
33. Corcoran, O., Mortensen, R. W., Hansen, S. H., Troke, J., and Nicholson, J. K.: HPLC/^{1}H NMR spectroscopic studies of reactive α-1-*O*-acyl isomer formed during acyl migration of *S*-naproxen β-1-*O*-acyl glucuronide. *Chem. Res. Toxicol.* 2001. **14**, 1363–1370.
34. Keun, H. C., Ebbels, T. M. D., Antti, H., Bollard, M. E., Beckonert, O., Schlotterbeck, G., Senn, H., Niederhauser, U., Holmes, E., Lindon, J. C. and Nicholson, J. K.: Analytical reproducibility in ^{1}H NMR-based metabonomic urinalysis. *Chem. Res. Toxicol.* 2002, **15**, 1380–1386.
35. Timbrell, J. A.: Biomarkers in toxicology. *Toxicology*, 1998, **129**, 1–12.
36. Vermeersch, G., Marko, J., Cartigny, B., Leclerc, F., Roussell, P. and Lhermitte, M.: Salicylate poisoning detected by ^{1}H NMR spectroscopy. *Clin. Chem.* 1988, **34**, 1003.
37. Bales, J. R., Nicholson, J. K. and Sadler, P. J.: Two-dimensional proton nuclear magnetic resonance "maps" of acetaminophen metabolites in human urine. *Clin. Chem.* 1985, **31**, 757.
38. Cartigny, B., Azaroual, N., Imbenotte, M., Sadeg, N., Testart, F., Richecoeur, J., Vermeersch, G. and Lhermitte, M.: ^{1}H NMR spectroscopy investigation of serum and urine in a case of acute tetrahydrofuran poisoning. *J. Anal. Toxicol.* 2001, **25**, 270–274.
39. Imbenotte, M., Azaroual, N., Mathieu, D., Cartigny, B., Vermeersch, G. and Lhermitte, M.: Determination by ^{1}H NMR spectroscopy of paraquat in urine from acutely poisoned patients: comparison with second-derivative spectroscopy method. *J. Anal. Toxicol.* 1999, **23**, 586–590.
40. Harada, H., Shimizu, H. and Maeiwa, M.: ^{1}H NMR of human saliva: an application of NMR spectroscopy in forensic science. *Forensic Sci. Int.* 1987, **34**, 189–195.
41. Cartigny, B., Azaroual, N., Mille-Hamard, L., Imbenotte, M., Kintz, P., Vermeersch, G. and Lhermitte, M.: 1H NMR urine analysis as an effective tool to detect creatine supplementation. *J. Anal. Toxicol.* 2002, **26**, 355–359.
42. Schlager, J. J., Sabourin, C. L. K., Johnston, D. S., Midboe, E. G. and Dillman, J. F.: Application of genomics, proteomics, and metabonomics technologies to the development of medical countermeasures against chemical warfare agents. Army Science Conference, Dec 2–5, 2002, http://www.asc2002.com/summaries/d/DP-04.pdf.
43. Gibb, J. O. T., Svendsen, C., Weeks, J. M. and Nicholson, J. K.: Spectroscopic investigations of tissue metabolite biomarker response to Cu(II) exposure in terrestrial invertebrates: identification of free histidine as a novel biomarker of exposure

to copper in earthworms. *Biomarkers*, 1997, **2**, 295–302.

44. Bundy, J. G., Osborn, D., Weeks, J. M., Lindon, J. C and Nicholson, J. K.: An NMR-based metabonomic approach to the investigation of coelomic fluid biochemistry in earthworms under toxic stress. *FEBS Lett.* 2001, **500**, 31–35.

45. Bailey, N. J. C., Oven, M., Holmes, E., Nicholson, J. K. and Zenk, M. H.: Metabolomic analysis of the consequences of cadmium exposure in *Silene cucubalus* cell cultures via ^{1}H NMR spectroscopy and chemometrics. *Phytochemistry* 2003, **62**, 851–858.

46. Corcoran, O., Wilson, I. D. and Nicholson, J. K.: Rapid multi-component detection of fluorinated drug metabolites in whole urine from a 'cassette' dose study using high resolution ^{19}F NMR spectroscopy. *Anal. Commun.* 1999, **36**, 259–261.

47. Corcoran, O., Lindon, J. C., Hall, R., Ismail, I. M. and Nicholson, J. K.: The potential of ^{19}F NMR spectroscopy for rapid screening of cell cultures for models of mammalian drug metabolism. *Analyst*, 2001, **126**, 2103–2106.

48. Keun, H. C., Beckonert, O., Griffin, J. L., Richter, C., Moskau, D., Lindon, J. C. and Nicholson, J. K.: Cryogenic probe ^{13}C NMR spectroscopy of urine for metabonomic studies. *Anal. Chem.* 2002, **74**, 4588–4593.

49. Spraul, M., Freund, A. S., Nast, R. E., Withers, R. S., Maas, W. E. and Corcoran, O.: Advancing NMR sensitivity for LC–NMR–MS using a cryoflow probe: application to the analysis of acetaminophen metabolites in urine. *Anal. Chem.* 2003, **75**, 1536–1541.

50. Corcoran, O., Wilkinson, P. S., Godejohann, M., Braumann, U., Hofmann, M. and Spraul, M.: Advancing sensitivity for flow NMR spectroscopy: LC–SPE–NMR and capillary scale LC–NMR. *Am. Lab. Chrom. Perspectives*, 2002, **34**, 18–21.

51. Bruker BioSpin, INCA system, www.bruker-biospin.com/nmr/products/av_inca.html.

52. Griffin, J. L., Williams, H. J., Sang, E., Clarke, K., Rae, C. and Nicholson, J. K.: Metabolic profiling of genetic disorders: a multitissue ^{1}H nuclear magnetic resonance spectroscopic and pattern recognition study into dystrophic tissue. *Anal. Biochem.* 2001, **293**, 16–21.

53. Biological Atlas of Insulin Resistance Project, www.bair.org.uk.

Bioinformatic Tools in Toxicogenomics

Handbook of Toxicogenomics: Strategies and Applications. Edited by Jürgen Borlak

ISBN: 3-527-30342-1

9
Generation and Validation of a Reference System for Toxicogenomics DNA Microarray Experiments

Jürgen Cox, Hans Gmünder, Andreas Hohn, and Hubert Rehrauer

9.1
Genomics and DNA Microarrays

Drugs generally exert therapeutic effects by interacting with proteins, the drug targets, to restore the normal function of the cell or to compensate for abnormalities. A compound may be designed to optimally bind to a certain protein. The effects of a compound are then assessed in a live model organism. In many instances the precise effects of a drug in an organism may not be understood. As long as the drug's beneficial effects clearly outweigh potential adverse side effects, the drug is passed for further development. However, a detailed insight into the mechanisms triggered by a compound might help to better predict the viability of a drug in an earlier development phase. Conventional methods have not allowed scientists to fully explore the mechanism of action of a drug in relation to gene expression patterns and pathways, because the complex multidimensional relationships that exist in biological systems cannot be addressed by traditional gene-by-gene analysis.

Genomics has the potential to provide far more detailed insight into a compound's MOA. The goal of genomics is to systematically describe primary DNA sequence in coding and regulatory regions, single nucleotide polymorphisms (SNPs) within species or subgroups, temporary changes in gene expression patterns during development as a consequence of physiological responses or diseases, and subcellular localization and intermolecular interaction of protein products. DNA microarrays are a prime example of a genomics technology. They offer a possibility to establish global views at the gene expression level by systematically measuring DNA and RNA variations [1]. DNA microarrays allow for a parallel analysis of the expression of many genes – ideally the entire gene set of an organism – and for observation of the state of a biological system at a given time and environmental condition. Therefore, expression analysis can be used as a highly sensitive indicator for the activity and the effects of a drug. Modern DNA microarrays are straightforward to employ, gene expression studies using microarrays are at the forefront of genomics research, and the technology is sufficiently mature to be used by toxicology laboratories with stringent standardization requirements [2, 3].

Handbook of Toxicogenomics: Strategies and Applications. Edited by Jürgen Borlak

ISBN: 3-527-30342-1

9.2 Toxicogenomics

9.2.1 Challenges of Conventional Toxicology Approaches

Although a drug candidate's beneficial effects are discovered relatively early, potential toxic effects are assessed by classical toxicology only later during drug development. Conventional drug safety evaluations involving histopathology, haematology, and blood chemistry are expensive and time-consuming. Furthermore, scaling up the chemistry to provide the quantity of compound material required often further delays the start of toxicological tests. However, as a result of more identified targets, high-throughput screening of thousands of compounds, and smarter lead optimization, toxicologists today are confronted with more compounds to analyze and, in turn, the need to increase their throughput capabilities.

9.2.2 Opportunities for Genomics

Toxicogenomics, which deals primarily with the effects of compounds on gene expression patterns in target cells or tissues, is emerging as a key approach in screening new drug candidates. Toxicogenomics reveals genetic signatures that can be used to predict the short- and long-term biological effects of exposure to a drug and to identify potential toxic mechanisms with small amounts of compound material at an early stage during drug discovery. Such assessments reduce the costs for expensive late-stage drug development processes and allow more rapid stop/go decisions during early development stages. In addition, toxicogenomics is set to complement traditional pathology and toxicity studies, especially when the drug itself is difficult to track by conventional detection methods or when its clinical outcome takes a long time to become manifest. Toxicogenomics is a process (Figure 9.1) that requires three key steps – the establishment of reference compendia with compounds from different toxicological classes, the classification of drug candidates based on the reference compendia, and the prediction of the toxicity of these compounds [4–6].

9.3 Processes and Methods for Toxicogenomics

9.3.1 Experimental Design

Before starting microarray experiments for toxicogenomics, some critical points concerning the experimental setup must be addressed. Detecting rare transcripts is one major challenge; therefore, the arrays used should allow for the measurement of transcripts across several orders of magnitude, down to just a few copies per cell. It is

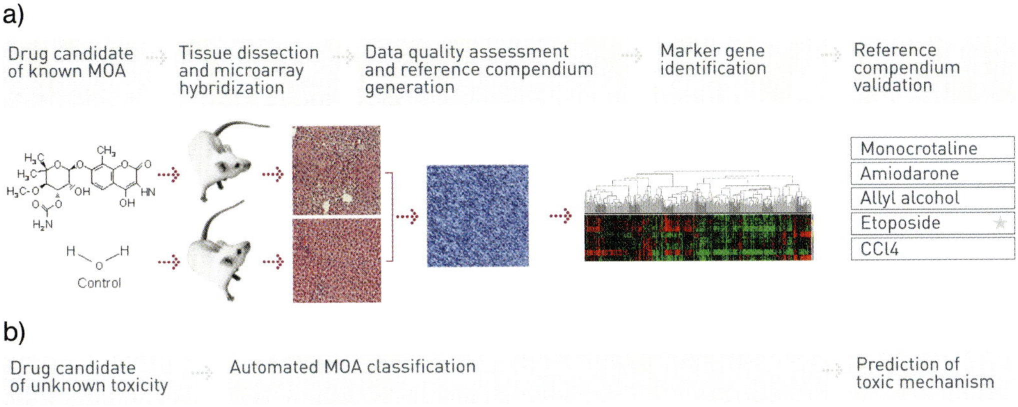

Fig. 9.1 Predictive in silico toxicology. (a) Reference compendium generation. Well characterized compounds are used to generate a library of expression fingerprints. In a first data analysis step, the data quality is checked, outlier chips are removed, and the data are normalized. Subsequently, well characterized compounds and supervised learning methods are used to create the reference compendium. As a next step, statistical methods are applied to identify genes with high discriminating power, and a refined reference compendium is generated. Finally, removing and reintroducing compounds or compound classes validates the reference compendium. (b) Automated classification of novel compounds. The validated reference compendium is used to classify novel compounds and predict their toxicity, as well as the toxic MOA. New compounds can be used to further enhance the reference compendium and gradually build a large, comprehensive reference system.

indispensable for a complete global view to detect these low-abundance genes, because the detection of quantitative changes of such rare transcripts may give an indication of when and how signal cascades were initiated. Performing replicate experiments helps to increase the reliability and sensitivity for detecting rare transcripts. However, as there are economical reasons for limiting the numbers of replicas, assuring the quality of isolated RNA and eliminating experiments with poor quality are important activities. Before starting extensive experimental series, it is also necessary to determine time points and compound concentrations at which changes in gene expression are anticipated. Determining optimal parameters, along with reducing the effects of unrelated environmental influences on gene expression, greatly helps to optimize the predictive value of mRNA signatures. Finally, suitable positive and negative controls, for example, stress or vehicles, must also be included. Laboratory protocols for RNA isolation, cRNA preparation, hybridization, staining, scanning, and imaging must also be standardized to increase the reliability of experiments [7].

9.3.2 Data Quality Assessment

Assessing the data quality of experiments is essential for building a reference database with predictive value. That microarrays can contain small defects is well known.

Additionally, small changes in the experimental procedure may lead to deviations in data quality. Changes in the scanner setting or misalignment of the scanner may lead to faulty quantification of chip images (see Section 9.4). If unnoticed, erroneous data from such experiments can affect the quality of the toxicological reference compendium and reduce its robustness. A critical aspect of data quality assessment (and by the same token, of all the ensuing analysis steps) is the guaranteed reproducibility of all applied methods. Judgments based on visual inspection of microarrays are not sufficient and should be avoided in favour of well characterized automated computational methods [8].

9.3.3
Reference Compendium Generation

Once the expression data is confirmed to be of optimal quality, the next step is to build a database of mRNA signatures for known compounds. Novel compounds are profiled against the compendium; therefore, several members of each toxicological class must be included. An unlimited number of compounds can be profiled, and as long as the experimental procedure and the type of chips used are not changed, more compounds can be added to improve and enhance the compendium's predictive quality. Along with the gene expression patterns, the database should also store additional information from blood samples, phenotypic observations, tissue sections, clinical outcomes, and so forth. This information is very useful in building classes for the supervised classification and interpretation of gene expression patterns (see Section 9.3.4).

Two basic methods are available for building the reference compendium. The first method uses all the available expression data, whereas the second method employs only a limited number of previously determined marker genes. The advantage of using a method with no restriction on the number of genes is that more genes and pathways can be utilized for toxicological predictions as the list of compounds in the database grows. Therefore, to get as much information as possible, such 'unlimited' approaches should be preferred whenever possible. However, not every laboratory has the resources for large arrays with thousands of genes, and some toxicology laboratories may turn to smaller, customized chips for large-scale studies. A compromise may be to use large arrays to determine an optimal set of genes that allow for classifications of a large variety of compounds and to switch to a smaller customized array for that particular set of genes. Marker gene selection should be based on unbiased computational methods employing algorithms to select genes with high discriminatory power between different compounds. With this method, uncharacterized pathways are taken into account. However, previously acquired knowledge on the effects of compounds on cellular pathways can be used to enrich the set of statistically found marker genes [9–11].

9.3.4
Classification

Once established and validated, the reference compendium can be used to classify novel compounds. Matching the gene expression profile of a new drug candidate to profiles of known compounds reveals in a very early phase whether the compound is suited for further development or whether it will most probably show undesired side effects in later phases. Novel compounds that have been unequivocally classified and properly annotated can then be added to the reference compendium, provided that the quality of the experiments matches that of the experiments used to construct the reference compendium. The cycle is repeated until the compendium achieves robustness for reliably classifying novel compounds or even compound mixtures.

9.4
Diagnosis of Microarray Data Quality

Genedata's strategy for detecting errors in gene expression measurements is outlined in this section. Although microarray technology is astonishingly precise and reliable, its routine application in toxicology and pharmacology requires process control that takes all errors into account that may have a significant impact on the results.

The accuracy of microarray measurements depends on a high signal-to-noise ratio. Although frequently expressed genes are relatively easy to measure, rare transcripts can no longer be accurately measured if their expression falls within the range of technical noise. As many genes involved in regulatory systems are expressed at relatively low levels, data quality assessment is essential for generating meaningful data.

Errors can occur at each step of a hybridization experiment, for example, during extraction of the genetic material, microarray hybridization, or quantification of the scanned image [12, 13]. Data quality control must include quality measures that cover the entire process – from sample extraction to the digital quantification of expression signals. Some examples of potential errors and their corresponding quality measures are discussed below and demonstrated in Figure 9.2.

9.4.1
Sample Preparation

Degradation processes during mRNA extraction or incomplete reverse transcription of purified mRNA leads to the partial representation of transcripts. Incomplete reverse transcripts can be analyzed by measuring the 3′/5′ ratios of probe pairs targeted at the 3′ end or the 5′ end, respectively, of a gene.

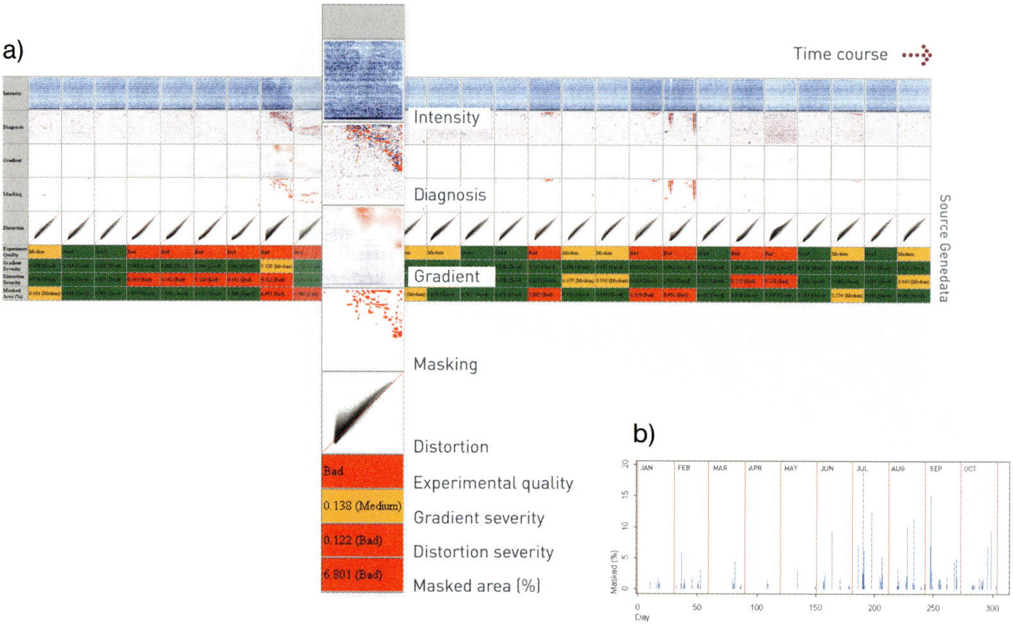

Fig. 9.2 Data quality assessment. The quality of the reference compendium depends on the accuracy of the underlying measurements. The Genedata Expressionist Refiner software program introduces objective criteria for the identification and elimination of faulty microarrays and automates and standardizes the process of data generation. (a) Detailed data quality assessment of a subset of microarrays. The Expressionist Refiner program identifies the three critical quality parameters – gradients, distortions, and defects – and provides criteria for experimental acceptance, rescue, or elimination. (b) Chronology of data quality issues. In the example shown, the percentage of masked arrays is displayed for 650 Affymetrix GeneChip® microarrays processed over a period of 300 days.

9.4.2 Dye Incorporation

Two-channel arrays (microarrays that are simultaneously hybridized with an experimental and a control sample) are less prone to local signal variations. However, such experiments require the incorporation of two different dye labels in the two samples. These experiments produce reliable results only if the dyes are incorporated at comparable rates. Successful incorporation of both dyes is assessed by measuring the balance of the signals from both dyes.

9.4.3 Distortion

Two-channel arrays are scanned at two wavelengths that have different backgrounds [14]. The background has to be removed for each channel separately. Inappropriate background correction for one of the channels results in a nonlinear relationship between the two channels – referred to as distortion. The amount of distortion is quantified according to the average deviation from a linear fit of the two channels. The presence of distortion indicates a failure in background correction.

9.4.4 Impurities

Impurities in the hybridization medium or dust particles on the array surface prevent successful specific hybridization in local areas on an array. This condition results in abnormally low or high hybridization signals. These types of defects are identified by either comparing the signals from replicate spots at different locations on the array or by comparing the signals against a reference signal computed from a large number of array experiments. Affected regions must be masked and excluded from further analysis. Whether an array is usable or not depends on the percentage of the total area that is affected by defects.

9.4.5 Scanner Settings

The scanned image of an array suffers from saturation or low contrast if the scanner settings are inappropriately chosen. A dataset has to be excluded if major parts of the array are either saturated or show low signals that cannot be distinguished from the background.

9.4.6 Automation of Data Quality Control

Subjective measures for assessing data quality provide an added bias, are not scalable, and should therefore be avoided. Software such as the Genedata Expressionist Refiner program uses objective criteria to measure a variety of quality parameters. Based on an automated analysis it is then possible to decide which experiments can be retained for further processing.

9.4.7 Preprocessing of Microarray Data

Before microarray data can be used in expression analysis they must be standardized so that they can be compared with other experiments. If in an experiment the expression of a gene is measured multiple times, these replicate measurements must be summarized in a single value that can then be compared to measurements from other experiments. Furthermore, microarray data represent measurements with a finite precision that have a measurement uncertainty or error. Computing this error is indispensable if the significance of an observed expression change has to be quantified later. A related quantity is the p value, which is factored in as the probability that a value has actually been generated by gene expression and not by an artefact. Summarizing replicate signals is a prerequisite for comparing expression data at the gene level. Computing the corresponding measurement errors and *p* values allows for differentiating the true expression changes from artefacts in subsequent analyses.

In summary, data quality assessment ensures that only high-fidelity measurements are fed into the expression database and used for building a reference compendium. Automation of data quality control should be favoured over subjective criteria. Gene expression measurements should be provided together with measures of an error, such as a *p* value. It is important to store those quality parameters together with the actual measurements in the expression database so that they can be considered in later analyses.

9.5 Generating a Reference Compendium of Compounds

For a given toxicological endpoint, such as liver necrosis, replicate experiments are performed for a multitude of compound dosages and treatment times. Therefore, analyses of several compounds generate large, complex datasets that require sophisticated, automatic structuring methods. Two basic approaches exist for structuring the large and complex datasets that occur in toxicogenomics experiments – unsupervised learning methods and supervised learning methods.

In unsupervised learning methods, no assumption is made about the structure of the data. Two-dimensional hierarchical clustering is an example of unsupervised learning. If genes that distinguish between toxic MOAs have been carefully selected, the results of such analyses can be displayed as 'toxic fingerprints'. However, this approach may lead to unsatisfactory results if effects due to the experimental setup (technical or biological influences that result in experimental noise) override compound-specific effects.

The second method, supervised learning, takes into account the available information from well established compounds. This approach has been shown to structure toxicogenomics data meaningfully. A typical example of a supervised learning method is the 'classifiers' [15]. Automated determination of toxicity relies on classification algorithms that use the expression data obtained from treated tissues to make reliable predictions. Furthermore, sophisticated gene selection algorithms allow researchers to focus on genes that are indicative of the toxic effects of interest, thereby optimizing the predictive strength.

Microarray classification can follow two different strategies. The first strategy uses as many genes as possible – preferably all available genes on a microarray. A classification algorithm is applied that works well in high-dimensional spaces, is robust, and remains insensitive to experimental noise. A prominent example of such a classifier is the support vector machine algorithm [16, 17]. Generalized forms of linear discriminant analysis can also be included as examples [18]. The second strategy employs a simpler classification algorithm but places emphasis on careful gene selection. Genes can be selected manually according to biological knowledge or with the help of statistical algorithms.

There is no universal answer to the question of which of the two strategies, focusing on the classifier or on the gene selection, is better. Concentrating on the classifier and dispensing altogether with gene selection is certainly the concept that is easier to extend, because, when a restricted set of marker genes is used, an update of the reference compendium will probably change the marker gene set significantly. On the other hand, the gene selection approach might give further insight into the nature of the cellular processes involved. A rigid decision for the first or second strategy is not recommended. Instead, it is recommended to work with a substantial arsenal of classification algorithms and gene selection methods and to experimentally determine the strategy and the algorithms that best suit the data.

Experience has shown that employing the first strategy – using all the genes and then subsequently reducing the number of genes until an optimal gene set is found – is the best approach. For gene selection, a standardized algorithmic approach is less biased than a subjective gene selection based on established knowledge of marker genes. Gene selection algorithms range from simple univariate tests, such as one-way analysis of variance (ANOVA), to highly sophisticated ones, for example, genetic programming-based algorithms.

9.5.1 Cross Validation

Cross-validation is an important technique for deciding which algorithms are optimal. Furthermore, cross-validation can help to discover unexpected relationships between mechanisms of actions. The basic ideas behind the principles of supervised learning methods and cross-validation are sketched in Figure 9.3. A classifier separates, based on training data, the gene expression space into regions, the domains of the different groups. In Figure 9.3 a gene space has been divided into three parts, each belonging to a different mode of toxicity. In a cross-validation step, one or several microarrays are taken out of the training data set (triangle marked 'A' in Figure 9.3 a), and the classifier is recomputed. If the experiment that was excluded is reassigned to its original MOA class (as shown in Figure 9.3 b), the assignment is considered stable under cross-validation.

A second example demonstrates the detection of a cross-validation error. For this purpose, another experiment is removed and the classifier is recomputed again. Figure 9.3 c indicates that the recomputed boundaries after the removal of the experiment marked with an arrow deviate significantly. This time the experiment is assigned to a different MOA class, indicating a cross-validation error.

Several methods of cross-validation are available. The 'leave-one-out' cross-validation method removes one experiment at a time. With '*n*-fold' cross-validation, a randomly selected fraction of experiments is omitted and reclassified. For toxicological experiments, subgroup cross-validation can be employed when additionally categorizing and classifying further experiments. An example of subgroup classification is to classify in the first round according to histopathological endpoints, and in the second round according to compound MOA classes. In cross-validation methods, the experiments that fail to classify correctly are used to calculate the cross-validation error rate.

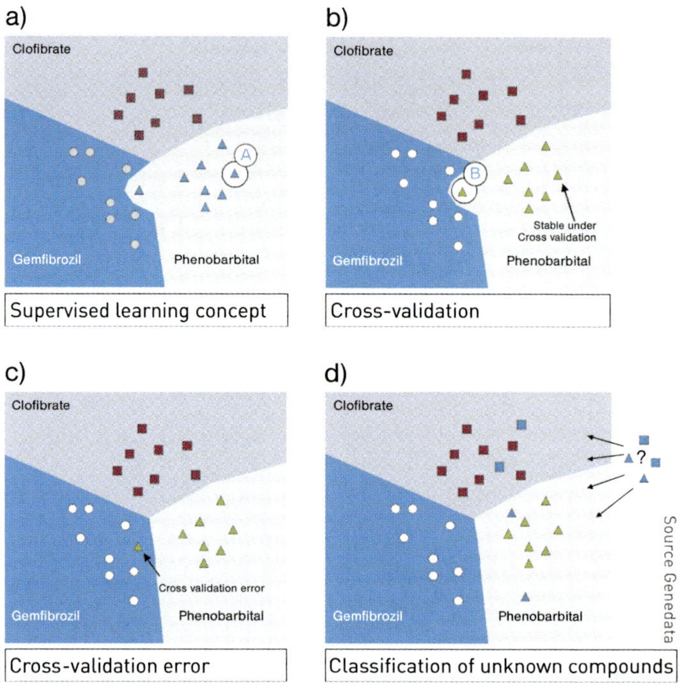

Fig. 9.3 Reference compendium generation and validation. Principle of supervised learning methods: (a) When processing a high-dimensional gene space, the algorithm selects planes that optimally separate the compound classes. The classifier then removes one or more experiments at a time and recomputes the reference compendium. (b) The classifier reintroduces the experiment that was removed. If the experiment is reassigned to the same MOA class (as shown in this example), the assignment is considered to be stable under cross-validation. A second example demonstrates the detection of a cross-validation error. For this purpose, another experiment was removed and the reference compendium was recomputed. (c) As the experiment that was removed represented an outlier experiment, the separation planes are slightly different than in the previously cited example. This time the experiment is assigned to a different MOA class, indicating a cross-validation error. (d) The reference compendium derived from an optimal set of marker genes and proven reliable with cross-validation can be used to classify novel compounds.

By systematically assessing various classification and gene selection methods, one is now in the position to find the combination of classifier and gene selection method, as well as the size of the gene set, with the optimal predictive power. The reference compendium derived from an optimal set of marker genes and an optimal classification algorithm can then be used to classify novel compounds (Figure 9.3 d).

An example of the classification of compounds according to MOA classes is shown in Figure 9.4. The classification results are shown for all the genes from a microarray (Figure 9.4 a) and after optimizing the set of marker genes (Figure 9.4 b). Figure 9.4 c shows the cross-validation error as a function of the number of top-discriminating genes (according to ANOVA). Different lines represent the different classification algorithms that were applied. The higher error rate for small numbers of marker genes is explained

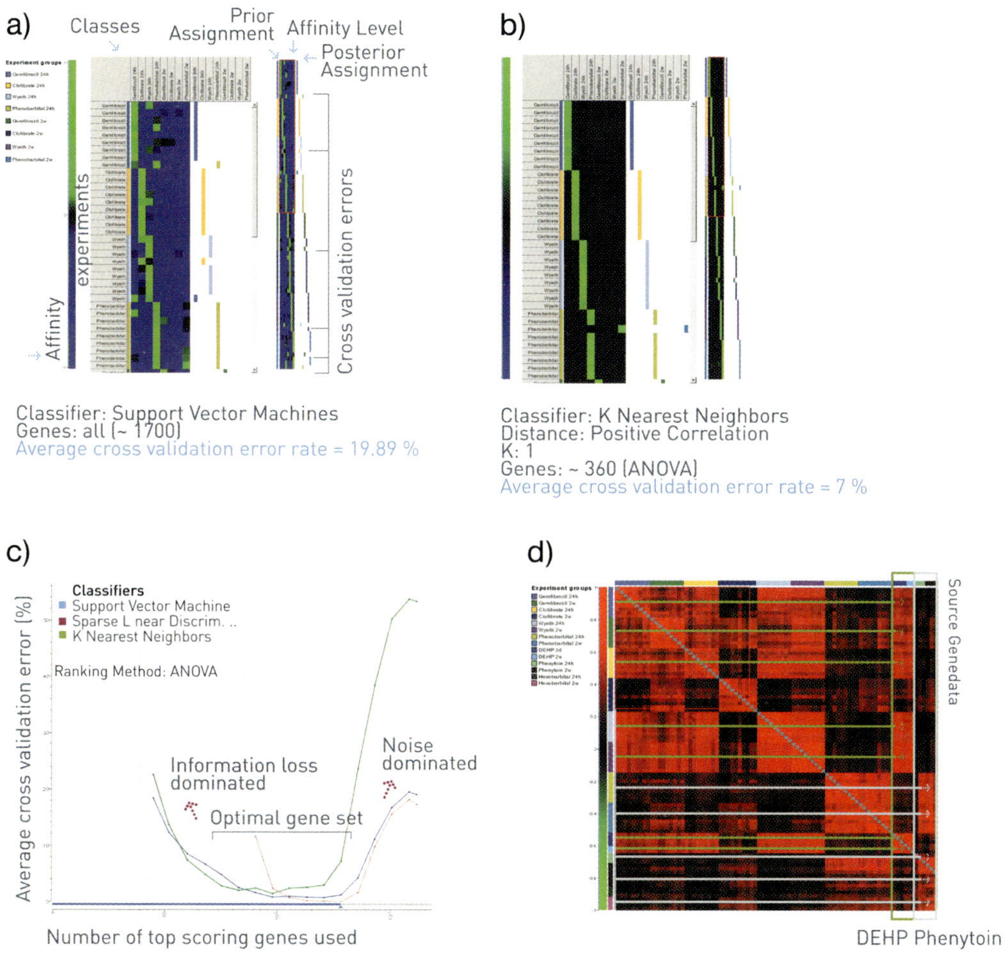

Fig. 9.4 Reference compendium generation of toxic MOA fingerprints. (a) Classification of compounds using all 1700 genes of a microarray. Rows indicate different experiments; columns indicate MOA class assignments. The affinity to a given class is shown on a colour scale (reproduced here as shades of grey). The prior assignment of MOA classes and the assignment under cross-validation are also displayed. The experiment reveals a high percentage of correct classifications (error rate less than 20%). (b) Classification of experiments using only the top 360 marker genes. Note that the error rate has dropped to 7%. (c) Determination of the optimal set of marker genes for discrimination. The graph shows the cross-validation error as a function of the number of top-discriminating genes. Different lines represent the different statistical algorithms that were used. The higher error rate for a small numbers of marker genes is explained by the loss of information, whereas the higher error rate with very large numbers of marker genes is explained by the noise rate of nonessential marker genes. The optimal number of marker genes depends on the classifier used. (d) Classification of unknown and known compounds into MOA classes with the optimized set of marker genes. Results show that newly classified compounds as well as established compounds strongly correlate with the appropriate MOA classes.

by the loss of information, whereas the higher error rate with very large numbers of marker genes is explained by the noise rate of nonessential genes. In the example, the highest degree of prediction is reached with about 400 top-scoring genes. If optimal classification of novel compounds is all that matters, one should follow this recommendation. However, it is interesting to note that the error rate stays low when going to smaller marker gene sets, to sizes of approximately 30 genes. When one is interested in uncovering the responsible cellular processes, this short list of genes is a good starting point. This set of genes may be sufficient for designing an assay to distinguish a certain number of compounds. However, one needs to keep in mind that, if compounds that belong to novel MOA classes are added to the reference compendium, the list of genes will very likely have to be extended. Finally, the validated and optimized reference compendium can be used to categorize novel compounds into MOA classes (Figure 9.4 d).

9.6
Mechanism of Action

Although generation of a validated reference compendium is sufficient for the classification of novel compounds, the marker genes identified are also a valuable resource for further characterizing the MOA of compounds and compound classes. For this purpose a detailed and comprehensive description of the genes' functions, as well as of their involvement in cellular pathways, is essential. Bioinformatics will have a major influence on improving our understanding of such diverse areas as the regulation of gene expression, protein structure determination, protein–protein interactions, and cross-species comparisons. Information about exons, introns, regulators, transcription factor binding sites, splicing variants, and SNPs can be accessed and used to enlarge the knowledge about the structure and function of genes. Protein structures and motifs, functional annotations, and information about protein–protein interactions and protein–DNA interactions can be included in more wide-reaching analyses. Metabolite data from tissues and fluids treated with compounds provide further indication of the drug's effects on a system, and such data can be correlated with gene expression and protein expression data.

Although a comprehensive discussion of the possibilities of genomics is outside the scope of this chapter, the following section outlines a few examples of MOA studies that immediately can follow the profiling of mRNA data.

9.6.1
Alternative Structuring of Profiling Data

The data provided by large-scale profiling studies can be structured in various ways. One angle, as described above, is to structure the data according to compounds, concentrations, and time points. One alternative is to summarize compounds into MOA classes, thus providing genes that distinguish MOA classes as well as genes that distinguish compounds within a class. Another possibility is to classify according to histopathological endpoints.

9.6.2
Promoter Analysis

The analysis of transcription factor binding sites gives further insight into the regulatory pathways stimulated by compounds. To answer the question of whether there is a characteristic, modular structure of transcription factor binding sites, the upstream genomic regions of such coregulated genes are selected and an automated analysis is performed to identify putative (novel) transcription factor binding sites. Those putative sites can then be mapped onto the entire genome to identify further genes that may have been missed by gene expression analysis.

9.6.3
Pathways

To analyze regulatory and metabolic networks based on mRNA profiles, mapping of gene expression data onto editable standard and custom biochemical pathway maps results in classification of the expressed genes into superior classes and, at the same time, leads to a deeper understanding of the drug effects. Such pathway analysis of expression data should also allow the mapping of entire gene expression experiment sets, such as time series or concentration series. Experiments in which drugs are applied at different time points and concentrations help to differentiate between primary and secondary drug effects.

9.6.4
Mapping Gene Expression Profiles onto Genomes

Genomic clustering of genes is commonly found in prokaryotes, due to the presence of transcriptional operons; however, clustering may also occur to a lesser extent for pathway members in eukaryotic genomes. Therefore, gene expression patterns mapped onto whole genomes may detect potential chromosomal clustering of functionally related genes. If such an association exists, it reduces the complexity of gene expression patterns, because considering only a representative gene of clusters may be sufficient for predicting potential toxic effects of a drug candidate.

9.6.5
In silico Comparative Genomics

One needs to keep in mind that animal models may not always reflect the behaviour of a drug in humans. Targets may be sufficiently different in humans to elicit disparate binding behaviour in a drug, the drug may bind to other targets, or cellular pathways may be regulated in an alternative fashion. However, experiments on humans are largely restricted. Comparative genomics analysis *in silico* helps to extrapolate from an animal model to humans. With the help of *in silico* comparative genomics, the corresponding genes (orthologs) in humans are identified, SNP or haplotype analysis stratifies human populations having different responses to a drug, and splice variants give an indication of other mechanisms that are affected [19, 20].

9.7
Outlook

Generation of a reference library of compounds is a very effective tool for characterizing novel compounds. However, to gain mechanistic insights into a drug's action, a multitude of genomics data is required to fully explore functional networks. With the generation of microarray data, proteomics data, and metabonomics data, a comprehensive analysis of the effects of drugs on regulatory and metabolic pathways will become possible.

References

1. E. S. Lander, The new genomics: global views of biology, *Science* **274**, 536–539 (1996).
2. K. V. Chin, and A. N. Kong, Application of DNA microarrays in pharmacogenomics and toxicogenomics, *Pharm Res* **19**, 1773–1778 (2002).
3. E. S. Lander, Array of hope, *Nat Genet Suppl* **21**, 3–4 (1999).
4. H. K. Hamadeh et al., An overview of toxicogenomics, *Curr Issues Mol Biol* **4**, 45–56 (2002).
5. R. Ulrich and S. H. Friend, Toxicogenomics and drug discovery: will new technologies help us produce better drugs? *Nat Rev Drug Discov* **1**, 84–88 (2002).
6. J. F. Waring, J. F. and D. N. Halbert, The promise of toxicogenomics, *Curr Opin Mol Ther* **4**, 229–235 (2002).
7. G. A. Churchill, Fundamentals of experimental design for cDNA microarrays, *Nat Genet* **32** (Suppl 2), 490–495 (2002).
8. J. Quackenbush, Microarray data normalization and transformation, *Nat Genet* **32** (Suppl 2), 496–501 (2002).
9. T. R. Hughes et al., Functional discovery via a compendium of expression profiles, *Cell* **102**, 109–126 (2000).
10. H. K. Hamadeh et al., Gene expression analysis reveals chemical-specific profiles, *Toxicol Sci* **67**, 219–231 (2002).
11. H. K. Hamadeh et al., Prediction of compound signature using high density gene expression profiling, *Toxicol Sci* **67**, 232–240 (2002).
12. K. Johnson and S. Lin, QA/QC as a pressing need for microarray analysis: meeting report from CAMDA'02, *BioTechniques* **34**, S62–S63 (2003).
13. D. V. Nguyen, A. B. Arpat, N. Wang, and R. J. Carroll, DNA microarray experiments: biological and technological aspects, *Biometrics*, **58**, 701–717 (2002).
14. A. B. Goryachev, P. F. MacGregor, A. M. Edwards, Unfolding of microarray data, *J Comput Biol*, **8**:4, 443–461 (2001).
15. S. Dudoit, J. Fridlyand, and T. Speed, Comparison of discrimination methods for the classification of tumors using gene expression data, *J Am Stat Assoc* **97**, 77–87 (2002).
16. N. Cristianini and J. Shawe-Taylor, *An Introduction to Support Vector Machines and other Kernel-based Learning Methods*, Cambridge University Press, 2000.
17. S. Ramaswamy, et al., Multiclass cancer diagnosis using tumor gene expression signatures, *Proc Natl Acad Sci USA* **98**, 15149–15154 (2001).
18. J. Cox, Sparse linear discriminant analysis for microarray data, in preparation.
19. D. K. Slonim, From patterns to pathways: gene expression data analysis comes of age, *Nat Genet* **32** (Suppl 2), 502–508 (2002).
20. E. F. Petricoin et al., Medical applications of microarray technologies: a regulatory science perspective, *Nat Genet* **32** (Suppl 2), 474–479 (2002).

10 The Chemical Effects in Biological Systems (CEBS) Knowledge Base

Michael Waters, Gary Boorman, Pierre Bushel, Michael Cunningham, Rick Irwin, Alex Merrick, Kenneth Olden, Richard Paules, James Selkirk, Stanley Stasiewicz, Brenda Weis, Ben Van Houten, Nigel Walker, Honghui Wan, and Raymond Tennant

"Where is the wisdom we have lost in knowledge?
Where is the knowledge we have lost in information?"

T. S. Elliott

10.1 Overview

Toxicogenomics is a new scientific field that studies how the genome responds to environmental stressors or toxicants (Nuwaysir et al. 1999; Burchiel et al. 2001; Fielden and Zacharewski 2001; Thomas et al. 2001; Aardema and MacGregor 2002; Afshari 2002; Hamadeh et al. 2002; Olden 2002; Tennant 2002; Ulrich and Friend 2002). It combines studies of genetics, genomic-scale mRNA expression (transcriptomics), cell and tissue-wide protein expression (proteomics), metabolite profiling (metabonomics), and bioinformatics with conventional toxicology in an effort to understand the role of gene–environment interactions in disease. New molecular technologies, such as DNA microarray analysis and protein chips, can measure the expression of hundreds to thousands of genes and proteins at a time, providing the potential to accelerate discovery of toxicant pathways and specific chemical and drug targets. The power and potential of these new toxicogenomics methods are capable of revolutionizing the field of toxicology. In recognition of this, NIEHS has created the National Center for Toxicogenomics (NCT; http://www.niehs.nih.gov/nct/concept.htm). The NCT has five major goals:

1. to facilitate the application of gene and protein expression technology;
2. to understand the relationship between environmental exposures and human disease susceptibility;
3. to identify useful biomarkers of disease and exposure to toxic substances;
4. to improve computational methods for understanding the biological consequences of exposure and responses to exposure;

Handbook of Toxicogenomics: Strategies and Applications. Edited by Jürgen Borlak

ISBN: 3-527-30342-1

5. to create a public database of environmental effects of toxic substances in biological systems.

The NCT was formally established in September of 2000 and is working to implement a strategy through which these goals can be achieved. This chapter and a recently published paper from the NCT (Waters et al. 2003) is a response to goal 5. It delineates the conceptual framework and some major design considerations for the proposed Chemical Effects in Biological Systems (CEBS) knowledge base. Ideker et al. (2001) have used the phrase 'systems biology' to describe the integrated study of biological systems at the molecular level – involving perturbation of systems, monitoring molecular expression, integrating response data, and modelling the system structure and function. Here we similarly use the phrase 'systems toxicology' to describe the toxicogenomics evaluation of biological systems, involving perturbation by toxicants and stressors, monitoring molecular expression and conventional toxicological parameters, and iteratively integrating response data. CEBS will incorporate high-quality datasets from each of the new toxicogenomics technologies, as well as from contemporary molecular and cellular toxicology.

The CEBS goals are (1) to create a reference toxicogenomic information system of studies on environmental chemicals/stressors and their effects; (2) to develop relational and descriptive compendia on toxicologically important genes, groups of genes, single nucleotide polymorphisms (SNPs), and mutant and knockout phenotypes in animal models that are relevant to human health and environmental disease; and (3) to support hypothesis-driven research and discovery research in environmental toxicology. The CEBS goals must be approached in an incremental fashion, recognizing that, in the face of rapid technological change, it is impossible to anticipate all of the opportunities and problems that can develop.

The conceptual design framework for CEBS is based upon functional genomics approaches that have been used successfully in analyzing yeast gene expression datasets (Hughes et al. 2000). The proposed framework is illustrated in Figure 10.1.

Because CEBS will contain data on global gene expression, protein expression, metabolite profiles, and associated chemical/stressor induced effects in multiple species (e.g., from yeast to humans), it will be possible to derive functional pathway and network information based on cross-species homology. CEBS datasets will be fully documented in experimental protocols and therefore searchable by compound, structure, toxicity endpoint, pathology endpoint, gene, gene group, etc., as a function of dose, time, and the condition of the target tissue. Controlled vocabularies, dictionaries, and descriptive explanatory text or metadata (that can be processed by a computer) will guide researchers in understanding toxicogenomics datasets. A knowledge base will be developed by carefully assimilating toxicological, biological, and chemical information from multiple public domain databases and by progressively refining that information about classes of chemicals and their biological effects in various species (Zweiger 1999; Tennant 2002). By analogy to the GenBank database for genome sequences, ultimately it will be possible to query CEBS globally using a transcriptome of a tissue of interest (or a list of outliers from a gene expression analysis) to BLAST (Altschul et al. 1990) the knowledge base and have it return information on genes, groups of

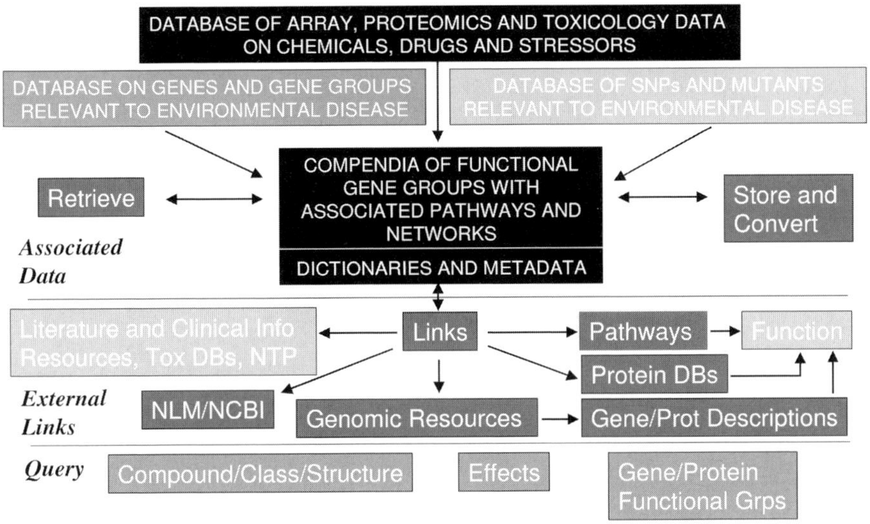

Fig. 10.1 Conceptual framework of the CEBS knowledge base – a cross-species reference toxicogenomic information system on chemicals/stressors and their effects.

genes, metabolic and toxicological pathways, and associated phenotypic information, observed in datasets for hits (i.e., compounds that display similar effects in multiple tissues and species, and the dose, time, and phenotypic severity with which these effects are observed). This will be possible because all probe sets and analytically determined proteins for each gene represented in the knowledge will be sequence-aligned to gene models. With the expected high quality data content, CEBS will rapidly become an important scientific resource that provides users with the suite of tools needed to interpret toxicogenomics data and a toxicological reference information system with which to model biological responses across species.

As compendia of expression profiles are indexed and compared in order to discern diagnostic signatures, it will become increasingly possible to characterize an unknown physical or chemical exposure by comparing its gene or protein expression profile to profiles in the database. Joint research by scientists at the NIEHS Microarray Group (NMG) and Boehringer-Ingelheim Pharmaceuticals has shown that global gene expression profiles for chemicals from different mode-of-action classes can provide gene expression 'signatures' of chemical exposures in male rats (Hamadeh et al. 2002b, a). These studies were performed on acutely exposed animals, and the expression patterns appear to be representative of the adaptive or pharmacologic activity of the chemicals. Using a small training set, Hamadeh et al. (2002b) were able to correctly ascertain chemical class signatures based on pattern recognition of acutely induced genes. This study, in essence, validated the toxicogenomics hypothesis that knowledge can be gained regarding the nature of blinded samples using an initial training set of chemicals.

10.2
NCT Intramural Research

Current NCT research aims to formally discriminate between 'chemical signatures' reflecting early adaptive or pharmacological responses with no ensuing pathology and 'effects signatures' that entail altered tissue steady state, toxicity, histopathology, or disease (Bartosiewicz et al. 2001). We are therefore in the process of developing learning sets of genomic profiling data for various classes of agents, with doses ranging from those that are pharmacologic to those that are toxic. We also intend to perform comparative studies that address cross-species differences in toxicological responses as well as susceptibility differences in human subgroups.

The combined and integrated data on gene/protein/metabolite changes collected in the context of dose, time, target tissue, and phenotypic severity across species will provide the interpretive information needed to define the molecular basis for chemical toxicity and to model the resulting toxicological and pathological outcomes (Boorman et al. 2002). It should then be feasible to search for evidence of exposure or injury prior to any clinical or pathological manifestation, facilitating identification of early biomarkers of exposure, toxic injury, or susceptibility. It is anticipated that toxicogenomics research will lead to the identification, measurement, and evaluation of biomarkers that are more accurate, quantitative, and specific. These biomarkers will be recognized as important factors in a sequence of key events that will help to define the way in which specific chemicals or environmental exposures cause disease. In other words, toxicogenomics should help to delineate the mode of action of various classes of agents and the unique attributes of certain species and population subgroups that make them susceptible to toxicants, as an important step in comparatively assessing potential human health risk (Farland 1992).

NCT intramural scientists are now performing additional proof-of-concept experiments that are designed to establish how 'effects signatures' can be defined and to link the patterns of altered gene expression to specific parameters of well defined conventional indices of toxicity. For example, experiments can be designed to correlate gene expression patterns with liver pathologies such as hepatomegaly, hepatocellular necrosis, or inflammation. It is also possible to look for correlative patterns, for example, in enzyme levels in liver and other tissues or cells such as blood. Changes in serum enzymes provide diagnostic markers of organ function that are commonly used in medicine and toxicology. This 'phenotypic anchoring' of gene expression data to conventional indices removes some of the subjectivity of conventional molecular expression analyses and helps to distinguish the toxicological signal from other gene expression changes that may be unrelated to toxicity, such as the varied pharmacological or therapeutic effects of a compound (Tennant 2002).

Future NCT studies will define molecular perturbations caused by environmental chemicals in terms of phenotypic severity, dose, and time (Hamadeh 2002 c). We will explore quantitative or absolute gene expression profiling (Dudley et al. 2002) and consider combining such an approach with physiologically based pharmacokinetic (PB/PK) and pharmacodynamic modelling. PB/PK modelling can be used to derive a quantitative estimate of target tissue dose at any time after treatment, thus creating the possibility to anchor molecular expression profiles in internal dose, as well as in time and phenotypic severity. Relationships among gene, protein, and metabolite expression may then be described as a function of the applied dose of an agent and the ensuing kinetic and dynamic dose–response behaviour in various tissue compartments. In addition, the species under study and interspecies interindividual differences must be taken into account. With the aid of the knowledge systematically generated and assembled (Zweiger 1999) through literature mining, comparative analysis, and iterative biological modelling of molecular expression datasets over time, the adaptive responses of biological systems will be differentiated from those changes that are associated with or precede clinical or visible adverse effects. We anticipate that our understanding of mechanisms of toxicity and disease will improve as these new methods are used more extensively and toxicogenomics databases are developed more fully. The expected result will be the emergence of toxicology as an information science that will enable thorough analysis, iterative modelling, and discovery across biological species and chemical classes. CEBS will be designed to meet the information and modelling requirements of an integrated systems toxicology, as illustrated conceptually in Figure 10.2.

Key priorities for NCT intramural toxicogenomics studies are the profiling of specific compounds and disease processes that lead to target organ toxicities (e.g., hepato- and nephrotoxicity). These studies will entertain the following considerations, and emphasis will be placed on the early steps in the disease processes. Multiple compounds that elicit a particular hepato- or nephrotoxicity will be studied at mul-

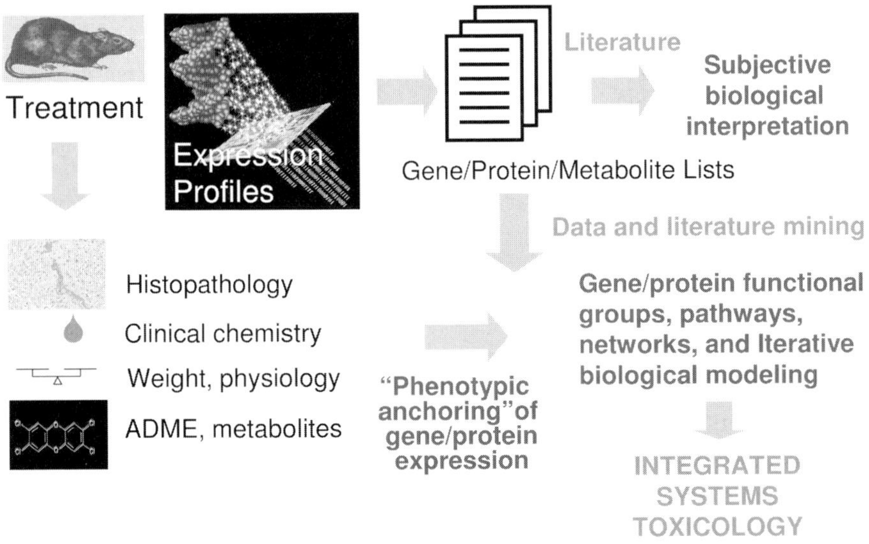

Fig. 10.2 Interpretation of molecular expression profiles with literature mining, phenotypic anchoring, and iterative biological modelling for systems toxicology. ADME refers to absorption, distribution, metabolism and excretion.

tiple sampling times following exposure. Subtoxic as well as toxic doses will be used, and nontoxic isomers and related compounds will be included to assess the specificity of effects observed. Drugs and chemicals will be selected for study based on criteria such as human exposure and recent toxicology studies demonstrating consistent cross-species effects. Ideally, a drug will show a therapeutic effect and chemicals will display mechanism(s) of toxicity that are prototypical for other agents, including those in our proof-of-concept studies. For example, acetaminophen or paracetamol is the first agent to be studied comprehensively by the NCT. Its selection was based on an extensive literature (Bessems and Vermeulen 2001) showing that its liver toxicity is a common response in rodents and in humans, its metabolism is similar in rodents and in humans, it displays both therapeutic and toxic effects, and there are opportunities for clinical investigation. Furthermore, it has been studied using toxicogenomic methods by several laboratories (Cunningham et al. 2000; Reilly et al. 2001 a,b; Ruepp et al. 2002; Yamazaki et al. 2002), offering the possibility of comparative assessment of observed molecular expression, toxicology, and pathology.

10.3
Toxicogenomics Research Partnerships

The magnitude and complexity of the science underlying the broad goals of the NCT is such that no one organization has the technical, fiscal, or intellectual resources with which to solely accomplish them. A central strategy of the NCT is therefore the development of partnerships with universities, other federal research and regulatory agencies, and the private sector through the formation of consortia that will address critical scientific challenges in toxicogenomics. The NCT is in fact a synergistic collaboration between intramural and extramural scientists based on research partnerships.

Operating under a National Institutes of Health cooperative agreement mechanism, the Toxicogenomics Research Consortium (TRC) is a key model for achieving the strategic objectives of the NCT. The TRC consists of five academic centres in addition to the NMG. They are Duke University, the Frederick Hutchinson Cancer Research Center of the University of Washington, Massachusetts Institute of Technology, the Oregon Health and Science University, and the University of North Carolina at Chapel Hill. The consortium members provide specialized expertise in gene expression profiling and bioinformatics; they will perform both independent and cooperative research on various aspects of toxicogenomics. In the current state of gene expression technology, there are various methodologies for arraying genes and for assessing mRNA expression and multiple bioinformatics tools that are being applied in the analysis and management of such data. Therefore, an initial goal of the TRC is to perform a series of standardization experiments for gene expression, to address sources of variation, to develop standard practices, and to establish data quality criteria and bioinformatics standards. Initial proof-of-concept experiments are being performed to assess the ability of the consortium members to perform standardized toxicogenomics experiments and to exchange and interpret data across multiple microarray platforms. Data generated from such experiments will be incorporated into the CEBS knowledge base and ultimately will be used to design further hypothesis-driven research. The TRC will build on these standardization experiments in performing additional collaborative studies to investigate molecular responses to various environmental stressors. The TRC is now fully operational and is presently receiving database support through the NCT's CEBS knowledge base contractor, Science Applications International Corporation (SAIC), and microarray analysis and bioinformatics support through Paradigm Genetics. SAIC has begun to receive datasets from the TRC and from Paradigm Genetics for deposition into CEBS. These efforts of the TRC and CEBS contractors will make a unique contribution to the field of toxicogenomics and to the quality of the CEBS knowledge base. CEBS will house data from NIEHS intramural and extramural research programs and will accept high-quality datasets from other federal, academic, and industrial partners.

The NCT is also participating in a second consortium that deals with many of the same platform and bioinformatics issues as the TRC, with the Health and Environmental Sciences Institute of the International Life Sciences Institute (ILSI HESI; http://hesi.ilsi.org/). ILSI HESI is coordinating the efforts of approximately 30 pharmaceutical companies in a worldwide effort to harmonize cross-platform gene expression data and analysis methods. The ILSI Genomics Project has focused on three categories of toxicants: *in vivo* hepatotoxins, *in vivo* nephrotoxins, and *in vitro* genotoxins. The NCT has been involved in the former two categories of study in which animals were dosed, tissues were taken for histopathology and RNA extraction, and RNA samples were then distributed to participating laboratories for microarray analysis using methods chosen by the respective participating laboratories. This type of collaboration has minimized problems associated with RNA extraction and quality control issues and provided a basis for direct comparisons among various microarray platforms.

10.4 Microarray Analysis

Microarray data resulting from intramural NCT toxicogenomics experiments are currently captured in the NIEHS MicroArray Project System (MAPS). MAPS is a laboratory management information system developed at NIEHS (Bushel et al. 2001) in which ~40 data fields are defined to manage microarray project information; detail experimental design; track clones, sample preparation, labelling, and hybridization; and survey the quality control and assurance of processed microarray chips. The NMG currently produces a Yeast Chip v. 1 (6.2 K clones) and four mammalian chips: the Human ToxChip v. 3. (2.2 K clones), the Rat ToxChip v. 2. (6.8 K clones), and human and mouse oligonucleotide discovery chips (17.0 K and 16.0 K oligonucleotides, respectively). Gene accession numbers for each gene or EST on each chip are automatically updated biweekly at http://www.ncbi.nlm.nih.gov/UniGene/to reflect the current build of the National Center for Biotechnology Information (NCBI) Uni-

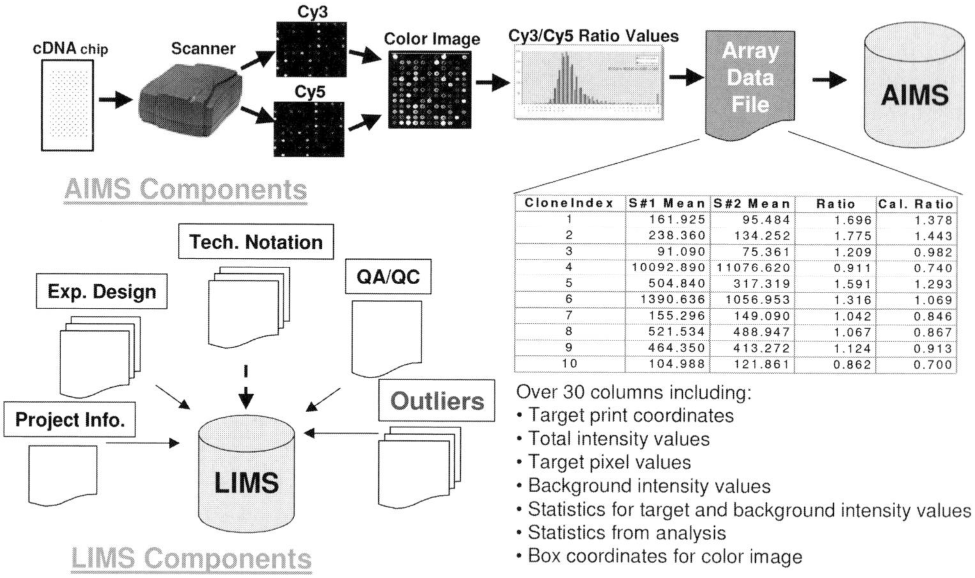

Fig. 10.3 Components of the microarray image and data analysis process. AIMS = analysis information management system; LIMS = laboratory information management system

Gene. Hundreds of thousands of novel EST sequences have been included in NCBI's UniGene. NMG cDNA chips include a substantial proportion of ESTs, thus offering the potential to discover novel genes involved in important biological or toxicological outcomes and disease processes. To provide some perspective on the information management requirements of gene expression analysis, the image and data analysis processes for microarray experiments are illustrated in Figure 10.3.

10.5 Implementation of a CEBS Prototype

With the assistance of the NIEHS Computer Technology Branch, the NCT has implemented a prototype version of the CEBS database through the application and integration of software developed for the NMG and the National Toxicology Program (NTP). Toxicology and pathology data from intramural NCT toxicogenomics experiments are currently being captured in an Oracle database by the NTP's Toxicology Database Management System (TDMS) and are being integrated with microarray gene expression data (Figure 10.4).

Prototype CEBS (Model A, Figure 10.4) is a temporary workbench for concept definition and systems integration in the development of CEBS. Nevertheless, this model provides early Internet access to NCT datasets and will implement software applications and statistical server routines required to analyze microarray data and

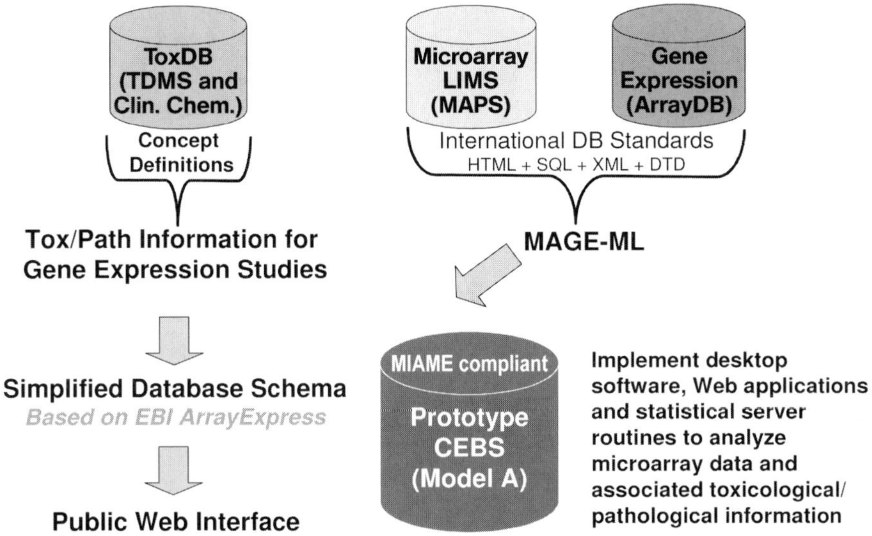

Fig. 10.4 Prototype CEBS (model A).
TDMS = toxicology database management system, MAPS = microarray project system, HTML = hypertext markup language, SQL = structured query language, XML = extensible markup language, DTD = document type definition, MAGE–ML = microarray gene expression markup language, MIAME = minimum information about a micro array experiment.

associated toxicological information. It will provide minimal information about a microarray experiment (Brazma et al. 2001) and support the MIAME 1.1 specification (http://www.mged.org/Workgroups/MIAME/miame_1.1.html) of the Microarray Gene Expression Database (MGED) Society (http://www.mged.org/). Many additional database standards are under review for use in the development of CEBS, but perhaps the most important ones are those under the purview of MGED. MGED has expert working groups on: (1) experimental description and data representation standards; (2) microarray data XML exchange format (CEBS will use MGED MAGE-ML data exchange formats based on the MAGE-OM object model); (3) ontology (Karp 2000) for sample description (CEBS will follow the MGED core ontology and the gene ontologies of the Gene Ontology Consortium at http://www.geneontology.org/ for biological process, molecular function, and cellular component); (4) normalization, quality markup control, and cross-platform comparison; and (5) future user group queries, query language, and data mining, all of which are providing important input for the development of CEBS.

In embracing the MGED standards, the NCT has partnered with the European Bioinformatics Institute (EBI; http://www.ebi.ac.uk/microarray/) in the UK, the International Life Sciences Institute's Health and Environmental Sciences Institute (ILSI HESI; http://hesi.ilsi.org/) in the USA, and the Technical Committee on the Application of Genomics to Mechanism Based Risk Assessment to initiate the development of guidelines for describing toxicogenomics experiments (MIAME/Tox). The

MIAME/Tox document (available at http://www.mged.org/) has been drafted by the three partners and is based on the MIAME 1.1 (minimum information about microarray experiments) specification produced by the MGED Society. The goal of MIAME 1.1 (http://www.mged.org/Workgroups/MIAME/miame_1.1.html) is to outline the minimum annotation required to unambiguously interpret and potentially reproduce and verify array-based gene expression experiments. MIAME concentrates on information and provides a conceptual framework for microarray experiment descriptions. MIAME/Tox extends MIAME to provide a toxicogenomics annotation framework that captures sufficient and structured information for toxicogenomics experiments to correctly retrieve, analyze, and interpret the data or to replicate the experiments. MIAME/Tox annotation information for gene expression experiments includes fields for free text format along with information to be provided by maximum use of controlled vocabularies or external ontologies (such as species taxonomy, cell types, anatomy terms, histopathology, clinical chemistry, toxicology, and chemical compound nomenclature). A major additional objective of MIAME/Tox is to guide the development of toxicogenomics databases and data management software.

10.6
Systems Toxicology: Bioinformatics and Interpretive Challenges

To develop a toxicogenomics knowledge base that will support the requirements of systems toxicology, we must address bioinformatics and interpretive challenges at multiple levels of biological organization and phenotypic severity. Figure 10.5 illustrates some of these challenges as molecular expression analysis is used to monitor, after exposure to a chemical, the sequential adaptive, pharmacological, toxicological, and pathological events that are observable in biological systems.

The lower levels of complexity (genes, gene groups, functional pathways) reflect our current levels of understanding and our ability to describe and package that knowledge using what might be termed linear bioinformatics. In fact, risk assessors seek to define a sequence of key events and common (linear) modes of action for environmental chemicals and drugs (Farland 1992, 1996; Larsen et al. 2000). The networks and systems level of biological organization reflects global bioinformatics challenges,

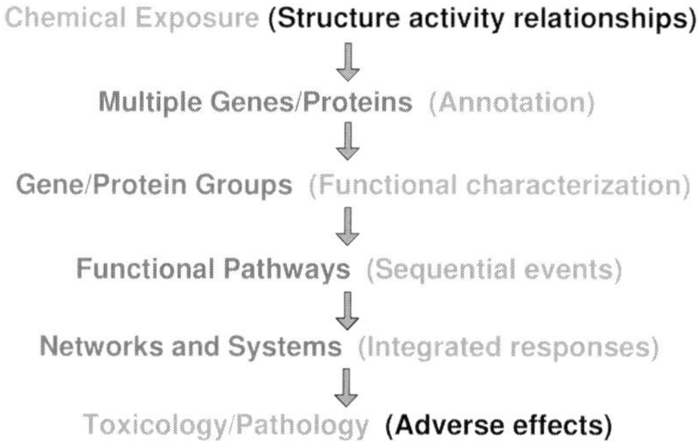

Fig. 10.5 Interpretive bioinformatics challenges at levels of increasing biological complexity in a paradigm leading from chemical exposure to adverse outcomes.

wherein the cell expresses global changes constantly in response to environmental stimuli. This is a systems biology reality that can be addressed only by using fully context-documented toxicogenomics datasets properly assembled with appropriate statistical and mathematical modelling to develop an integrated systems toxicology. There is, however, a substantial amount of data entry, data processing, and knowledge building that must be performed before such advanced bioinformatics approaches can be applied. It should be recognized that the development of a knowledge base to accurately reflect global molecular expression and to aid to systems biological interpretation is a complex issue that is dealt with only superficially in the present discussion. Keeping these challenges and concepts in mind, below we present some conceptual arguments regarding the phased development of the CEBS knowledge base – a process that undoubtedly will require a decade or more to complete. Progress in the development of CEBS can be monitored at http://www.niehs. nih.gov/nct/.

However, we first need to present information in the area of understanding the function of biomarkers of toxic outcomes that may become apparent in global gene expression studies. The next section reflects our current thinking about ways to address this problem.

10.7 Understanding Functions of Biomarkers

Microarray technology provides investigators with powerful methods for identifying biomarkers and potential new targets for experimental therapeutics. However, many of the biomarkers and new targets are unvalidated genes/ESTs or hypothetical proteins. A novel bioinformatics tool will be developed with the CEBS for understanding functions of unvalidated genes and hypothetical proteins, using an integrated approach to five types of biomedical information resources: (1) microarray expression profile comparison, (2) coevolutionary profile comparison, (3) domain fusion analysis, (4) structural analysis, and (5) text mining in MEDLINE. The general strategy is demonstrated in Figure 10.6.

10.7.1 Microarray Expression Profile Analysis

There is a reasonably large amount of microarray expression data available in the public domain. Gene expression clustering is useful in addressing these datasets in at least three ways: (1) extraction of regulatory motifs (coregulation from coexpression); (2) inference of functional annotation; and (3) as a molecular signature in distinguishing cell or tissue types. In this approach, the gene expression data are utilized to find functional hits for an unvalidated gene or a hypothetical protein through expression profile comparison across all experiments. An expression profile is usually a 2D or 3D matrix associated with time points, doses, and chemicals. Functional hits (close neighbours) can be detected by comparing the expression profile of a query with that of all other known genes.

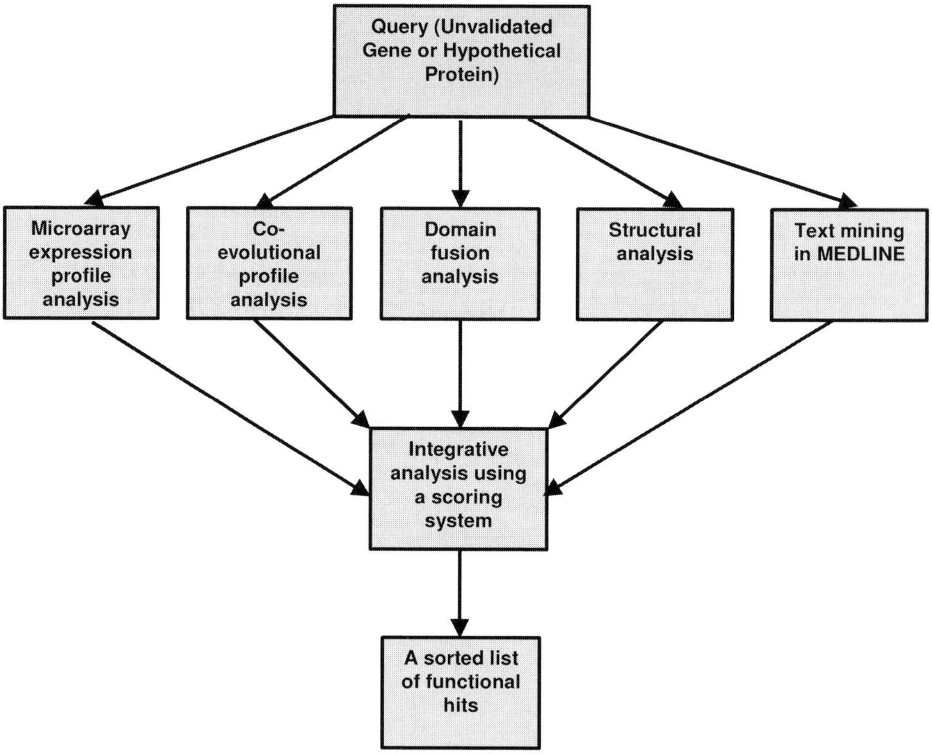

Fig. 10.6 The architecture of the novel bioinformatics system for annotating (invalidated genes) and hypothetical proteins.

10.7.2
Coevolutional Profile Analysis

Functional hits (close neighbours) can be obtained by comparing the coevolutionary profile of the hypothetical gene and that of all other known genes. A coevolutionary profile of a gene is a positive vector, in which the value of each coordinate is $\frac{1}{\log^2 E}$, where E is the lowest E value reported by BLAST in a search against a complete genome. Two genes in an organism can have similar coevolutionary profiles for one of two reasons. First, genes with a high level of sequence similarity will have, by definition, similar coevolutionary profiles: the Euclidean distance (the sum of squares) between the coevolutionary profile vector of two genes is less than a cutoff value. Second, for two genes that lack sequence similarity, a similarity in coevolutionary profiles reflects a similar pattern of occurrence of their homologs across species. This coupled inheritance may indicate a functional link between the genes, on the hypothesis that the genes are always present together or always both absent because they cannot function independently of one another. The profiles in CEBS will be constructed using complete genomes, collected from the NCBI's COGs website (http://www.ncbi.nlm.nih.gov/COG/).

10.7.3 Domain Fusion Analysis

Functional hits will be found for inferring gene function and interactions from genome sequences based on the observation that some pairs of interacting genes have homologs in another organism fused into a single gene chain (domain with unknown functions fused with other known domains, especially in microbial genomes). Fusion links between genes can be found by a BLAST search of the translated sequences against nrdb90 (http://www.ebi.ac.uk/~holm/nrdb90/), a representative composite of major protein sequence databases in which no two sequences have sequence identity $\geq 90\%$. Two genes are considered to be fusion-linked if each has an alignment of at least 70 residues to the same nrdb90 protein with a maximum expectation value of 10^{-10} and with a maximum overlap of 15 residues between the two alignments.

10.7.4 Structural Analysis

The following powerful protein structure prediction software tools will be applied to predict the structure of a query:

- Threader (http://www.hgmp.mrc.ac.uk/Registered/Option/threader.html).
- LIBRA I (http://www.ddbj.nig.ac.jp/E-mail/libra/LIBRA_I.html).
- PEDANT (http://pedant.gsf.de/).
- SAPS (http://www.isrec.isb-sib.ch/software/SAPS_form.html).

Then an 'integrated' structure will be detected based on four predicted structures by using the computational geometry technique. Functional hits of the query will be obtained by a VAST search (a vector alignment search tool; http://www.ncbi.nlm.nih.gov/Structure/VAST/vast.shtml) against the PDB database.

10.7.5 Text Mining in MEDLINE Based on Literature Profile Comparison

A 'literature profile' of a query is defined by the information indexed from its SwissProt record. The description, comments, and keywords in the record will be gathered. Then, the record's MEDLINE cross references will be retrieved. The literature of the query is defined as the concatenation of these unstructured texts. After literature is gathered for each sequence, a list of domain-specific stop words will be generated; these are words containing little information for identifying the sequences. The classic vector–cosine model of text retrieval is employed and is also part of the algorithm used to compute 'related articles' for PubMed (http://ncbi.nlm.nih.gov/PubMed/). That is, the similarity score between the literature profiles of two genes is computed using a vector cosine measure. In this model, texts are represented as a vector in which each coordinate corresponds to the number of frequencies a word occurs in a text. Texts are tokenized utilizing all nonalphanumeric characters as delimiters. All words that are not stop words are then converted to lowercased tokens. The distance between two texts X and Y is defined as the cosine of the angle between their word vectors $\mathbf{v}(X)$ and $\mathbf{v}(Y)$: $d(X,Y) = 1 - \cos\theta\,(\mathbf{v}(X), \mathbf{v}(Y))$. Then functional hits will be detected by comparing the literature profiles of the query with that of all known genes.

10.7.6
Integrative Analysis

A global evaluating procedure will be designed for the tool to determine a final ranked list of hits in accordance with an intuition that those hits that appear on multiple lists and are located in the upper level of each list are more significant and meaningful. Finally, a sorting order of significant, meaningful, functional hits will be given and users can select the top 5–30 hits on the list for their further curation and annotation (see Figure 10.6).

10.8
Phased Development of the CEBS Knowledge Base

The CEBS knowledge base will be developed in four substantially overlapping phases: Phase I involves the gathering of microarray gene expression and toxicology/pathology data and the development of gene and protein annotation and bioinformatics tools. Phase II incorporates corresponding proteomics datasets with similar annotation and bioinformatics tools and develops a temporary proteomics database. Phase III integrates gene, protein and, ideally, metabolite databases and links them with numerous Internet resources for metabolic and functional pathway discovery. Phase IV adds two additional databases, one for gene/protein groups and one for SNPs to what is described above. The three databases then are integrated with a series of bioinformatics tools (data and literature mining) and computational algorithms designed to generate new knowledge.

10.8.1
CEBS Phase I: Microarray/Gene Expression Data, Toxicology/Pathology Data and Associated Analysis Tools

CEBS Phase I will be a public toxicogenomics database containing datasets from the TRC, the intramural NCT research program, and industrial and governmental partners. It will be composed mainly of microarray and toxicology data and information. To assist the TRC in populating CEBS with microarray data, the NCT awarded a resource contract to provide access to high-throughput microarray gene expression analysis. As illustrated in Figure 10.7, CEBS Phase I will track all microarray techni-

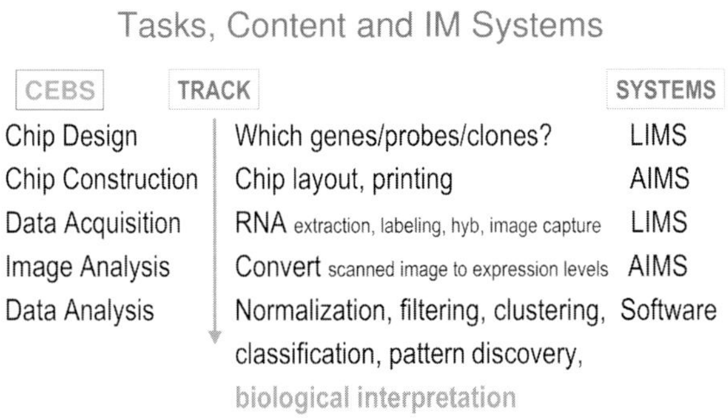

Fig. 10.7 Microarray experimental components – information management (IM) systems for data acquisition and biological interpretation.

cal and experimental components relating to chip design and construction, data acquisition, image analysis, and data analysis. It will also track clone set gene sequences, descriptors, and other genomic annotations, as well as associated toxicological/pathological endpoints, and will provide basic bioinformatics tools for data analysis and biological interpretation.

CEBS Phase I will be protocol-driven. All datasets within CEBS will be linked by reference to an experimental protocol number and metadata that will specify standard operating procedures, observations, and measurements to be recorded. CEBS Phase I will include complete sample annotation (e. g., sample name, organism, biosource provider, sample source, developmental stage, age and units, time points, organ/tissue, growth conditions, medium, culture temperature, genetic variation, individual name or ID, disease state, additional clinical information and units, target cell type, cell line, treatment application, treatment type, separation technique, sample extraction method, amplification method, label, etc.). All the data types (numbers, graphs, observations, images, etc.) will be related by the experimental protocol. The data to be stored and their location will be similarly identified in the process of defining the experimental protocol, as will reports to be generated and analyses to be performed. The purpose of this high degree of context documentation is to facilitate extensive query and biological interpretation. Domain-specific metadata will introduce experimental datasets in each analytical domain: transcriptomics, toxicology, pathology, etc. CEBS Phase I will incorporate raw microarray image files as well as fully processed outlier gene lists, together with appropriate visualization tools. Results will be displayed or juxtaposed in various views or graphic user interfaces that will provide insights, facilitate further analysis, and suggest new hypotheses to test.

CEBS also will access biological, chemical, and toxicological resources in public domain databases, as well as pathway information such as that available in the Kyoto Encyclopedia of Genes and Genomes (KEGG) at http://www.genome.ad.jp/kegg/ (Ogata et al. 1999) and in "What Is There?" (WIT) at http://wit.mcs.anl.gov/WIT2/ (Selkov et al. 1998). Links will be built to other databases such as the European Bioinformatics Institute ArrayExpress database (http://www.ebi.ac.uk/microarray/

ArrayExpress/arrayexpress.html), the National Library of Medicine's GEO Database or Gene Expression Omnibus at http://www.ncbi.nlm.nih.gov/geo/(Edgar et al. 2002), and the NTP's new Oracle toxicology information bank.

To address the first of the bioinformatics and interpretive challenges mentioned above, basic gene annotation in CEBS Phase I will be largely automated, and annotation resources will be routinely consulted to provide a complete range of updated gene/protein information. The process of gene annotation is illustrated in Figure 10.8, and some major biological data and information resources for gene annotation are shown in Table 10.1. The links for these annotation resources were operational at the time of writing this chapter. However, please consult the NCT website at http://www.niehs.nih.gov/nct/for a current list of links.

Continuous refinement of gene annotation and sequence definition will improve the interoperability of cross-platform datasets (Zweiger 1999). Steps for keeping sequence data current can be as follows: (1) sequence all cDNA clone sets and refer to the known sequences of oligonucleotide sets, (2) reference GenBank accession numbers and UniGene ID numbers for genes and GenBank accession numbers and dbEST cluster ID numbers for ESTs, (3) reference TIGR gene indices (http://www.tigr.org/tdb/tgi.shtml) Quackenbush et al. 2001) for EST or oligonucleotide consensus sequence and perform a MegaBLAST against trace archives for genomes of interest. Performing a MegaBLAST against trace archives means to compare nucleotide sequence data against the current raw data underlying first-pass sequences generated by various genome sequencing centres. This is particularly important for the rat genome, which is presently very incomplete. This effort to derive new information about incomplete genomes will substantially enhance the discovery value of ESTs on cDNA chips and will facilitate cross-species investigation of gene/protein functional analogies, as will be discussed.

Functional characterization presents a second bioinformatics and interpretive challenge. Functional characterization can involve the grouping of similar genes and

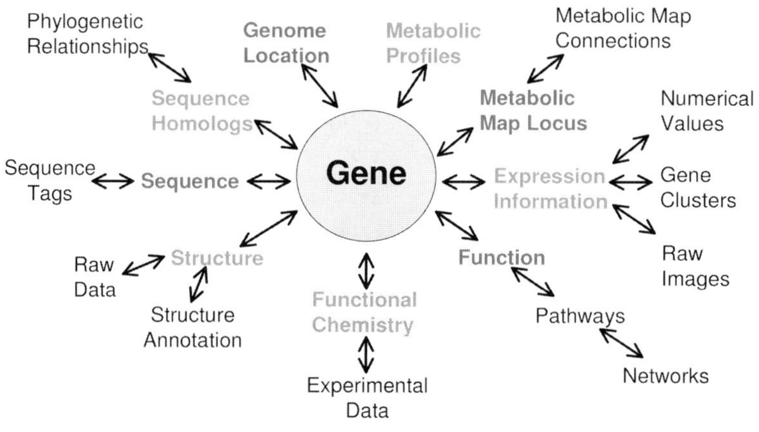

Fig. 10.8 Information (annotation) associated with a single gene (adapted from Gibas and Jambeck 2001).

Tab. 10.1 Some major biological data and information resources for gene annotation.

Subject	*Source*	*URL*
Biomedical literature	PubMed	http://www.ncbi.nlm.nih.gov/entrez/query.fcgil
Nucleic acid sequence (e.g., for the rat)	GenBank	http://www.ncbi.nlm.nih.gov/entrez/query.fcgi?db=nucleotide
	RGD	http://rgd.mcw.edu/ebEST http://rgd.mcw.edu/EBEST/
Annotation		http://www.tigr.org/ http://biodas.org/
Genome sequence	GenBank	http://www.ncbi.nlm.nih.gov/entrez/query.fcgi?db=genome http://www.ncbi.nih.gov/PMGifs/Genomes/euk_g.html
	TIGR	http://www.tigr.org/tdb/ http://www.tigr.org/tdb/tgi/
Protein sequence	GenBank SwissProt	http://www.ncbi.nlm.nih.gov/entrez/query.fcgi?db=protein http://www.expasy.ch/sprot/
Protein structure	Protein DB PIR	http://www.rcsb.org/pdb/ http://www-nbrf.georgetown.edu
Protein mass spectra	PROWL	http://prowl.rockefeller.edu
Post-translational modifications	RESID	http://www-nbrf.georgetown.edu/pirwww/search/textresid.html
Biochemical pathways	KEGG WIT PathDB	http://www.genome.ad.jp/kegg/ http://wit.mcs.anl.gov/WIT2/ http://emp.mcs.anl.gov http://www.ncgr.org/software/pathdb/

gene products. There are a number of conventional means to accomplish this, including supervised and unsupervised classification/predicttion, artificial intelligence, various genetic algorithms, as well as a number of annotation resources, as just discussed. We propose to use these methods and resources in concert with querying the scientific literature to develop knowledge of the function of genes and gene products.

Literature queries can facilitate gene annotation as well as biological interpretation of microarray expression results. The challenge is to deal not only with accepted microarray gene annotation names but also with legacy data in the earlier scientific literature, with the ultimate objective of making linkages of gene and protein annotations with literature based on sequence information. MEDLINE is the most widely accessible repository of biomedical literature, currently containing over 11 million abstracts and growing rapidly. Unfortunately, it is difficult to use the gene name found in a nucleotide sequence database record (or as presented in a list of outliers) to search the biomedical literature effectively.

The generation of names for genes and gene products based on sequence information is a significant challenge. Ultimately, genes and gene products must be linked by sequence data. Sequence-based synonym naming requires expertise in both data extraction and bioinformatics. Expertise in bioinformatics is required, since much of the searching will need to be done using BLAST (http://www.ncbi.nlm.nih.gov/BLAST/) (Altschul et al. 1990). Genomic BLAST pages are available for human, mouse, rat, zebra fish, and other eukaryotic and microbial genomes at the NCBI's BLAST website.

Nucleotide sequence databases, e.g., GenBank and UniGene, do not contain a 'gene product' name field. Instead, the name is imbedded in other information. For example, the GenBank nucleotide definition for 'Estrogen Receptor 1' (the HUGO recognized name for this receptor) is 'Homo sapiens estrogen receptor 1 (ESR1), mRNA'. Extraction of the appropriate search terms 'Estrogen Receptor 1' and 'ESR1' from the GenBank definition is a trivial task, but one that becomes intractable when a large number of genes or protein products are being searched in the literature or when the process is being automated, as is being contemplated in the development of the CEBS knowledge base.

To improve the interoperability between microarray gene annotation and the scientific literature, all genes in the clone lists are being provided with vetted name lists. By vetting, we mean that each gene name is searched in MEDLINE, and the way in which MEDLINE parses the name is examined to ensure that it is being searched in the desired manner. For example, searching MEDLINE via Entrez (http://www.ncbi.nlm.nih.gov/Entrez/) with the query phrase 'Estrogen Receptor 1' does not return any abstracts. Closer inspection of the search results indicates that this is because this phrase does not occur in the MEDLINE phrase index. The vast literature (more than 10 000 abstracts) concerning this receptor is only accessible with the legacy names of 'Estrogen Receptor' and 'Estrogen Receptor alpha'.

Once name lists suitable for searching MEDLINE are available, we have two tools to help mine the literature data, OmniViz and PDQ_MED. OmniViz (Battelle Memorial Laboratory, Columbus, OH, USA) is a global literature search and visualization software package that can be of great help in obtaining an overview of relevant biomedical publications. The proximity-of-data query software, InPharmix's PDQ_MED (Sluka 2002), can facilitate rapid access to relevant abstracts in MEDLINE for multiple genes (e.g., from a list of outliers).

In CEBS Phase I, a database of gene identifiers, gene sequences, and synonym names suitable for searching the scientific literature will be available; such a database is currently in beta test at NIEHS for human, mouse, rat, and yeast chips printed at the NMG. An Internet interface to the database will be provided, allowing CEBS users to enter a chip name and a list of gene IDs or GenBank accession numbers. The output from the interface will be a list of names suitable for searching in MEDLINE or for use with literature-mining tools such as PDQ_MED or OmniViz. This is an important step toward improving the interoperability between microarray gene annotations and the scientific literature and, ultimately, toward building knowledge in CEBS. We have only begun to determine the optimal approaches to tackle the problems at hand that impede progress in functional annotation.

10.8.2
CEBS Phase II: Protein Expression Database and Metabolomics Datasets

The proteomics efforts within the NCT consist of an intramural research program, a proteomics resource contract, and extramural and innovative research grant awards in proteomics. The close association of the NCT Microarray and Proteomics research groups and the NTP provides a unique opportunity for integrating genomics, proteomics, and toxicology datasets. The Proteomics Group and Mass Spectrometry Group perform hypothesis-driven research on differentially expressed proteins in key tissues and biological fluids of interest to toxicogenomics. A primary platform for separating and identifying proteins used by NCT Proteomics research groups is two-dimensional (2D) gel separation of proteins and mass spectrometry (MS) or 2D-MS. Analysis by 2D-MS creates protein maps in which proteins for a specific tissue are organized by isoelectric point (pI) and molecular weight (MW). To assist the NCT in populating CEBS with proteomics data, the NCT has awarded a proteomics resource contract to Large Scale Biology Corporation that will allow access to high-throughput 2D-MS capabilities on an industrial scale. Critical target tissue and serum from toxicology studies will be analyzed for differential protein expression. As discussed earlier, a primary goal of NCT intramural and contract proteomic studies is biomarker discovery for proteins (including serum/plasma proteins) that are indicative of chemical exposure and/or provide mechanistic insight into chemical toxicity. Therefore, concurrent analysis of serum/plasma will be performed in addition to specific target organs for each study.

In addition to 2D-MS proteomics, a new platform called SELDI or surface-enhanced laser desorption ionization is being developed intramurally to screen serum from experimental animals and clinical sources to find new biomarkers (Issaq et al. 2002). Serum proteins are selectively bound to chemically active surfaces on SELDI 'biochips' and rapidly scanned with high mass accuracy. The normalized serum mass spectra from chemical-treatment or disease groups can be compared for differences in specific proteins or in key clusters of protein masses, to find appropriate biomarkers for chemical exposure or a disease process. Two other important aspects of NCT proteomics are the extramural proteomics granting activities through the Division of Extramural Research (DERT) and the Small Business Innovation Research (SBIR) awards that will engage promising academic research projects in proteomics and also harness new innovative proteomics technologies for toxicology.

Many of the standards and practices used in the interpretation of microarray and gene expression are also applicable to the interpretation of protein expression datasets. Thus, the object model, MAGE-OM, built by MGED for microarray gene expression databases also will be applicable to proteomics and possibly metabonomics. Proteomics objects that will be linked in a linear chain by one-to-many relationships include the biological sample, raw 2D stained gel image, enzyme digest, feature number (protein spot), MW, pI, mass spectrum for MALDI MS, m/z ions for protein fingerprint identification, sequence tag from tandem MS analysis, MS search data results, and protein identification search results. The derived objects that will be included are the study parameters including experimental, biological, and toxicological details; processed gel images; annotated master gel images for each specific tissue or biological fluid; list of differentially expressed proteins determined from image analysis; and feature (protein spot) table of estimated pI, MW, accession numbers, and protein functional groups. As an important contribution to the development of toxicogenomics database infrastructure, the NCT has just released the CEBS MAGE Proteomics-OM (http://cebs.niehs.nih.gov/protein/), which is able to capture proteomics domain information analogous to that specified by MIAME. SAIC has extended the MAGE-OM to model proteomic data and has integrated elements of the protein expression model PEDRo (http://pedrodownload.man.ac.uk/) developed to capture minimum information for protein expression datasets. It is believed that making gene expression and proteomics data accessible via a uniform, cross-technology object model will facilitate the development and reuse of software to analyze and display data across disciplines. The model should be extended easily to capture new types of expression experiments in other biological disciplines.

10.8.3 CEBS Phase III: Integrate Microarray/Gene Expression and Protein Expression Databases using a Gene/Protein Group Strategy

The integration of microarray/gene expression and protein expression data is a critical step that will require development of knowledge of gene/protein functional relationships and gene/protein groups and the development of algorithms that will increase our knowledge of the functions of these groups through actual experimentation. To build knowledge, we will mine the published literature for genes and groups of functionally related genes or protein products that are relevant to known endpoints in toxicology, pathology, cell regulatory processes, metabolism, and the like. This literature mining and analysis process will utilize vetted gene names, and the output will be groups of genes/proteins that represent putative functional groups based on the literature. We will then develop algorithms to test these putative functional gene groups derived from the literature against treatment-related expression profiles and against clustered genes (and coregulated ESTs) to confirm gene grouping based on phenotype, as illustrated in Figure 10.9.

This literature-based functional classification of gene groups and their association with known toxicant-responsive pathways will begin to define the relationships between gene and protein expression and our conventional understanding of metabolism, toxicology/pathology, modulation and homeostasis, cell regulation, and cell signalling. It will also offer an opportunity for discovery of yet-unidentified genes (ESTs) that are coregulated with known genes.

To the extent possible, we will confirm gene group membership by sequence analysis, and we will develop statistical procedures and algorithms (Wolfinger et al. 2001) to continually refine our knowledge of gene/protein groups and their relationship to functional pathways. With full sequence definition of all genes, proteins, and gene/protein group members, it will be possible to begin to BLAST outlier genes and proteins from new experimental datasets against datasets already contained in the CEBS database. This will begin to facilitate and inform the integration of transcriptomics

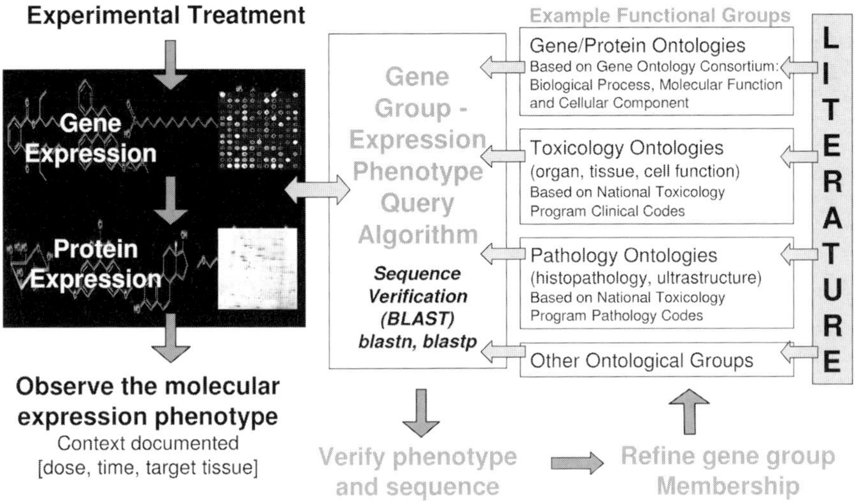

Fig. 10.9 Literature-derived putative functional gene groups validated against actual expression profiles of known toxicant-responsive pathways.

and proteomics datasets across treatment, dose, time, tissue type, and phenotypic severity. We also propose to integrate metabonomics datasets into CEBS Phase III, because of the pivotal role that metabolism plays in experimental and clinical toxicology as well as in hazard identification and risk assessment (Nicholson et al. 1999; Holmes et al. 2000; Holmes et al. 2001; Bundy et al. 2002; Nicholson et al. 2002).

10.8.4
CEBS Phase IV: Knowledge Technology

The development of a knowledge base for systems toxicology will require merging several different knowledge-building strategies: In addition to mining the literature for chemical-specific functionally characterized gene/protein groups, testing putative functional gene/protein groups against treatment-related gene and protein expression profiles, and determining the relationships of these gene/protein groups to functional pathways, we will consult gene ontologies from the GO Consortium (http://www.geneontology.org/) to guide naming these gene groups and to verify the accuracy of the ontologies in terms of biological process, molecular function, and cellular component. This standard hierarchical vocabulary reflects broad biological goals accomplished by ordered assemblies of molecular functions, tasks performed by individual gene products, and subcellular structures, locations, and macromolecular complexes.

Standardized gene and protein ontological relationships are significant, in that they can help to define functional relationships among genes and groups of genes and proteins. Therefore, we will attempt to confirm the putative functional relationships across multiple molecular expression datasets in the evolving knowledge base. Gene/protein ontology is an important corollary to the gene/protein group strategy and may prove to be an effective approach to the integration of gene and protein expression datasets, especially if it can effectively be converted to a heuristic process.

As a further adjunct to the building of knowledge, a more complete and heuristic data compendium strategy will be devised, based on statistical classification and clustering algorithms (to look for coregulation) of genes and proteins as a function of dose, time, and target site (Figure 10.10). Here, the experimental protocol defines the doses and the time course as well as the bioassays and biological measurements that will be made. The bioinformatics protocol specifies the various statistical and clustering algorithms that will be applied to look for correlated and coregulated genes. Ontologies will be used as described above. Note that an ontology lists similar elements, while a pathway describes an interaction among diverse elements. Using literature-derived putative gene groups (ideally vetted in appropriate gene ontologies), an iterative and heuristic gene/protein group phenotype analysis is expected to yield validated gene/protein groups that map to known functional pathways and, in terms of toxicology, to define the sequence of key events and common modes of action for environmental chemicals and drugs. Compendia of data will be assembled within each toxicogenomic and toxicological/pathological domain.

Thus, CEBS Phase IV will enable query by compound, structure, class, toxic or pathologic effects, gene annotation, gene/protein group, and functional (e.g., metabolic and toxicological) pathways that lead to toxicity and disease. To facilitate integration of compound-specific datasets, all genes, proteins, and gene/protein groups, will be linked to the gene/protein name and sequence database that was described

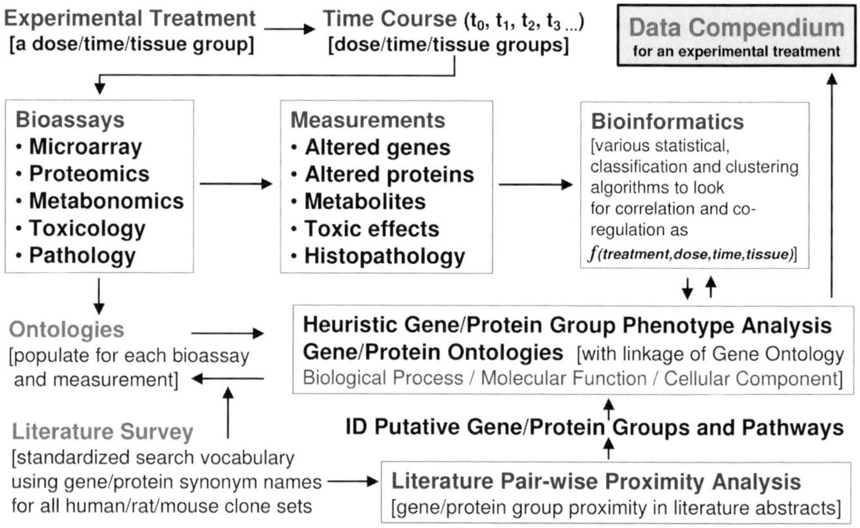

Fig. 10.10 Heuristic gene/protein functional analysis including ontological and literature orientation to describe biological process, molecular function, and cellular component.

earlier. This will facilitate query by any of the query categories listed above. Ultimately, one will globally query (or BLAST) CEBS using a transcriptome of a tissue of interest (or a list of outliers from gene expression or proteins from proteomics analysis) and have the knowledge base return all similar toxicogenomics data and datasets as well as contextually associated phenotypic information for compounds tested in various species and tissues represented in the knowledge base. This will be possible because of the derivation and maintenance of up-to-date sequence information on all genes and proteins represented in the knowledge base. In a sequence-driven knowledge base, a global query can return comparative genomic information (discussed below) based on BLAST cutoff values selected by the user. For example, a BLAST $-\log_{10}(E\,\text{value})$ cutoff for human-to-human comparisons might be 250, whereas for rat-to-human it might be 150, and for yeast-to-human as low as 100 or less, i.e., the cutoff values are significantly organism-related and might not be related to the assigned names of genes. The actual cutoffs used must also take into account the nature of the query sequence; in particular, 3′ tails (containing poly-A) are more difficult to match across species than are full-length coding sequences.

10.8.4.1 A Dose–Phenotype Strategy

Another strategy that must be carefully considered in the development of the CEBS knowledge base is one based on the lowest effective dose required to produce a particular molecular expression phenotype or phenotype severity. We believe that quantitative structure–activity relationships (QSARs) can be developed only for discrete toxicogenomic events and outcomes that can be anchored in an effective dose and a particular toxicological/pathological response or outcome. Precise phenotypic anchoring of discrete toxicogenomic events (derivation of unique gene/protein group signatures) at their lowest effective dose will be possible only if the internal dose can be established or modelled for the particular agent or its metabolites in the target tissue. This lowest effective dose, 'toxicant signature' strategy has been employed successfully in the development of the Environmental Protection Agency/International Agency for Research on Cancer genetic activity profile database (Waters et al. 1991). Graphic profiles and corresponding data listings of lowest effective/highest ineffective doses for genotoxic agents in various cell types and organisms and for various endpoints are available in this database of approximately 700 compounds. To develop a similar database for toxicogenomic endpoints, one annotates and organizes gene expression datasets as a function of compound, organism, endpoint, dose, and time, for select verified gene groups and coregulated ESTs. One then plots, for example as a histogram, outlier up-regulated and down-regulated genes for any appropriate toxicological or pathological endpoint as a function of lowest effective dose. Note that unidentified but coregulated ESTs (i.e., ESTs associated with other genes that are seen to be up- or down-regulated in response to an environmental toxicant) can contribute to the histogram and potentially to the generation of new knowledge about the mechanism of action of the compound. We should note that there will be primary, secondary, and tertiary effects of the same toxicant that will be distinguished from one another based on the molecular and toxicological/pathological phenotypes described and documented in the knowledge base.

Resulting histogram plots are phenotypically anchored in dose and condition of target tissue and facilitate ready development of global QSARs for the compounds and specific endpoints under consideration. Such a quantitative endpoint-profiling approach can readily be combined with physiologically based pharmacokinetic (PB/PK) and pharmacodynamic modelling (in fact, such modelling can be used to derive an estimate of internal dose in the target tissue). One then has the possibility to develop quantitative descriptions of the relationships among gene, protein, and metabolite expression profiles as a function of applied dose of the agent under consideration and to model the ensuing kinetic and dynamic dose–response parameters in various tissue compartments. This is an important strategy for CEBS, as it will contribute directly to future advancements in PB/PK and pharmacodynamic modelling and support a formal quantitative risk-assessment process (Simmons and Portier 2002).

10.8.4.2 **Cross-species Gene/Protein Comparative Expression Profiling**

With the availability of full genome sequences for several model organisms, there is intensive research toward the prediction, annotation, and mapping of genes across species. Of particular interest are the protein coding genes and the intracellular signalling networks and their interactions. Similarities among novel protein sequences in model organisms have become an important and extremely useful source for hypotheses concerning protein function. *Drosophila melanogaster* and *Caenorhabditis elegans* are attractive animal model systems for studying human genes because of their genetic tractability and their phenotypically well characterized genes (Chervitz et al. 1998; Nelson 1999 a; Culetto and Sattelle 2000; Rubin and Merchant 2000).

The genome database at the NCBI has assembled Clusters of Orthologous Groups (http://www.ncbi.nlm.nih.gov/COG/) for homologous nucleotide sequences in more than 40 species, mainly microbial, but including *D. melanogaster, C. elegans,* and *Saccharomyces cerevisiae*. The functional analysis of homologous genes in diverse genetic models is particularly relevant for proteins involved in human diseases, to gain rapid understanding of human disease mechanisms and to enhance the probability for development of novel therapies (Rubin et al. 2000).

Many cell functions are regulated by similar gene families across organisms (e.g., genes for the regulation of the cell cycle, cytoskeleton, cell adhesion, cell signalling, and apoptosis). This conservation of essential genes is also observed for transcription factors and many downstream signalling processes. It is believed that the completion of mouse, rat, and zebra fish genome sequencing efforts will provide information not only for the characterization of novel genes but also on the existence of homologous genes involved in every aspect of cell growth and functional differentiation. Gaining an understanding of the evolution and function of stress-response genes from yeasts to humans, for example, could be extremely valuable. Thus, we propose to provide within CEBS links to appropriate genome information resources and, eventually, to develop a comprehensive inventory of homologous genes/proteins across species from yeast to humans that may be important in toxicology and human disease. We anticipate that many of these homologous genes may be expressed similarly in response to environmental exposures that display similar modes of action. Strategically, these stress-responsive genes and gene clusters could be crucial for the interpretation of cross-genome expression profiles in an integrated health and ecological risk assessment. A core set of homologous genes should include genes involved in xenobiotic activation/detoxification mechanisms, perturbations of cell homeostasis mechanisms, oxidative damage, cell injury, death, and regeneration and genes controlling critical signalling mediator molecules for these biological processes. Phase I and Phase II enzymes metabolize most environmental xenobiotic chemicals, and much is known about their chemical substrates, inducers, and inhibitors. Phase I enzymes, the cytochromes P450 (CYPs), both bioactivate and also detoxify xenobiotics. The primary step involved in the activation process mediated by CYP proteins is oxidation, or bioactivation of xenobiotics to electrophiles. Phase II enzymes conjugate some of these oxidized metabolites to form water-soluble excretable substances. We propose to begin our compilation of cross-species gene/protein comparative expression analysis by focusing on the xenobiotic metabolic enzymes, the CYPs. Approximately 2500 *CYP* genes have been characterized in many organisms (http://drnelson.utmem.edu/CytochromeP450.html), including bacteria and mammalian systems (Nebert and McKinnon 1994; Nelson et al. 1996; Nelson 1999b), and their substrate, inducer, and inhibitor specificities must be studied in relation to alterations in molecular expression across species and across classes of xenobiotics.

We anticipate that, as homologous genes are identified, as compendia of gene/protein expression profiles are developed, and as functional pathways are derived and studied across species, we will be able to begin defining the networks and systems level of biological organization, wherein the cell expresses global changes in response to environmental stimuli. Again, we believe that fully context-documented toxicogenomics datasets and mathematical modelling will enable development of an integrated systems toxicology and bioinformatics. In summary, CEBS Phase IV can create the capability to assess the global toxicogenomic responses of biological systems to environmental stressors and to relationally link toxicogenomics data to conventional effects data. Since CEBS Phase IV will include datasets on multiple experimental organisms, cross-species comparisons and extrapolations will be possible on molecular, subcellular, cellular, organ, and systems levels.

10.8.4.3 Further Development of the Phase IV CEBS Knowledge Base

Based on the forgoing discussion and advances in the field, we have attempted to describe the basic strategies for the development of the core of the CEBS knowledge base as it is now conceptualized. Two additional CEBS Phase IV modules are envisioned for the future. One is a transcription module that may be used to make a priori predictions of the expression of genes and the other a haplotype linkage-disequilibrium module that may be used to predict the differential expression of genes in human haplotypes and to estimate the relative sensitivity of population subgroups. The transcription module will build upon rapidly developing knowledge of transcription factors and their pivotal importance in gene regulation. Since the number of transcription factors appears limited (around 2000 for humans), their study, to include sequence definition and binding sites, can be developed into a predictive science as related to gene and protein expression (Wingender et al. 2000; Wingender et al. 2001; Forde et al. 2002; Schrem et al. 2002). The haplotype linkage-disequilibrium module, on the other hand, will take advantage of our evolving knowledge of human haplotypes and associated SNPs that confer differential responses within human population subgroups to various classes of environmental toxicants and stressors (Li 2001). This module will require the addition of an SNP database. NIEHS has for some time been engaged in the development of the Gene SNPs Database (http://www.genome.utah.edu/genesnps/). We should note that SNPs represent only ~90% of all DNA sequence variants. The remainder include insertions, deletions, inversions, and duplications (one base or many bases or kilobases). Any or all of these can be important in any gene being studied. Addition of an SNP database is anticipated to enable an understanding of the relationship between environmental exposures and human disease susceptibility (Li 2001). This module is important, therefore, in both a toxicological and a risk-assessment context.

Field and clinical research applications of toxicogenomics methods are anticipated by the NCT. It is well known that a single nucleotide polymorphism, a single base change in the information of a gene, can cause a protein to malfunction. Experimentally, it is possible to construct panels of mutants that enable discovery of the impacts of malfunctions in transcription and translation. Preliminary data indicate that gene expression profiles will be useful as diagnostic tools for identifying early stages of various pathologies including cancer (Golub et al. 1999; Perou et al. 2000; Alizadeh et al. 2001, 2002; Alaiya et al. 2002). If this approach enables earlier detection of disease than is currently possible through other approaches, it may allow earlier initiation of therapeutic interventions. Additionally, gene expression profiling may become an important tool for predicting therapeutic outcome and may be particularly useful in addressing the significant variability that has been observed in how well patients respond to different types of drug therapy. Such patterns of variability have been studied using expression profiling and, in some instances, expression signatures have been seen to be associated with individuals who are responders or nonresponders to a particular type of drug therapy. Once this kind of result is validated, it may be possible to use expression profiling to optimize the therapeutic regimen for individual patients, thus increasing the chance of a good treatment outcome. It may also be possible to identify susceptible subpopulations for purposes of quantitative risk assessment.

10.9 Conclusions

The NCT and other organizations (Waring et al. 2001; Castle et al. 2002; Pennie and Kimber 2002) are performing experiments to validate the concept of gene expression profiles as 'signatures' of toxicant classes, disease subtypes, or other biological endpoints. Initial studies indicate that classes of toxicants and toxic responses can be recognized as gene expression signatures using microarray technology. Such experiments have begun to correlate gene expression profiles with other well defined parameters, including toxicant class, chemical structure, pathological or physiological response, or other validated indices of toxicity. For example, experiments have been designed to correlate gene expression patterns with liver pathologies such as necrosis, apoptosis, fibrosis, or inflammation. It is also possible to look for correlative patterns in surrogate tissues, such as blood. Changes in serum enzymes provide diagnostic markers of organ function that are routinely used in medicine and toxicology. Such phenotypic anchoring of gene expression data using conventional indices will distinguish the toxicological signal from other gene expression changes that may be unrelated to toxicity, such as the adaptive, pharmacological, or therapeutic effects of a compound.

By constructing and populating CEBS, the NCT is assisting the field of environmental health research to evolve into an information science in which experimental gene and protein expression datasets are compiled and made readily available to the scientific community. The analysis of these expression profiles for different chemicals from different classes over dose and time can be used to identify expression profiles that are consistently and mechanistically linked to specific exposures and disease outcomes. Once enough high-quality data have been accumulated and assimilated, it will become possible to characterize an unknown biological or physical sample by comparing its gene and/or protein expression profile to compendia of expression profiles in the database (Hughes et al. 2000). The NCT will develop the capacity to use gene expression signatures to facilitate toxicological characterization of toxicants and their biological effects. As the field of toxicogenomics evolves, toxicogenomics databases will begin to support predictive toxicology and hazard assessment. This will help scientists predict the toxicological impact of suspected toxicants and calculate how much of a hazard these toxicants actually represent to human and environmental health.

Infrastructure development is essential to facilitate the integration of the existing public toxicology and structure–activity databases with those under development in toxicogenomics (Richard and Williams 2002). In this way, both conventional toxicology and structure–activity databases and the CEBS public knowledge base can realize their full potential in supporting mechanistic interpretations and risk assessment (Simmons and Portier 2002) in the future. Concomitant with development of the databases must be the evolution of bioinformatics and data-mining tools and the training of individuals to use them.

The NIEHS is committed to the development of the CEBS knowledge base with which to initiate this evolutionary process. This chapter has attempted to provide a vision of what CEBS will offer and how, in general terms, it might be constructed. The magnitude of the effort required to develop and populate such a knowledge base requires a collective will and collaborative efforts. Therefore, we will pursue the interoperability of CEBS with other databases elsewhere (e.g., those on cell signalling, protein–protein interactions, and biological and metabolic pathways) to enhance our ability to interpret toxicogenomic datasets. We will seek to develop additional mechanisms through which partnerships with scientists in academia, the private sector, and other governmental organizations can be created, and we welcome advice, criticism, and participation in this enterprise.

As the CEBS knowledge base expands to include structurally or functionally related agents and as gene identification and annotation progresses, it will be possible to search in a comprehensive way for common, critical, or causal relationships. It will then become possible to create pathway maps of common cellular processes, to map partial genome arrays to pathways, and to link such changes to known phenotypic markers of toxicity. The knowledge base and its relational linkages must grow incrementally, and the developers and users must have the patience and dedication to stay the course. Such incremental growth will eventually become exponential growth, and the field of toxicology will be profoundly changed.

In the realm of molecular epidemiology, our growing understanding of genomic anatomy (gene sequence and polymorphisms) will form the basis for characterizing person-to-person and ethnogeographic sequence variations in genes that affect responses to drugs and chemicals that affect human susceptibility and vulnerability. Eventually, gene and protein expression profiles from exposed humans (and from organisms in the environment) will be compared to reference expression profiles based on national or international gene expression databases (Ermolaeva et al. 1998). Studying and analyzing patterns of gene expression across species will help us to understand the relationship between DNA sequence variation and the phenotype, which will in turn help us to understand and integrate the assessment of human and ecological risks.

Given the vast numbers and diversity of drugs, chemicals, and environmental agents, the diversity of species in which they act, the time and dose factors that are critical to the induction of beneficial and adverse effects, the diversity of phenotypic consequences of exposures, etc., it is only through the development of a profound knowledge base that toxicology and environmental health can rapidly advance. Toxicogenomics has the potential to change the way in which environmental toxicology is performed. It will contribute new methods, new data, and new interpretation to the field. The ultimate goal of the NCT is to create a knowledge base that allows environmental health scientists and practitioners to understand and prevent adverse environmental exposures in the 21st century.

Acknowledgments

We thank the following scientists for valuable discussions on the development of the CEBS knowledge base: Drs. Cynthia Afshari on basic design characteristics, Rob DeWoskin on PB/PK modelling, Hisham Hamadeh on user interfaces and gene annotation, Paul H. M. Lohman on dose profiling, dynamic linkage, and P450 metabolism, Srikanth Nadadur on comparative genomics, Nancy Stegman, Jerry Nehls, and John Doherty on database design and information technology, and James Sluka on literature mining and PDQ_MED. We also thank Drs. Amal Abu-Shakra, Neal Cariello, Skip Eastin, John Grovenstein, Paul Nettesheim, Lorenzo Tomatis, Susanna Sansone, and Larry Wright for their many helpful ideas and comments on the manuscript. We are indebted to Drs. Samuel Wilson and Lutz Birnbaumer for their continuing support of the NCT program.

Abbreviations

ADME	absorption, distribution, metabolism, and excretion
AIMS	Analysis Information Management System
BLAST,	Basic Local Alignment Search Tool
CEBS	Chemical Effects in Biological Systems
DTD	document type definition
GO	gene ontology
HTML	hypertext markup language
ILS HESI	Health and Environmental Sciences Institute of the International Life Sciences Institute
LIMS	Laboratory Information Management System
MAGE-ML	microarray gene expression markup language
MAGE-OM	microarray gene expression object model
MAPS	Microarray Project System
MGED	Microarray Gene Expression Database Society
MIAME	minimum information about a microarray experiment
NCT	National Center for Toxicogenomics
NMG	NIEHS Microarray Group
NTP	National Toxicology Program
PB/PK	physiologically based pharmacokinetic
PED	Protein Expression Database
SNPs	single nucleotide polymorphisms
SQL	structured query language
TDMS,	Toxicology Database Management System
TRC	Toxicogenomics Research Consortium
XML	extensible markup language

References

Aardema MJ, MacGregor JT. 2002. Toxicology and genetic toxicology in the new era of 'toxicogenomics': impact of '-omics' technologies. Mutat Res 499: 13–25.

Afshari CA. 2002. Perspective: microarray technology, seeing more than spots. Endocrinology 143: 1983–1989.

Alaiya AA, Franzen B, Hagman A, Dysvik B, Roblick UJ, Becker S, et al. 2002. Molecular classification of borderline ovarian tumors using hierarchical cluster analysis of protein expression profiles. Int J Cancer 98: 895–899.

Alizadeh AA, Ross DT, Perou CM, Van de Rijn M. 2001. Towards a novel classification of human malignancies based on gene expression patterns. J Pathol 195: 41–52.

Altschul SF, Gish W, Miller W, Myers EW, Lipman DJ. 1990. Basic local alignment search tool. J Mol Biol 215: 403–410.

Bartosiewicz MJ, Jenkins D, Penn S, Emery J, Buckpitt A. 2001. Unique gene expression patterns in liver and kidney associated with exposure to chemical toxicants. J Pharmacol Exp Ther 297: 895–905.

Bessems JG, Vermeulen NP. 2001. Paracetamol (acetaminophen)-induced toxicity: molecular and biochemical mechanisms, analogues and protective approaches. Crit Rev Toxicol 31: 55–138.

Boorman GA, Anderson SP, Casey WM, Brown RH, Crosby LM, Gottschalk K, et al.

2002. Toxicogenomics, drug discovery, and the pathologist. Toxicol Pathol 30: 15–27.

Brazma A, Hingamp P, Quackenbush J, Sherlock G, Spellman P, Stoeckert C, et al. 2001. Minimum information about a microarray experiment (MIAME): toward standards for microarray data. Nat Genet 29: 365–371.

Bundy JG, Spurgeon DJ, Svendsen C, Hankard PK, Osborn D, Lindon JC, et al. 2002. Earthworm species of the genus *Eisenia* can be phenotypically differentiated by metabolic profiling. FEBS Lett 521: 115–120.

Burchiel SW, Knall CM, Davis JW II, Paules RS, Boggs SE, Afshari CA. 2001. Analysis of genetic and epigenetic mechanisms of toxicity: potential roles of toxicogenomics and proteomics in toxicology. Toxicol Sci 59: 193–195.

Bushel PR, Hamadeh H, Bennett L, Sieber S, Martin K, Nuwaysir EF, et al. 2001. MAPS: a microarray project system for gene expression experiment information and data validation. Bioinformatics 17: 564–565.

Castle AL, Carver MP, Mendrick DL. 2002. Toxicogenomics: a new revolution in drug safety. Drug Discov Today 7: 728–736.

Chervitz SA, Aravind L, Sherlock G, Ball CA, Koonin EV, Dwight SS, et al. 1998. Comparison of the complete protein sets of worm and yeast: orthology and divergence. Science 282: 2022–2028.

Culetto E, Sattelle DB. 2000. A role for *Caenorhabditis elegans* in understanding the function and interactions of human disease genes. Hum Mol Genet 9: 869–877.

Cunningham MJ, Liang S, Fuhrman S, Seilhamer JJ, Somogyi R. 2000. Gene expression microarray data analysis for toxicology profiling. Ann NY Acad Sci 919: 52–67.

Dudley AM, Aach J, Steffen MA, Church GM. 2002. Measuring absolute expression with microarrays with a calibrated reference sample and an extended signal intensity range. Proc Natl Acad Sci USA 99: 7554–7559.

Edgar R, Domrachev M, Lash AE. 2002. Gene expression omnibus: NCBI gene expression and hybridization array data repository. Nucleic Acids Res 30: 207–210.

Ermolaeva O, Rastogi M, Pruitt KD, Schuler GD, Bittner ML, Chen Y, et al. 1998. Data management and analysis for gene expression arrays. Nat Genet 20: 19–23.

Farland WH. 1992. The U.S. Environmental Protection Agency's Risk Assessment Guidelines: current status and future directions. Toxicol Ind Health 8: 205–212.

Farland WH. 1996. Cancer risk assessment: evolution of the process. Prev Med 25: 24–25.

Fielden MR, Zacharewski TR. 2001. Challenges and limitations of gene expression profiling in mechanistic and predictive toxicology. Toxicol Sci 60: 6–10.

Forde CE, Gonzales AD, Smessaert JM, Murphy GA, Shields SJ, Fitch JP, et al. 2002. A rapid method to capture and screen for transcription factors by SELDI mass spectrometry. Biochem Biophys Res Commun 290: 1328–1335.

Gibas C, Jambeck P (2001), Developing Bioinformatics Computer Skills, Sebastopol, CA: O'Reilly.

Golub TR, Slonim DK, Tamayo P, Huard C, Gaasenbeek M, Mesirov JP, et al. 1999. Molecular classification of cancer: class discovery and class prediction by gene expression monitoring. Science 286: 531–537.

Hamadeh HK, Amin RP, Paules RS, Afshari CA. 2002. An overview of toxicogenomics. Curr Issues Mol Biol 4: 45–56.

Hamadeh HK, Bushel PR, Jayadev S, Martin K, DiSorbo O, Sieber S, et al. 2002a. Gene expression analysis reveals chemical-specific profiles. Toxicol Sci 67: 219–231.

Hamadeh HK, Bushel PR, Jayadev S, DiSorbo O, Bennett L, Li L, et al. 2002b. Prediction of compound signature using high density gene expression profiling. Toxicol Sci 67: 232–240.

Hamadeh HK, Knight, B.L., Haugen, A.C., Sieber, S., Amin, R.P., Bushel, P.R., Stoll, R., Blanchard, K., Jayadev, S., Tennant, R.W., Cunningham, M.L., Afshari, C.A., and Paules, R.S. 2002c. Methapyrilene toxicity: anchorage of pathologic observations to gene expression alterations. Toxicol Pathol 30: 470–482.

Holmes E, Nicholls AW, Lindon JC, Connor SC, Connelly JC, Haselden JN, et al. 2000. Chemometric models for toxicity classification based on NMR spectra of biofluids. Chem Res Toxicol 13: 471–478.

Holmes E, Nicholson JK, Tranter G. 2001. Metabonomic characterization of genetic variations in toxicological and metabolic responses using probabilistic neural networks. Chem Res Toxicol 14: 182–191.

Hughes TR, Marton MJ, Jones AR, Roberts CJ, Stoughton R, Armour CD, et al. 2000.

Functional discovery via a compendium of expression profiles. Cell 102: 109–126.

IDEKER T, GALITSKI T, HOOD L. 2001. A new approach to decoding life: systems biology. Annu Rev Genomics Hum Genet 2: 343–372.

ISSAQ HJ, VEENSTRA TD, CONRADS TP, FELSCHOW D. 2002. The SELDI–TOF MS approach to proteomics: protein profiling and biomarker identification. Biochem Biophys Res Commun 292: 587–592.

KARP PD. 2000. An ontology for biological function based on molecular interactions. Bioinformatics 16: 269–285.

LARSEN JC, FARLAND W, WINTERS D. 2000. Current risk assessment approaches in different countries. Food Addit Contam 17: 359–369.

LI H. 2001. A permutation procedure for the haplotype method for identification of disease-predisposing variants. Ann Hum Genet 65: 189–196.

NEBERT DW, MCKINNON RA. 1994. Cytochrome P450: evolution and functional diversity. Prog Liver Dis 12: 63–97.

NELSON DR. 1999a. Cytochrome P450 and the individuality of species. Arch Biochem Biophys 369: 1–10.

NELSON DR. 1999b. A second CYP26 P450 in humans and zebrafish: CYP26B1. Arch Biochem Biophys 371: 345–347.

NELSON DR, KOYMANS L, KAMATAKI T, STEGEMAN JJ, FEYEREISEN R, WAXMAN DJ, et al. 1996. P450 superfamily: update on new sequences, gene mapping, accession numbers and nomenclature. Pharmacogenetics 6: 1–42.

NICHOLSON JK, LINDON JC, HOLMES E. 1999. 'Metabonomics': understanding the metabolic responses of living systems to pathophysiological stimuli via multivariate statistical analysis of biological NMR spectroscopic data. Xenobiotica 29: 1181–1189.

NICHOLSON JK, CONNELLY J, LINDON JC, HOLMES E. 2002. Metabonomics: a platform for studying drug toxicity and gene function. Nat Rev Drug Discov 1: 153–161.

NUWAYSIR EF, BITTNER M, TRENT J, BARRETT JC, AFSHARI CA. 1999. Microarrays and toxicology: the advent of toxicogenomics. Mol Carcinog 24: 153–159.

OGATA H, GOTO S, SATO K, FUJIBUCHI W, BONO H, KANEHISA M. 1999. KEGG: Kyoto Encyclopedia of Genes and Genomes. Nucleic Acids Res 27: 29–34.

OLDEN K. 2002. New opportunities in toxicology in the post-genomic era. Drug Discov Today 7: 273–276.

PENNIE WD, KIMBER I. 2002. Toxicogenomics; transcript profiling and potential application to chemical allergy. Toxicol In Vitro 16: 319–326.

PEROU CM, SORLIE T, EISEN MB, VAN DE RIJN M, JEFFREY SS, REES CA, et al. 2000. Molecular portraits of human breast tumours. Nature 406: 747–752.

QUACKENBUSH J, CHO J, LEE D, LIANG F, HOLT I, KARAMYCHEVA S, et al. 2001. The TIGR gene indices: analysis of gene transcript sequences in highly sampled eukaryotic species. Nucleic Acids Res 29: 159–164.

REILLY TP, BOURDI M, BRADY JN, PISE-MASISON CA, RADONOVICH MF, GEORGE JW, et al. 2001a. Expression profiling of acetaminophen liver toxicity in mice using microarray technology. Biochem Biophys Res Commun 282: 321–328.

REILLY TP, BRADY JN, MARCHICK MR, BOURDI M, GEORGE JW, RADONOVICH MF, et al. 2001b. A protective role for cyclooxygenase-2 in drug-induced liver injury in mice. Chem Res Toxicol 14: 1620–1628.

RICHARD AM, WILLIAMS CR. 2002. Distributed structure-searchable toxicity (DSSTox) public database network: a proposal. Mutat Res 499: 27–52.

RUBIN GM, YANDELL MD, WORTMAN JR, GABOR MIKLOS GL, NELSON CR, HARIHARAN IK, et al. 2000. Comparative genomics of the eukaryotes. Science 287: 2204–2215.

RUBIN RB, MERCHANT M. 2000. A rapid protein profiling system that speeds study of cancer and other diseases. Am Clin Lab 19(8):28–29.

RUEPP SU, TONGE RP, SHAW J, WALLIS N, POGNAN F. 2002. Genomics and proteomics analysis of acetaminophen toxicity in mouse liver. Toxicol Sci 65: 135–150.

SCHREM H, KLEMPNAUER J, BORLAK J. 2002. Liver-enriched transcription factors in liver function and development. I. The hepatocyte nuclear factor network and liver-specific gene expression. Pharmacol Rev 54: 129–158.

SELKOV E, JR., GRECHKIN Y, MIKHAILOVA N, SELKOV E. 1998. MPW: the Metabolic Pathways Database. Nucleic Acids Res 26: 43–45.

SIMMONS PT, PORTIER CJ. 2002. Toxicogenomics: the new frontier in risk analysis. Carcinogenesis 23: 903–905.

SLUKA JP. 2002. Extracting knowledge from genomic experiments by incorporating the biomedical literature. In: *Methods of Microarray Data Analysis II* (S.M. Lin and K.F. Johnson E, ed). Boston: Kluwer.

TENNANT RW. 2002. The National Center for Toxicogenomics: using new technologies to inform mechanistic toxicology. Environ Health Perspect 110: A8–10.

THOMAS RS, RANK DR, PENN SG, ZASTROW GM, HAYES KR, PANDE K, et al. 2001. Identification of toxicologically predictive gene sets using cDNA microarrays. Mol Pharmacol 60: 1189–1194.

ULRICH R, FRIEND SH. 2002. Toxicogenomics and drug discovery: will new technologies help us produce better drugs? Nat Rev Drug Discov 1: 84–88.

WARING JF, JOLLY RA, CIURLIONIS R, LUM PY, PRAESTGAARD JT, MORFITT DC, et al. 2001. Clustering of hepatotoxins based on mechanism of toxicity using gene expression profiles. Toxicol Appl Pharmacol 175: 28–42.

WATERS MD, STACK HF, GARRETT NE, JACKSON MA. 1991. The Genetic Activity Profile database. Environ Health Perspect 96: 41–45.

WATERS MD, BOORMAN G, BUSHEL P, CUNNINGHAM, IRWIN R, MERRICK A, et al. 2003. Systems toxicology and the chemical effects in biological systems knowledge base, Environmental Health Perspectives 111: 811–824.

WINGENDER E, CHEN X, HEHL R, KARAS H, LIEBICH I, MATYS V, et al. 2000. TRANSFAC: an integrated system for gene expression regulation. Nucleic Acids Res 28: 316–319.

WINGENDER E, CHEN X, FRICKE E, GEFFERS R, HEHL R, LIEBICH I, et al. 2001. The TRANSFAC system on gene expression regulation. Nucleic Acids Res 29: 281–283.

WOLFINGER RD, GIBSON G, WOLFINGER ED, BENNETT L, HAMADEH H, BUSHEL P, et al. 2001. Assessing gene significance from cDNA microarray expression data via mixed models. J Comput Biol 8: 625–637.

YAMAZAKI K, KUROMITSU J, TANAKA I. 2002. Microarray analysis of gene expression changes in mouse liver induced by peroxisome proliferator-activated receptor alpha agonists. Biochem Biophys Res Commun 290: 1114–1122.

ZWEIGER G. 1999. Knowledge discovery in gene-expression–microarray data: mining the information output of the genome. Trends Biotechnol 17: 429–436.

11
Investigating the Effective Range of Agents by Using Integrative Modelling

Andreas Freier, Ralf Hofestädt, and Thoralf Toepel

11.1
Introduction

The analysis of pharmaceutical mechanisms, one of the tasks of pharmacology, is based on knowledge about physiological and biophysical processes in the cell. However, the understanding of qualitative statements requires the study of complex cellular networks. In this context, metabolic pathways are chains of enzymatically [1] and genetically [2] controlled biochemical reactions that consume nutrients, release energy, and synthesize cellular substances (amino acids, lipids, etc.). The energy is used by several endergonic processes, e. g., biosynthesis, cell division, endocytosis and exocytosis, production of ion gradients, and cellular movements. Interference with these regulatory systems often causes metabolic diseases.

Drugs are substances that influence regulatory systems. The World Health Organization (WHO) defines a drug as "any substance or product that is used or intended to be used to modify or explore physiological systems or pathological states for the benefit of the recipient." This implies that drugs positively affect cellular systems, for example, by promoting inhibited reactions or activating alternative pathways. Of course, any drug can also have negative effects, for example, if it is overdosed. Here, the toxicology of the substance has to be analysed [3].

The interactions of drugs and receptor molecules are often studied. Receptors mainly have one binding site, where only one specific substance or kind of substance can bind. Once the substance has been bound to the receptor, the conformation of the receptor changes, resulting in transfer of information. Various classes and subclasses of receptors exist, e. g., ligand-controlled ion channels, receptors coupled with guanyl nucleotide–binding proteins (G proteins), receptors showing the activity of the enzyme Tyrosine kinase, and receptors regulating DNA transcription.

The mechanism of receptor protein interaction with G proteins is, briefly, as follows: a transmembrane receptor protein made up of several peptide chains arranged as a cylinder has a binding site in the centre of the cylinder. G proteins, which are responsible for signal transduction, are located close to the receptor on the inner site of the membrane. The binding of a ligand to the receptor results in activation of a

Handbook of Toxicogenomics: Strategies and Applications. Edited by Jürgen Borlak

ISBN: 3-527-30342-1

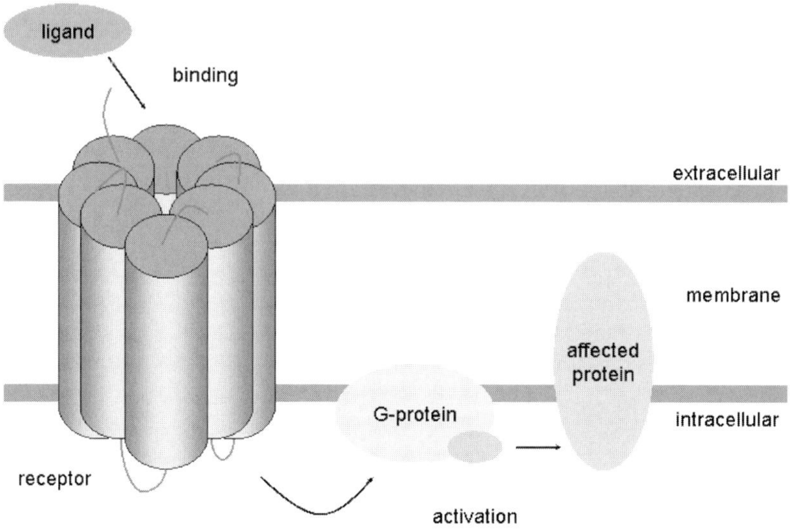

Fig. 11.1 Domain-specific notation of a receptor with interacting G-protein.

subunit of the G protein, which transmits a signal to affected proteins nearby. The strength of the signal depends on the duration of ligand binding and the number of activated G proteins. After certain time, the system returns into its initial state. Figure 11.1 shows the mechanism of a receptor using a domain specific notation.

Biophysical processes can often, but not always, be classified by describing patterns of processes, which may involve computational modelling of biochemical networks. Classic methods for investigating biological networks use mathematical models [4]. Experimental approches combined with modelling start at the biological problem and create a hypothesis about the mechanism and the structure of the studied system. Based upon the hypothesis the experimental design as well as a mathematical model will be developed in parallel. Validating the observations gained by experiments against the computational prediction will lead to a modification of the experimental design, the model, or the hypothesis (Figure 11.2) [5]. Finally, the optimized model will give a dynamic representation of the biological system.

Classes or patterns of molecular objects and processes can often be identified in molecular databases. The use of different databases while doing computational modelling leads to the problem of dynamically integrating the data into mathematical models. This chapter presents an approach combining mathematical modelling with the integration of molecular databases. We introduce novel methods of deriving mathematical models from data, in which data structures of molecular objects are directly combined with mathematical equations. The application of these models and methods will facilitate or enable the integrative and large scale analysis of, for example, the action of drugs.

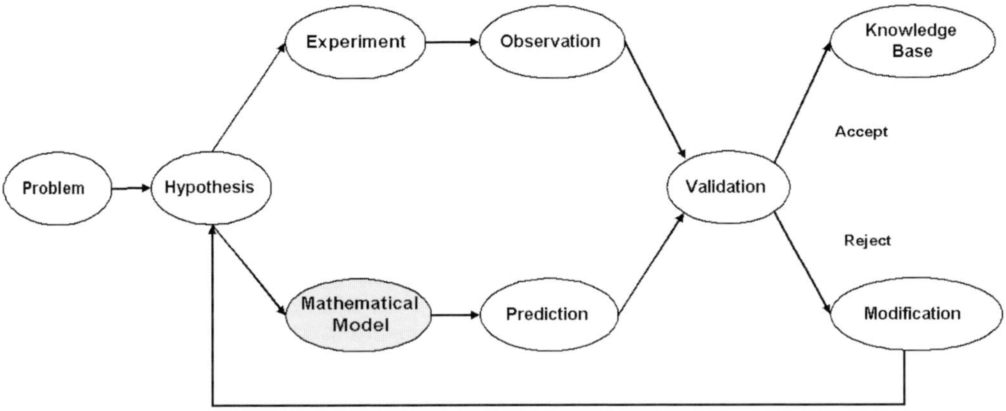

Fig. 11.2 Process of modelling biological systems [4].

11.2 Mathematical Models

Models are limited or simplified representations of real systems and they are used to study the complexity of their real counterparts. Today, the area of modelling biological systems is dominated by approaches referred to as classic methods, such as mathematical modelling [4].

Quantitative analysis of the dynamics of biological networks often requires differential equations [6], which determine the rates of the flows in the system under various conditions. Most of biological systems are very complex and show nonlinear behaviours, which makes it hard to solve them analytically. While universal mathematical software packages with numerical equation-solving capabilities exist, specific tools have been developed in the field of metabolic networks, including Gepasi [7], WinSAAM [4] and DBSolve [8].

In addition, tools for modelling biochemical systems using Petri nets (PN) [9, 10] and stochastic simulation [28, 29] are available. An advantage on Petri nets is that equations are visualized graphically so that the user can construct and modify them very easily. PN are bipartite graphs built from four types of elements: places, transitions, arcs, and tokens. Each equation is directly modelled using a transition which is graphically represented by a vertical or horizontal bar. Places are circles containing information about concentrations of substances represented by tokens (dots). Arcs are directed edges indicating the flow of materials consumed and produced by each transition. Actually, a transition will consume tokens from places connected as input and produce tokens at places connected as output. To define reaction rates, transitions can be associated with equations which are computed in a continous or discrete manner at runtime. Furthermore, stoichiometric coefficients can be assigned to arcs to determine the number of tokens processes in each transition. The configuration of tokens represents the state of the system.

In the early stages of the modelling process, the modeller analyzes the mechanism of the real system under study. As mentioned in Section 11.1, these mechanisms can describe classes of processes. Figure 11.3 shows a simplified example of a Petri-net model for the interaction of receptors with G protein, based on the example shown in Figure 11.1. The displayed network represents a pattern, which is applicable to every receptor of its type, e.g., the activation of adenylate cyclase or of phospholipase C. For each application, the identities of places and transitions have to be substituted by the objects of the real system. The configuration of the system is given mythe initial number of tokens. In the example signal, receptor, G protein, and effector are present which one element each.

Representing sets of equations by Petri nets makes it clear that biological systems can be interpreted as special types of graphs. Graph theory has been applied to metabolic networks in the past [11, 12]; in principle, it enables us to analyse the complexity of biological networks. For many problems, the total state of systems, details of the system, and the kinetics of the system processes are unknown. In addition, detailed information can be hidden within large datasets, which have to be mined. Additionally, biological models can be very complex and need to be verified to avoid inconsistencies, which are not easily detectable. However, an advantage of graph theory is that previous work in this broad area has provided a robust library of directly applicable methods for calculating qualitative information about the effective range of agents.

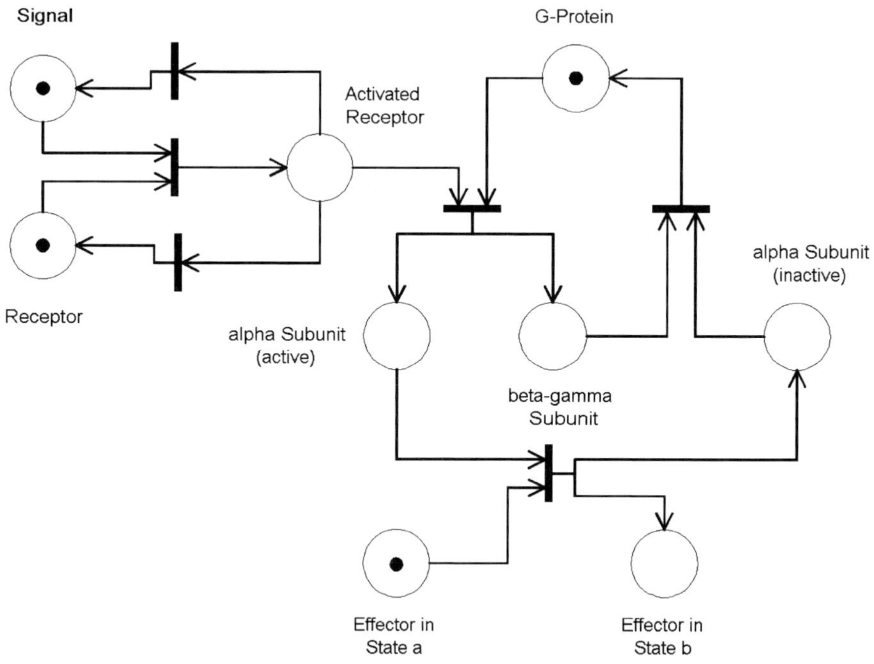

Fig. 11.3 The mechanism of G-protein interacting with a receptor, visualized as a Petri net.

11.3 Modelling Molecular Databases

Today, in addition to performing laboratory experiments and searching the literature, researchers increasingly rely on databases for aid in modelling biological systems. As mentioned in Section 11.1, many molecular databases relevant to biochemical substances and reactions already exist. To incorporate remote data into one's own analyses automatically, it should be integrated with local databases; however, this procedure frequently results in various types of conflicts, owing to semantic overlapping, differences in description, structural differences, and heterogeneity. In practice, most of the time spent integrating databases is consumed by paying attention to these problems. In the following sections the characteristics of molecular databases are discussed using several case studies.

11.3.1 Drug Databases

Although database systems that cover metabolic and gene regulation networks are already available and mostly freely accessible for academic research, drug databases are not, and recent data has to be acquired from proprietary data sources, e. g., literature databases or lists of agents and medical products. In addition, public databases of medical products do not contain the real names of the agents but the trademarks (more than 9000 products are registered in Germany alone). To analyze drug actions in the context of metabolic and gene regulation networks, modelling and implementing of custom databases is necessary. This section will give an overview about the modelling of static relationships in the certain domains.

Corresponding to our inhouse database DrugDB, the first case study is a drug database which provides data about biochemical mechanisms of drug action and their direct targets, as well as the resulting effects. Because of the highly complex relationships in DrugDB, only a subset its structure is summarized in Figure 11.4. In fact, the database is finely granulated and contains a total of 53 classes. In a static conceptual schema a classes defines a special type of objects having well defined properties. Edges between the classes of objects indicate that the two classes are related to each other. Naming the relationship will define its semantics. Different types of relationships can be defined, e. g. association, aggregation or inheritance. In the following examples only aggregations and associations are included.

Most drugs have a designated target, which is often highly specific to the drug. Administration of the drug results in activation or deactivation of the target entity. The mechanisms of action of each drug are stored in the database and linked to the resulting changes in metabolic systems, which are often the actual goal of administering the drug. The goal of this database is to classify and reveal the activities of different drugs and to link to the biochemical networks that they influence.

The access to drug databases integrated with metabolic data gives us information about the activation of alternative pathways around metabolic blocks. The possibility

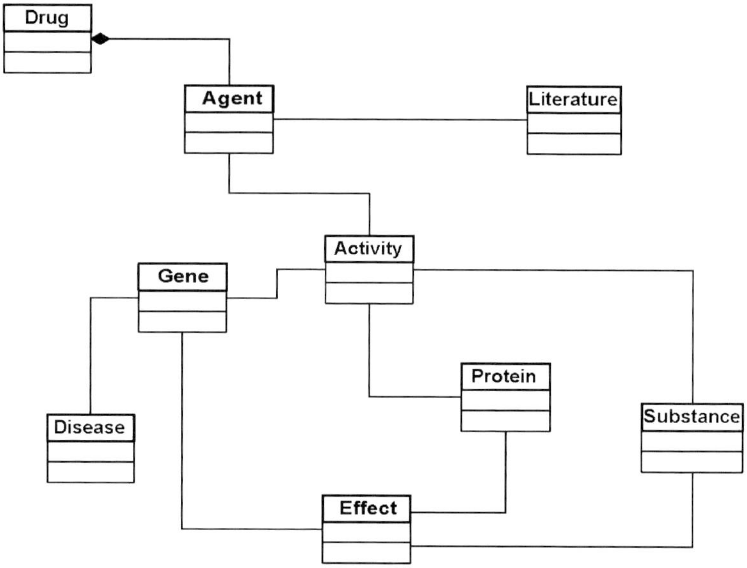

Fig. 11.4 Conceptual scheme of a drug database.

of searching for drugs that can modulate these pathways at different biochemical levels should offer new possibilities for the treatment of metabolic diseases.

11.3.2 Pathway Databases

In a second example we show elements of databases containing data about pathways, which are, as mentioned in the introduction, at least one of the main targets of drug action. Pathway databases are freely available for academic purposes and, in comparing them with other types of molecular databases, we can see that they offer data of relatively high quality. Typical pathway databases include BRENDA [13], KEGG [14], and EcoCyc [15]. In this section we discuss the structure and application of pathway databases.

The first element of our simplified example (Figure 11.5) is the class *metabolism*, which contains at least all pathways of an organism. Currently, more than 80 pathways are annotated and published in databases. Pathways consist of elementary reactions that are specifically catalyzed by enzymes (>4000). For example, the glycolysis pathway, a central pathway, includes 10 reactions and occurs in many eukaryotic and prokaryotic organisms. The pathway shows complex dynamics (periodic, chaotic), which are caused by several nonlinear reactions. To give an example, one of these reactions is catalyzed irreversibly by the enzyme phosphofructokinase (PFK). PFK consumes the metabolite D-fructose 6-phosphate and produces D-fructose 1,6-bisphosphate. At the same time ATP is converted to ADP, the substrate (ATP) inhibits the reaction, and ADP acts as activator. Pathway data is highly specific for different organisms and tissues and needs to be stored adequately.

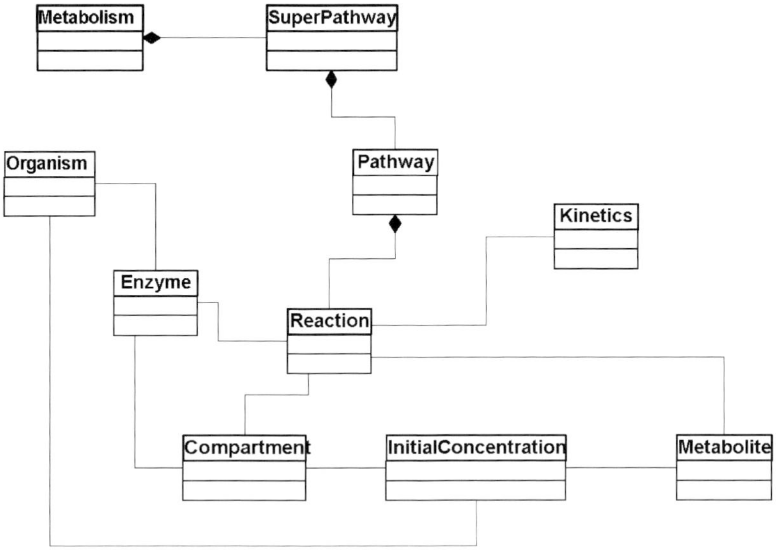

Fig. 11.5 Conceptual scheme of a pathway database.

11.3.3 Gene Expression Databases and Others

The control of protein synthesis has been an object of study since the middle of the last century. The initial analyses [16] showed the basic mechanisms of gene regulation in bacteria. Available databases concerning gene regulation and expression include TRANSFAC [17] and RegulonDB [18]. A limited version of TRANSFAC is available, and the professional version can be acquired with an academic license. RegulonDB contains data about bacteria and is freely available.

Our example handles regulatory mechanisms and gene expression processes. The simplified schema shown in Figure 11.6 is related to regulation in prokaryotes and contains ten classes that reference each other. Beginning at the class *protein*, for each protein the binding to enhancing and repressing binding sites is stored in *interaction* objects. An enhanced or repressed promoter controls transcription units (operons) containing a set of genes to be expressed. Final products of gene expression are polypeptides that function as either signals or enzymes. Sequence information can be used to predict hypothetical promoters and binding sites. Detailed information about the annotation of sequences in terms of genes and proteins can be gained from EMBL [19] and SwissProt [20].

The increasing number of databases requires efficient methods to access and integrate recent data mostly automatically. In addition, currently existing databases are growing rapidly, and integration methods have to be as generic as possible to be useful. Furthermore, molecular databases can be queried for information about static relationships between molecular objects. Obviously, the networks of objects created by

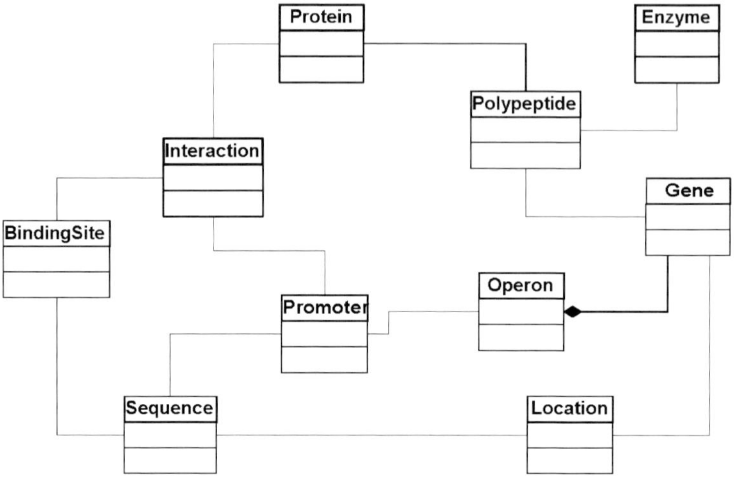

Fig. 11.6 Conceptual scheme of a gene regulatory database.

static relationships cannot be translated directly into mathematical models without additional modelling and mapping efforts.

11.4
Integrative Modelling

In the above sections we presented models and methodologies for the representation of static and dynamic aspects of biochemical networks. Actually, two main problems have been pointed out: (1) recent data is spread over dozens of heterogeneous, distributed, and evolving databases and data cleaning is important to ensure the consistency of data; (2) most of the work of modelling systems is still done manually, that is, single processes have to be designed and linked with each other. Nevertheless, the above sections did also show that conceptual modelling of static and dynamic views is important to understand the structure behind complex biological systems. We now want to apply computational methods to conceptual models to reconstruct models from available data sources systematically.

The main idea of integrative modelling is to include all aspects of modelling in a sequential and incremental process. Figure 11.7 shows the different levels of this cycle, whereby the modeller is controlling and responsible to decide the following questions:

- Which data sources should be used to obtain data?
- What type of objects are part of my system?
- In what type of processes these objects are involved?
- Which objects and processes are parts of a system and how does the system behave?

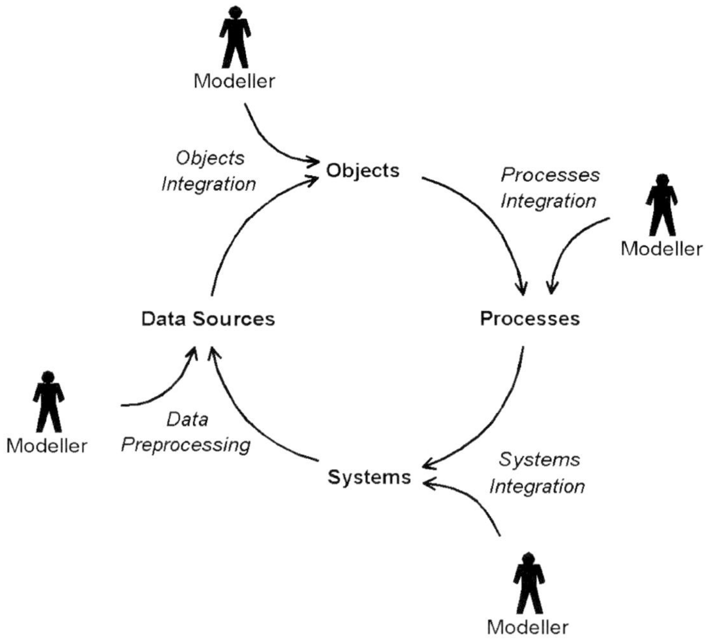

Fig. 11.7 The cycle of integrative modelling.

While these questions are part of the conceptual modelling, the modeller can be supported by computational methods, which are summarized under the categories data preprocessing, objects integration, process integration and systems integration.

11.4.1
Data Preprocessing

We enter the workflow at the preprocessing of data, where we prefer to prepare all data sources separately storing their content in a primarily relational database. If this should not be possible in event of proprietary systems, we apply the tool BioDataServer [ISB], which is a mediator system developed by our group providing online access to various molecular data sources. The tool is capable to emulate a virtual relational database over proprietary systems, e. g. websites and flat files, and it can be used to extract data from data sources to transform and load it into relational databases.

11.4.2
Object Oriented Models and Data Integration

In the second step of our workflow molecular objects are collected together with their properties and relationships. Actually, we use the object-oriented approach to specify these models and include information about from which datasources the objects stem from. Here we have to answer at first the question of which objects participate in our system. Classes of objects which appear in different data sources are semantically integrated and represented by a unique class in the model. Furthermore, classes which should be included in the model but do not appear in any data source can also be added.

The specification of models implies that software is required to implement databases which are capable to store objects related to the model persistently. Adding or removing classes from the conceptual schema causes classes and objects in the storage layer to be modified. Adding an object class to the database allows the user to both store objects of this class persistently in the database and to retrieve selected objects from the database by using database queries.

The integrative aspects of database modelling consist of (1) integrating classes from different data sources into the model and (2) importing objects from the content stored in these data sources. Figure 11.8 shows by example a conceptual schema

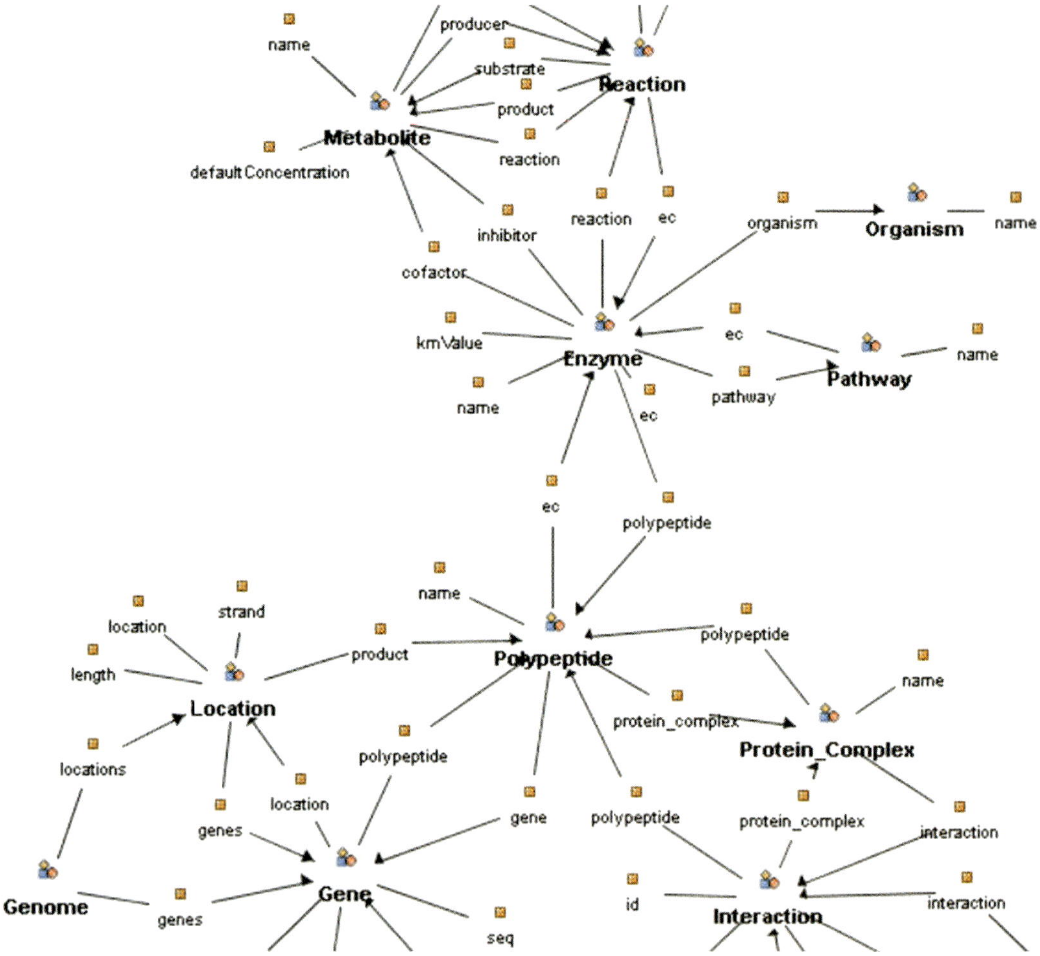

Fig. 11.8 Conceptual modelling of static properties and relationships

containing classes from different domains drawn by our tool iUDB[ISB], which enables the modeller to edit specifications interactively and implements databases automatically based upon the specifications modelled. The conceptual model includes classes at metabolic level (reactions, metabolites, enzymes, ...), as well as classes from gene regulatory level (genes, polypeptides, regulatory interactions, ...). In this drawing attributes of classes are directly linked to the a class, e. g. the class *pathway* has an attribute *name*, which means that for each pathway a name is stored as value. Attributes which are additionally linked to other classes determine directed relationships between objects of these classes. In the example shown in Figure 11.8 pathways are related to enzymes, expressed by the attribute *ec*. These directed relationships are also called references.

With the modelling of processes by means of object-oriented modelling, recent objects participating at processes should be modelled as a separate class. Even if supported by modelling tools, the identification of object classes is conceptual work, it requires knowledge of the biochemical background and it cannot be automated. Nevertheless, we can automate the integration of objects using data integration. One important aspect here is the adequate specification of object keys, which are attributes that uniquely identify objects, so that it is impossible to store two objects that have the same values for all of key attributes.

Figure 11.9 shows how the specification of object keys directly influence the object space. In the example an object class Enzyme is shown which is uniquely identified not only by the attribute *EC* (EC classification), but also by *Organism* and *Tissue*. With this three-dimensional object space, enzymes having the EC number "3.5.3.1" occupy the plane defined by *Tissue* and *Organism* at the point where *ec_number* = 3.5.3.1.

When integrating data from relational data sources into a model defined by a conceptual schema object keys become important as integrity constraints for assigning external data to local objects. In general, a set of these assertions is called mapping, whereby in the approach described here for each datasource the modelling of a separate mapping to an object class is necessary. By that, there are no dependencies between different the mappings of different data sources.

The process of object integration will be briefly explained. As mentioned before, the integration of objects requires the modelling of mappings between classes and data sources (Figure 11.10). These mappings contain assertions between the attributes specified with the class and the columns of the related tables. In most cases, different attributes will be mapped to different tables. In the figure above, three col-

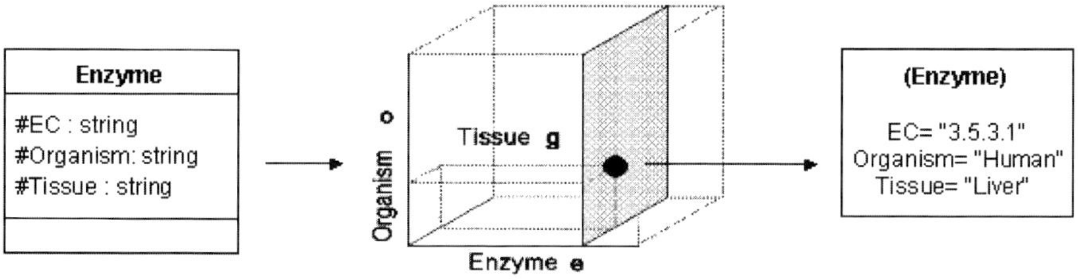

Fig. 11.9 Definition of object spaces by object keys.

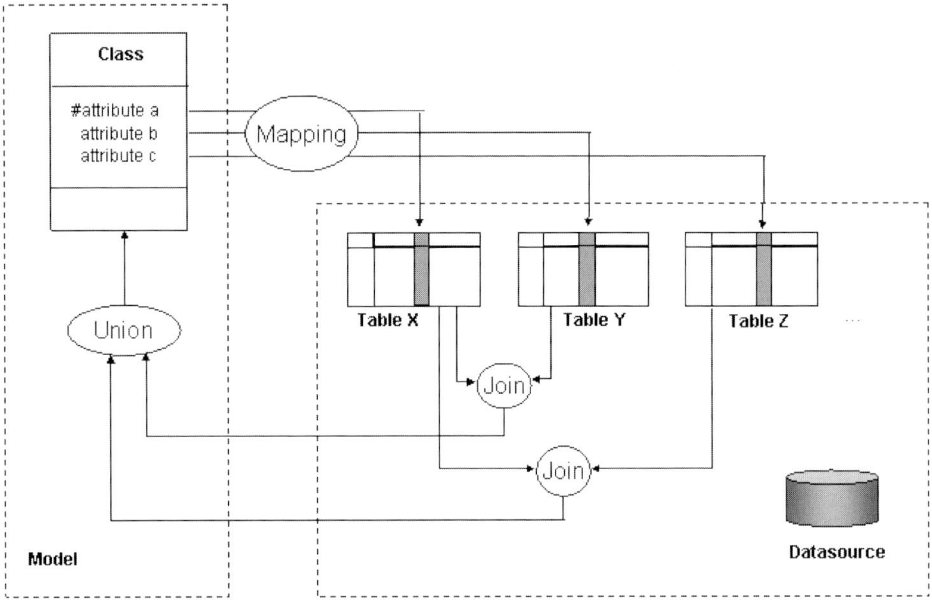

Fig. 11.10 Integration of objects from relational tables

umns of the tables *X*, *Y* and *Z* assigned to the attributes *a*, *b* and *c* have been marked. After all assertions have been defined by the modeller, an integration mechanism will apply them in order to select values from the assigned columns. To organize the results in an object-oriented format, relational *join* operations are computed to combine the columns. Finally, the result has to be inserted into the model. A *union* operation is now storing all values within the associated objects. Object keys are used here to locate the objects in the model.

11.4.2
Process Oriented Modelling Using Views

With the modelling of objects discussed in the last section we have been integrating and storing data locally as objects in our model. We next have to analyse and clean the content of integrated databases empirically in a mostly time-consuming and application-specific procedure. The following step in our workflow is the modelling of bioprocesses based on the principle of modelling patterns of processes described in Section 11.1.

Our method focuses at the static relationships of object oriented models. To give an example, Figure 11.11 shows a subset of the schema drawn in Figure 11.8, where we now try to identify object classes which represent dynamic processes. Actually, the classes *Enzyme* and *Reaction* are candidates for representing the catalysis of biochemical reactions. We intuitively decide to model processes of the type catalysis including all objects of the class *Reaction*. The class has been marked with a circle to

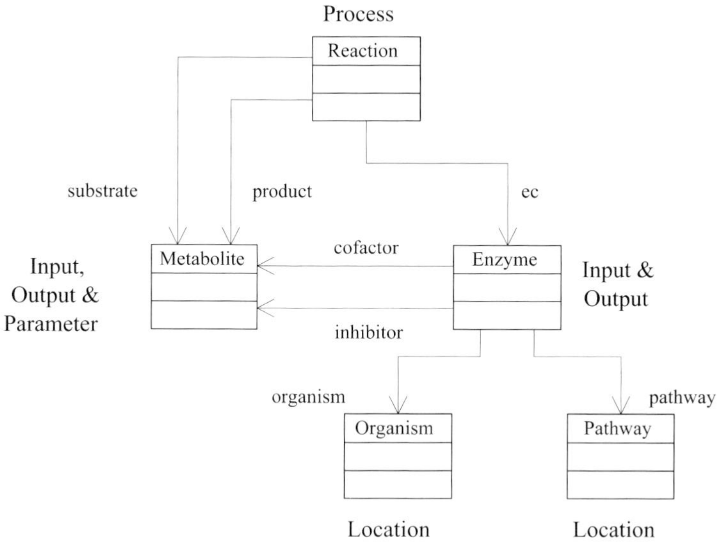

Fig. 11.11 Modelling patterns of processes using paths of static relationships.

determine the starting point for the further operations. As next we model all objects participating at our processes. Therefore, we define paths in the schema starting at *Reaction* and leading to each participant. The first path contains the reference *substrate* pointing to the class *Metabolite*. The path constitutes that all metabolite objects reachable by the path will take part at processes of the type catalysis. Additionally, there is a path to *Metabolite* using the reference *product*. Here we see, that it is necessary to differ between the roles of a path. In our approach four roles can be assigned:

- Input,
- Output,
- Parameter and
- Location.

There are multiple roles assignable to each path. Input and output roles are used to define the flow of material. Parameters are objects influencing the process, e. g. as inhibitors or cofactors. Paths leading to locations determine where the processes can be observed. In the example we defined at least defined six paths. Different metabolites act as input, as output and as parameter. The same enzymes are defined as input and as output of the process, while organisms and pathways give us information about the location.

Actually, the construction of a path is very simple, but once defined such a pattern of a process can act as a rule to calculate instances of processes from object-oriented models. For each object of the class *Reaction* a single processes will be created and the paths defined in the pattern will be traced starting at the current object. All objects found at the end of the traced paths are then assigned to the processes in the role in which they have been defined in the model.

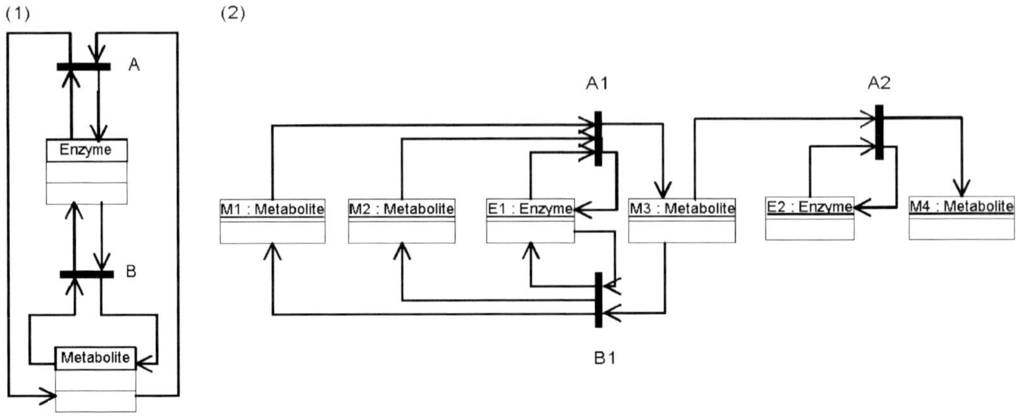

Fig. 11.12 Relationship between conceptual mode (1) and objects level (2).

The combination of classes of processes leads to conceptual process oriented models, which are bipartite graphs containing classes of processes and classes objects. Figure 11.12 shows the relationship between a conceptual model (1) and the instances defined by the model (2). The example contains two object classes *Metabolite* and *Enzyme* and two classes of processes *A* and *B* which are consuming and producing objects of the classes *Metabolite* and *Enzyme* in different directions. In fact, these two patterns could describe the catalysis as a reversible and discrete process.

In the second part of Figure 11.12 we see a process oriented network including different types of objects and processes. It is clear that a conceptual model with a relatively low number of elements can describe the structure behind a very complex network. The advantage of the approach consists in the automation of building the instances from conceptual models. The remaining task for the modeller is to identify the types of processes and to model the patterns. Depending on the size of the object oriented model, the automated reconstruction of processes produces a large number of element which are interconnected in large scale networks. For performance enhancements in the further analysis of the, we materialize all of the computed processes, which means that they are stored directly within the model in a database.

11.4.3
System Oriented Modelling and Simulation

Actually, the application of conceptual process oriented modelling leads to very large and complex networks. For each of the molecular objects the model provides information about processes that consume and produce it. Each process provides information about its materials flow, parameters and location. The motivation the last step in our workflow, called systems integration, is to discover networks formed by different models and to use these networks in the modelling of dynamic systems.

To enable the discussion about the occurrence of objects as potential agents, we have to model them conceptually as participants at processes in the model. Furthermore, recent information is hidden in the complexity of the total network. The task is now to analyse the network and to extract the parts of interest, while unnecessary parts will be hidden. A first reduction will be achieved by filtering the total network for location specific processes. Actually, modelling of organisms and pathways as locations of bioprocesses will result in networks of organism specific pathways, e. g. the Glycolysis pathway in the organism rat. Based upon the conceptual schema of Figure 11.12, the next Figure 11.13 visualizes the network of all biochemical reactions in the organism rat as a graph.

It is obvious that the filtering of networks by their location will still produce complex information, while it is not clear that the network is a closed graph. A first approach is the exploration of the network by hand by recursively traversing the database. Another is approach uses graph theory to discover complex relationships automatically.

What can we expect from this approach are qualitative statements. Simple knockout experiments can be executed by computing shortest and alternative pathways, while added and deleting molecular objects in the network. Furthermore, graph theory can be applied for the modelling of systems. To differ the elements of a system from its environment, closed networks need to be computed interconnecting an initial set of objects and processes. The automated reconstruction of networks can be used to compute the topology of a dynamic system. In cases where only a low amount information networks of similar biological systems can be merged. To continue the workflow with third party tools, e. g. visualization and simulation tools, the discovered networks can be stored within the model and exported into common graph based and systems biology file formats.

As explained in Section 11.1, the quantitative modelling of dynamic systems includes equations for each process, e. g. differential, difference or stochastic equations. Solving them as equation systems aims at the computation of initial state or optimisation problems. Actually, adding dynamics to a process requires the specifica-

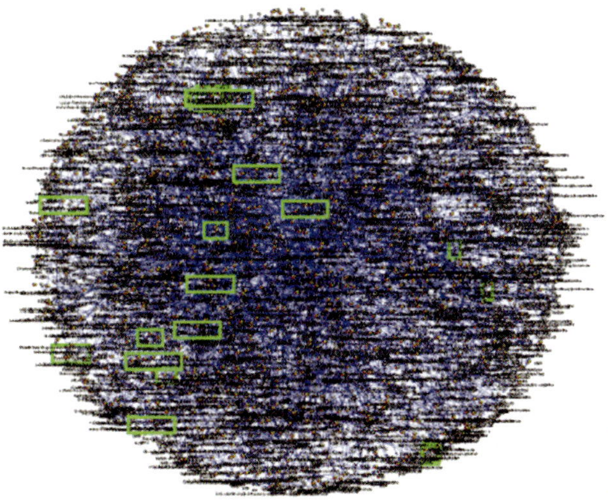

Fig. 11.13 Visualization and exploration of materialized views.

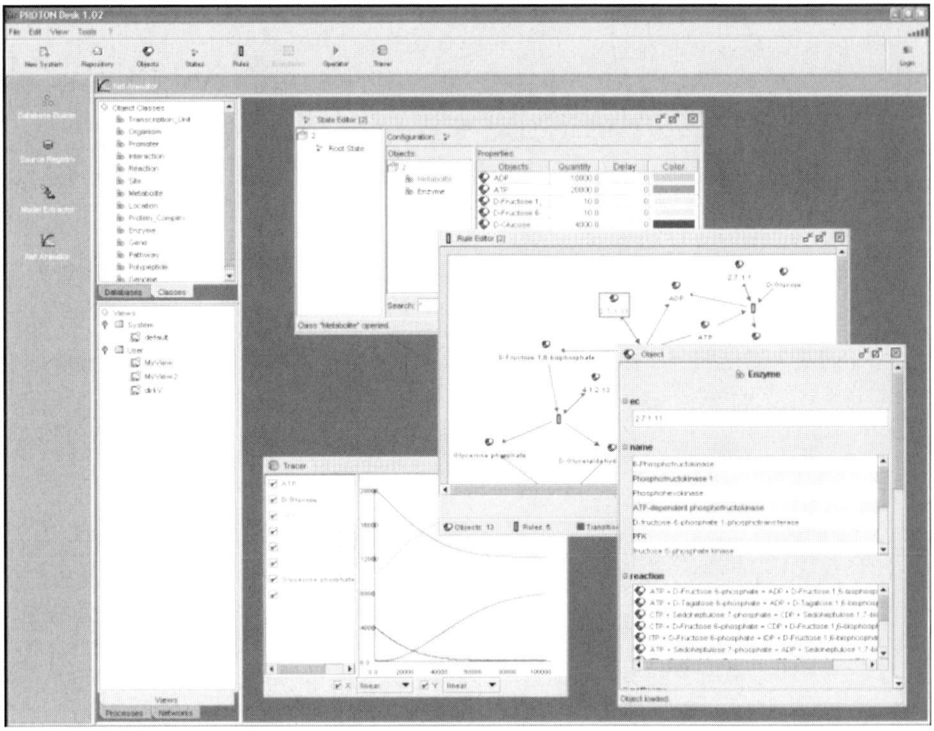

Fig. 11.14 Quantitative simulation of integratively modelled systems.

tion of the equation itself, as well as the specification of the concentrations of the participating objects and the estimated parameters.

11.4.4 Implementation

The approach of integrative modelling covers different fields of computer science. At this point we give a short overview of our implementation of the methods discussed. The basic idea of the PROTON system (Figure 11.15) is to enable the modeller to control the modelling cycle interactively. At our point of view a centralized and service oriented architecture is suitable to handle the many different operations. In this approach a model is represented by a service providing the content of the model as well as the methods operating at the model: preprocessing of data, objects integration, processes integration and systems integration.

The right choice of the underlying database system is essential for the approach. Our module *Proton Server*, which is hosting the models of different users makes internally use of the database management system *FastObjects t7* from Versant. The system has been completely developed in the Java programming language. Consequently, the graphical modelling environment ProtonDesk has been implemented as

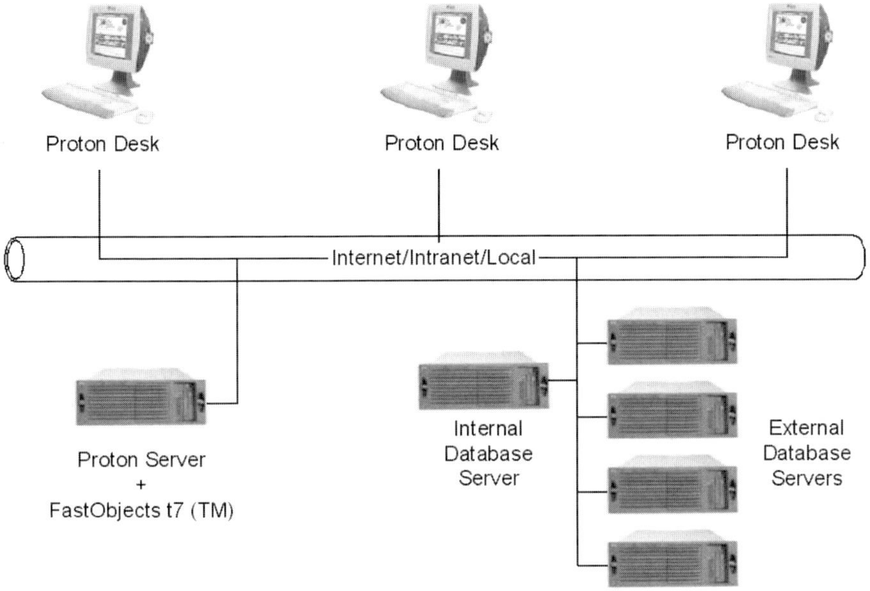

Fig. 11.15 PROTON integrates methods and data using a service based architecture.

a so-called smart client, which is an autonomous application making use of the models and methods implemented in the server.

11.5 Summary

This chapter has introduced novel methods of using computational approaches in integratively modelling biological systems. Within the growing amount of data, more and more intelligent and integrated computational systems are required to enable the user to control the networks contained in molecular databases. Modelling remains time consuming work and there are tasks, especially those related to tuning the dynamics of systems, that still need human interaction and cannot be done automatically. Nevertheless, we have progressed from modelling of instances to conceptual modelling techniques. In addition, hands-on approaches were discussed at different levels from modelling to implementation to enable and motivate our readers to transfer them into their own developments.

References

1. McMurry, J. (1996) *Organic Chemistry*, 4th edn. Brooks/Cole Publishing Company, California.
2. Russel, P. J. (1996) *Genetics*, 4th edn. Harper Collins, New York.
3. Rang, H. P., Dale, M. M. and Ritter, J. M. (2003) *Pharmacology*, Churchill Livingstone, Edinburgh.
4. Wastney, M. E., Patterson, B.H., Linares, O.A., Greif, P.C. and Boston, R.C. (1999) *Investigating Biological Systems Using Modeling*, Academic Press., California.
5. Baxevanis, A. D. (2001) *The Molecular Biology Database Collection: an update compilation of biological database resources.* Nucleic Acids Res, 29, 1–10.
6. Boyce, W. E. and DiPrima, R. C. (2000) *Elementary Differential Equations.* Wiley, New York.
7. Mendes, P. (1997) *Biochemistry by numbers: simulation of biochemical pathways with Gepasi 3.* Trends Biochem Sci, 22, 361–363.
8. Goryanin, I., Hodgman, T. C. and Selkov, E. (1999) *Mathematical simulation and analysis of cellular metabolism and regulation.* Bioinformatics 15, 749–758.
9. Drath, R. (1998) Hybrid Object Nets: An object-oriented concept for modeling complex hybrid systems. In: *Hybrid Dynamical Systems. 3rd International Conference on Automation of Mixed Processes*, ADPM'98, pp. 437–42.
10. Masao Nagasaki, Atsushi Doi, Hiroshi Matsuno, Satoru Miyano, *A Versatile Petri Net Based Architecture for Modeling and Simulation of Complex Biological Processes*, Genome Informatics, 15(1), pp. 180–197.
11. Kohn, M. C. and Letzkus, W. (1982) A graph-theoretical analysis of metabolic regulation. Journal of Theoretical Biology, 100, 293–304.
12. Kohn, M. C. and Lemieux, D. R. (1991) *Identification of regulatory properties of metabolic networks by graph theoretical modeling.* Journal ofTheoretical Biology, 150, 3–25.
13. Schomburg, I., Chang, A. and Schomburg, D. (2002) *BRENDA, enzyme data and metabolic information. Nucleic Acids Res.*, **30**, 47–49.
14. Kanehisa, M. and Goto, S. (2000). *KEGG: Kyoto Encyclopedia of Genes and Genome.* Nucleic Acids Res, 28, 27–30.
15. Karp, P.D., Riley, M., Saier, M., Paulsen, I.T., Paley, S., Pellegrini-Toole, A. (2002) The Ecocyc database. *Nucleic Acids Res*, 30, 56.
16. Jacob, F. and Monod, J. (1961) Genetic regulatory mechanism in the synthesis of proteins. *J Mol Biol*, 3, 318–356.
17. Matys, V., Fricke, E., Geffers, R., Gösling, E., Haubrock, M., Hehl, R., Hornischer, K., Karas, D., Kel, A. E., Kel-Margoulis, O. V., Kloos, D.-U., Land, S., Lewicki-Potapov, H., Michael, B., Münch, R., Reuter, S., Rotert, I., Saxel, H., Scheer, M., Thiele, S. and Wingender, E. (2003) TRANSFAC: transcriptional regulation, from patterns to profiles. *Nucleic Acids Res*, 31, 374–378.
18. Huerta, A.M., Salgado, H., Thieffry, D. and Collado-Vides, J. (1998) RegulonDB: a database on transcription regulation in *Escherichia coli. Nucleic Acids Res*, 26, 55–60.
19. Baker, W., van den Broek, A., Camon, E., Hingamp, P., Sterk, P., Stoesser, G. and Tuli, M. A. (2000) The EMBL nucleotide sequence database. *Nucleic Acid Res*, 28, 19–23.
20. Boeckmann, B., Bairoch, A., Apweiler, R., Blatter, M.-C., Estreicher, A., Gasteiger, E., Martin, M. J., Michoud, K., O'Donovan, C., Phan, I., Pilbout, S. and Schneider, M. (2003) The SwissProt protein sequence database and its supplement TrEMBL in 2003. *Nucleic Acids Res*, 31, 365–370.
22. Zhang, C. and Zhang, S. (2002) *Association Rule Mining.* Springer-Verlag, Berlin.
23. Booch, G. (1996) *Object-Oriented Analysis and Design.* Addison-Wesley.

24. Etzold, T. and Argos, P. (1993) SRS: an indexing and retrieval tools for flat file data libraries. *CABIOS*, 9, 49–57.

25. Freier, A., Hofestädt, R., Lange, M. and Scholz, U. (2002) BioDataServer: a SQL-based service for the online integration of life science data. *In Silico Biology*, 2.

26. Karp, P. and Paley, S. (1996) Integrated access to metabolic and genomic data. *J Comp Biol*, 3, 191–212.

27. Krull, M., Voss, N., Choi, C., Pistor, S., Potapov, A. and Wingender, E. (2003) *TRANSPATH: an integrated database on signal transduction and a tool for array analysis.* Nucleic Acids Res. 2003 Jan 1; 31(1):97–100.

28. Shimizu TS and Le Novere N (2001) *STOCHSIM: modelling of stochastic biomolecular processes* Bioinformatics 17, 575–576.

29. Kierzek A.M., Zaim J. and Zielenkiewicz P., (2001) *The effect of transcription and translation initiation frequencies on the stochastic fluctuations in prokaryotic gene expression.* Journal of Biology Chemistry. 276, 8165–8172.

12
Databases and Tools for *in silico* Analysis of Regulation of Gene Expression

Alexander Kel, Olga Kel-Margoulis, Jürgen Borlak, Dimitry Tchekmenev, and Edgar Wingender

12.1
Introduction

Regulation of gene expression is the key problem of the era of functional genomics. Now we know that genes in genomes of higher eukaryotic organisms are regulated mainly by means of multiple regulatory proteins – transcription factors (TF) – acting through specific regulatory sequences (TF binding sites) that are usually located near the genes when they act as a promoter or at more remote locations when they are part of an enhancer. Having genomic sequences available on one hand and the massive, albeit phenomenological, amount of gene-expression data on the other hand, the challenge is to understand the regulatory mechanisms affecting every single gene in the genome by computer analysis of the gene regulatory sequences and by integrating these data with biological knowledge of gene signal transduction and metabolic and physiological networks. Sophisticated computational tools for regulatory sequence analysis that employ powerful statistical and machine-learning algorithms driven by the rich databases that collect biological facts enable us to make profound *in silico* predictions and to formulate experimentally testable hypotheses. Such *in silico*-driven experiments can greatly accelerate our understanding of gene regulatory mechanisms and the identification of new target genes. Understanding how gene regulation mechanisms are encoded in the genomic regulatory sequences will give us a powerful means for deciphering causes of major human diseases.

12.2
Concepts of Gene Regulation

In multicellular organisms the number of different possible intracellular molecular states is extremely large. These states correspond to different stages of cellular ontogenesis in different tissues, organs, and cell types, to many developmental stages and cell cycle phases, to the huge number of cell responses, and to various external

Handbook of Toxicogenomics: Strategies and Applications. Edited by Jürgen Borlak

ISBN: 3-527-30342-1

and internal signals and influences. Each state is characterized and precisely organized by differential expressions of specific sets of genes. To generate this huge diversity of cellular molecular states, the expressions of most of the genes in a genome are organized in multiple ways, producing a complex pattern of gene expression in various cellular conditions. Gene expression is regulated at several stages, namely transcription (including initiation, elongation, and termination), splicing, translation, and protein degradation. Often, transcription initiation is the most important and closely regulated level of regulating gene expression. A multiplicity of gene-expression patterns on the transcription level is provided by means of combinatorial regulation. Combinatorial regulation of transcription is organized through binding of a multiplicity of transcription factors (TFs) to their target sites (cis elements) in regulatory regions. Corresponding TFs interact with each other and with particular components of the basal transcription complex, as well as with coactivators and corepressors, histone acetyltransferases and deacetylases, thereby forming function-specific multiprotein complexes, which are often referred to as enhanceosomes.

12.2.1
Transcription Factors

Transcriptional regulation is achieved by a functionally defined large family of proteins: the transcription factors (McKnight and Yamamoto, 1992; Wingender, 1993). These proteins interact with the DNA of promoters and enhancers in a more or less sequence-specific manner, recognizing defined sequence patterns and/or structural features. In contrast to prokaryotes, where the major control mechanism is to repress a generally active transcription machinery, eukaryotes have to meet much more complex requirements to coordinate the execution of genetic programs. This is achieved by directed activation of those genes whose products are needed under certain cellular conditions, in general, only a few percent of all genes of the genome. Once bound to the DNA, these factors may influence transcription by several mechanisms.

- Most TFs enhance the formation of the preinitiation complex at the TATA box/initiator element through interaction of a transactivation domain with the components of the basal transcription complex, either directly or through coactivators or mediators.
- Some TFs cause changes in the chromosome architecture, making the chromatin more accessible to RNA polymerase(s).
- Some TFs are auxiliary factors, optimizing the DNA conformation to favour the activity of another TF.
- Some TFs exert repressing influences, either directly by an active inhibiting domain or by disturbing the required ensemble of TFs within a regulatory array (promoter, enhancer).
- One group of TFs do not directly bind to DNA but rather assemble into higher-order complexes through protein–protein interactions.

A definition of 'transcription factor' was proposed earlier (Wingender, 1997): a transcription factor is a protein that regulates transcription after nuclear translocation by specific interaction with DNA or by stoichiometric interaction with a protein that can be assembled into a sequence-specific DNA–protein complex.

Most transcription factors are modular. They may include:

- A DNA-binding domain (DBD).
- An oligomerization domain, because most factors bind to DNA as dimers, but some as higher-order complexes. This region usually forms a functional unit with the DBD.
- A transactivation (or transrepressing) domain, which is frequently characterized by a significant overrepresentation of a certain type of amino acid residue (e.g., glutamine-rich, proline-rich, serine/threonine-rich, or acidic).
- A modulating region that is often the target of modifying enzymes, mostly protein kinases.
- A ligand-binding domain.

Except for the last domain type, these domains may be redundantly present in a single polypeptide chain.

12.2.2 Modern Concepts of the Structure and Function of the Gene-regulation Regions in the Genome

Blueprints for gene regulation are encoded in the structure of gene regulatory sequences. It is generally accepted that the gene-regulation regions of eukaryotic organisms have a modular structure. The fundamental principle of how molecular genetics systems are organized can be described as a hierarchy of modules (Ratner, 1990), for example, the modular structure of genomic DNA in both its structural and regulatory parts (Ratner, 1990). Recently, much attention has been paid to studying the modular structure of regulatory regions that control transcription of eukaryotic genes (Dynan, 1989; Johnson and McKnight 1989; Struhl, 1999; Werner, 1999). Modularity is a very important principle for understanding the molecular mechanisms of function of these regions and their evolution and especially for deciphering the complex mechanisms of differential gene expression in multicellular organisms.

12.2.2.1 Modular Hierarchical Structure of Gene-regulation Regions

Regulatory DNA is characterized by a modular hierarchical structure. An elementary module corresponds to a single TF binding site. Next, hierarchical levels are occupied by composite elements, promoters and enhancers, and finally by an integral system for regulation of gene transcription.

The regulatory regions of every gene contain a number of binding sites for structurally and functionally different transcription factors, thus providing combinatorial regulation – one of the major principles of genome structure and functioning. Gene-specific regulation in many cellular situations is achieved through the formation of multicomponent protein complexes on regulatory DNA. Both specific protein–DNA and protein–protein interactions contribute to gene-specific transcriptional regulation.

We consider several levels of structural hierarchy.

1. The minimal functional modules are the *binding sites for transcription factors.* These are short DNA elements (5–20 bp) that can be specifically recognized by certain transcription factors. There are many different TF binding sites, in accord with the great variety of transcription factors. As of now, >1300 human TFs have been collected in the TRANSFAC® database. As an example, a collection of binding sites for AhR factors is shown in Figure 12.1. The function of DNA binding sites is the specific binding of TFs and their tethering in a particular orientation relative to the other components of multiprotein complexes. Binding sites for the

Site sequence	acc	site ID	gene	from	to
cacgtg**gcgtg**tcttgt	R02649	MOUSE$CYTOP_01	CYP1A1 (cytochrome P450 1A1)	-1227	-1146
cagcta**gcgtg**acagca	R02650	MOUSE$CYTOP_02	CYP1A1 (cytochrome P450 1A1)	-1076	-1048
ggagtt**gcgtg**agaaga	R02651	MOUSE$CYTOP_03	CYP1A1 (cytochrome P450 1A1)	-1066	-977
ccgaat**gcgtg**cgatcg	R02652	MOUSE$CYTOP_04	CYP1A1 (cytochrome P450 1A1)	-933	-869
tgtctc**gcgtg**gatcct	R02653	MOUSE$CYTOP_05	CYP1A1 (cytochrome P450 1A1)	-893	-641
aagctc**gcgtg**agaagc	R02654	MOUSE$CYTOP_06	CYP1A1 (cytochrome P450 1A1)	-509	-448
gtcgag**gcgtg**cgttcc	R13150	MOUSE$CYP1B1_01	Cyp1B1 (cytochrome P-450 1B1)	-870	-841
cgctgg**gcgtg**cagatg	R13159	HS$CYP1A1_01	CYP1A1 (cytochrome P450 1A1)	-401	-391
tagctt**gcgtg**cgccgg	R13161	HS$CYP1A1_03	CYP1A1 (cytochrome P450 1A1)	-900	-890
ggcgtt**gcgtg**agaagg	R13162	HS$CYP1A1_04	CYP1A1 (cytochrome P450 1A1)	-988	-978
cccctc**gcgtg**actgcg	R13163	HS$CYP1A1_05	CYP1A1 (cytochrome P450 1A1)	-1061	-1051
cgagtt**gcgtg**agaaga	R00270	RAT$CYTOP_04	CYP1A1 (cytochrome P450, 1a1)	-1029	-1005
ctgctc**gcgtg**agaagc	R13271	RABBIT$CYP1A1_01	CYP1A1 (cytochrome P450 1A1)	-1012	-984
cggctc**gcgtg**ctgggg	R13226	MOUSE$AhRR_01	AhRR (Aryl hydrocarbon receptor repressor)	-59	-55
gactta**gcgtg**ttcctc	R13227	MOUSE$AhRR_02	AhRR (Aryl hydrocarbon receptor repressor)	-393	-387
ttaaag**gcgtg**agccgt	R13228	MOUSE$AhRR_03	AhRR (Aryl hydrocarbon receptor repressor)	-1302	-1296
cggccg**gcgtg**cgcggg	R13260	HS$CATHD_02	CATH-D (cathepsin D)	-130	-126
tgcctt**gcgtg**tttgtg	R13262	MOUSE$POLK_01	Polk (polymerase (DNA directed), kappa)		
agagtt**gcgtg**cccctt	R13263	MOUSE$POLK_02	Polk (polymerase (DNA directed), kappa)		
gaatgt**gcgtg**acaagg	R13264	RAT$UGT1A1_01	Ugt1 (UDP-glucuronosyltransferase 1 family, member 1)	-134	-129
ttatgt**gcgtg**tgtata	R13237	Mouse$IL2_15	IL-2 (interleukin-2)	-860	-831
gcatgt**gcgtg**cacatg	R13238	Mouse$IL2_16	IL-2 (interleukin-2)	-823	-794
aagttc**gcgtg**acgaag	R13240	MOUSE$ALDH3A1_01	Aldh3a1 (aldehyde dehydrogenase 3a1)	-98	-74
tggggg**gcgtg**gcacac	R13248	HS$CFOS_28	c-fos	-1163	-1159
gaactc**gcgtg**cagcag	R13268	HS$UGT1A6_01	UGT1A6 (UDP glycosyltransferase 1 family, polypeptide A6)	-1502	-1498
attaca**gcgtg**agccac	R13274	HS$PS2_02	PS2	-530	-508

Fig. 12.1 A collection of binding sites for AhR transcription factors. The sequence of each site, accession number, and site ID in the TRANSFAC database, gene name, and position of the site relative to the start of transcription are shown. The core part of the site is shown in bold.

same TF can be found in regulatory regions of several different genes and therefore can be considered to be standard modules constituting a regulatory region. But these sites may differ in one or several positions, which makes the problem of recognizing such sites by computer programs extremely difficult.

2. Regulatory modules of the second hierarchical level are *composite regulatory elements*. The term 'composite element' (CE) was introduced during studies of the glucocorticoid response element in the mouse proliferin promoter, in which a glucocorticoid receptor binding site is adjacent to an AP-1 site (Diamond et al., 1990). In addition, this term was applied to very different pairs of interacting sites and factors (Gutman and Wasylyk, 1990; Du et al., 1993; Jackson et al., 1993; Rooney et al., 1995, and others). Based on these examples, we define a composite element as a minimal functional unit within which both protein–DNA and protein–protein interactions contribute to a highly specific pattern of regulation of gene transcription (Kel. et al., 1995 b, 1997). A specialized database, TRANSCompel (Kel-Margoulis et al., 2000, 2002), contains information about known CEs.

Binding of a TF to the regulatory region is determined not only by the structure of the cis element, but also by the possible protein–protein interactions; in other words, by its ability to specifically contact – directly or indirectly – the factors binding to other sites of the given regulatory region. Two or three closely situated binding sites for different TFs in combination form a CE, which is a functional unit with new regulatory advantages. Structurally similar elements are present in very different genes, which seems to imply that such regulatory modules are functionally significant.

CEs are composed of the modules of the previous hierarchical level, the individual binding sites (Figure 12.2). Similar binding sites may constitute parts of functionally different CEs. For instance, AP-1 binding sites are parts of the AP1/ETS composite elements, NFAT/AP1, NF-κB/AP1, and AP1/Oct. CEs of the AP1/ETS type provide gene activation in response to a variety of proliferative signals and constitute the so-called Ras and oncogene response units (Wasylyk et al., 1993). NFAT/AP1 CEs provide cross coupling of Ca^{2+}-dependent and Ras/Raf/MEK signalling pathways (Rao et al., 1997). NF-κB/AP1 CEs contribute to gene activation in response to hypoxia. In turn, TFs of the ETS family cooperate within CEs not only with AP-1 factors, but also with a variety of different TFs, for example, CBFα, SRF, Sp1, and ETS. Factors of the NF-κB family can be found within CEs with C/EBP, STAT, Sp1, IRF, HMG I, etc.

At this hierarchical level, the potential variability is considerably higher than that of individual binding sites. Within a set of similar CEs, several parameters can vary: individual binding sites themselves, sequence and distance between individual sites, and sometimes, mutual orientation of individual sites. For instance, CEs of the AP1/ETS type differ in terms of the mutual location of individual sites (Figure 12.2, compare N 1 and 2). Individual binding sites can be immediately adjacent (Figure 12.2, N 1), overlapping (Figure 12.2, N 4), or separated by several

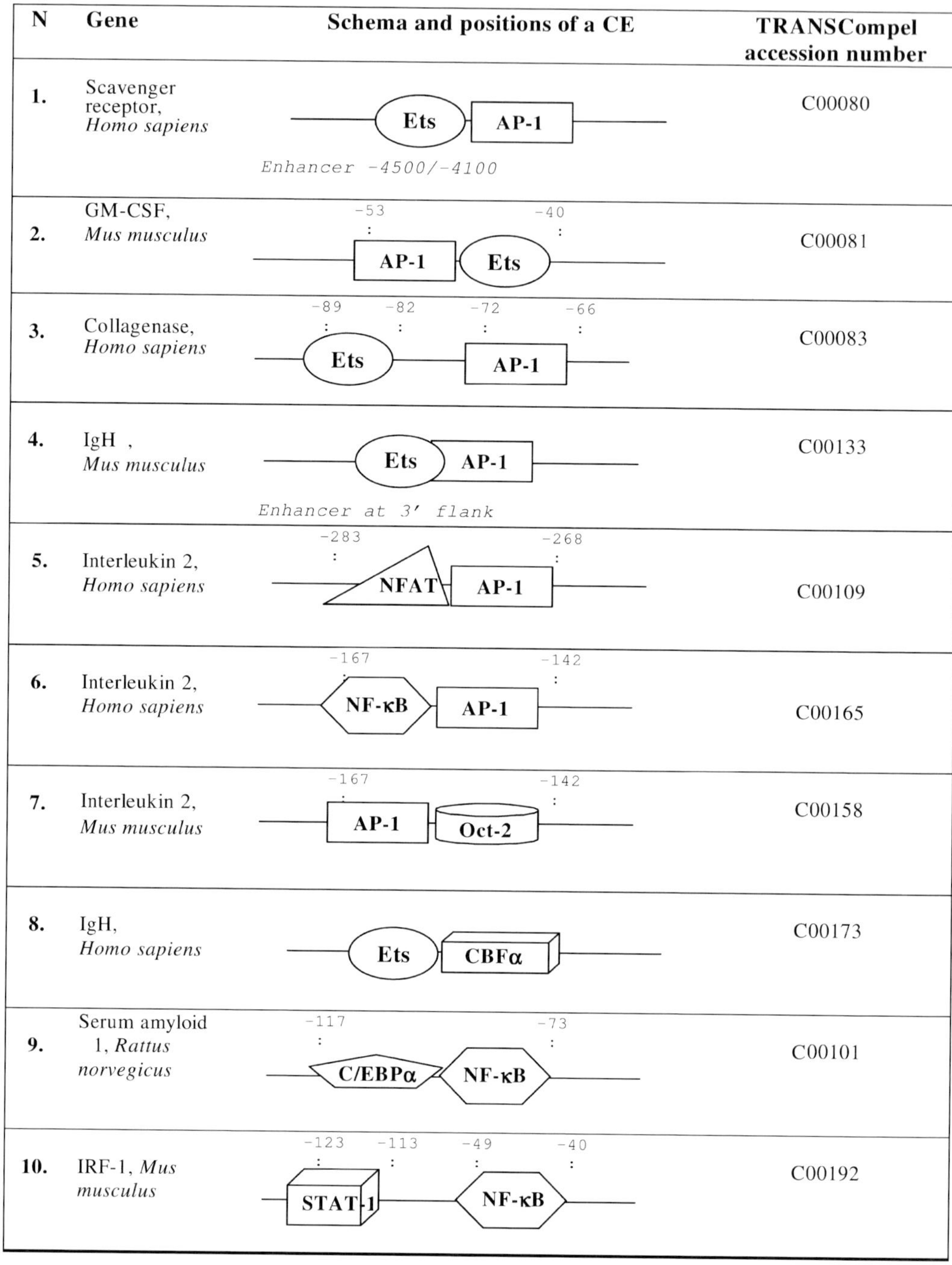

Fig. 12.2 Composite regulatory elements as the second level of hierarchical structure of gene regulatory regions.

nucleotides (Figure 12.2, N 3). Thus, composite regulatory elements, as modules of the second hierarchical level, display some new functions that cannot be provided by individual binding sites. New functions resulting from protein–protein interactions, along with DNA–protein interactions, include the following:

- Stabilization of DNA–protein complex by direct or indirect interactions between the corresponding TFs (Chen et al., 1998, and others).
- Cross-coupling of intracellular signal-transduction pathways and, as a result, new functions in gene transcription regulation (considered in detail below).

3. The next level in the hierarchical organization of gene regulatory regions is formed by promoters, enhancers, and distal regulatory regions. The structural similarity between promoters and enhancers is that both are composed of the modules of the previous hierarchical levels – CEs and individual binding sites for TFs. A crucial difference between promoters and enhancers is that basic promoter elements – the TATA box, Inr-element, and some others – are responsible for formation of the basal transcription complex, the precise definition of the starting point, and the direction of transcription. Enhancers and distal regulatory regions modulate the rate of transcription initiation, often resulting in tissue-specific or inducible regulation, as well as some other features. Within eukaryotic genes, enhancers can have various locations.

   - Immediately upstream of promoters, for example, in the human interleukin-2 gene and the human apolipoprotein AI gene.
   - In far upstream regions: for example, the T-cell–specific inducible enhancer in the human GM-CSF gene is located at –3500 bp, and in the human IL-3 gene at –13 000 bp.
   - In introns: for instance, the cell cycle-dependent enhancer of the human *pcna p120* gene is located in the first intron. The liver-specific enhancer of the human apolipoprotein B gene is located in the first intron, and a liver/small intestine-specific enhancer is in the second intron. A p53-inducible enhancer is located in the third intron of the human GADD45 gene.
   - In 3′ gene flanks, for example, in the human and mouse IgH genes.

   Promoters and enhancers are formed by several modules of the previous hierarchical levels: CEs and individual binding sites. Many parameters are required to describe the structure of the promoters and enhancers: the number and set of individual binding sites and CEs, their variations, mutual location, and orientation, as well as the distance between them. The consequence of the variability is that each promoter or enhancer is practically unique. In addition, some of the promoters or enhancers are similar in terms of sets of individual binding sites.

4. Finally, the highest level of hierarchy is represented by *the integration of all regulatory regions* of a gene. On the basis of known examples, the following functions of the integrated system of gene regulatory regions can be considered.

   - Determining the local chromatin structure, which influences the accessibility of particular DNA regions to TFs.

- Overall control of the transcription at all stages, including initiation, elongation, and termination.
- Contributing to the 3-dimensional DNA structure.
- Providing a unique expression pattern for each gene.
- Providing coordinated gene expression.

12.3 Databases Relating to Gene Regulation

Despite the fact that gene regulation is one of the focuses of functional genomics, there are currently only a few databases that store data on gene regulation (Table 12.1). The reason is that the molecular mechanisms of gene regulation appear to be very complex, which leads to a wide variety of experimental techniques for analysis of gene regulation. Laborious manual annotation of the scientific literature is needed to systematize all this information and store it in a computer-readable form. The recently appearing masses of data from microarray gene expression experiments are very useful for understanding gene regulation and can be more easily organized in a database. But these phenomenological data only partly meet the needs of the biological community working on functional genomics, because data regarding the details of molecular mechanisms of gene regulation are necessary to understand the causality of the observed gene expression.

Tab. 12.1 Databases that contain information on various aspects of gene regulation.

N	*Database*	*Information on gene regulation*	*URL*
1.	EMBL Nucleotide Sequence Database	For some genes there is information on location of transcription start site, TATA box, CAAT box, and some TF binding sites.	http://www.ebi.ac.uk/embl.html
2.	GenBank		http://www.ncbi.nlm.nih.gov/Web/Genbank/
3.	SwissProt	Structure of TFs, domain structure, short functional description. For many proteins there is information on tissue-specific expression.	http://www.expasy.ch/
4.	PIR: Protein Information Resource		http://www-nbrf.georgetown.edu/pir
6.	EPD: Eukaryotic Promoter Database	Location of transcription starts; some information on gene expression; functional classification of gene products.	http://www.epd.isb-sib.ch/
7.	DBTSS	Transcription start sites; genomic sequences (human and mouse); predicted TF binding sites.	http://dbtss.hgc.jp/
8.	TRANSFAC	TFs, TF classification, their binding sites, weight matrices, structure of gene regulatory regions, gene expression.	http://www.biobase.de/ http://www.gene-regulation.com/

Tab. 12.1 (continued)

N	Database	Information on gene regulation	URL
9.	TRRD	Structure of transcription regulatory regions of genes; binding sites for TFs, gene expression.	http://www.bionet.nsc.ru/trrd/
10.	COMPEL, TRANSCompel	Composite regulatory elements; TF protein–protein interaction.	http://compel.bionet.nsc.ru/ http://www.biobase.de/
11.	TFD	Sites of TF binding; consensi.	http://www.ifti.org/
12.	RegulonDB	Transcription regulation of *E. coli* genes. TFs and their binding sites, consensi, weight matrices.	http://www.cifn.unam.mx/Computational_Biology/regulondb
13.	PRODORIC	Information on prokaryotic gene expression; TFs; genomic TF binding sites; regulatory networks.	http://prodoric.tu-bs.de/
14.	SCPD, The Promoter Database of *Saccharomyces cerevisiae*	Genes, promoters, TFs, sites, consensi, weight matrices.	http://cgsigma.cshl.org/jian/
15.	Muscle-Specific Regulation of Transcription	Description of regulatory regions of muscle-specific genes; sites.	http://agave.humgen.upenn.edu/MTIR/HomePage.html
16.	EpoDB	Database of genes that relate to vertebrate red blood cells.	http://agave.hum-gen.upenn.edu/epodb/
17.	GeNet	Information on functional organization of regulatory gene networks acting at embryogenesis.	http://www.csa.ru/Inst/gorb_dep/inbios/genet/genet.htm
18.	PlantCARE	Transcription regulation in plants; regulatory cis elements; TFs.	http://sphinx.rug.ac.be:8080/PlantCARE/
19.	PLACE		http://www.dna.affrc.go.jp/htdocs/PLACE/
20.	TRANSPATH	Information on molecules and reactions involved in signal transduction in the cell.	http://www.biobase.de/
21.	GeneNet	Object-oriented databases that include information on a number of gene regulatory networks.	http://wwwmgs.bionet.nsc.ru/systems/MGL/GeneNet/
22.	CSNDB: Cell Signaling Networks Database	Information on signal transduction reactions and signalling molecules.	http://athos.is.s.u-tokyo.ac.jp/ace/
23.	SPAD: Signaling Pathway Database	Integrated database for genetic information and signal transduction systems.	http://www.grt.kyushu-u.ac.jp/spad/
24.	KEGG: Kyoto Encyclopedia of Genes and Genomes	Information on some signalling molecules; graphical representation of several signal transduction networks.	http://www.genome.ad.jp/kegg/

Common nucleotide sequence databases and genomic databases such as GenBank, EMBL, Ensembl, and RefSeq contain some pieces of information relating to the regulation of gene expression. First, some types of gene regulatory sequences, such as promoters, enhancers, LCR, S/MARs, translation 5′UTR and 3′UTRs, translation enhancers, and TF binding sites, are represented in EMBL and GenBank. But this information is very sporadic, suffers from nonuniformity in the format of description, and is sometimes even contradictory. This information is not the main focus of these databases. Very important sources of information on gene regulation are the protein databases PIR and SwissProt. Structural and functional descriptions of TFs can be found in these databases. These protein databases also contain valuable information about tissue-specific expression of many genes.

Recently developed genomic databases, such as Ensembl (http://www.ensembl.org/) and the UCSC genome browser (http://genome.ucsc.edu/), put a great deal of emphasis on storing structural information about genes. Users of these resources can obtain any kind of functional information, including information on gene regulation, through links to the corresponding entries in the sequence databases mentioned above.

Three major groups of specialized databases deal with gene regulation. The first group comprises databases that store information on regulatory sequences, including gene regulatory regions and promoters, and information about transcription factors and their binding sites. The most recognized databases in this group are EPD and TRANSFAC. Another group of databases includes regulatory networks and signal-transduction pathways. Among them, the most popular databases are CSNDB and TRANSPATH. The third group includes databases that store information about gene expression that is based primarily on microarray data.

Two ontology databases: GO (Gene Ontology) and CYTOMER are becoming very important sources of information in studies of gene regulation. With GO, genes can be classified into many different functional categories, thus providing a way to study correlations between gene expression and gene function. CYTOMER is a database of physiological systems, developmental stages, anatomical structures and substructures, and their constituent cell types for particular organisms (Chen et al., 1999; Fricke et al., 2001).

12.3.1 TRANSFAC Database

The TRANSFAC database on eukaryotic transcriptional regulation consists of data on transcription factors, their target genes, and regulatory binding sites. TRANSFAC contains data from a wide variety of eukaryotic organisms, from humans to yeast.

At the core of the database is the interaction of TFs (FACTOR table) with their DNA binding sites (SITE table), through which they regulate their target genes (GENE table). In addition to genomic sites, 'artificial' sites, which have been synthesized in the laboratory without any known relation to a gene, e.g., random oligonucleotides and IUPAC consensus sequences, are also stored in the SITE table. Sites must be experimentally verified to be included in the database. Experimental evi-

Tab. 12.2 Total number of entries in each table of the TRANSFAC database, release 8.2.

Table name	*Number of entries*
FACTOR	5597
SITE	13934
GENE	3989
MATRIX	722
CELL	1598
CLASS	53
METHOD	94
REFERENCE	10511
JOURNALS	385

dence for interaction with a factor is given in the SITE entry in the form of the method that was used (gel shift, footprint analysis, etc.) and the cell from which the factor was derived (factor source). Based on the method and cell, a quality value is given to describe the confidence with which an observed DNA binding activity can be assigned to a specific factor. From a collection of binding sites for a factor, nucleotide weight matrices are derived (MATRIX table).

According to their DNA binding domain, TFs are assigned to a certain class (CLASS). In addition to the 2-dimensional CLASS table, a hierarchical factor-classification system was proposed, as was also done some time ago (Wingender, 1997). Table 12.2 shows the number of entries in the various tables and flat files for the current release of TRANSFAC.

12.4
Regulatory Sequence-analysis Tools and Approaches

The achievements in developing rich databases in which various information on gene regulation is compiled has accelerated the development of computer programs for analyzing gene regulatory sequences. The ultimate goal of the computational approaches is to reconstruct in silico the structural organization of the regulatory genomic regions by analyzing only the DNA sequence, thus providing computer methods for predicting the full spectrum of their regulatory functions. All hierarchical elements of these regions (single TF binding sites, CEs, promoters and enhancers, long regulatory regions, S/MARs, LCRs, etc.) are to be categorized and modelled so that we will be able to recognize them in genomic sequences. This allows us to make reasonable *in silico* predictions of the regulatory function of sequences being studied.

Over several years, many computational tools for analyzing regulatory sequences have been developed (Bucher, 1999; Fickett and Wasserman, 2000). They include rather simple tools as well as sophisticated systems that employ powerful statistical and machine-learning algorithms. In all these approaches two major strategies are used, which we call 'top–down' and 'bottom–up' strategies. In the top–down strategy, researchers analyze the structure of higher hierarchical elements such as promoters or full regulatory regions without making a strong a priori hypothesis about their internal structure (black-box approach). In such strategies oligonucleotide frequencies, as well as many other calculable parameters of DNA sequences, are used in the analysis, without focusing on the biological and physical properties of such parameters. In the bottom–up strategy, researchers make models of the complex units, using the lower hierarchical elements as building blocks. The structure of promoters is analyzed on the basis of their elements, including specific TF binding sites and other signals. The top–down strategy is useful during the initial steps of an analysis when there is limited knowledge about the internal structure of the regulatory units. The bottom–up strategy makes sense in knowledge-rich areas and is the next logical step in the analysis of regulatory genomic regions. Let us consider some of these approaches in more detail.

12.4.1 Motif Analysis

The first methods that appeared for analyzing regulatory sequences were various methods of motif analysis, which is a top–down strategy.

As described above, regulatory regions in genomes are not uniform in internal structure. They contain DNA signals, most of which are short contiguous stretches of nucleotides that serve a particular type of regulatory function, such as target sites for binding of transcription factors, DNA bending sites of a particular type, heteroduplex formation signals, regions of Z and H forms of DNA, etc. Signals of the same type can be grouped into an ideal pattern called a motif, and the observed signals in sequences are different instances of the given motif.

Several 'languages' are used to describe motifs:

1. A motif can be described by a *consensus* sequence of length l, which contains the most frequent nucleotide in each position of the observed signals. The particular number (or percentage) of positions k that can mismatch the consensus are typically given. Such (l, k) models for describing motifs are suitable for many different DNA signals, but they usually fail to properly describe the TF binding sites, where different nucleotide positions have completely different degrees of variability and cannot be described by a single parameter k.

2. A motif can be described by a single sequence that allows for several letters at each position in the motif. For example, the sequence AWCTTB describes a motif that allows letters A and T at the second position (W = A/T) and letters T, G, or C at the last position (B = not-A). Sometimes this description is complemented by a mismatch parameter k as in the first description, which may be different for exact nucleotides and ambiguous nucleotides.

3. A more biologically relevant representation of a motif is a probability matrix that assigns a different probability to each possible letter at each position in the motif (Schneider et al., 1986).

12.4.1.1 Motif-finding Algorithms

The goal of motif finding, given a set of sequences, is to identify new motifs that are common to all or most of the sequences in the set. These new motifs are believed to correspond to some a priori unknown DNA signals that are important for the function of the given set of sequences.

Motif-discovery algorithms make use of two major strategies. The first is called the pattern-driven (PD) approach. It looks through all possible motif representations in a given solution space and finds the one that best fits the set of sequences being analyzed. The second is called the sequence-driven approach (SD), which comprises algorithms that compare sequences to each other, trying to find local similarities between them to build motifs (Brazma et al., 1997). PD algorithms can find the most optimal motifs, but they are slow and only practical for short motifs. SD algorithms are fast but do not guarantee finding optimal motifs. Both types of algorithms are used in analyzing regulatory genomic sequences. Let us consider some of them in more detail.

Many approaches have been developed for automatic motif discovery, which apply SD and PD strategies, as well as combinations of them. Among the best-performing are the Gibbs sampler (Lowrence et al., 1993), MEME (Bailey and Elkan, 1995), CONSENSUS (Hertz and Stormo, 1999), PROJECTION (Buhler and Tompa, 2002), and combinatorial approaches (Pevzner and Sze, 2000).

Pioneering work in this field was carried out by Gribskov et al. (1990), who introduced a scoring matrix called 'profile'. This method was applied first for finding motifs in protein sequences in the form of weight matrices. It was further developed and applied to regulatory DNA sequences as well. Stormo and Hartzell (1989) used a greedy algorithm that was later improved by applying expectation maximization (EM) (Lawrence and Reilly, 1990).

Still later, an iterative Gibbs sampling algorithm (Lawrence et al., 1993) was introduced, which became the most frequently used algorithm for searching motifs. It can discover multiple motifs, but the number of occurrences of each motif in each sequence in the dataset must be specified in the input. Many other algorithms have been developed for revealing multiple motifs by the PD approach, such as MOTIF (Smith et al., 1990), which searches for words consisting of three letters separated by a certain distance. Another algorithm was developed which discovers multiple motifs by clustering words of length k and which have at least r matches (Saqi and Sternberg, 1994; similar to Smith et al., 1990). Clustering is applied to the most frequently occurring patterns to combine related patterns and obtain a reduced set of motifs. Exhaustive PD approaches were used for analyzing DNA motifs in promoter sequences. Van Helden et al. (1998) compared the frequency of conserved words in a given set of promoters with the frequencies in a reference set, thus revealing promoter-specific motifs. This approach was further developed by Kielbasa et al. (2001). In the recent work of Sinha (2002), the search for overrepresented motifs in a 'positive' set of sequences (typically, promoters of coregulated genes) versus a 'negative' set of sequences is supported by a powerful formalism of computing p values for the motifs. Kel et al. (1998) proposed another approach to finding overrepresented motifs by using genetic algorithms (GA).

12.4.1.2 Heterogeneity: Search for Multiple Motifs

Ideally, every transcription factor is characterized by a specific DNA motif implicated in its target sites. In reality, such a unique motif is difficult to find and sometimes does not exist. First, *in vivo* transcription factors bind to DNA in a complex with other factors, coactivators, and nucleosome components, and these complexes may be very different at different places in the genome. So the local interaction environments impose specific constraints that certainly influence the DNA binding specificity of the transcription factor. Thus, we should talk about an *in vivo* TF motif that can be rather sparse or even split into several complex-specific motifs for the same TF.

Moreover, in reality, sets of binding sites that can be retrieved from a database or collected from the literature typically include sites for a certain family of TFs rather than for a single TF. These facts makes it very important for a computational method to be able to find subsets of sites in a mixture of many local subtypes.

Recently we developed a powerful new algorithm to search for multiple motifs in one set by using kernel functions (Tikunov and Kel, 2002). The method is able to reveal several motifs (in the form of weight matrices) in a set of unaligned sequences. Every weight matrix characterizes a pattern that can be found in a significant subset of sequences under analysis. Comparison with results obtained with CONSENSUS and Gibbs sampling shows that the kernel method is clearly superior at identifying several motifs from noisy data (Kel et al., 2004).

The high sensitivity of the kernel method results from the fact that the estimation of sequence distribution probabilities is mainly built on the basis of sequences located near the consensus, whereas all other methods estimate the background probabilities based on the complete set of sequences.

Heterogeneity of TF binding sites was taken into account in several other approaches, always yielding better recognition accuracy (Kel et al., 1995 b; Shelest et al., 2003).

12.4.2
Recognition of TF Binding Sites

Several thousand different TFs function in human cells. More than 1000 TFs have been well studied and are included in databases such as SwissProt and TRANSFAC. Even though TRANSFAC contains information about more than 5000 genomic sites (see above; about 1500 in human genes), it is far from complete. Taking into account 33 000 genes in the human genome and the fact that every gene might have up to 100 functioning sites in all regulatory regions (including promoters, enhancers, and far-upstream regulatory regions), we can expect millions of sites in the human genome. Knowledge about the number, sequence, and position of all these sites in the genome will bring us to a new level of understanding of how genes are regulated during development, how they function in the organism, and how genes are deregulated is disease states.

Computer analysis of genome sequences provides the means for predicting binding sites for different TFs. Most TFs can be characterized by a specific DNA motif that is common to most of their binding sites. Given a known motif, there are many different methods of searching for the motif in DNA sequences.

12.4.2.1 Search by Consensus or Pattern

In an early stage of analysis of binding sites for a new TF, only a few examples of known sites for this factor are available. These known examples are used as patterns in the search for new potential binding sites for these TFs. Because information on the variability of the positions in the pattern is extremely limited, the simple pattern-search methods usually allow for a certain percentage of mismatches in any position of the pattern. When more examples of the known sites become available, consensi are created that describe the observed variability of nucleotides in different positions of the sites with the ambiguous-letter code (e. g., the letter S marks a position where nucleotides G and C are equally observed, W corresponds to either A or T). Pattern-search tools such as SIGNAL SCAN (Prestridge, 1991; Prestridge and Stormo, 1993), PatSearch (Wingender et al., 1996), and SITE (Solovyev and Rogozin, 1986) can use consensi in the search and assign different mismatch penalties to the different letters of the ambiguous code. Pattern-search methods are useful for finding new potential sites, but they are rather inaccurate and characterized by relatively high false-negative and false-positive rates.

12.4.2.2 Weight Matrices: MatInspector, Match, and Other Programs

Weight matrices are used to describe highly degenerate TF binding sites. The basis of any weight matrix is the counts of the observed nucleotides in the corresponding position of known sites. To build a reliable weight matrix, one needs a collection of a few known binding sites for a certain TF. The most up-to-date collection of weight matrices is contained in the TRANSFAC database (http://www.biobase.de/). Several weight matrix-based search programs have been developed, e. g., ConsInspector (Frech et al., 1993), MATRIX SEARCH (Chen et al., 1995), MatInspector (Quandt et al., 1995), Match (Gössling et al., 2001), and TRANSPLORER (http://www.biobase.de/). Different programs use different formalisms for calculating weight matrices from the nucleotide counts, based on thermodynamic considerations (Berg and von Hippel, 1987, 1988), information theory (Stormo, 1998), application of pseudocounts (Henikoff and Henikoff, 1996), and consideration of forbidden nucleotides (Tronche et al., 1997). The search algorithms are greatly accelerated by using hash tables (Goessling et al., 2001). These tools have been applied intensively over the past several years for analyzing the regulatory regions of many functional classes of genes, including globin genes (Hardison et al, 1997), muscle- and liver-specific genes (Wasserman and Fickett, 1998), and genes involved in the regulation of the cell cycle (Kel et al., 2001).

12.4.2.3 Match Algorithm

The match algorithm uses two score values: the matrix similarity score (weight) and the core similarity score (Goessling et al., 2001), which resembles the algorithm previously published by Quandt et al., (1995). The matrix similarity score denotes the quality of match between the sequence and the whole matrix, and the core similarity score is a weight for the quality of match between the sequence and the matrix core (the five most-conserved consecutive positions in a matrix). Both scores range from 0 to 1, where 1 denotes an exact match.

The main steps of the algorithm are:

1. For each matrix, all possible core matches in sequence s are identified. Because the length of a core is defined as 5, all subsequences x of length 5 within the sequence s are found.

2. For each of these subsequences, its start position in the sequence s and its core similarity score are stored in a table.

3. For each entry with a core similarity score higher than a certain cutoff, each occurrence of this subsequence is looked up in the sequence s and is extended at both ends so that it fits the matrix length. Then the matrix similarity score is calculated, and those matches with a matrix similarity score higher than a certain cutoff are output by the program.

The score for the matrix similarity of a subsequence x of sequence s of length L is calculated as follows (Kel et al., 1999):

$$\text{mat\_sim} = \text{mat\_sim}\,(x) = \frac{\text{Current} - \text{Min}}{\text{Max} - \text{Min}} \tag{1}$$

where $\text{Current} = \sum_{i=1}^{L} I(i) f_{i,b_i}$, $\text{Min} = \sum_{i=1}^{L} I(i) f_i^{\min}$, $\text{Max} = \sum_{i=1}^{L} I(i) f_i^{\max}$, $f_{i,B}$ = frequency of nucleotide B occurring at position i of the matrix ($\mathbf{B} \in \{A,C,G,T\}$), and $f_i^{\min}$ and $f_i^{\max}$ are the frequencies of the nucleotides that are the rarest and the most frequent in position i in the matrix.

The information vector $\mathbf{I}(i) = \sum_{\mathbf{B} \in \{A,T,G,C\}} f_{i,B} \ln(4 \times f_{i,B})$ describes the conservation of the positions i in a matrix (Quandt et al., 1995). Multiplication of the frequencies by the information vector leads to higher acceptance of mismatches in less-conserved regions and less acceptance of mismatches in highly conserved regions.

The core similarity score is calculated in the same way as the matrix similarity score, but only the 5-nucleotide core part of the matrix is taken into account.

We call the collection of known binding sites that is used for building a weight matrix a 'training set' of positive examples. We need a 'test set' of negative examples (or a control set) to estimate the rate of false positives (FP); that is, to estimate how often the considered matrix will wrongly predict that a site is a binding site for the TF when in reality it is not. We often use a set of second and third exons as a test set of negative examples. Alternatively, different kinds of computationally randomized sequences are used as a test set. Of course, we cannot guarantee that all predicted sites in such sequences are negative, but usually we believe that number of real sites in the sequences is minimal.

Ideally, in addition to the training set, a separate set of sites for the same TF should be used to estimate the potential rate of false negatives (FN). This is a test set of positive examples. Estimations of the FN rate that are done on the basis of the training set are usually more optimistic and farther from reality than estimations based on an independent test set. Unfortunately, the number of known examples is often very limited and all of them are used for building the matrix, so it is impossible to create a separate test set.

Different kinds of bootstrap methods are used to overcome this problem by reusing randomly selected subsets of sites from the training set. A special kind of bootstrap is the so-called jackknife method, which is most often used for evaluating weight matrices. For a set of N sites we sample a new subset N times; the new subset contains all but one sequence from the original set. A new weight matrix is built on the basis of this subset. This new matrix is applied to the site that was left out and was not used for matrix construction. The results of N corresponding recognitions are averaged, so that the FN rate is estimated.

Application of the jackknife method produces more realistic results, although it often gives estimations that are a bit too pessimistic, because the matrix is always changing during the test, thus adding some additional variability to the method.

Matrix methods have been successful in the recognition of binding sites of many transcription factors, such as CREB, AP-1, and E2F (Kel et al., 1999, 2001). Nevertheless, it is still weak in recognizing target sites for some other factors that are characterized by a very vague motif or by a complex motif that contains several conserved modules at variable distances from each other (for example, NF-1 and C/EBP sites, and sites for some nuclear receptors).

12.4.2.4 TRANSPLORER

TRANSPLORER (TRANScription exPLORER) is a software package for analyzing transcription regulatory sequences. It includes a tool for predicting potential binding sites for TFs in any sequence that may be of interest. Currently, the TRANSPLORER site prediction tool uses collections of position weight matrices (PWM). It can use several matrix sources: the largest and most up-to-date library of matrices is derived from the TRANSFAC Professional database (http://www.biobase.de/pages/products/databases), but other matrix libraries, as well as any user-developed matrix libraries can also be invoked. This means that it provides an opportunity to search for a great variety of TF binding sites. A search can be made using all the matrices or subsets of matrices from the libraries.

TRANSPLORER has an advanced user interface (Figure 12.3) and comes with many filtering options, which allow you to specify what kinds of sites you want to see in the program output. You can view the results as a table or in an elaborate graphical representation, in which specific colour schemes are helpful for visualizing different kinds of information about the sites found. TRANSPLORER provides a variety of options that allow you to tailor the program output to your personal preferences.

As an additional feature, TRANSPLORER allows you to specify your search with 'profiles', which are each a specific subset of matrices from one or several libraries, with optimized cutoffs for each matrix. TRANSPLORER provides a tool for creating (editing, deleting) matrix profiles. In addition, TRANSPLORER includes several optimized tissue-specific profiles.

The cutoffs in TRANSPLORER are thresholds that the scores of a match must exceed to be shown in the output. Appropriate cutoff selection for TRANSPLORER depends largely on your objectives. We have precalculated three different cutoffs for each matrix presented in the library, designed to:

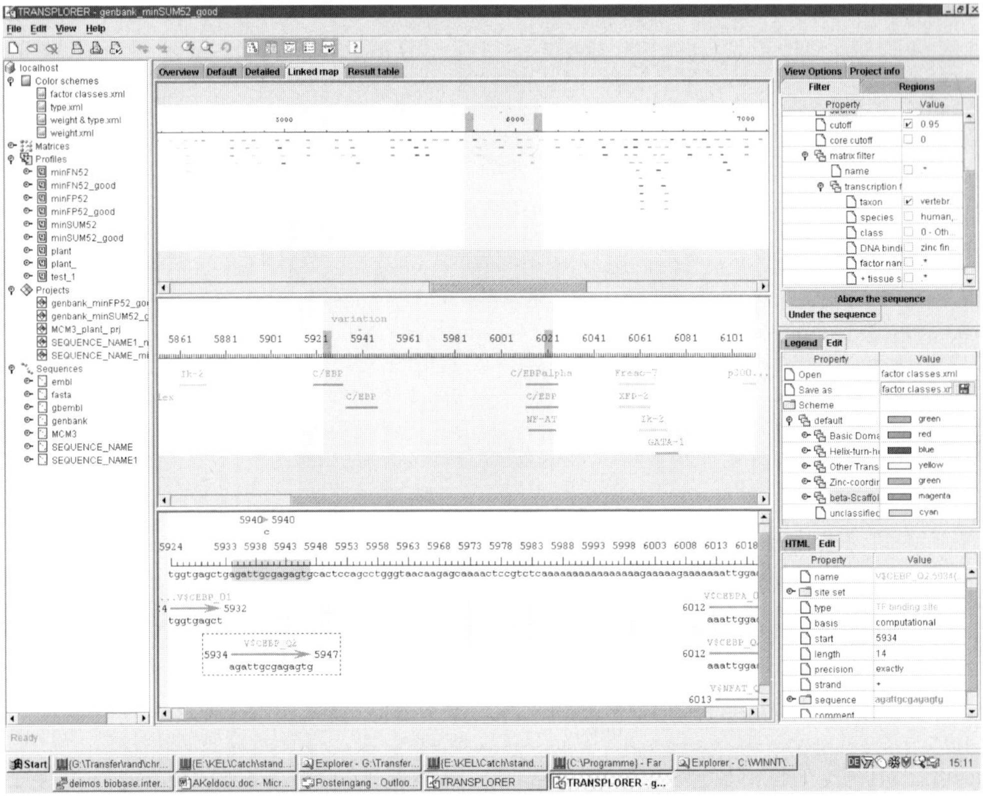

Fig. 12.3 The output window of TRANSPLORER. Three different panels represent three scales to see potential TF binding sites (central part). Sites for factors of different families are represented in different colours as defined by the user (right, middle panel). Numerous filter options allow the user to focus on results of particular interest (right, top panel). Database links and details of single pieces of information can be selectively expanded (right, bottom panel).

- minimize the false positive (over-prediction error) rate,
- minimize the false negative (under-prediction error) rate,
- minimize the sum of both errors.

12.4.2.5 Correlation between Positions: Dinucleotide Weight Matrices

In the classical weight matrix method, individual positions are considered to be independent and their contributions to the binding energy to be additive (Berg and von Hippel, 1987). Neither assumption is quite correct for the binding sites of TFs. To deal with the nonadditive effects of different positions, an information measure was suggested, which assigns higher weights to the more-conserved positions (Quandt et al., 1995).

To consider the correlation between neighbouring site positions, hidden Markov model (HMM) approaches were applied (Ehret et al., 2001). HMMs calculate the probability of nucleotides in a certain position, depending on the preceding nucleotide(s). Another approach is based on di- and trinucleotide matrices that consist of frequencies of all doublets or triplets occurring at a given position (Kondrakhin et al., 1994). Long-distance correlation between nucleotides in non-neighbouring positions can also contribute to the recognition of sites (Kel et al., 1995 a).

Dinucleotide weight matrices were used for the recognition of a vast number of TF binding sites (Kel et al., 1995 b). Usually, dinucleotide matrices showed sufficiently better recognition accuracy than mononucleotide matrices constructed under the same conditions. Dinucleotide matrices can take into account the correlation among neighbouring site positions, thus providing better recognition. Further confirmation of the importance of correlation between neighbouring positions in TF binding sites was provided recently by experimental work with oligonucleotide microarrays (Bulyk et al, 2002).

12.4.2.6 **Influence of Site Flanks: Local Context. SITEVIDEO System**

A weight matrix captures position-specific preferences in a short region only, which often corresponds to the most-conserved part of the site; however, the weight matrix does not cover regularities in the flanking regions of the sites. Therefore, new methods were developed that take flanking regions of the sites into account. The program ConsInspector makes a pairwise alignment of a sequence to the set of sites that includes the core of the sites as well as the flanking regions (Frech et al., 1993). Similarities found in the flanks are used for supporting the site recognition. Various artificial-intelligence approaches are used to develop new methods for the recognizing cis-elements, with the aim of revealing additional features in the flanking regions of sites. An application of the perception method was developed for recognition of GREs (glucocorticoid regulatory elements; Seledtsov et al., 1991). It creates a model that includes 30 bp on each flank of the GRE sites.

The pattern-recognition program SITEVIDEO (Kel et al., 1993) was used to build recognition programs for TF binding sites (Kel et al, 1995 b). The SITEVIDEO system allows an analysis of a set of sites including their flanking regions and the design of high-accuracy recognition methods by using several standard multidimensional discriminating methods and approaches from the field of artificial intelligence, such as perceptron, neural networks, and others (Minsky and Papert, 1969; Bolch and Huang, 1974). SITEVIDEO considers quantitative characteristics such as (1) statistical properties: characteristics related to the frequencies of mono- or oligonucleotides and their uneven location in the functional sites; (2) physical properties: charge, stacking energy, mass, volume, polarity, and hydrophobicity; and (3) chemical properties: presence of certain atomic groups in the nucleotides and certain other distinctive features of their chemical structures. In addition, a new approach to visually monitoring recurrent design by the recognition methods has been applied (Kel et al., 1993). Recently this technique was used for building a new recognition method for binding sites of E2F TFs – the key regulators of the cell cycle. An exhaustive search for contextual motifs was made in the flanking regions of these sites.

Evaluating found vs. represented motifs, a 'score of context' was defined that is used in addition to the weight matrix search. As a result, the new method of E2F site recognition provides a level of accuracy that is 5 times that of the conventional weight matrix method (Kel et al., 2001).

Thus, many reliable methods have been developed that can be used for recognition of TF binding sites. Unfortunately, the best approaches usually need to be trained with valuable training samples, and therefore, until now have been applied only to a limited number of TFs for which many binding sites are already known.

Searches for individual TF binding sites in DNA sequences, although widely used (for review see Frech et al., 1997), can hardly be applied directly to the characterization of transcriptional regulation of individual or sets of genes, for three main reasons: (1) the poor recognition ability of most programs currently being used (high rates of false positives and false negatives); (2) very incomplete lists of TF binding sites being searched; and (3) incomplete definition of the specificity of transcriptional regulation of a gene by correctly determined individual sites, because of the combinatorial nature of regulation.

12.4.3
Recognition of Composite Regulatory Elements

Combinatorial regulation is the basic mechanism of gene-expression control in eukaryotic organisms. The pattern of expression of eukaryotic genes is encoded in the structure of their transcription regulatory regions, mainly by the combination of TF binding sites. During the past several years, several computational approaches have appeared addressing the problem of combinatorial regulation of transcription. Specific TF binding site combinations were used for identifying muscle-specific promoters (Frech et al., 1998; Wasserman and Fickett, 1998), liver-enriched genes (Tronche et al., 1997), and yeast genes (Brazma et al., 1997).

As described in the introduction, the first and most important level of combinatorial regulation is provided by composite regulatory elements (CEs) – combinations of target sites for two different transcription factors that interact with each other, resulting in a particular expression pattern common to genes that contain this CE (Kel et al., 1995). Several examples of CEs have been collected in the TRANSCompel database (Kel-Margoulis et al., 2001).

12.4.3.1 Motif-finding Techniques for Analysis of Composite Elements

The 'ab initio' motif-finding techniques, which do not take into account any previous knowledge about possible known motifs, often have problems in finding TF binding sites that are 'too weak'. These are instances of sites that differ significantly from their consensus while still serving as targets for the TFs. As described before, such 'weak' sites can function due to synergism with other sites in CEs. Usually the binding of transcription factors to such weak sites is stabilized by protein–protein interactions of this TF with other TFs that bind to nearby sites. Because traditional motif-finding algorithms usually find one (or a few) high-scoring patterns, they often fail to find CEs that consist of pairs of weak TF sites. One or both sites in such pairs may

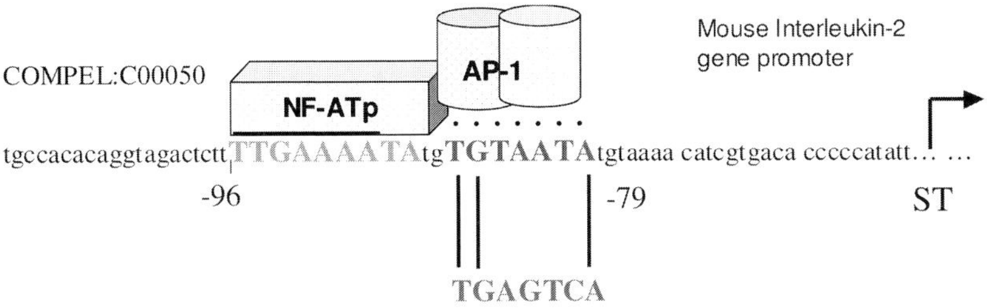

Fig. 12.4 An example of NF-AT/AP-1 CE in the promoter of the mouse interleukin-2 gene. The AP-1 site differs from the canonical AP-1 consensus.

not be statistically significant on its own. An example of such a composite element is shown in Figure 12.4.

We can see in this composite element that the AP-1 site differs very much from the canonical AP-1 consensus (shown below). It is clear that such a site cannot be found alone.

Recently, a couple of new approaches have appeared for revealing such composite motifs in sets of sequences: BioProspector (Liu et al., 2001), Co-Bind (GuhaThakurta and Stormo, 2001), and MITRA (Eskin and Pevzner, 2002). The first two are based on an extension of the Gibbs sampling techniques for finding significant motifs consisting of two modules that have some flexible distance between them. The algorithm maximizes the joint likelihood of co-occurrence of two motifs. The MITRA approach is a pattern-driven approach based on enumeration of l-mers. The algorithm uses a mismatch tree data structure to split the space of all possible patterns into disjoint subspaces that start with a given prefix. It thus avoids an 'explosion' of the search space for long composite motifs consisting of two parts.

All these approaches have proved their efficiency for some examples of composite motifs in yeast and bacterial genomes.

12.4.3.2 Matching Algorithms for Searching Composite Elements

Several tools have been designed for searching known CEs directly in nucleotide sequences. With the FastM program (Frech et al., 1998), you can specify a pair of weight matrices and set a preferable distance range between corresponding sites in the CE. Another tool, called Catch (http://www.biobase.de/), searches for CEs with the pattern-matching approach. CEs from the TRANSCompel database are used as patterns for the Catch program. Several parameters can be set to restrict the search, such as maximum mismatches in the cores of site1 and site2 comprising the CEs, maximum variation of the distance between the two sites (as a percentage), and a cutoff value for a general score for the CE. The CE score reflects how well the match coincides with the known example of the CE in TRANSCompel. Score function takes into account the number of mismatches in both sites and the distance between them. All found matches are directly linked to the TRANSCompel entries containing the corresponding CEs.

We have applied the Catch program to 5′ regions of genes expressed in activated T cells (T genes). For this analysis we chose a set of CEs that are located in the regula-

Tab. 12.3 Frequency of potential CEs that provide various aspects of lymphoid- and myeloid-restricted transcriptional regulation within various sequences.

Sequences studied	*Frequency of potential CEs in 1000 bp*
T genes	1.636
5′ regions of T genes	2.894
Random [A] = [T] = [C] = [G] = 0.25.	0.832
Random (nucleotide composition as in 5′-regions of T genes) [A] = 0.2865; [T] = 0.2615; [G] = 0.2196; [C] = 0.2323	0.938

tory regions of genes expressed in activated T, B, and myeloid cells and contained in the TRANSCompel database. The set included the following types of CEs: AP-1/NF-κB, AP-1/Oct, AP-1/NFAT, AP-1/Ets, NF-κB/HMG, NF-κB/IRF, C/EBP-α/AML, C/EBP-α/PU.1, Ets/AML. The frequency of the potential CEs in the 5′ regions of T genes is 3 times that in random sequences having the same nucleotide composition (Table 12.3). (Kel-Margoulis et al., 2000)

It is clear that the list of known composite elements is far from complete. To find new types of CEs, some statistical estimations were made for finding pairs of TF binding sites that are close to each other in a sequence and can participate in a CE. Application of χ^2 statistics allows pairs of sites to be revealed that often can be found at a short distance from each other (Kel et al., 1995 a). By using this tool, unknown pairs were revealed, such as CREB/SP-1 and GATA/NF-κB, which may be new potential composite regulatory element types.

12.4.3.3 **Composite Score**

A method called ‘composite score’ was developed for revealing NFAT/AP-1 CEs (Kel et al., 1999). It includes two matrices, for two corresponding TFs. The range of allowed distances between matrix matches and their mutual orientation are taken into account, as well as the coordinate variation of the matrix scores for the two factors. A low score of one matrix is compensated by a high score of another matrix, thus providing optimal binding energy for the protein–DNA complex on the CE.

A set of 13 NFAT/AP-1 CEs was extracted from the COMPEL database (release 2.1). For each CE we used the Match™ program and computed two scores: q_{NFAT} and q_{AP-1} for the two corresponding binding sites constituting the CE. From these scores two parameters, $\pi_{NFAT} = \log(1 - q_{NFAT})$ and $\pi_{AP\text{-}1} = \log(1 - q_{AP-1})$, were calculated, estimating the binding energy for these two factors with their binding sites. To model the synergistic binding of two factors to DNA, we combined two parameters: π_{NFATp} and π_{AP-1} and designed a method for recognition of CEs. For combining these two parameters into one recognition function, we used the SITEVIDEO software (Kel et al., 1993), which provides a means of obtaining the best discrimination between a training set of CEs and control data (random sequences).

We found that identifying composite elements with this method is very effective for predicting gene-expression patterns, as demonstrated for promoters of genes

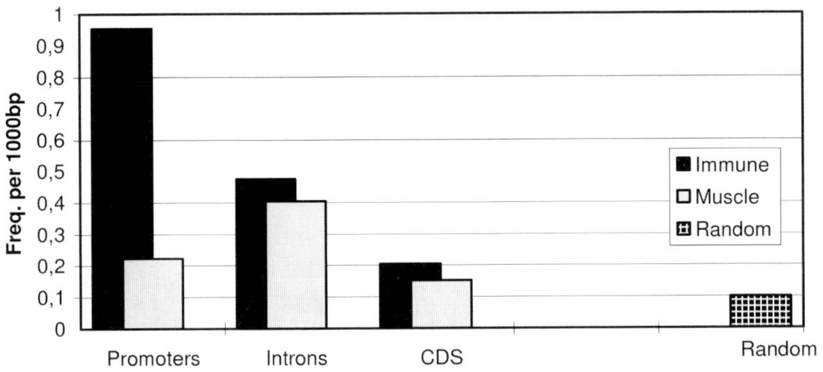

Fig. 12.5 Frequencies of NFAT/AP-1 composite elements (q_{CE} >10.0) in the functional parts of immune cell–specific genes and muscle-specific genes and in random sequences.

highly induced upon immune response. NFAT/AP-1 composite elements were found in high concentration in the promoters of genes that are induced upon immune cell activation. (Figure 12.5).

Clusters of these composite elements provide a good landmark for identifying promoters of immune-specific genes. Several genes potentially regulated by this mechanism were revealed by genome search and suggested for experimental verification (Kel et al., 1999).

12.4.4
Analysis of Promoters

Computer-assisted prediction of eukaryotic promoters is one of the most straightforward approaches to the analysis of transcription regulation with sequence data (Bucher, 1990).

12.4.4.1 Types of Promoters: Core Promoter Recognition

A promoter can be defined as a structural part of a gene that defines its transcription starting point and mediates and controls the initiation of transcription. Promoter sequences may include a TATA box, the initiator region (Inr), upstream activating elements, and downstream elements. However, not all of these elements are always required. This means that the DNA pattern that defines a so-called core promoter (around –50 to +10) can vary significantly in different genes and can be divided into four classes (reviewed in Werner, 1999). Briefly, these classes comprise (1) core promoters, which consist of a TATA box only, which directs transcriptional initiation at a position about 30 bp downstream; (2) core promoters, which do not contain any TATA box and therefore are referred to as TATA-less – in these promoters, the exact position of the transcriptional starting point is controlled mainly by an initiator element Inr (Smale, 1994; and Smale, 1997); (3) composite promoters consisting of both a TATA box and an initiator element; and (4) so-called null promoters, which have neither a TATA box nor an initiator and rely exclusively on upstream and downstream promoter elements (PDE) (Smale, 1994; Novina and Roy, 1996).

12.4.4.2 **Brief Survey of Promoter-recognition Programs**

Two different approaches have been applied so far to promoter recognition. The first approach is purely *sequence-based*, making use of different statistics of nucleotides and oligonucleotides in the promoter sequences without considering known promoter signals and cis-elements. Specific features of the distribution of nucleotides and oligonucleotides of different lengths (di-, tri-, and longer oligonucleotides) are revealed in the training set of known promoters, and these features are then used to build recognition procedures. In most of the applications that use the sequence-based approach, the authors have not paid much attention to the biological meaning of the found high- or low-frequency oligonucleotides and their distribution in promoter sequences. We call this approach top–down (see above).

In contrast, in the *signal-based* approach (bottom–up), authors build their tools on the basis of features and signals (such as TATA, CAAT boxes, consensi of TF binding sites, and physical and chemical properties of DNA) that are known to have high biological significance for promoter structures.

Both approaches have their merits. Using known signals makes much more sense than simple oligonucleotide counting, because it can capture crucial features of promoter structure that may be unresolved by the total oligonucleotide approach. On the other hand, oligonucleotide analysis provides a general sketch of all possible signals that might still be unknown and therefore might be missed by procedures that are based on known signals only.

In Table 12.4, we survey several promoter-recognition programs now available.

Testing of the promoter-prediction tools has demonstrated that nearly all the available tools have a rather low level of recognition accuracy (specificity vs. sensitivity) (Fickett and Hatzigeorgiou, 1997). The accuracy of some more recently developed tools, however, is much higher – mainly because of larger training sets, better signal databases, and powerful new techniques of machine learning and pattern recognition. But the recognition accuracy is still relatively low, so these programs cannot really be used for direct annotation of a genome without additional information. It has become obvious that prediction of a 'general promoter structure' is not just a difficult task but also a misleading one, and that each promoter must be described on the basis of its specific composition of regulatory elements. Addressing more specifically the biological features of promoters, the most promising trend is to identify specific promoter structures that are common to a group of functionally related promoters (e.g., tissue-specific promoters). Identification of composite regulatory elements is now very important for the recognition of promoters and for prediction of their structure.

Tab. 12.4 Promoter recognition programs.

Program name	***Description***	***Ref/URL***
Sequence-based		
Autogen Promoter	The first program for recognition of eukaryotic promoters. Based on distinctive features of dinucleotide distribution in a sample of promoters from EPD database.	Kel et al. (1993 b)
PromFind	The algorithm operates by scoring the sequence with a differential hexamer measure. The author suggests searching for a peak score (independent of an absolute threshold) and has shown that it is more accurate than a search based on a fixed scoring threshold.	Hutchinson (1996) http://iubio.bio.indiana.edu/soft/molbio/mswin/mswin-or-dos/profin11.exe
NNPP	Applies several neural networks for analysis of nucleotide composition of the core promoter region that includes TSS (transcription start site) and TATA box.	Reese and Eeckman (1997) http://www.fruitfly.org/seq_tools/promoter.html
Promoter 2.0	The neural network uses as input a window of DNA sequence, as well as the output of other neural networks. Genetic algorithms are used for optimization of the weights in the neural networks to discriminate maximally between promoters and nonpromoters	Knudsen (1999) http://www.cbs.dtu.dk/services/promoter
McPromoter V3.0	A neural network is used to combine features of nucleotide context, features describing CpG islands, and some selected physicochemical parameters of DNA.	Ohler et al. (2001) http://promoter.informatik.uni-erlangen.de/
CorePromoter	Implements a stepwise strategy based on initial localization of a functional promoter in 1- to 2-kb (extended promoter) region and further localization of a transcriptional start site in 50- to 100-bp (core promoter) region covering the interval –60 to +40. The method uses a position-dependent 5-tuple measure that is analyzed with the help of a quadratic discriminant analysis technique (QDA).	Zhang (1998) http://argon.cshl.org/genefinder/CPROMOTER/
PromoterInspector	The program is based purely on libraries of IUPAC words extracted from training sequences by an unsupervised learning approach.	Scherf et al. (2000) http://genomatix.gsf.de/cgi-bin/promoterinspector/promoterinspector.pl

Tab. 12.4 (continued)

Program name	***Description***	***Ref/URL***
FirstEF	Uses a set of discriminant functions that can recognize structural and compositional features such as CpG islands, promoter regions, and first splice-donor sites. The core of this algorithm is a decision tree that processes results of these discriminant functions.	Davuluri et al. (2001) http://www.cshl.org/mzhanglab/
Dragon Promoter Finder	Identifies TSS positions by using five independent promoter-recognition models with artificial neuron networks.	Bajic et al. (2002) http://sdmc.lit.org.sg/promoter/ and http://www.biobase.de/
Dragon Gene Start Finder	Currently the best-performing program. Assesses the gene start in mammalian genomes and predicts a region that should overlap the first exon of the gene or be close to it.	Bajic and Seah (2003) http://sdmc.lit.org.sg/promoter/ and http://www.biobase.de/
Signal-based		
PromoterScan	TF binding sites are searched with a pattern-matching algorithm based on the TFD database. The combined individual density ratios of all binding sites are then used to build a scoring profile. This profile, in combination with a weight matrix for TATA box, is used by the program to predict TSS locations.	Prestridge (1995) http://bimas.dcrt.nih.gov/molbio/proscan/
TSSG and TSSW	The algorithm predicts potential transcription start positions by a linear discriminant function, combining characteristics that describe functional motifs and oligonucleotide composition of promoters.	Solovyev et al. (1997) http://www.softberry.com/
FunSiteP	Based on localization of binding sites of TFs. Because distribution of TF sites is uneven, the authors constructed a weight matrix of binding site localization. FunSiteP recognizes promoters in nucleotide sequences and tentatively identifies the functional class the promoters must belong to (according to Bucher's specifications).	Kondrakhin et al. (1995) http://compel.bionet.nsc.ru/FunSite/fsp.html

12.4.5
Functional Classification of Promoters and Prediction of Gene Regulation

12.4.5.1 Functional Classification Based on Combinations of Binding Sites

During the past several years, several computational approaches have appeared that address the problem of combinatorial regulation of transcription. Specific TF binding site combinations were used for the identification of muscle-specific promoters (Frech et al., 1998; Wasserman and Fickett, 1998), for liver-enriched genes (Tronche et al., 1997), for yeast genes (Brazma et al., 1997), and for immune-specific genes (Kel et al., 1999) (see Section 12.4.3.3). Promoters of genes regulated during the cell cycle could be recognized by the combination of E2F binding sites with a dozen of additional oligonucleotide motifs (Kel et al., 2001). It becomes clear that TF site combinations provide a key to functional classification of promoters and to the annotation of regulatory regions in genomes.

12.4.5.2 Decision Tree

For automatic annotation of genomic regulatory regions, methods of classifying promoters into different functional groups are necessary.

We developed a decision tree classifier for the seven functional classes of promoters using combinations of TF binding sites (Kel-Margoulis et al., 2002). The bottom nodes of the tree contain seven different promoter classes. The training set of 212 promoters was used to optimize the decision tree structure with the help of genetic algorithms. The topology of the decision tree obtained in the analysis is shown in Figure 12.6.

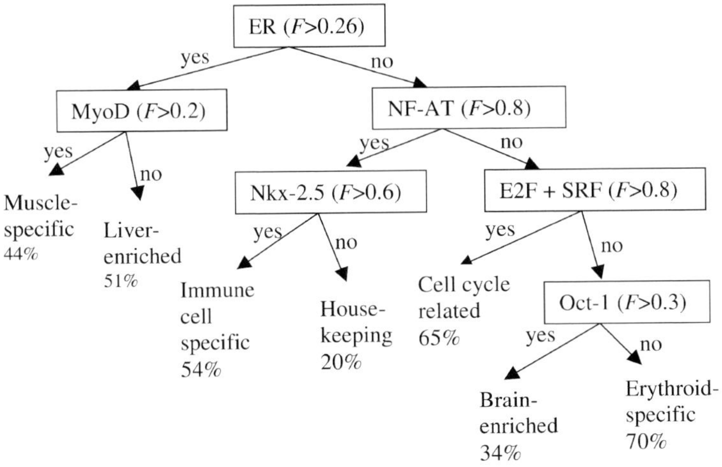

Fig. 12.6 A decision tree for classification of promoters into seven functional classes. To classify a new promoter, the sequence (x) is passed down the tree beginning at the top. If the functional score $F(x)$ is $> F_{cutoff}$, the sequence is passed down to the left, otherwise to the right. The functions $F(x)$ and the cutoffs were optimized by a genetic algorithm.

The following set of TF binding sites appeared to be the most effective for classification of the mentioned sets of promoters: E2F, Oct-1, NF-AT, MyoD, SRF, and ER.

The percentages of the promoters correctly classified by the tree are shown below each bottom node. You can see that cell cycle-related and erythroid-specific promoters are classified best (65%–70% of correct classifications). In contrast, promoters of housekeeping genes and brain-enriched genes are the most difficult to classify (34% and 20% of correct classifications, respectively). It is known that these two classes contain genes with very heterogeneous functions and expression. More effort should be expended in the initial grouping of promoters into functionally unified classes.

12.4.5.3 Clusters of Sites: Composite Clusters

Most TF target sites are located in 5′ regions of genes. We assume that binding sites for TFs that bind together to a regulatory region of a gene tend to be colocalized in a relatively short region inside the 5′ regulatory region, so as to provide the possibility for protein–protein interactions between these factors. Therefore, we expect that such sites for many different factors are clustered into 5′ regulatory regions that we call composite clusters (or heteroclusters). The presence of such composite clusters in genomic sequences might be a good indication of regulatory regions of genes. The structure of composite clusters can tell us much about regulatory mechanisms.

Clusters of binding sites for the same TFs (homoclusters) are believed to help to increase the probability of binding these factors to their target regions in the genome. Statistical estimations made by Karlin and Macken (1991) are used for revealing statistically significant homoclusters of TF binding sites in nucleotide sequences (Kel et al., 1999). The Match™ program includes functionality for revealing such clusters. By applying this tool, clusters of E2F binding sites were found in the sequences of human chromosomes 21 and 22 (Kel-Margoulis et al., 2001 b).

A new statistical technique has recently appeared, which is suitable for identifying statistically significant homoclusters and heteroclusters (Wagner, 1999). The technique was applied to two transcription factors, Mcm1 and Stel2, involved in cell cycle and mating control in the yeast *Saccharomyces cerevisiae*. Clusters of binding sites for these factors were revealed in the yeast genome (Wagner, 1999).

A tool called Cister was developed for revealing heteroclusters (Frith et al., 2001). It uses a hidden Markov model–based method for searching for clusters of cis-elements (TFs). The found clusters are considered to be landmarks for detecting promoters and other regulatory regions in DNA sequences. According to the estimation given by the authors, the program achieves a sensitivity of promoter predictions of 67%, while making one prediction per 33 kb of nonrepetitive human genomic sequences. A web interface is available at http://sullivan.bu.edu/~mfrith/cister.shtml. You can search for site clusters in a sequence and adjust the search parameters.

To reveal site clusters it is absolutely necessary to set correct cutoff parameters for searching TF sites by the weight matrices. Some sites that are part of CEs often differ significantly from the consensus; for these, the lack of binding energy for a TF is compensated for by protein–protein interactions with other factors. To find such cryptic sites as parts of heteroclusters (or composite clusters), a program called ClusterScan was developed (Kel et al., 2001 b). It uses a genetic algorithm that can find optimal parameters for searching composite clusters of TF sites in regulatory genomic sequences. The composition of the identified clusters can tell us much about regulatory mechanisms and provide a means for functional classification of regulatory regions and for automatic annotation of regulatory regions in genomes (Kel-Margoulis et al., 2001 b)

12.4.6 Phylogenetic Footprinting

Phylogenetic footprinting is a new approach to reveal potential TF binding sites in promoter sequences. The idea is based on the assumption that functional sites in promoters should evolve much more slowly than other regions that do not carry any conservative function. Therefore, potential TF binding sites that are found in the evolutionarily conserved regions of promoters have a higher chance of being considered as 'real' sites.

Global comparison of human and mouse genomes is now possible, and several groups are systematically working on this. One of the available resources for the global comparison of human and mouse genomes is the Berkeley Genome Pipeline (http://pipeline.lbl.gov/). They use a system called VISTA (Mayor et al., 2000) for handling global alignment and for revealing so-called conservative noncoding sequences (CNS) that are good landmarks in genomes for finding functionally important promoters, enhancers, and silencers (Duret and Bucher, 1997).

The most difficult step of phylogenetic footprinting is the alignment of promoter sequences between different organisms. Conventional alignment methods often cannot align promoters, because of the high level of sequence variability. We developed a new alignment method that takes into account the similarity in distribution of potential binding sites (Cheremushkin and Kel, 2002; http://compel.bionet.nsc.ru/FunSite/footprint/).

This method has been used effectively for alignment of human/mouse CNS as revealed by the Berkeley Genome Pipeline. New potential binding sites for various TFs were revealed. Binding sites for TFs that belong to the same family and have overlapping locations on the alignment are considered to be a positive match in the phylogenetic footprint. A list of 17 117 CNS with a total length of alignment of 2 418 267 bp was analyzed. We applied a set of 240 weight matrices from TRANSFAC (release 5.3) with cutoffs optimized to minimize the sum of false-positive and false-negative errors. We found 58 106 conserved TF binding sites.

12.5 Analysis of Gene Expression Data

Functionally related genes involved in the same molecular genetic, biochemical, or physiological process are often regulated co-ordinately. This co-ordination is maintained by TFs which, after being activated, are able to switch on or off several target genes by binding to their binding sites in the regulatory regions of the co-ordinately expressed genes. Therefore, it is tempting to look for TF binding sites that regularly appear in the regulatory regions of co-expressed genes. Our knowledge of the functioning of the corresponding TFs can then be used for generating working hypotheses about the molecular mechanisms of co-ordinate gene regulation.

12.5.1
Analysis of the Promoters of Co-regulated Genes

The masses of data on gene expression coming from microarray experiments provide valuable information for deducing gene regulatory mechanisms. Groups of co-expressed genes can be revealed from this data by various clustering techniques. Several techniques are used for analysis of regulatory regions of co-expressed genes in clusters. First, motif-finding algorithms are used to search for oligonucleotide motifs that are overrepresented in the promoters of co-expressed genes. The found motifs may correspond to binding sites for TFs. Approaches that have been described above include Gibbs sampling, MEME, Consensus, ClustalW, and AlignACE, all of which are applied to this task. Another approach is to search for potential TF binding sites, using a collection of known weight matrices. Finally, the most promising techniques of searching for specific combinations of TF binding sites that correlate with gene expression patterns have to be applied as well.

Recently, an analysis of pairs of TF binding sites in correlation with gene expression data was done for yeast genes (Pilpel et al., 2001). The authors searched for so called 'synergistic' pairs of TF sites, for which the expression coherence score (EC) of genes containing both sites in their promoters was significantly greater than that of genes containing either motif alone. The EC score for a set of K genes is defined as p/P, where $P = 0.5\ K\ (K-1)$ is the number of all gene pairs and p is the number of gene pairs that have very similar expression patterns (similar expression values in all measured conditions). A number of synergistic pairs were revealed that regulate expression of yeast genes in the cell cycle and during sporulation (Pilpel et al, 2001). A general motif synergy map was proposed that shows a network of functional interactions between different pairs of TFs.

ClusterScan (Kel et al., 2001 b) provides a means for analyzing more complex combinations of TF binding sites. Several new methods have appeared recently for revealing composite modules in sets of co-regulated promoters (Frith et al., 2002; Hannenhalli and Levy, 2002; Sharan et al., 2003). They are based on different statistics. Let us consider in some more detail the most effective method that is based on a genetic algorithm (Kel et al., 2001 b).

12.5.1.1 Genetic Algorithm to Determine Composite Regulatory Modules

We define a composite module (CM) as a set of TF weight matrices with given matrix cutoffs and other parameters, which is associated with a specific functional type of gene regulatory region. We have developed a new computational method to determine CMs in a set of promoter (or other regulatory) sequences of co-expressed genes. This method is based on a genetic algorithm (a prototype of this method is implemented in the tool package ClusterScan; Kel et al., 2001 b). The CMs are characterized by the following parameters: K – number of PWMs in the module (typically 6 to 12). The program selects these K matrices from a library of all considered matrices. We use different profiles including the profile vertebrate_minFN62.prf, which includes 410 matrices for different transcription factors of vertebrate organisms (TRANSFAC release 6.4). A certain cutoff value $q^{(k)}_{\text{cuttoff}}$, relative importance value $\phi^{(k)}$, and maximum number of best matches $\kappa^{(k)}$ are assigned to every weight matrix k $(k = 1, K)$ in the CM. Some matrices are organized in pairs. A parameter R is defined which puts a limit on the distance between matches of these matrix pairs (at least one pair of matches should be found fitting this limit). When all these parameters are defined, we can calculate a 'composite module score' (CM score) for any sequence X, with the following equation:

$$F_{\text{CM}}(X) = \sum_{k=1,K} \phi^{(k)} \times \sum_{i=1}^{\kappa^{(k)}} q_i^{(k)}(X) \tag{2}$$

where $q_i^{(k)}(X)$ are the $\kappa^{(k)}$ best-scoring sites found in sequence X by matrix (k). An implementation of the genetic algorithm is used to determine the parameters of CMs that are specific to a particular set of promoters. A general description of genetic algorithms is available elsewhere.

We define the goal function G as a weighted sum of false-negative and false-positive errors and the value of T-test that are calculated over several random iterations of bootstrap procedures of splitting of the initial set into training and testing subsets. In addition, we test the normal-likeness of the distributions of the F function over the set of positive and negative sequences. This algorithm for calculating the goal function gives us evidence for the usability of the obtained solutions for classification of individual sequences.

The program implementation of the method is called CompositeModuleFinder. It takes as input two sets of sequences (the set that is analyzed and a background set) and a set of weight matrices for TFs. For defined parameters K and R, over a number of iterations, the program optimizes the set of matrices selected, their quantity, their cutoffs, and the relative importance and maximum number of best matches. You can vary the parameters K and R and compare the results. The output of the program is a profile ready to be run in Match or TRANSPLORER.

12.5.1.2 Analysis of Promoters of Ah Receptor–Regulated Genes

The aryl hydrocarbon receptor (AhR) is a ligand-activated nuclear transcription factor that mediates responses to a variety of toxins. Among them are halogenated aromatic toxins such as 2,3,7,8-tetrachlorodibenzo-*p*-dioxin (TCDD), polynuclear aromatic hydrocarbons, combustion products, and numerous phytochemicals such as flavonoids and indole-3-carbinol (I3C). Experimental data obtained by RT–PCR on AhR-responsive genes were investigated with the CompositeModuleFinder to reveal TF binding sites and their specific combinations related to AhR-responsiveness (Kel et al., 2004 b).

Several matrices in various combinations were revealed in the 5′ regions of these genes. Among the most discriminative matrices were those for the following TFs:

HNF1, AhR, GR, OCT, and C/EBP. Among the most prominent matrix pairs selected by the algorithm were HNF-1/Sp-1 and AP-1/NF-1 for the maximum distance $R = 100$ bp; E2F/NF-1, AhR/Myb, HNF3/NFY, HNF6/NF-κB, and Sp-1/Myb for the maximum distance $R = 50$ bp; and HNF-1/GR for the maximum distance $R = 40$ bp. It was interesting to observe that not all matrices found individually were also found in pairs and that not only discriminating individual TFs appear in pairs. This gives

Tab. 12.5 Composite module CM_{AhR} constructed for the (–2000 +2000) set of AhR-regulated promoters.

Factor or pair of factors (distance)	***φ (see Eq. 2)***
E2F	0.105086
OCT1	0.084289
GR	0.077050
YY1	–0.169821
IRF/SRY (50)	0.213636
HNF3/SRY (50)	0.164787
AP1/NF1 (100)	0.149481
SP1/MYB (50)	0.138358
GR/HNF1 (40)	0.137571
AHR/MYB (50)	0.124308
HNF1/SP1 (100)	0.110810
E2F/ROR (100)	–0.115593
AHR/CREB (100)	–0.086788

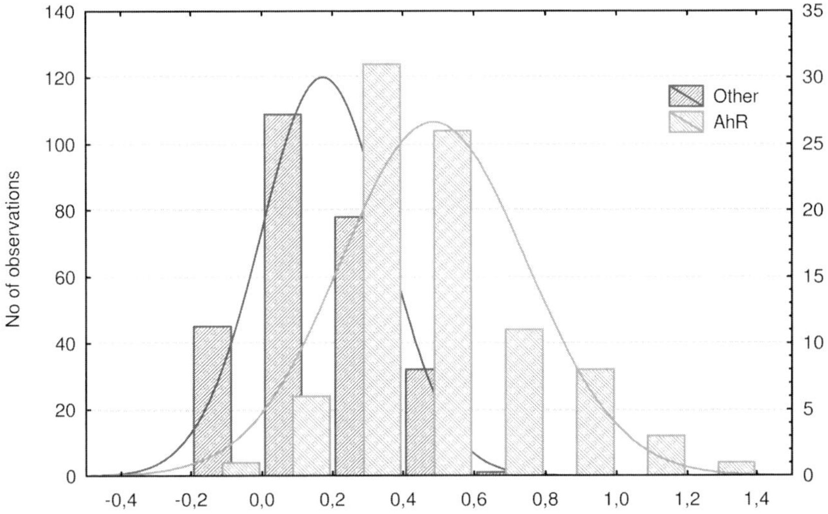

Fig. 12.7 Discrimination between (–2000 +2000) promoters (light gray) and background promoters from chromosome 21 (PR: –2000 +2000) (dark gray) by the composite module CM_{AhR}. The composite module score F_{CM} is given on the abscissa.

us an additional idea of the composite structure of the promoters being studied. In Table 12.5 we present a combination of individual matrices and matrix pairs that give one of the best discriminations of the set of promoters of AhR-regulated genes (–2000 +2000) from other promoters. We call this set of matrices AhR-associated composite regulatory modules (CM_{AhR}) of the promoters being studied.

As can be seen in Figure 12.7, the distribution of the composite module scores F_{CM} is clearly different in these two sets of promoters (T-test value is 12.12, p value = 1.7 10^{-28}). The AhR-responsive promoters have clearly higher F_{CM} scores than the background promoters.

Acknowledgments

The authors are indebted to Dmitri Tchekmenev, Volker Matys (BIOBASE GmbH), Yuri Tikunov (Institut Cytology and Genetics, Novosibirsk), and Susanne Reymann (Fraunhofer Institute (Fh-ITEM)) for their great contributions to the preparation of this manuscript and to Aida G. Romashchenko and Vadim A. Ratner (Institut Cytology and Genetics, Novosibirsk) for fruitful discussions of the results presented in the manuscript. Parts of this work were supported by the Siberian Branch of the Russian Academy of Sciences, by a grant from the European Commission (BIO4-95-0226), by a grant from Volkswagen-Stiftung (I/75941) and by grant of INTAS (03-51-5218).

References

Bailey T.L., Elkan C. (1995) Unsupervised learning of multiple motifs in biopolymers using expectation maximization. *Machine Learning*, **21**, 51.

Bajic VB, Seah SH. (2003) Dragon Gene Start Finder identifies approximate locations of the 5′ ends of genes. Nucleic Acids Res. **31**, 3560–3563.

Bajic V.B., Seah S.H., Chong A., Zhang G., Koh J.L.Y., Brusic V. (2002) Dragon Promoter Finder: recognition of vertebrate RNA polymerase II promoters. *Bioinformatics*, **18**, 198–199.

Berg, O.G., von Hippel, P. H. (1987) Selection of DNA binding sites by regulatory proteins: statistical-mechanical theory and application to operators and promoters. *J. Mol. Biol.* **193**, 723–750.

Berg, O. G., von Hippel, P. H. (1988) Selection of DNA binding sites by regulatory proteins. II. The binding specificity of cyclic AMP receptor protein to recognition sites. *J. Mol. Biol.* **200**, 709–723.

Bolch B.W., Huang C.J. (1974) Multivariate statistical methods for business and economics, Prentice-Hall, Englewood Cliffs, NJ, USA.

Brazma A., Jonassen I. Eidhammer I., Gilbert D. (1998) Approaches to the automatic discovery of patterns in biosequences. Technical Report *Journal of Computational Biology* **5**, 279–305.

Brazma, A., Vilo, J., Ukkonen, E. (1997 b) Finding transcription factor binding site combinations in the yeast genome. In *Proceedings of the German Conference on Bioinformatics* GCB'97, Kloster Irsee, Bavaria, Sept. 22–24, 1997 (H.W. Mewes, D. Frishman, eds.), 57–60.

Bucher P. (1990) Weight matrix descriptions of four eukaryotic RNA polymerase II promoter elements derived from 502 unrelated promoter sequences. *J Mol Biol* **212**, 563–278.

Bucher P. (1999) Regulatory elements and expression profiles. *Curr Opin Struct Biol* **9**, 400–407.

Buhler J, Tompa M. (2002) Finding motifs using random projections. *J Comput Biol* **9**, 225–242.

Bulyk M.L., Johnson P.L., Church G.M. (2002) Nucleotides of transcription factor binding sites exert interdependent effects on the binding affinities of transcription factors. *Nucleic Acids Res* **30**, 1255–1261.

Chen L., Glover J.N., Hogan P.G., Rao A., Harrison S.C. (1998) Structure of the DNA-binding domains from NFAT, Fos and Jun bound specifically to DNA. *Nature* **392**, 42–48.

Chen Q.K., Hertz G.Z., Stormo G.D. (1995) MATRIX SEARCH 1.0: a computer program that scans DNA sequences for transcriptional elements using a database of weight matrices. *Comput Appl Biosci* **11**, 563–566.

Chen, X., Dress, A., Karas, H., Reuter, I., Wingender, E. (1999) A database framework for mapping expression patterns. In *Proceedings of the German Conference on Bioinformatics GCB'99*. Hanover, Germany, pp. 174–178

Cheremushkin E., Kel A. (2002) Promoter-Footprint: a new method for alignment of regulatory genomic sequences: phylogenetic footprinting of TF binding sites. In L. Florea, B. Walenz, S. Hannenhalli (eds) *Currents in Computational Molecular Biology 2002. RECOMB 2002*, Washington DC, USA, pp. 40–41.

Davuluri R.V., Grosse I., Zhang M.Q. (2001) Computational identification of promoters and first exons in the human genome. *Nat Genet* **29**, 412–417.

Diamond M.I., Miner J.N., Yoshinaga S.K., Yamamoto K.R. (1990) Transcription factor interactions: selectors of positive or negative regulation from a single DNA element. *Science* **249**, 1266–1272.

Du W., Thanos D., Maniatis T. (1993) Mechanisms of transcriptional synergism between distinct virus-inducible enhancer elements. *Cell* **74**, 887–898.

Duret, L., Bucher, P. (1997) Searching for regulatory elements in human noncoding sequences. *Curr Opin Struct Biol* **7**, 399–406.

Dynan W.S. (1989) Modularity in promoters and enhancers. *Cell* **58**, 1–4.

Ehret G.B., Reichenbach P., Schindler U., Horvath C.M., Fritz S., Nabholz M., Bucher P. (2001) *J Biol Chem* **276**, 6675–6688.

Fickett J.W., Hatzigeorgiou A.G. (1997) Eukaryotic promoter recognition. *Genome Res* **7**, 861–878.

Fickett J.W., Wasserman W.W. (2000) Discovery and modeling of transcriptional regulatory regions. *Curr Opin Biotechnol* **11**, 19–24.

Frech K., Herrmann G., Werner T. (1993) Computer-assisted prediction, classification, and delimitation of protein binding sites in nucleic acids. *Nucleic Acids Res* **21**, 3117–3118.

Frech K, Quandt K, Werner T. (1997) Finding protein-binding sites in DNA sequences: the next generation. *Trends Biochem Sci* **22**, 103–104.

Frech, K., Quandt, K., Werner, T. (1998) Muscle actin genes: a first step towards computational classification of tissue specific promoters. *In Silico Biology* 1, 0005, http://www.bioinfo.de/isb/1998/01/0005/

Fricke, E., Land, S., Rotert, S., Karas, D., Wingender, E. (2001) Cytomer: a database on gene expression sources. Proceedings of the *German Conference on Bioinformatics GCB'01*. Braunschweig, Germany, pp. 149–151.

Frith M.C., Hansen U., Weng Z. (2001) Detection of cis-element clusters in higher eukaryotic DNA, *Bioinformatics* **17**, 878–889.

Frith M.C., Spouge J.L., Hansen U., Weng Z. (2002) Statistical significance of clusters of motifs represented by position specific scoring matrices in nucleotide sequences. *Nucleic Acids Res* **30**, 3214–3224.

Goessling E., Kel-Margoulis O.V., Kel A.E., Wingender E. (2001) MATCH^{TM}: a tool for searching transcription factor binding sites in DNA sequences: application for the analysis of human chromosomes. In: *Proceedings of the German Conference on Bioinformatics (GCB2001)*, October 7–10, 2001, Braunschweig, pp. 158–160.

Gribskov M., Luthy R., Eisenberg D. (1990) Profile analysis. *Methods Enzymol*, **183**, 146–159.

Guhathakurta D., Stormo G.D. (2001) Identifying target sites for cooperatively binding factors. *Bioinformatics* **17**, 608–621.

Gutman A., Wasylyk B. (1990) The collagenase gene promoter contains a TPA and oncogene-responsive unit encompassing the PEA3 and AP-1 binding sites. *EMBO J* **9**, 2241–2246.

Hannenhalli S, Levy S. (2002) Predicting transcription factor synergism. *Nucleic Acids Res* **30**, 4278–4284.

HARDISON R.C., OELTJEN J., MILLER W. (1997) Long human–mouse sequence alignments reveal novel regulatory elements: a reason to sequence the mouse genome. *Genome Res* **7**, 959–966

HERTZ G.Z., STORMO G.D. (1999) Identifying DNA and protein patterns with statistically significant alignments of multiple sequences. *Bioinformatics* **15**, 563–577.

JACKSON D.A., ROWADER K.E., STEVENS K., JIANG C., MILOS P., ZARET K.S. (1993) Modulation of liver-specific transcription by interactions between hepatocyte nuclear factor 3 and nuclear factor 1 binding DNA in close apposition. *Mol Cell Biol* **13**, 2401–2410.

JOHNSON P.F., MCKNIGHT S.L. (1989) Eukaryotic transcriptional regulatory proteins. *Annu Rev Biochem* **58**, 799–839.

KARLIN, S., MACKEN, C. (1991) Assessment of inhomogeneities in an *E. coli* physical map. *Nucleic Acids Res* **19**, 4241–4246.

KEL A.E., PONOMARENKO M.P., LIKHACHEV E.A., ORLOV Y.L., ISCHENKO I.V., MILANESI L., KOLCHANOV N.A. (1993 a) SITEVIDEO: a computer system for functional site analysis and recognition: investigation of the human splice sites. *Comput Appl Biosci* **9**, 617–627.

KEL A.E., KOLCHANOV N.A., KAPITONOV V.V., PONOMARENKO M.P., LIKHACHEV E.A., LIM H.A , MILANESI L. (1993 b) Computer analysis and recognition of functional sites on the base of oligonucleotide patterns distributions. In: Cantor, C.R., Lim H.A. (eds) *Proceedings of the Second International Conference on Electrophoresis, Supercomputing and the Human Genome*, June 1992, St. Petersburg, FL, USA., 521–544.

KEL A., KONDRAKHIN YU., KOLPAKOV PH., PONOMARENKO M., WINGENDER E., KOLCHANOV N. (1995 a) Computer analysis of the structure of transcription factor binding sites, *SAMS*, **18–19**, 819–822.

KEL A.E., KONDRAKHIN Y.V., KOLPAKOV P.A., KEL O.V., ROMASHENKO A.G., WINGENDER E., MILANESI L., KOLCHANOV N.A. (1995 b) Computer tool FUNSITE for analysis of eukaryotic regulatory genomic sequences. *In: Proc. 3rd Intern. Conf. Intelligent Systems for Molecular Biology, AAAI Press, California, 1995*, pp. 197–205.

KEL A., PTITSYN A., BABENKO V., MEIER-EWERT S., LEHRACH H. (1998) A genetic algorithm for designing gene family-specific oligonucleotide sets used for hybridization: the G protein-coupled receptor protein superfamily *Bioinformatics* **14**, 259–270.

KEL A., KEL-MARGOULIS O., BABENKO V., WINGENDER E. (1999) Recognition of NFATp/AP-1 composite elements within genes induced upon the activation of immune cells *J Mol Biol* **288**, 353–376.

KEL A.E., KEL-MARGOULIS O.V., FARNHAM P.J., BARTLEY S.M., WINGENDER E., ZHANG M.Q. (2001 a) Computer-assisted identification of cell-cycle related genes: new targets for E2F transcription factors. *J Mol Biol* **309**, 99–120.

KEL A., KEL-MARGOULIS O., IVANOVA T., WINGENDER E. (2001 b) ClusterScan: a tool for automatic annotation of genomic regulatory sequences by searching for composite clusters. In: *Proceedings of the German Conference on Bioinformatics GCB 2001*, Braunschweig, Germany, October 7–10, 2001, pp. 96–101.

KEL, A., REYMANN, S., MATYS,V., NETTESHEIM, P., WINGENDER, E., BORLAK, J. (2004) A novel computational approach for the prediction of networked transcription factors of Ah-receptor regulated genes. *Mol. Pharmacol.* Sep1 [Epub ahead of print].

KEL, A., TIKUNOV Y., VOSS N., WINGENDER E. (2004) Recognition of multiple patterns in unaligned sets of sequences: comparison of kernel clustering method with other methods. *Bioinformatics* **20**, 1512–1516.

KEL O.V., ROMASCHENKO A.G., KEL A.E., WINGENDER E., KOLCHANOV N.A. (1995) A compilation of composite regulatory elements affecting gene transcription in vertebrates. *Nucleic Acids Res* **23**, 4097–4103.

KEL, O.V., KEL, A.E., ROMASCHENKO, A.G., WINGENDER, E., KOLCHANOV, N.A. (1997) Composite regulatory elements: classification and description in the COMPEL database. *Mol Biol (Mosk)* **31**, 498–512.

KEL-MARGOULIS, O. (2001) Automatic annotation of the regulatory regions of cell cycle related genes on human chromosomes. In: *Genome Sequencing and Biology. Cold Spring Harbor Symposia*, 2001

KEL-MARGOULIS, O.V., ROMASCHENKO, A.G., KOLCHANOV, N.A., WINGENDER, E., KEL, A.E. (2000 a) TRANSCompel: a database on composite regulatory elements providing combinatorial transcriptional regulation. *Nucleic Acids Res* **28**, 311–315.

KEL-MARGOULIS O.V., ROMASCHENKO A.G., DEINEKO I.V., KOLCHANOV N.A., WINGENDER E., KEL A.E., Database on composite regulatory elements in eukaryotic genes (COMPEL) (2000 b) In: *Proceedings of the Second International Conference on Bioinformatics of Gene Regulation and Structure BGRS 2000*, August 7–11, 2000, Novosibirsk, Vol. 1, pp. 45–48.

Kel-Margoulis O.V, Kel A.E., Reuter I., Deineko I.V., Wingender E. (2002 a) TRANSCompel: a database on composite regulatory elements in eukaryotic genes. *Nucleic Acids Res* **30**, 332–334.

Kel-Margoulis O.V., Ivanova T.G., Wingender E., Kel A.E. (2002 b) Automatic annotation of genomic regulatory sequences by searching for composite clusters. *Pac Symp Biocomput* 2002, 187–198

Kielbasa S.M., Korbel J.O., Beule D., Schuchhardt J., Herzel H. (2001) Combining frequency and positional information to predict transcription factor binding sites. *Bioinformatics* **17**, 1019–1026.

Knudsen S. (1999) Promoter 2.0: for the recognition of PolII promoter sequences *Bioinformatics* **15**, 356–361.

Kolchanov N.A., Rogozin I.B., Kel A.E., Ponomarenko M.P., Lihachov J., Milanesi L. (1991) In: Kanehisa, M. (ed), *Proc. Genome Informatics Workshop II. Japan*, pp. 104–107.

Kondrakhin Y.V., Shamin V.V., Kolchanov N.A. (1994) Construction of a generalized consensus matrix for recognition of vertebrate pre-mRNA 3′-terminal processing sites. *Comput Appl Biosci* **10**, 597–603.

Kondrakhin Y.V., Kel A.E., Kolchanov N.A., Romashchenko A.G., Milanesi L. (1995) Eukaryotic promoter recognition by binding sites for transcription factors. *Comput Appl Biosci* **11**, 477–488.

Lawrence C. E., Reilly A. A. (1990) An expectation maximization (EM) algorithm for the identification and characterization of common sites in unaligned biopolymer sequences. *Proteins: Structure Function and Genetics* **7**, 41–51.

Lawrence C.E., Altschul S.F., Boguski M.S., Liu J.S., Neuwald A.F., Wootton J.C. (1993) Detecting subtle sequence signals: a Gibbs sampling strategy for multiple alignment. *Science* **262**, 208–214.

Liu X., Brutlag D.L., Liu J.S. (2001) BioProspector: discovering conserved DNA motifs in upstream regulatory regions of co-expressed genes. *Pac Symp Biocomput* 127–138.

Mayor C., Brudno M., Schwartz J. R., Poliakov A., Rubin E. M., Frazer K. A., Pachter L. S., Dubchak I. (2000) VISTA: visualizing global DNA sequence alignments of arbitrary length. *Bioinformatics* **16**, 1046.

McKnight S. L., Yamamoto K. R. (1992) *Transcriptional Regulation*. Cold Spring Harbor Laboratory Press, Cold Spring Harbor, NY.

Minsky M., Papert S. (1969) *Perceptrones*, MIT Press, Cambridge MA, USA.

Novina C.D., Roy A.L. (1996) Core promoters and transcriptional control. *Trends Genet* **12**, 351–355.

Ohler U., Niemann H., Liao G., Rubin G.M. (2001) Joint modeling of DNA sequence and physical properties to improve eukaryotic promoter recognition. *Bioinformatics* **17**, 199–206.

Pevzner P.A., Sze S. (2000) Combinatorial approaches to finding subtle signals in DNA sequences. In: *Proceedings of the Eighth International Conference on Intelligent Systems for Molecular Biology*, pp. 269–278.

Pilpel Y., Sudarsanam P., Church G.M. (2001) Identifying regulatory networks by combinatorial analysis of promoter elements. *Nat Genet* **29**, 153–159.

Prestridge D. S. (1995) Predicting pol II promoter sequences using transcription factor binding sites. *J Mol Biol* **249**, 923–932.

Prestridge, D. S., Stormo, G. (1993) SIGNAL SCAN 3.0: new database and program features. *Comput Appl Biosci* **9**, 113–115.

Ptitsyn A.A., Rogozin I.B., Grigorovich D.A., Strelets V.B., Kel A.E., Milanesi L., Kolchanov N.A. (1996) AutoGene: a computer system for nucleotide sequence analysis. *Mol Biol (Mosk)* **30**, 258–264.

Quandt, K., Frech, K., Karas, H., Wingender, E., Werner, T. (1995) *Nucleic Acids Res* **23**, 4878–4884.

Rao A., Luo C., Hogan P.G. (1997) Transcription factors of the NFAT family: regulation and function. *Annu Rev Immunol* **15**, 707–747.

Ratner V.A. (1990) Towards the unified theory of molecular evolution (TME). *Theor Popul Biol* **38**, 233–261.

Reese, M.G., Eeckman, F.H., Kulp, D., Haussler, D. (1997) Improved splice site detection in Genie, *J Comput Biol* **4**, 311–323.

Reuter, I. (2000) Dissertation, http://www.biblio.tu-bs.de/ediss/data/20000317a/20000317a.html

Rooney J.W., Hoey T., Glimcher L.H. (1995) Coordinate and cooperative roles for NF-AT and AP-1 in the regulation of the murine IL-4 gene. *Immunity* **2**, 473–483.

Saqi M. A., Sternberg M. J. (1994) Identification of sequence motifs from a set of proteins with related function. *Protein Engineering* **7**, 165–171.

Scherf, M., Klingenhoff, A., Werner, T. (2000) Highly specific localization of promoter regions in large genomic sequences by PromoterInspector: a novel context analysis approach. *J Mol Biol* **297**, 599–606.

Schneider T. D., Stormo G. D., Gold L., Ehrenfeucht A. (1986) Information content of binding sites on nucleotide sequences. *J Mol Biol* **188**, 415–431.

Seledtsov, I. A., Solovyev, V. V., Merkulova, T. I. (1991) New elements of glucocorticoid-receptor binding sites of hormone-regulated genes. *Biochim Biophys Acta* **1089**, 367–376.

Sharan R, Ovcharenko I, Ben-Hur A, Karp R.M. (2003) CREME: a framework for identifying cis-regulatory modules in human–mouse conserved segments. *Bioinformatics* Suppl 1, I283–I291.

Shelest, E., Kel, A.E., Gössling, E., Wingender, E. (2003) Prediction of potential C/EBP/NF-kappaB composite elements using matrix-based search methods. *In Silico Biol.* **3**, 71–79.

Sinha S. (2002) Discriminative motifs. In *RECOMB2002 Proceedings of the Sixth Annual International Conference on Computational Biology*, pages 291–298. Washington, DC, USA, April 18–21, 2002.

Smale S.T. (1994) Core promoter architecture for eukaryotic protein-coding genes. In: Conaway, R.C. Conaway, J.W. (eds) *Transcription: Mechanisms and Regulation*. Raven Press, New York, 63–81.

Smale, S.T. (1997) Transcription initiation from TATA-less promoters within eukaryotic protein-encoding genes. *Biochim Biophys Acta* **1351**, 73–88.

Smith H. O., Annau T. M., Chandrasegaran S. (1990) Finding sequence motifs in groups of functionally related proteins. *Proc Natl Acad Sci USA* **87**, 826–830,.

Solovyev V.V., Rogozin I.B. (1986) The program package of the context analysis of DNA, RNA and protein sequences. 1. Search for homology and functional sites. Institute Cytology and Genetics of the USSR Academy of Science, Novosibirsk, (Russ.), 1–70.

Solovyev V.V. et al. (1997) In: *Proceedings of the Fifth International Conference on Intelligent Systems for Molecular Biology* (Gaasterland, T., Karp P., Karpus K., Ouzounis C., Sander C., Valencia A., eds), pp. 294–302.

Stormo G.D. (1998) Information content and free energy in DNA–protein interactions. *J Theor Biol* **195**, 135–137.

Stormo G.D., Hartzell G.W. (1989) A tool for multiple sequence alignment. *Proc Natl Acad Sci USA* **86**, 1183–1187.

Struhl K. (1999) Fundamentally different logic of gene regulation in eukaryotes and prokaryotes. *Cell* **98**, 1–4.

Tikunov Y., Kel A. (2000) Kernel method for estimation of functional site local consensi: classification of transcription initiation sites in eukaryotic genes In: *Proceedings of the German Conference on Bioinformatics (GCB00)*, October 5–7, 2000, Heidelberg, Germany, p. 83–88

Tikunov Y., Kel A. (2002) Kernel method for identification of local patterns in unaligned sets of functional sites. In *The Third International Conference on Bioinformatics of Genome Regulation and Structure (BGRS'2002)*, Novosibirsk, p. 57–60.

Tronche, F., Ringeisen, F., Blumenfeld, M., Yaniv, M., Pontoglio, M. (1997) Analysis of the distribution of binding sites for a tissue-specific transcription factor in the vertebrate genome. *J Mol Biol* **266**, 231–245.

van Helden, J., Andre, B., Collado-Vides, J. (1998) Extracting regulatory sites from the upstream regions of yeast genes by computational analysis of oligonucleotide frequencies. *J Mol Biol* **281**, 827–842.

Wagner A. (1999) Genes regulated cooperatively by one or more transcription factors and their identification in whole eukaryotic genomes. *Bioinformatics* **15**, 776–784.

Wasserman W.W., Fickett J.W. (1998) Identification of regulatory regions which confer muscle-specific gene expression. *J Mol Biol* **278**, 167–181.

Wasylyk B., Hahn S.L., Giovane A. (1993) The Ets family of transcription factors. *Eur J Biochem* **211**, 7–18.

Werner, T. (1999) Models for prediction and recognition of eukaryotic promoters. *Mammalian Genome* **10**, 168–175.

Wingender E. (1993) *Gene Regulation in Eukaryotes*. VCH, Weinheim.

WINGENDER, E. (1997) Classification scheme of eukaryotic transcription factors. *Mol Biol (Mosk)* **31**, 483–497.

WINGENDER E., KARAS H., KNUEPPEL, R. (1996) TRANSFAC database as a bridge between sequence data libraries and biological function. *Pacific Symposium on Biocomputing '97 (PSB'97)*, R. B. Altman, A. K. Dunker, L. Hunter, T. E. Klein (eds.). World Scientific, pp. 477–485.

ZHANG M.Q. (1998 a) Identification of human gene core promoters in silico, *Genome Res* **8**, 319–326.

ZHANG M.Q. (1998 b) Statistical features of human exons and their flanking regions, *Hum Mol Genet* **7**, 919–932.

13
Systems Biology Applied to Toxicogenomics

Klaus Prank, Matthias Höchsmann, Björn Oleson, Thomas Schmidt, Leila Taher, and Dion Whitehead

13.1
Introduction to Systems Biology

As we enter the post-genomics era, systems biology is emerging as a powerful formalism for identification of system structure and simulation of complex biological behaviour. A systems biology approach attempts to integrate experimental, computational, and theoretical biology to understand biological systems. The aim is to develop a system-level analysis that provides a deep understanding of system structure and dynamics. The application of systems biology depends on cross-disciplinary teams of researchers working together to develop high-throughput technologies for data acquisition and storage and sophisticated computational methods for analysis and simulation (Figure 13.1). An immediate aim of systems biology is to build a common language that links experimental biological scientists with engineers, and computer scientists, and mathematicians. The long term goal is to integrate these technologies

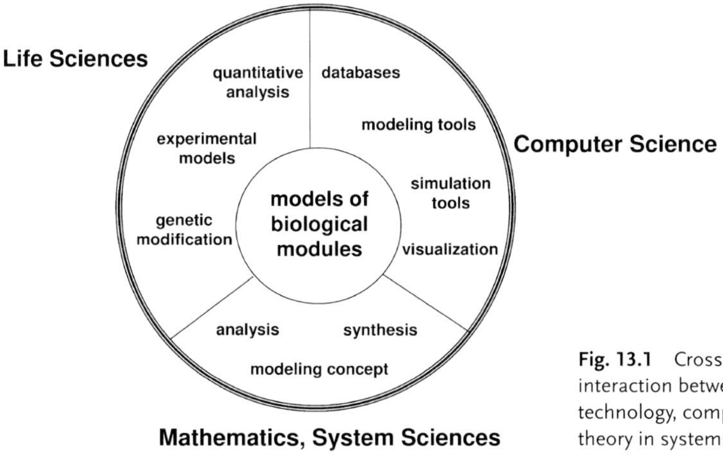

Fig. 13.1 Cross-disciplinary interaction between experiments, technology, computation, and theory in systems biology.

Handbook of Toxicogenomics: Strategies and Applications. Edited by Jürgen Borlak

ISBN: 3-527-30342-1

and biological knowledge to create a new paradigm for biological research, driven by a robust interaction between experiments, technology, computation, and theory [1, 2].

Systems biology is a young, emerging field that aims at system-level understanding of biological systems. Since the days of Wiener [3], system-level understanding has been a long-standing goal of biological sciences. Cybernetics, for example, aims at describing animals and machines from control and communication theory. Unfortunately, molecular biology had just started at that time, so only phenomenological analysis was possible. It only recently became possible for system-level analysis to be grounded on discoveries at the molecular level. With the progress of genome sequencing projects and of other molecular biology projects that accumulate in-depth knowledge of the molecular nature of biological systems, we are now at the stage to seriously look into the possibility of system-level understanding solidly grounded on molecular-level understanding (Figure 13.2).

What does it mean to understand at the system level? Unlike molecular biology, which focuses on molecules, including the sequences of nucleotide acids and proteins, systems biology focuses on systems that are composed of molecular components. Although systems are composed of materials, the essence of a system lies in its dynamics, so it cannot be described merely by enumerating its components. At the same time, it is misleading to believe that only system structure, such as network topologies, is important without paying sufficient attention to the diversity and functionalities of components. Both the structure of the system and its components play an indispensable role in forming the state of the system as a whole. Within this context, understanding the structure of a system, such as gene regulatory or biochemical networks, as well as the physical structures; understanding the dynamics of a system, by both quantitative and qualitative analysis as well as by constructing a theory/

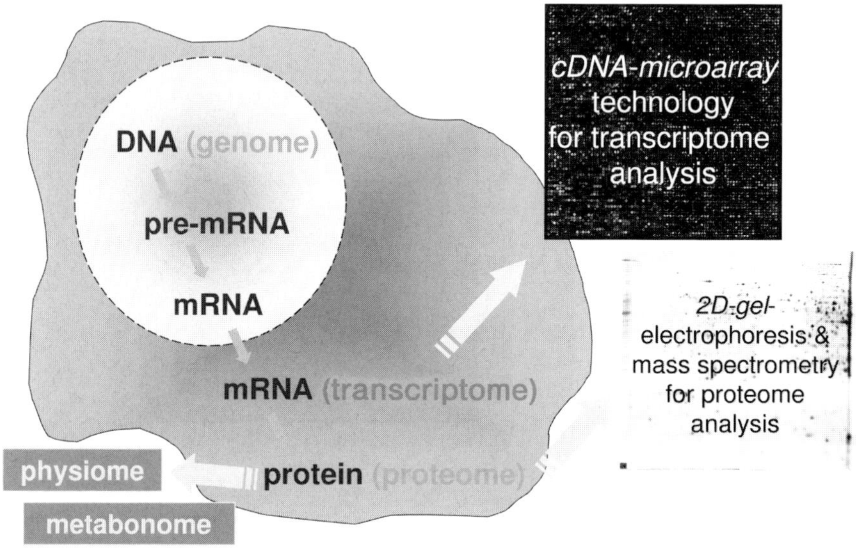

Fig. 13.2 System level understanding of a biological system.

model with powerful prediction capability; understanding the control mechanisms in the system; and understanding the design of the system – are all key milestones for judging how well we understand the system (Figure 13.3).

New high-throughput technologies in genomics, transcriptomics, proteomics, and metabonomics allow for deciphering the intracellular signalling machinery in great detail (Figure 13.2). In contrast to conventional approaches in toxicology that use single gene and protein expression patterns as indicators for the toxicity of well established model toxins, the genome, transcriptome, proteome, and metabolome can now be tested in parallel to explore the disruption of regulatory processes on a system-wide level. This experimental approach generates large, high-dimensional datasets for the identification of regulatory processes by data-processing techniques. A meaningful understanding of the regulatory processes and networks being identified requires subsequent mathematical modelling and simulation. Making *in silico* predictions requires that current knowledge from numerous public and proprietary databases be integrated. These computationally very demanding methods of data analysis and simulation require intensive use of high-performance computing. The *in silico* predictions need to be validated in *in vivo* as well as *in vitro* experiments to close the iterative research cycle of systems biology of toxicity testing in many cell types. The long-range perspective of the systems biology approach will lead to more rational drug design through the identification of organ-specific toxic side effects with *in silico* simulations. This will lead to more rational and cost-effective R&D of new drugs by helping to significantly reduce the attrition rate of new drugs in the late phase-III and post-market periods.

Many exciting and profound issues are being actively investigated, including the robustness of biological systems, network structures, and dynamics and applications to drug discovery. Systems biology is in its infancy, but this is the area that has to be explored and the area that we believe will be the mainstream of biological sciences in this century.

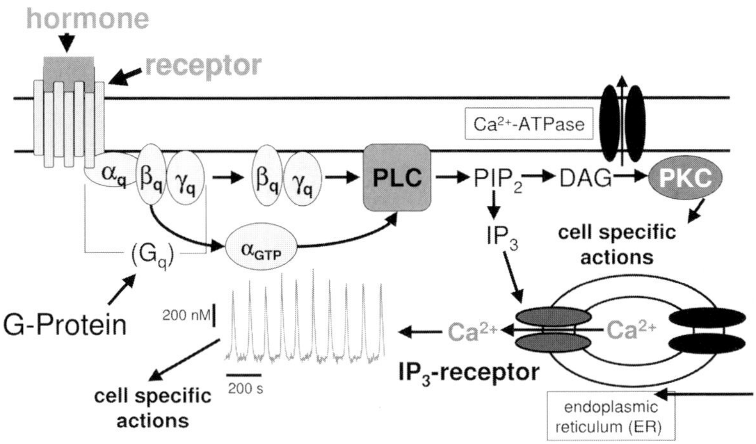

Fig. 13.3 Biochemical model for intracellular Ca^{2+} dynamics.

13.1.1 System-level Understanding of Biological Systems

13.1.1.1 System Structure Identification

Bottom–Up Approach

The bottom–up approach of systems structure identification tries to construct a biological regulatory network, such as a gene regulatory or metabolic network, based on the compilation of independent experimental data, mostly through literature searches and also through specific experiments to obtain data concerning very specific aspects of the network of interest. This approach is appropriate when most of the elements of the networks, e.g., genes, metabolites, and their regulatory relationships, are well understood. The bottom–up approach might thus help to find the last few pieces when most of the pieces of the system are known. In some cases, biochemical constants can be measured so that very precise simulations can be performed. If most of the parameters of the system under study are known, the main purpose of research is to build a precise simulation model that can be used to analyze the dynamic properties of the system by changing the parameters that cannot be changed in the actual system and to confirm that available knowledge generates simulation results that are consistent with available experimental data. This is demonstrated by the experimental measurement and mathematical modelling and simulation of intracellular calcium dynamics in hepatocytes upon endocrine stimulation (Figure 13.4) [4, 5]. Some preliminary attempts have also been made to predict unknown genes and their interactions [6, 7], by manually searching for possible unknown interactions to obtain simulation results consistent with experimental data; exhaustive searches of all possible spaces of network structures were not done.

Top–Down Approach

The top–down approach takes the view of functionality from the top, such as a complete tissue or organ and its function, e.g., a heart beating or endocrine organs secreting. With the top–down approach one tries to break things down into their components on each level. The hope is to connect at some level with the bottom–up approach. Thus, we end up with different elements at the next level. There are many ways to break up such a multilevel structure. Given that we now know that genes play roles in many different functionalities, we do not have a unique way of going up. The most obvious difficulty with the top–down approach is that we do not know what is the best way of breaking the upper level into components at a lower level, so that it can meet any of the bottom–up approaches. Thus, a middle–out approach is absolutely necessary. Brenner and Noble discuss in the book listed under [8] in the discussion part of the book at several places about the middle-out approach.

Middle–Out Approach

Brenner argues that his definition of middle–out requires starting between the organism and the genes, i.e., the cells [8], because it allows for going 'outward' to physiology and 'inward' to molecules. Thus, the discussion of cell types is very important.

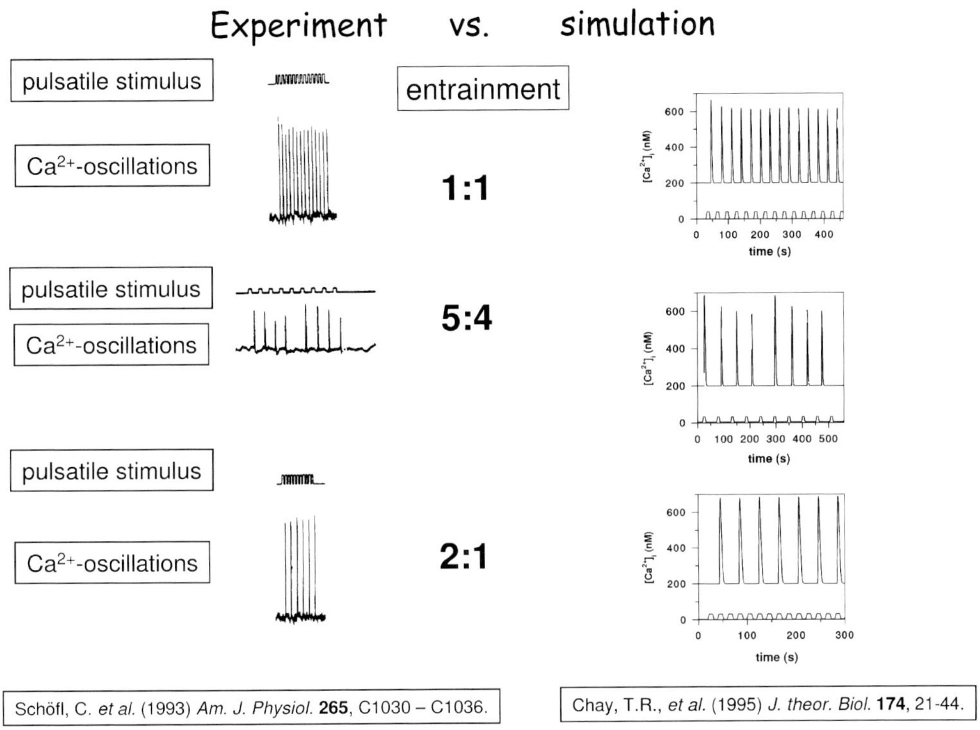

Fig. 13.4 Experiment and simulation. Stimulation of alpha 1-receptor by periodic pulses affects the amplitude and frequency of calcium transients. The experimentally found entrainment between extracellular pulses and intracellular calcium spikes is reproduced in the computer simulations (nonexcitable cell models).

Parameter Identification

To understand a system, it is important to identify not only the structure of the network under study, but a set of parameters, because all computational results have to be matched and tested again actual experimental results. Additionally, the identified network is used for simulating a quantitative analysis of the system's response and behavioural profile. Very often, the parameter set has to be estimated on the basis of experimental data. Various parameter optimization methods, such as genetic algorithms and simulated annealing, are used to find a set of parameters that can generate simulation results consistent with experimental data [9]. In finding a parameter set, one needs to remember that there may be multiple parameter sets that generate simulation results that fit equally well to experimental data. An important feature of parameter optimization algorithms used for this purpose is the ability to find as many local minima as possible, rather than to find a single global minimum. This ability needs to be combined with a method to indicate specific experiments needed to identify which one of such parameter sets is the correct parameter set.

Although it is important to accurately measure and estimate the genuine parameter values, in some instances exact parameters are not critical. For example, it was shown through an extensive simulation that the segment polarity network in *Drosophila* exhibits a high level of robustness against parameter change [10]. For certain networks that are essential for survival, the networks need to be robust to various changes in parameters for the biological species to cope with genetic variations and external disturbances. For this kind of network, the essence is embedded into the structure of the network, rather than in specific parameters of the network. This is particularly true when feedback control is used to ensure robustness of circuits, as seen in bacterial chemotaxis [11].

Thus, parameter estimation and measurement may need to be combined with theoretical analysis on the sensitivity of the circuit to changes in certain parameters.

13.1.1.2 System Behaviour Analysis

Once the structures of a system are understood, the next task is to understand the dynamic behaviour of the system. How does it adapt to and resist perturbations from the environment? To understand this on the system level, it is essential to understand the mechanisms behind (1) the robustness and stability of the system, and (2) the functionalities of the circuits.

The task of understanding the behaviours of complex biological networks is not trivial. Computer simulations and theoretical analyses are essential to provide in-depth understanding of the mechanisms behind the circuits.

Simulation

Simulating the behaviour of genetic and metabolic networks plays an important role in systems biology research, and several efforts in development of simulators are ongoing [13–17]. The complexity of network behaviour and the large number of components involved do not enable an intuitive understanding of the behaviour of such networks. Accurate simulation models are a prerequisite for analyzing the dynamics of a system by changing the parameters and structure of the genetic and metabolic networks. Although such analysis is necessary for understanding dynamic behaviour, these operations are not possible with actual biological systems. Simulation is an essential tool not only for understanding the behaviour, but also for design processes. For the design of engineering systems, several forms of simulation are used. It is unthinkable today for any serious engineering system to be designed and built without simulation. VLSI (very large scale integrated) design of computer chips requires major design simulation, thus creating one of the major markets for supercomputers. Commercial aviation is another example. The Boeing 777 was designed almost entirely based on simulation and digital prefabrication. Once we enter that stage of designing and actively controlling biological systems, simulation will be the core of the design process.

To be a viable methodology for the study of biological systems, highly functional, accurate, and user-friendly simulator systems have to be developed. The computational power required by such simulators is rather high and requires highly parallel hardware and software systems such as cluster and vector computing. Although some simulators already exist, no system sufficiently covers the needs of a broad range of biology research, to be able to simulate gene expression, metabolism, and signal transduction for single and multiple cells. It must be able to simulate both high concentrations of proteins, which can be described by differential equations, and low concentrations of proteins, which need to be handled by stochastic process simulation.

A set of software systems needs to be developed and integrated to assist systems biology research. Such software includes:

- a database for storing experimental data,
- a cell and tissue simulator,
- parameter optimization software,
- bifurcation and system analysis software,
- hypotheses generator and experiment planning advisor software,
- data visualization software.

13.1.1.3 System Control

The *robustness* of a system refers to how the system maintains its functional properties despite external or internal disturbances. In biology, it relates to nondetectable or minor changes in the phenotype or in the function subsequent to changes in the environment (nutritional deprivation, exposure to chemical agents, change in temperature) or to internal failures (DNA damage, genetic disease).

In engineering systems, robustness is accomplished by using:

- *redundancy*, multiple elements perform equivalent functions,
- *modular design*, subsystems are separated to prevent failure spreading from one module to others,
- *structural stability*, stability is promoted by the intrinsic properties of the system,
- a form of *system control*, negative feedback or feedforward control.

The rest of this section discusses how these four principles of engineering robustness apply – with logical differences arising from the nature of the two kinds of systems – also to biological systems [20, 21].

Redundancy and Degeneracy

A common means of identifying the function of a gene is to perform a knockout experiment, in which that gene is removed or silenced early in development. The resultant phenotype should in principle allow inference of the putative function of the knocked-out gene. However, in many such experiments, the knockout phenotype appears to be the same as the wild-type phenotype, often because the target gene is one of at least two genes contributing to the phenotype and because its removal is automatically compensated for by the remaining members of that set of genes. This phenomenon is known as *degeneracy* and is a property of biological systems present at all levels of organization [22]. In immunology, different antibodies can bind to the same antigen. On the cellular level, different codons code for the same amino acids, and multiple pathways of signal transduction and metabolic circuits can be functionally complementary under unlike conditions. On the tissue level, many distinct patterns of muscle contraction yield equivalent outcomes.

Formally, the concept of degeneracy involves *structurally different elements* yielding the same or different functions depending on the context in which they are expressed.

In engineering, electric or mechanical circuits often contain duplicate elements to provide additional protection from failure. Analogously in communications technology, messages are normally repeated to decrease transmission errors. This presence of *identical elements* performing exactly the same function is referred as *redundancy* [23]. However, this distinction is very rarely observed in biology, the concepts of redundancy and degeneracy being frequently used as synonyms.

Both redundancy and degeneracy improve the system's robustness against damage to its components by using multiple pathways to accomplish one or several functions [24].

Modular Design

When designing a system, engineers normally build separate modules for specific functions and keep interactions between them to a necessary minimum [25]. This policy generally meets both economic and design constraints. Modular design prevents damage from spreading limitlessly, making the system function robust to change. Also, it facilitates evolutionary changes in some of the components, changes in one module do not affect the others.

In biological systems, modules can be defined as discrete identities with an identifiable function that distinguishes them from other modules. Separation of modules is achieved by chemical isolation or the specificity of the module components, and the modules can interact or not, according to the function that they perform. Modules need not be rigid structures; one component can belong to different modules at different times. Many modules have been successfully reconstituted *in vitro*.

Cellular systems are typical examples of modular systems. The system that governs chemotaxis in bacteria and the machinery for protein synthesis or DNA replication in any cell are specific examples. In genetics, modules are formed by sets of genes contributing to one complex or trait (for example, an organ system). These modular genetic systems are found in different genomic contexts performing a similar function.

In biology, modularity implies that the phenotype is not directly affected by the modification of only one module component, providing a path for evolution. In fact, proteins whose function is restricted to one module are modified much more easily than proteins like histones, which interact with many other proteins in different modules [26].

Structural Stability

A system is said to be stable if it has a tendency to remain close to a steady state, despite the influence of perturbations – transient changes in the input. The more quickly a system returns to its original state after a transient input is applied to it, the more stable it is. This means that the production and decay rates are balanced.

When the input to a stable system is suddenly changed from one constant value to another or from one periodic function to another, the output undergoes a temporary adjustment (transient) period until it reaches a new steady state. In contrast, if a perturbation is applied to an unstable system, the output signal may remain at a constant value different from the original value, may oscillate continuously at constant amplitude, or may decrease indefinitely with or without oscillation until the system is destroyed.

Some gene regulatory circuits are built to be stable for a broad range of parameter variations and genetic polymorphisms [27].

System Control

A system can generally be defined as a physical, chemical, and/or biological process in which an input signal is transformed into an output signal. This implies that the output is merely the result of the interaction of the input with the internal components of the system, and that therefore, when the input is varied in a particular way, the output is also caused to vary in a particular way. The output depends on the input according to the properties of the system (Figure 13.5), which ideally can be expressed in the form of mathematical equations (a model).

A system input is called a control if it can be chosen in such a way as to induce the system to conform to some desired behaviour. In general, process control refers to an engineering operation by which a system 'makes decisions' about how to best manipulate available variables to obtain a desired output. Control theory has been instrumental in the successful design of most man-made complex systems.

Although control theory can also contribute to the understanding of biological systems, they are rarely analyzed mathematically. This is due partly to the complexity of the estimation of numerical parameters and partly to the numerous interlocking control loops that biological system normally include, which make it difficult to study one system in isolation.

Characteristics of biological systems include:

- extremely complex, efficient, robust, and high-performance,
- control systems overrule,
- networks dominated by feedback loops arranged in a hierarchy,
- relevant variables are often difficult to measure, control, or even identify,
- virtually impossible to isolate.

Various control schemes used in complex engineering systems are also found in biological systems. Among them, feedforward control and feedback control – which are two major control schemes – are nearly ubiquitous in biological systems.

Feedforward control is a control strategy by which the controller measures a process variable representing the disturbances that can affect the process. An example

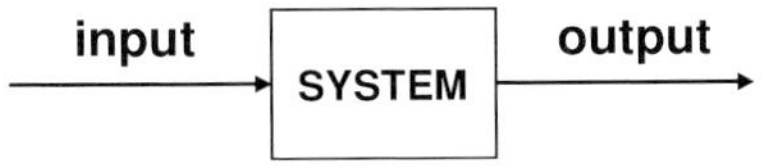

Fig. 13.5 General system block diagram.

of feedforward control in an engineering system is to regulate the temperature inside a room by installing a temperature sensor outside the room – if the outside temperature decreases, then a thermostat would begin heating the room before the inside temperature is affected, independent of what is taking place inside the room (i. e., somebody may have turned on the oven). Examples of biological feedforward control systems abound. Much eukaryotic gene expression is regulated in this way, and consequently, the adverse effects of defective genes cannot be ameliorated much by the cell. For instance, the concentration of chloride inside epithelial cells is controlled by production of the protein responsible for its transport to the extracellular matrix, the CFTR (cystic fibrosis transmembrane conductance regulator). The CFTR gene encodes a membrane protein that works as a cyclic AMP-regulated chloride channel in epithelial cells. It also regulates epithelial sodium channels and controls the regulation of other transport pathways. These channels transport chloride ions out of the cell, thus making its surroundings saltier, which in turn draws water out of the cell by osmosis. In the lungs, for example, this fluid acts as disinfectant, inhibiting the growth of microorganisms. Under normal circumstances, cellular control mechanisms lead to the transcription and translation of the gene for this protein in pulmonary epithelial cells. However, as there is no mechanism to check whether this has actually been achieved, in people with the most common mutation causing cystic fibrosis, a defective protein is assembled and directed to the endoplasmic reticulum for degradation instead of to the cell membrane. In consequence, lung cells are unable to secrete water, and clots of mucus obstruct breathing, favouring chronic bacterial and viral infections.

Although, in principle, feedforward control can be made error-free, the fact that it does not verify that the outcome corresponds to the expected effect makes it prone to mistakes. With a good control system, such errors may be few, but they accumulate in time until they eventually destroy the system. The only way to avoid this accumulation is to use feedback control [28].

Feedback control compensates for errors or deviations from the reference value after they have happened. Control actions are determined by the state of the system. In the example of the thermoregulated room, the heating would be switched on after a drop in the temperature inside the room. Basically, the system detects the difference between the desired output and the actual output and corrects this difference. The disadvantage of feedback control is that the actions are taken after the error or deviation has occurred, and therefore this control scheme is by definition imperfect. Nevertheless, if the perturbations are continuous and develop gradually, the controller can intervene at an early stage when the deviation is still small, which makes feedback control effective. This explains why feedback control is one of the most widely used control methods in engineering design and why it is ubiquitously present in biological systems.

Feedback control systems require a reference value – the desired output – which provides a target to aim for. In biological control systems these targets are sometimes obscure. Biological reference values may be genetically determined, for example, via the amino acid sequences of regulatory proteins, which ultimately define their binding constants for allosteric effectors.

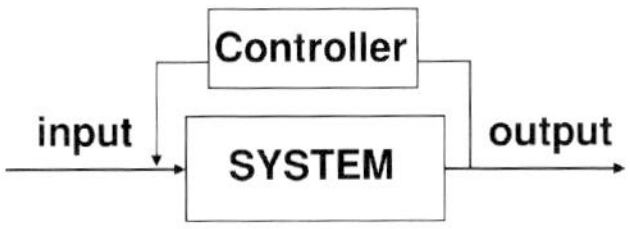

Fig. 13.6 System block diagram with feedback.

A system is subject to positive feedback if the output that is sent back to the input facilitates and accelerates the transformation in the same direction as the preceding results. If the output instead produces a result in the opposite direction to previous results, the system is said to be subjected to negative feedback. With positive feedback there is exponential growth or decline; with negative feedback there is maintenance of equilibrium (Figure 13.6). In this figure there is a general feedback loop, not specifically labelled as positive or negative. This description is only in the text!

Regulation of the level of glucose in the bloodstream is an example of negative feedback control. When the receptors in the pancreas detect a drop in the level of glucose in the blood, the alpha cells of the islets of Langerhans release the hormone glucagon to initiate a corrective response. Glucagon targets the liver, where it promotes the breakdown of glycogen to glucose. Thus, the lack of glucose in the bloodstream can be corrected by the secretion of glucose produced from glycogen. Conversely, when an increase in the level of glucose in the blood is detected, the beta cells of the islets of Langerhans release the hormone insulin to favour the conversion of glucose to glycogen.

13.1.2
Measurement Technology and Experimental Approaches

13.1.2.1 Experimental Measurements in Systems Biology

Although efforts to systematically obtain comprehensive and accurate datasets are under way, systems biology places many more demands on the experimental biologists than does the current practice of biology. It requires a comprehensive body of data and control of the quality of data produced so that they can be used as a reference point for simulation, modelling, and system identification. Eventually, many of the current experimental procedures must be automated to enable high-throughput experiments to be carried out with precise control of quality. Needless to say, not all biological experiments will be carried out in such an automated fashion, for important contributions will continue to be made by small-scale experiments. Nevertheless, large-scale experiments will lay the foundation for system-level understanding.

High-throughput, comprehensive, accurate measurement is the most essential part of biological science. Although expectations are high for a computational approach to overcome limitations in the traditional approach in biology, this approach will never generate serious results without experimental data upon which to ground the computational studies. For the computational and systems approach to be successful, measurement has to be (1) comprehensive, (2) quantitatively accurate, and (3) systematic.

Although the requirement for quantitative accuracy is obvious, the other two criteria need further clarification. Comprehensiveness can be further classified into three types:

- factor comprehensiveness,
- time-series comprehensiveness,
- item comprehensiveness.

13.1.2.2 **Next-generation Experimental Systems**

To cope with increasing demands for comprehensive and accurate measurement, a set of new technologies and instruments needs to be developed that offers a higher level of automation and high-precision measurement.

First, dramatic progress in the level of automation of experimental procedures for routine experiments is required to keep up with increasing demands for modelling and system-level analysis. High-throughput experiments may turn into a labour-intensive nightmare unless the level of automation is drastically improved. Further automation of experimental procedures would greatly benefit the reliability of experiments, throughput, and total cost of the whole operation in the long run.

Second, cutting-edge technologies such as microfluid systems, nanotechnology, and femtochemistry may need to be introduced to design and build next-generation experimental devices. The use of such technologies will enable us to measure and observe the activities of genes and proteins in a way that is not possible today. It may also drastically improve the speed and accuracy of measurement with existing devices.

In those fields in which there are obvious needs, such as sequencing and proteomics, the above goals are already being pursued. Beyond the development of high-throughput sequencers using high-density capillary array electrophoresis, efforts are being made to develop integrated microfabricated devices that enable PCR and capillary electrophoresis in a single microdevice [29, 30]. Such devices not only enable miniaturization and precision measurements, but will also allow significant increases in the level of automation.

In the developmental biology of *Caenorhabditis elegans*, identification of cell lineage is one of the major issues that needs to be met to assist analysis of the gene regulatory network for differentiation. The first attempt to identify cell lineage was carried out entirely manually [31, 32] and required several years to identify the lineage of the wild type. Four-dimensional microscopy allows multilayer confocal images to be collected at constant time intervals, but lineage identification is not automatic. With the availability of exhaustive RNAi knockout *C. elegans*, high-throughput cell lineage identification is essential for exploring the utility of the exhaustive RNAi. Efforts are under way to fully automate cell lineage identification, as well as acquisition of three-dimensional nuclear position data [33], fully utilizing advanced image-processing algorithms and massively parallel supercomputers. Such devices meet some of the criteria mentioned earlier and provide comprehensive measurement of cell positions with high accuracy. With automation, high-throughput data acquisition can be expected. If the project succeeds, it can be used to automatically identify the cell lineage of all RNAi knockout mutants for early embryogenesis. The technology may be augmented, but with major efforts, to automatically detect cell–cell contacts, protein localization, etc.

Combined with whole-mount in-situ hybridization and possible future single-cell expression profiling, these techniques may enable complete identification of the gene regulatory network of *C. elegans* in the near future.

Genomics, Transciptomics, and Proteomics

Genomics is a new, fast-paced scientific discipline. Within only a few years, tools and data provided by genomics have become the new basis of molecular life sciences.

Genomics comprises the generation and sequencing of DNA templates, the combination or assembly of the resulting DNA sequence data, and the interpretation or annotation of the assembled DNA sequence. Data acquired in genomics form the basis of subsequent functional analysis in transcriptomics and proteomics.

All branches of genomics rely on automated high-throughput procedures and robotic workstations. To obtain optimal results, automated workflows are complemented with manual or low-throughput techniques for special purposes.

Genomics depends on the continuous production, evaluation, and analysis of enormous amounts of samples and data. This requires state-of-the-art equipment and support in the bioinformatics field. An essential prerequisite for providing optimal genomics data is an experienced staff of scientists and technicians. Their continuous efforts permit the ongoing progress in methods application that is the groundwork for this fast-changing branch of modern science and technology.

Although deciphering of genome sequences is moving into ever higher gear, more than just experimental procedures for the investigation of biological functions of individual sequence elements and encoded gene products are important for further analyses. Experimental approaches to elucidating the complex interplay of gene products and regulatory sequences from a more global perspective become more and more crucial.

The aims of functional genomics are to derive as much information as possible about as many genes as possible, as quickly as possible. The analysis of global gene expression patterns (transcriptomics) is a key area, since the development and differentiation of a cell or an organism, as well as its adaptation to variable conditions, is determined in large part by the profile of gene expression. DNA array technology, in which thousands of different DNA sequences are arrayed in a defined matrix on a support (e. g., nylon or glass) in ever-growing densities, is rapidly becoming the method of choice for gene expression profiling. The applications of microarrays extend beyond the boundaries of basic research into environmental monitoring, pharmacology, and diagnostics. In recent years, DNA-microarray technology has overcome its initial problems and has emerged as an important tool for meeting many of these challenges.

Proteomics includes, not only the identification and quantification of proteins, but also the determination of their localization, modifications, interactions, activities, and, ultimately, function. Initially encompassing just two-dimensional (2D) gel electrophoresis for protein separation and identification, proteomics now refers to any procedure that characterizes large sets of proteins. The explosive growth of this field is driven by multiple forces: genomics and its revelation of more and more new proteins; powerful protein technologies, such as newly developed mass spectrometry approaches, global (yeast) two- hybrid techniques, and spin-offs from DNA arrays; and innovative computational tools and methods to process, analyze, and interpret prodigious amounts of data.

Metabonomics

The general aim of metabonomics is to identify, measure, and interpret the complex time-related concentration, activity, and flux of endogenous metabolites in cells, tissues, and biosamples such as blood, urine, and saliva. For the purposes of this chapter, 'metabolites' include not only small molecules that are the products and intermediates of metabolism, but also carbohydrates, peptides, and lipids. The need for innovative technologies for measuring and quantifying the metabolites involved in cellular pathways and networks is obvious. It is expected that the new technologies in metabonomics developed under this initiative will play a major role in transferring capabilities to laboratories and research institutes that are investigating the underlying pathways involved in cellular homeostasis, perturbation, development, and aging.

Many ongoing research programs focus on the development of new genomics and proteomics tools and the utilization of those approaches for studying cellular function. In contrast, relatively few research programs focus on metabonomics technology development and application. The aim of this initiative is to encourage the development of highly innovative and sensitive tools for identifying and quantifying cellular metabolites and their fluxes at high anatomical resolution – extending to subcellular – and at a temporal resolution that is appropriate to understanding cellular processes on biologically relevant timescales. The scope of projects that will be appropriate ranges from techniques for improving and refining the process of sample separation and processing; to new methods, reagents, or instrumentation for identifying and measuring metabolites and their fluxes; to the development and utilization of data reduction, management, and analysis tools needed to establish proof-of-concept for the technology. New technologies that, if successful, have the potential to be scalable, either as high-throughput applications or as advances that can be used in a large number of laboratories, are especially encouraged. Although it is also important to develop data storage, data mining, and pathway modelling capabilities for metabonomics, these issues are not explicitly included in this particular solicitation.

Physiomics and Toponomics

The physiome is the quantitative and integrated description of the functional behaviour of the physiological state of an individual or species. The physiome describes the physiological dynamics of the normal intact organism and is built upon information and structure (genome, proteome, and morphome). The term comes from 'physio' (life) and 'ome' (as a whole). In its broadest terms, it defines relationships from genome to organism and from functional behaviour to gene regulation. In the context of the Physiome Project, it includes integrated models of components of organisms, such as particular organs or cell systems and biochemical or endocrine systems.

The Physiome Project is a worldwide effort to define the physiome through the development of databases and models that will facilitate understanding the integrative function of cells, organs, and organisms. The project is focused on compiling and providing a central repository of databases, linking experimental information and computational models from many laboratories into a single, self-consistent framework. This coalescence of research efforts will promote the development of comprehensive databases and an integrative, analytical approach to the study of medicine and physiology.

The goals of the Physiome Project are:

- to develop and populate a database with observations of physiological phenomena and to interpret these in terms of mechanism (a fundamentally reductionist goal);
- to integrate experimental information into quantitative descriptions of the functioning of humans and other organisms (modern integrative biology glued together via modelling);
- to disseminate experimental data and integrative models for teaching and research;
- to foster collaboration amongst investigators worldwide, in an effort to speed up the discovery of how biological systems work;
- to determine the most effective targets (molecules or systems) for therapy, whether pharmaceutical or genomic;
- to provide information for the design of tissue-engineered, biocompatible implants.

13.2 Data Mining and Reverse Engineering of Regulatory Networks

13.2.1 Data Mining Techniques

The progress of information storage technologies in recent times has resulted in tremendous growth in the number and size of databases. In all areas, from business (e.g., credit card and supermarket transactions), science (e.g., molecular databases, astronomical data), and government (e.g., census data, birth records), more and more data are being stored. The massive amount of stored data promises to reveal previously unknown relationships and patterns, due to the size and scope of the datasets.

The discipline of data mining focuses on these emerging very large datasets, by developing techniques to deal with the problems usually present in these datasets. One of the difficulties is that the data under analysis have usually been collected for different purposes. For example, supermarket transaction records are recorded for the purpose of stocking and billing, not for the purpose of analyzing shopping *m measurements* →

n objects ↓

name	age	blood grp	income	...
bloggs, j	34	AB-	34000	
bliggs, k	67	O+	29000	
...				
...				

Fig. 13.7 Example matrix of patient data.

trends. In this respect, data mining is usually referred to as a secondary analysis, in contrast to statistics, for which the data is collected specifically for the purpose of analysis. Another difficulty in data mining is the aforementioned size of the datasets. Handling very large data sets imposes problems from the mundane, such as handling and storing the data, to the more conceptual, such as deciding if a relationship is due simply to chance or analyzing the data in a reasonable time.

By summarizing or presenting the datasets in novel ways, it is hoped that previously unsuspected or hidden relationships will be found. The relationships sought are referred to as models or patterns, and could be graphs, tree structures, linear equations describing the data, or patterns in a time series, for example.

Datasets can be conceptualized, in the simplest sense, as a collection of objects, with each object having some measurements. For n objects with m measurements, the dataset can be imagined as an $n \times m$ matrix. For instance, the n rows could be patients and the m columns could be patient medical data, e.g., age, weight, etc. (Figure 13.7). Measurements are of two types: categorical and quantitative. Quantitative data are numbers, e.g., birth weights, annual income, and categorical data falls into defined values, e.g., hair colour, blood group. Categorical data can be derived from numerical data, for example, defining the category 'minor' as between the ages 1–17 years. The types of data present in a dataset influence what analyses can be meaningfully performed. For example, linear regression, which models the relationship between two numerical measurements, is of little use for categorical data.

Data mining can be subdivided into different activities that serve different objectives:

1. Exploratory data analysis. This task is usually visual, in which charts and graphs are used to gain an impression of the data. Visualizing in more than three dimensions is not straightforward, and since data mining is often used to analyze high-dimensional datasets, techniques such as principle component analysis are often useful.

2. Descriptive modelling involves describing all the data. This can involve partitioning the data into groups, such as splitting marketing data into age groups, or calculating the overall probability distribution, or modelling the relationship between variables.

3. Predictive modelling differs from descriptive modelling in that predictive modelling attempts to predict an unknown variable (e.g., next week's price of some stock market share), whereas in descriptive modelling there is no unknown vari-

able. If the dataset contains patient data, the unknown variable could be prediction of an illness.

4. Rule and pattern discovery. The goal here is to find data points that differ significantly from the others, which can be difficult when the data exists in high-dimensional space. Human interpretation is very useful at this stage. An example is finding fraud in a set of transaction data.

5. Retrieval by content is a task performed by Internet search engines, such as Google. Here the user wants to find all patterns in a dataset that are similar in some way to a query pattern, e.g., finding relevant sentences in text mining, or similar pictures in an image database. Clearly, the success of the search depends in part on the defined similarity measure.

In regards to biology, the number and size of databases is already very large, and many are growing exponentially [34], especially in the 'omics' fields such as genomics, transcriptomics, and proteomics. Living systems are by nature dynamic and can exhibit variation both between individuals and within the same individual. On the other hand, existing biological databases represent only a snapshot of part of a system and are heterogeneous and numerous [35]. The result is that database integration becomes a crucial issue in biological data mining. However, this is not a trivial task.

13.2.2 Inferring Gene Regulatory Networks from Gene Expression Data

Inferring gene networks is predictive modelling based on biological data, in this case transcription levels of genes. The prediction here is the 'network' of gene regulation interactions that gives rise to the measured transcription levels. A promising use of this technology is the detection of toxic compounds early in the drug-discovery process, as toxicity is the major reason for rejected compounds [36], but toxicity is often addressed relatively late in the screening process.

The 'machines' that are used in measuring the data are called DNA microarrays. They consist of a chip with thousands of 'spots' (Figure 13.8). Each of these spots contains a small quantity of single-stranded DNA attached to the chip. The DNA in

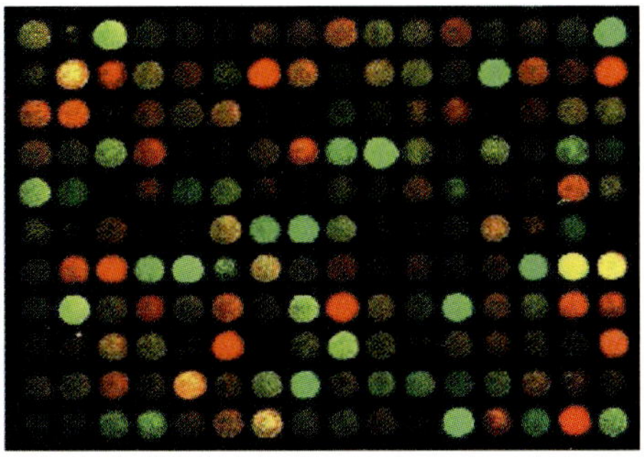

Fig. 13.8 DNA microarray chip. Each spot represents a single gene. The green spots indicate that cDNA from the wild type organism has bound, red indicates that cDNA from the knockout mutant has bound, and yellow means both have bound.

each spot is a specific sequence for a particular gene. The RNA transcripts in the sample are converted to cDNA and then labelled with a fluorescent dye. This is then washed over the chip, and if there is a cDNA whose sequence is complementary to a sequence on the chip, it binds and the label is detected with a photodetector. Usually control and test solutions are both washed over the same chip, each with different colour markers so that relative gene expression levels can be measured.

The gene expression levels are usually either time series or steady-state measurements. Time series are particularly difficult to construct, because the time intervals must be short with little noise in between steps, which is difficult in practice. In steady-state experiments, relationships are inferred by knocking out or over-expressing specific genes and comparing the expression levels in the mutant to those in the wild type.

The differences in gene expression levels between the wild type and, e.g., a knock-out mutant are then used to fit a model of gene regulation to the data. The interpretation of the results depends on how the gene interactions are represented. For example, in boolean networks genes are represented as simply on or off, but interactions involve switching other genes. This simplicity makes prediction and analysis somewhat easier but also difficult to interpret, as the model is not close to reality. Gene expression values in reality are continuous rather than on–off booleans.

Microarray technologies can theoretically measure the relative expression level of every gene, but even if the data were free of noise (which they are not), the transcriptome is still just a snapshot of one process. Thus expression data by themselves are difficult to interpret, being suggestive than conclusive, as there is a myriad of post-translational modifications that occur to regulate proteins. Thus, data mining and integration are integral to elucidating the reaction networks hidden behind the gene expression data.

13.2.3 Reverse Engineering of Metabolic and Signal-transduction Pathways

Metabolic and gene networks have been likened to electrical circuits, and this analogy contains interesting insights. Biological systems and advanced technologies are similar at the level of systems organization. They both have many levels of robustness and are designed/evolved to cope with uncertain external conditions.

Consider the bacterium *Escherichia coli*. The minimal number of genes needed for a cell to survive and replicate is estimated at around 300. *E. coli* has around 4000 genes, much more than the minimum. This large difference is needed to make the cell robust, not just in the face of fluctuating environmental conditions but also of failures in the reaction networks. This robustness comes with a price: complexity. For the cell to respond to many different external conditions and be resistant to failure, the internal environment develops a fragile homeostasis, as this stable internal environment enables quicker and more sophisticated responses. But the loss of internal homeostasis in usually catastrophic to the organism. Consider our obligatory use of oxygen as an electron acceptor. Oxygen is a very useful electron acceptor, but its use requires precision in the uptake, transport, and removal of CO_2. When this delicate system breaks down, the consequences are fatal. A comparison to *E. coli* is a Boeing 777 jumbo jet. The aircraft has 150 000 different subsystems that communicate through an elaborate system of protocols automated by about 1000 computers. This complexity is designed to be robust, i. e., to tolerate and respond to failures appropriately.

An important concept in both these systems is modularity. Modules are subsystems that have some independence with respect to modification or evolution. They maintain some form of identity when rearranged and use protocols to communicate with other modules. An example of a module in biology is the segmentation network in the fruit fly *Drosophila*. This module is robust to internal changes, in that most changes in the reaction rate of a protein or transcription factor do not disturb the module's function [37], i.e., setting up the segments in the fly embryo. Modules communicate through protocols, which are signals that have some agreed-upon meaning. In biological systems this could mean, e.g., that when the amount of some protein *X* increases, some module changes state. The protocols for feedback control in such systems are some of the more complex, because amplification systems are useful. However, without feedback mechanisms, it is relatively easy to build either uncertain high-gain amplifiers or precise low-gain ones, but prohibitively difficult to build precise high-gain amplifiers [38]. These protocols between modules must be fine-tuned, resulting in robust, sophisticated responses to external stimuli, but catastrophic failures in rare cases.

The concepts of robustness and modularity increase our understanding of complex systems. By regarding gene regulation networks and cell communication networks as many modules with switches, oscillators, and feedback mechanisms between them, the hope is to remove a subsystem and study its behaviour in isolation, which then may enable the construction of networks of systems [39].

Some genetic modules have been removed and analyzed. These form subsystems in gene regulation networks, and have analogies in, for example, electrical circuits:

1. Feedback loops, for example, where a protein modifies its own expression level. These systems have been shown to be more stable than genes without this regulation by both experimental and theoretical studies.

2. Switches, for which, after switching to a stable state after a stimulus, the system 'remembers' the stimulus.

3. Logic gates. Multiple repressors and activators enable 'IF *a* AND *b* THEN *c*' type switches. These can be stacked and joined to form complex decision-making subnetworks (Figure 13.9).

4. Oscillators: these are used by organisms to coordinate different systems and include circadian rhythms. However, the exact mechanism of biological clocks is not yet completely understood.

These basic components partly make up the gene regulatory networks that share many analogies to complex technology. However, the manner in which living systems respond to noise is often very different than that of constructed systems and

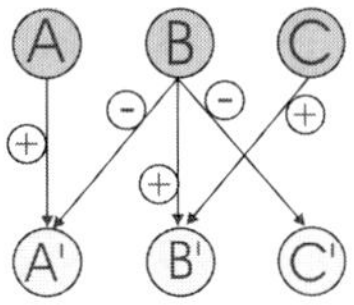

$A' = A \text{ or } \overline{B}$
$B' = B \text{ and } C$
$C' = \overline{B}$

Fig. 13.9 A simple Boolean network.

may provide insight into how human technologies can be improved. Understanding noise is crucial to understanding many biological systems, due in part to the inherent stochasicity in many systems, e. g., often the very small numbers of transcription factors, promoter sites, and tRNA molecules lead to high levels of random noise. Not only do living systems seem resistant to high levels of noise, for example, by using mechanisms like cascades of genes as attenuators, and positive and negative feedback loops, but some actually exploit noise. Haematopoietic stem cells, epigenetic inheritance, infection of a bacteria by a lambda phage – all these systems exploit noise. Some cellular processes can actually use noise to attenuate noise, in other words, noise can be used to *enhance* a signal when certain nonlinear effects are present [40].

By comparing complex biological systems and complex technologies, analogies are found. Electrical circuits give us metaphors for describing biological systems, nature in return rewards us with the need for more and better metaphors.

13.3 Modelling and Simulation Software

13.3.1 Automated Model Generation

In the past few decades the rapid increase in information about intracellular signal transduction and genetic networks has led to a view of regulatory biomolecular circuits as highly structured multicomponent systems that have evolved to perform optimally in very uncertain environments. This emerging complexity of biochemical regulation necessitates the development of novel tools for analysis, most notably, computer-assisted mathematical models. Computer modelling has proved to be of crucial importance in the analysis of genomic DNA sequences and molecular dynamics simulations and is likely to become an indispensable tool in biochemical and genetic research. Several platforms have been (or are being) developed (see Section 13.3.3) that enable biologists to do complex computational simulations of various aspects of cellular signalling and gene regulatory networks.

In spite of their promise, these new modelling environments have not been widely utilized by the biological research community. Arguably, among the reasons for this is the relative inaccessibility of the modelling interface to the typical classically trained geneticist or biochemist. Instead of schematic representations of signalling pathways, in which activation can be represented simply by an arrow connecting two molecular species, users are often asked to write specific differential equations or to chose among different modelling approximations. Even for fairly modest biomolecular circuits, such a technique requires explicitly writing dozens (or even hundreds) of differential equations, a job that can be tedious, difficult, and highly error prone, even for an experienced modeller. Thus, it would be extremely helpful to have a modelling interface that automatically converts a diagram- or reaction-based biochemical pathway description into a mathematical representation suitable for the solvers built into various currently existing software packages.

In addition to being more accessible to a broader research community, a tool allowing the automatic generation of mathematical models would facilitate the modelling of complex networks and interactions. For example, in intracellular signal transduction it is not uncommon to find multimolecular complexes of modifiable proteins. The number of different states that a multimolecular complex can have, along with the number of equations required to fully describe the dynamics of such a system, increases exponentially with the number of participating molecules or classes of molecules. It often occurs that the dynamics of each state is of interest. A modeller again faces the unpleasant and potentially error-prone task of writing dozens, if not hundreds, of equations. Automatic equation generation can significantly ease this task.

One tool developed for automatic model generation is Cellerator™ [41]. Cellerator is a Mathematica® package designed to facilitate biological modelling via automated equation generation. Cellerator was designed with the intent of simulating at least the following essential biological processes:

- signal transduction networks (STNs),
- cells that are represented by interacting signal transduction networks,
- multicellular tissues that are represented by interacting networks of cells that may themselves contain internal STNs.

These processes combine to form an obvious hierarchy that can be further subdivided for notational simplicity (e. g., STNs as elements of STNs, and so forth). In the past it was necessary to manually translate chemical networks from diagrams into chemical equations and then into ordinary differential equations. This process is tedious, highly error-prone, and impractical for all but the simplest of systems, because of the combinatorial increase in the number of equations with the number of chemical species. Cellerator provides a framework for generating, translating, and numerically solving a potentially unlimited number of biochemical interactions.

13.3.2 Parser

Very often, biochemical kinetics and signal transduction networks are written as a set of ordinary differential equations (ODE), which can be numerically integrated in a number of different simulators for deterministic modelling.

In many situations of biochemical interest, however, one is dealing with situations in which only a few reactants of some species are present. In these situations, the continuity assumption of the differential equation approach breaks down, and a numerical solution to the set of differential equations may lead to misleading results. An alternate approach is to perform a stochastic simulation of the system, in which each reaction that takes place is simulated by Monte Carlo methods. Following this approach is valid even when the reactant populations are very low, and indeed, one may see effects that are not apparent when the more traditional approach is used.

Very often, nevertheless, it is convenient to formulate the model in terms of differential equations, which biochemists are often used to working with. The program STODE [42, 43] takes a set of differential equations as input, extracts all necessary information, and performs a stochastic simulation of the system.

STODE is separated logically for the performance of two main tasks. The first consists of reading and processing the differential equations, and the second consists of running the simulation. In the first part, STODE takes as input a text file that specifies the set of differential equations to be parsed, as well as the rate constants, reactants (with their initial concentrations), and other constants needed to determine the system. This file is lexically analysed into tokens and fed to a parser that instantiates and assigns values to the various variables representing the reactants, constants, and differential equations. After this, STODE reconstructs the reactions associated with the differential equations, and if necessary, calculates the actual particle numbers from the given reactant concentrations.

The second task is that of performing the simulation. This is done according to Gillespie's algorithm, in which at each step the probability of each reaction being the next is calculated. This probability is proportional to the number of participating reactants and the rate constant for that reaction. Two random numbers are then generated, which in association with these probabilities, allow the next reaction and the time at which it occurs to be chosen. The time and particle numbers are then updated, and the probabilities for the next step are calculated.

The simulation proceeds in this way until a specified number of steps have been completed or a specified total time has been reached. During the course of execution, the particle numbers and time for each step are written to a file.

The program may be run in standalone mode or via a graphical interface. Generally, using an interface is somewhat slower, as the graphics have some overhead, but this allows the progress of the simulation to be viewed in real time and allows fine-tuning of the various parameters. For very long runs, you will probably prefer to use the standalone version.

When the graphical interface is invoked, you can specify the file to be used as input, or enter or modify the relevant data in an editor window. The results of the processed input can then be examined before beginning the simulation. As mentioned above, the simulation results are displayed in real time in a plotting window, which can be set to display results over the whole time frame or for a specifiable number of the most recent steps. As with the standalone version, the results are written to a file as the run proceeds. For both versions, a gnuplot command file is generated before exiting to enable easy viewing of the results with the gnuplot utility.

13.3.3 Systems Biology Workbench and Markup Languages

Efforts are being made to provide a common, versatile software platform for systems biology research. The Systems Biology Workbench project aims to provide a common middleware platform to which plug-in modules can be added to form a uniform software environment [18]. In addition to the software itself, the exchange of data and the interface between software modules is a critical issue in data-driven research tools. Systems Biology Markup Language (SBML) is a versatile and common open standard that enables the exchange of data and modelling information among a wide variety of software systems [19]. It is an extension of XML (extensible markup language) and is expected to become the industrial and academic standard format for data and model exchange. Another XML-based markup language is CellML, which is being developed by Physiome Science (Princeton, NJ, USA) in conjunction with the Bioengineering Research Group in the Department of Engineering Science at the University of Auckland.

The popularity of XML in the area of bioinformatics has clearly grown in the past few years. XML provides the capability of representing biological and medical data in a single as well as standardized data structure. However, the structure of XML documents defined using a XML DTD (document type definition) is limited to representing data in a hierarchical tree fashion. This approach imposes severe limitations upon both the data structure and the ability to validate an XML document. Utilization of the W3C's XML schema approach to document definition overcomes many of these limitations of the DTD approach. The biological XML definitions are freely available standards. Therefore, the DTDs and/or schemas are generally not protected by copyright laws and may be copied freely. Although the language definition draft document is copyrighted, its non-commercial use is often allowed. The XML applications and announced industry initiatives listed below have not been evaluated according to any serious criteria for quality and genuineness by the XML consortium. Since the various specification documents for XML/XLink/XSL are still somewhat in flux, it would often be unfair or difficult to make such a judgment. Obviously, many of these application areas provide exemplary models, having unquestioned integrity and high quality. Some already play a vital role in profitable commercial enterprises. It is also to be expected that some early XML/XLink/XSL applications may be merely demonstrations, toys, proof-of-concept applications; still others might be naive or ill-conceived. It may be necessary to regard some of these ideas as 'in draft', like some of the specification documents themselves (see http://www.xml.org/).

13.3.3.1 BIOML (BIOpolymer Markup Language)

The BIOpolymer Markup Language was developed by Proteometrics and Proteometrics Canada. Its major use is information annotation of biopolymer sequences. With BIOML the full specification of all experimental information known about molecular entities composed of biopolymers, for example, proteins, and genes, is possible. There is currently no general method for biopolymer sequence annotations in their biological context. With BIOML, the primary goal is to provide an extensible annotation framework and a common tool to exchange this information between scientists via the Internet. BIOML is slightly different to other markup languages, because the described document is not truly a document at all. Instead, a BIOML document describes a physical object, for example, a particular protein, in such a way that all known experimental information about that object can be associated with the object in a logical and meaningful way. A markup language has the advantage that the information is necessarily nested at different levels of complexity and assimilates very well with the inherent XML tree structure. Moreover, although BIOML's primary purpose is information transfer between computers, the additional style information available when using an XML-based approach simplifies the task of displaying that information in various types of browsing and display environments. BIOML was implemented and designed by Ron Beavis, with the help from David Fenyö (ProteoMetrics) and Brian Chait (Rockefeller University). David States (Washington University) assisted the DTD language definition editing (see http://www.bioml.com/BIOML/).

13.3.3.2 CML (Chemical Markup Language)

By intention, CML does not cover all chemistry but concentrates on polymers – discrete entities usually represented by a formula and a connection table. It supports a hierarchy for compound molecules, for example, clathrates and macromolecules. Several labelled numeric data types that can cover a wide range of requirements, in addition to physicochemical concepts, are supported. CML allows properties and quantities to be specifically attached to bonds, atoms, and molecules. It also supports reactions, as well as macromolecular structures and sequences. CML is designed to interact with several leading markup languages and XML protocols. It was tested with XHTML for text and images; SVG for line diagrams, graphs, reaction schemes, and phase diagrams; PlotML for graphs; MathML for equations; XLink for hypermedia, including atom spectral-peak assignments and reaction mapping; RDF and Dublin Core for metadata; and XML schemas for numeric and other data types. Often other generic tools are required in physical science, including units, multidimensional arrays with varied data types, terminology, and bibliography. There are no widely accepted standards (markup languages) for these at present. There is a CML development group effort continuing the development on their own, but they have stated that they will use other markup languages if they become widespread. An example is physiochemical data held as SELF (Henry Kehiaian, IUPAC+CODATA) and now converted to SELFML (PMR+HK) as an IUPAC/CODATA project. Many different organization types are adopting or have already adopted CML. A few examples are governmental and global agencies (e. g., drug regulatory agencies through the International Committee on Harmonization; ICH/M2) and the University of California San Diego, (UCSD), which has adopted CML as the chemical technology for its new terascale information and computing grid portals (see http://www.xml-cml.org/).

13.3.3.3 CellML

The CellML language is an XML-based markup language being developed by Physiome Sciences in Princeton, New Jersey, in conjunction with the Bioengineering Research Group at the University of Auckland's Department of Engineering Science and affiliated research groups. CellML's purpose is to store and exchange biological simulation models. It allows scientists to share models on any model-building software available. It also enables component reusability from one model to another, thus accelerating model design. CellML both includes model structure information (how the parts of a model are organizationally related to each another) and provides additional information (metadata) about the model that allows scientists to search for specific models or model components in a database or other repository. Mathematics and documentation are handed by other markup languages, such as MathML and (X)HTML. CellML will be expanded in future to enable it to use other existing languages to specify data and define simulation and rendering information.

The CellML project is closely connected with two other XML-based language projects currently being developed at the University of Auckland. Combined, these languages will provide a complete vocabulary for describing biological information over a range of resolutions from the microscopic subcellular to macroscopic organism level. One is AnatML, which aims at information exchange on the organ level and has been used at the University of Auckland to store geometric information and documentation that was generated during a skeleton digitization project. The other is FieldML, which can be used to describe spatially and temporally varying field information using finite elements. CellML is appropriate for storing geometry information inside AnatML, the distribution of spatial parameters inside compartments in CellML, or the distribution of spatial cellular model parameters across an entire organ. The first CellML models created were electrophysiological heart cell models. Since then, the language has been broadly generalized, and CellML can now be used to create virtually any type of biological model. CellML has been particularly successful at enabling modelling at the cellular level. Electrophysiological and signal-transduction network models have been created using CellML. Mechanical models, such as those that simulate heart muscle cell contraction, are another area of study. In the near future, it will be possible to express all three types of models with CellML.

13.3.3.4 GAME (Genome Annotation Markup Elements)

GAME was designed and developed by Suzanna E. Lewis and Erwin Frise at the University of California Berkeley. The goal of GAME is to provide an XML DTD and tools for annotating gene sequence features. GAME provides a group of DTDs for molecular biology. These DTDs can be combined to create more expressive DTDs. Annotations are collected features describing related sequences of genomic DNA, transcripts, mRNAs and cDNAs (which are treated as the logical equivalent of mRNAs), and proteins. Each of these molecules has regions along its length ('features') that are described in annotations. The features themselves are a combined summary of the results of both computational and genetic analysis of that DNA, RNA, or amino-acid sequence. Computational analyses are not considered features and are treated as primary data, as are the results of experimental analyses carried out at the bench. In other words, analytical results can be used to identify features, but are not considered features on their own in this context. Thus, each molecule is described in terms of both primary analytical results and expert-defined features that are supported by the preceding results. The combination of all these associated feature descriptions about the related molecules, from gene to protein, constitutes a statement that is called an 'annotation'. Noticeably, GAME does not actually include a sequence DTD. This is because sequence are treated in a separate DTD-let. So far, there is an XML DTD and an XSL stylesheet for bioxml:game0.2. Although the XSL stylesheet is outdated, it still enables the conversion of game1.001 documents into bioxml:game0.2 documents. This is very useful, since the *Drosophila* genome, for example, is available only in game1.001 format. Of course, GAME will be even more useful once there is a bioxml:game0.3 parser for bioPerl, bioPython, and bioJava. The current bioxml parser in bioPerl, used for parsing sequence elements, can already import data into bioPerl. The DTD is well commented for use in creating one's own interfaces (see http://www.bioxml.org/Projects/game/).

13.3.3.5 MoDL (Molecular Dynamics [Markup] Language)

MoDL – Molecular Dynamics Language (pronounced 'model') was designed and developed by the project team of Swami Manohar, Vijay Chandru, B. Arun, and A.D. Ganguly. Chemical simulations are an essential part of research in the field of toxicology. Enormous effort is involved in making sense of the huge amounts of data that these simulations provide. Visualization of simulation data is of great assistance in understanding chemical systems and acquiring new insights. MoDL provides simple constructs such as atoms, bonds, and molecules as simulation data entities. These constructs can be freely rotated. Atom and molecule types can be defined and then used to build a chemical compound. Plots can also be drawn in any position in a 3D scene (a MoDL file can be converted to VRML format with a program that uses the XML::Parser module of Perl). The visualizations can then be viewed in an Internet browser by using a VRML plug-in. A MoDL authoring tool that is still under development is available for download; the XML::Parser and XML::DOM modules of Perl have to be installed for it to work (see http://violet.csa.iisc.ernet.in/~modl/).

13.3.3.6 SBML (Systems Biology Markup Language)

The Caltech ERATO Kitano Systems Biology Project is developing Systems Biology Markup Language (SBML), using XML and UML (unified modelling language) for representation and modelling of the information components in cellular systems. SBML represents an attempt to specify a common, model-based description language for systems biology simulation software. The overall goal is to develop an open standard that will enable simulation software to communicate and exchange models, finally leading to the researchers' ability to run simulations and analyses across multiple software packages. SBML is the result of merging the most obvious modelling-language features of BioSpice, DBSolve, E-Cell, Gepasi, Jarnac, StochSim, and Virtual Cell. The XML encoding of the description language can define a file format. However, at this time, the main focus on using the XML-based description language is on its potential as a communication and interchange format between different programs. As XML schemas are difficult to read and absorb by human readers, the proposed data structures are defined by using a brief graphical notation based on a subset of UML. The SBML representation language is organized around five categories of information: model, compartment, geometry, species, and reaction. Not all of these are needed by every simulation package. The intent is rather to cover the range of data structures needed by collecting all the simulators examined so far (see http://www.sbml.org/).

13.3.4 Parameter Estimation

In real biological systems, metabolites, proteins, and mRNA concentrations are controlled by many parameters such as time, physicochemical properties, and the state of the environment around the system. The state of a cell thus depends on its temperature, on the kinetic constants of its various biochemical processes, and on the concentration of nutrients and other chemical compounds. In simulations, one does indeed start with parameters, such as kinetic constants and concentrations of external substrates and products, and uses the computer to calculate the changes in concentrations of the metabolites, proteins, and mRNAs with time. In contrast to this, what one does in an experiment is to measure the metabolites, proteins, and/or RNA, aiming to determine the values of the parameters. This is known as an inverse problem [44] and is similar to what happens in other areas of science and engineering, such as inverse kinematics (what forces to apply in a mechanical device to make it reach a certain point in space), and crystallography (given a X-ray diffraction pattern, how are the atoms arranged in the crystal).

This inverse problem of estimating the parameters of a large biochemical network from observations of concentrations is in essence not new. In enzymology the exact same problem has been routinely dealt with for a long time, where one uses time courses or initial rates of reaction to determine kinetic parameters of a single enzymatic reaction. The major difference to what is proposed here is the scale, because in whole-cell models we have not one but a large number of simultaneous biochemical reactions and thus a very high number of parameters to estimate.

Irrespective of scale and of whether one uses an automatic method or prefers to do things manually, parameter estimation is done according to this procedure:

1. Compare experimental with simulated values.
2. If the difference is small enough, stop; otherwise adjust parameters in the model.
3. Simulate the experiment.
4. Return to 1.

Step 2 is where all the action occurs, specifically, in the process of adjusting the parameters. In enzyme kinetics, step 2 can be performed by using linear regression if the rate equation can be linearized with respect to the parameters, such as in the double-reciprocal plot [45]. More recently, it had been argued [46, 47] that nonlinear regression is more appropriate. Here, one uses a numerical optimization method to carry out step 2 above, usually the Levenberg–Marquardt method [48, 49].

13.3.5
Simulators

In recent years a number of simulators for modelling and simulating cellular regulatory pathways and networks have been developed and are described in this section.

BioSpice simulates cellular pathways – pathways are graphically represented, and access to databases is provided. It represents cell dynamics as three-dimensional fluid–mechanical systems. It is written in Matlab/Java and is open source software. The people behind the project include Adam Arkin, project director of the Berkeley BioSpice Network Representation and Modeling System (NRMS).

Cellerator, mentioned above, models and simulates interacting signal transduction networks. Its main feature is biological modelling via automated equation generation by using (ordinary) differential equations. The language used for this program is Mathematica. The people behind this project are at the Jet Propulsion Laboratory, California Institute of Technology.

E-Cell aims at modelling and simulating the environment for biochemical and genetic processes. Features covered are functions of proteins, protein–protein interactions, protein–DNA interactions, regulation of gene expression, and other features of cellular metabolism. The mathematical models used in E-Cell comprise deterministic ODEs, discrete stochastic systems, and many components driven by multiple algorithms with different timescales. E-Cell was written in C++ in a project led by Masaru Tomita at the Institute for Advanced Biosciences, Keio University, Japan.

FluxAnalyzer is a graphical interface for Metabolic Flux Analysis (MFA). The features are stoichiometric analysis and determination of flux distributions in metabolic networks; it has abstract (symbolic) network representation and network graphics for visualizing the metabolic network (metabolic maps). FluxAnalyzer is written in MATLAB and is free for academic users. The people behind it include Steffen Klamt of the Systems Biology group of Ernst Dieter Gilles, MPI Dynamics of Complex Technical Systems, Magdeburg, Germany.

Gepasi allows for modelling biochemical systems. Its built-in features include the ability to model many compartments having different volumes; tools to fit models to data, to optimize any function of the model, and to perform metabolic control analysis, linear stability analysis, and parameter studies; and SBML support. The mathematics used include matrices and differential equations. Gepasi was developed in C, runs on Microsoft Windows, and is free. The software was developed by Pedro Mendes and his group at the Virginia Bioinformatics Institute (USA).

MCell is a general Monte Carlo simulator of cellular microphysiology. So far, its focus has been on one aspect of biological signal transduction, namely the microphysiology of synaptic transmission. Simulations are positioned on a biological scale above molecular dynamics but below whole-cell and higher-level studies. Diffusion of individual ligand molecules is simulated by a Brownian dynamics random-walk algorithm, and bulk solution rate constants are converted into Monte Carlo probabilities so that the diffusing ligands can undergo stochastic chemical interactions with individual binding sites, such as receptor proteins, enzymes, transporters, etc. Executables for MCell can be obtained as free software (copying and/or editing MCell without the authors' consent is expressly forbidden). The people who developed MCell include Tom Bartol of the Computational Neurobiology Laboratory (CLN) at the Salk Institute, San Diego (CA, USA) and Joel R. Stiles at Biomedical Applications, Pittsburgh Supercomputing Center (PA, USA).

Metabolizer. The aim is of Metabolizer is the simulation of complex biological systems. Its features include the integration of deterministic and stochastic simulation techniques of metabolic networks into a hybrid simulator and the provision of SBML support. The mathematical model behind Metabolizer is Gillespie's first-reaction method. ODE and PDE models are planed. Metabolizer is written in Java and was developed by Markus Schwehm in the Department of Computer Architecture, University of Tübingen.

ProMoT/DIVA. The aim of ProMoT/DIVA is to produce structured dynamic simulation models. It features symbolic transformations and optimization. The models behind it include differential and algebraic rate equations. ProMoT was written in Lisp/Java, is free software, and runs on Linux/Unix. The people behind the project are at the Virtual Biological Laboratory: Martin Ginkel, Andreas Kremling, Torsten Nutsch at MPI Dynamics of Complex Technical Systems, Magdeburg, Germany.

ScrumPy is a program for biochemical modelling. The features include steady-state determination, time-course simulation, MCA functions, and determination of elementary modes and enzyme subsets. The software is written in Python and is distributed as open-source software by the Metabolic Control Analysis Research Group, Oxford Brookes University, UK.

Stochastirator simulates chemical and biological reaction networks in a stochastic mathematical framework and was implemented in C++ by Eric Lyons and Larry Lok.

StochSim is a general-purpose biochemical simulator which features individual molecules or molecular complexes that are represented as individual software objects. Reactions between molecules occur stochastically (employing 'pseudomolecules'). It also allows for multiple states of molecules (conformational state, ligand binding, phosphorylation, methylation or other covalent modification). The model behind the simulator is based on random selection of two molecules. It was developed using a platform-independent core simulation engine by Carl Firth of the Computational Cell Biology group in the Department of Zoology of the University of Cambridge (USA).

STOCKS. The aim of STOCKS, which stands for STOChastic Kinetic Simulation of biochemical processes, is to simulate the time evolution of a system composed of a large number of first- and second-order chemical reactions. It enables several cellular generations by using a linearly growing volume of reaction environment and a simple model of cell division. Substances in equilibrium are modelled as random pools having a gaussian distribution. The mathematical model behind STOCKS is Gillespie's direct method. The software was developed in C++, runs under Unix/Linux, and is licensed as public-domain (GNU GPL) software by Andrzej M. Kierzek, Institute of Biochemistry and Biophysics, Warszawa, Poland.

Virtual Cell. Virtual Cell allows for remote users to model and simulate environment to create biological models of various types and run simulations on a remote server. A transparent general-purpose solver is used to translate the initial biological description into a set of concise mathematical problems. Virtual Cell is based on mathematical simplifications using pseudo-steady state approximations and mass conservation relationships. Virtual Cell uses a Java-based graphical interface and was developed by Jim Schaff and his group (Virtual Cell Developer) at the National Resource for Cell Analysis and Modeling, NRCAM, USA.

13.3.6 Visualization

As with simulators, in recent years a number of tools for visualizing metabolic, genetic, and signal-transduction networks have been developed.

GeneVis provides a visual environment for exploring the dynamics of gene regulation networks. Currently, gene regulation is the focus of intensive research worldwide, and computational aids are being called for to help in the study of factors that are difficult to observe directly. GeneVis provides a particle-based simulation of gene networks and visualizes the simulation process as it occurs. Two dynamic visualization techniques are provided: visualization of the movement of regulatory proteins and visualization of the relative concentrations of these proteins. Several interactive tools relate the dynamic visualizations to the underlying gene-network structure.

InterViewer3. Protein–protein interaction networks often consist of thousands or more nodes. This severely limits the utility of many graph-drawing tools because they become too slow for interactive analysis of the networks and because they produce cluttered drawings with many crossing edges. A new layout algorithm with complexity-management operations for visualizing a large-scale protein interaction network was developed and implemented in a program called InterViewer3. InterViewer3 simplifies a complex network by collapsing a group of nodes with the same interacting partners into a composite node and by replacing a clique with a star-shaped subgraph. InterViewer3 is 10 times faster than other drawing programs.

13.4 Toward Predictive *in silico* Toxicogenomics

13.4.1 A Systems Biology Approach to *ab initio* Hepatotoxicity Testing

Global transcription profiling and machine learning are a prerequisite for a systems biology approach to drug toxicity prediction. In contrast to what has been reported in the field of toxicogenomics, for the first time the accuracy and generality of a hepatotoxicity predicting model can be validated. This approach will not only have direct application in drug toxicity prediction but also may provide a stepping stone for the modelling of complicated biological systems.

13.4.2
In silico Toxicogenomics for Personalized Medicine

The goal of personalized medicine is to use the understanding of mechanisms and pathways of disease together with the unique characteristics of the individual to accelerate the prevention, detection, and cure of disease. Personalized medicine redefines diseases on the molecular level, so that diagnostics and therapeutics can be targeted to specific patient populations, thereby offering the right treatment to the right patient.

Personalized medicine represents a significant advance over most current diagnostic methods and therapies, which were developed to detect and treat symptoms and/or apparent causes of disease broadly across all patients. Conventional drug development approaches do not take into account that, due to genetic variations, a disease may manifest itself slightly differently in different patients and that drugs may exhibit different side effects and levels of toxicity.

Using genetic tools to define disease endpoints at the molecular rather than phenotypic (combined genetic and environmental) level has the goal of determining which groups and subgroups of patients will respond to a treatment being developed and which patients will fail to respond. In addition, a better understanding of the human genome allows us to better understand the mechanisms of drug toxicity, leading to the development of potentially superior drugs that minimize serious adverse reactions.

Although the ultimate goal of personalized medicine is to yield molecular-based diagnostic tests and therapeutics, personalized medicine is also employed as a way to increase the efficiency and reduce the risks of the drug development process. This is done by identifying novel drug targets that are linked to the fundamental mechanisms of disease and screening out compounds with toxicogenomic markers, thereby allowing for more careful selection for inclusion in clinical trials those patients who are genetically most likely to benefit from the treatment being tested, as well as those genetically least likely to experience serious side effects.

13.4.3
Future of Predictive *in silico* Toxicity Testing in the R&D Process

Currently, one of the major bottlenecks in bringing new drugs to market are late withdrawals in preclinical and clinical trials as well as post-market. Avoiding such withdrawals, which are due to unexpected side effects, requires a broader scope than studying drug–target protein interactions or drug–single cell transcriptional readout. It is likely that systems biology approaches will predict the intra- and intercellular regulatory processes in whole organs, such as the liver, which can be explored for in-silico drug toxicity testing. The integration of large, high-dimensional datasets from the new platform technologies is a major challenge to the R&D process in the pharmaceutical industry, for which no comprehensive solution has been found. Using toxicity testing in the liver as an example, we intend to develop in-silico solutions and transfer this knowledge to our partners in the pharmaceutical industry. This will lead to a significantly better approach to computational toxicity testing than data obtained from isolated *in vivo* and *in vitro* assays allow. In-silico approaches are likely to be requested in investigational and new drug applications (IND/NDA) by regulatory agencies such as the U.S. FDA. Mathematical models that predict the effects and side effects of new drugs in silico at the level of intra- and intercellular regulatory processes are therefore of high relevance for cutting R&D costs through more rational drug design and for improving the approval process through regulatory agencies. We can surely expect an exponential increase of the use of such models and predictive in-silico simulations as their complexity and predictive power grows. A number of pharmaceutical companies (Eli Lilly, Novartis, GSK) have established or will establish centres of systems biology to improve the current situation of R&D in the pharmaceutical industry.

References

1. Kitano H, Systems biology: a brief overview, *Science*, **295**: 1662–1664, 2002.
2. Kitano H, Computational systems biology, *Nature*, **420**: 206–210, 2002.
3. Wiener N, *Cybernetics or Control and Communication in the Animal and the Machine*, Hermann et Cie, Paris, 1948.
4. Schofl C, Brabant G, Hesch RD, von zur Muhlen A, Cobbold PH, Cuthbertson KS, Temporal patterns of alpha 1-receptor stimulation regulate amplitude and frequency of calcium transients. *Am. J. Physiol.*, **265**: C1030–1036,1993.
5. Chay TR, Lee YS, Fan YS, Appearance of phase-locked Wenckebach-like rhythms, devil's staircase and universality in intracellular calcium spikes in non-excitable cell models. *J. Theor. Biol.*, **174**: 21–44, 1995.
6. Morohashi M, Kitano H, A method for reconstructing genetic regulatory network for *Drosophila* eye formation. *Proc. 6th International Conference on Artificial Life*, pp. 72–80, 1998.
7. Kyoda K, Kitano H, Simulation of genetic interaction for *Drosophila* leg formation. *Proc. Pacific Symposium on Biocomputing '99*, pp. 77–89, 1999.
8. Bock G, Goode J, Complexity in biological information processing. *Novartis Foundation Symposium* **239**: 150–158, 2001.
9. Hamahashi S, Kitano H, Parameter optimization in hierarchical structure. *Proc. 5th European Conference on Artificial Life*, pp. 467–471, 1999.
10. von Dassow G, Meir E, Munro EM, Odell G, The segment polarity network is a robust developmental module. *Nature*, **406**: 188–192, 2000.
11. Yi T-M, Huang Y, Simon M, Doyle J, Robust perfect adaptation in bacterial chemotaxis through integral feedback control. *Proc. Natl. Acad. Sci. USA*, **97**: 4649–4653, 2000.
12. Tomita M, Shimizu K, Matsuzaki Y, Miyoshi F, Saito K, Tanida S, Yugi K, Venter C, Hutchison C, E-Cell: software environment for whole cell simulation. *Bioinformatics*, **15**: 72–84, 1999.
13. Mendes P, Kell D, Non-linear optimization of biochemical pathways: applications to metabolic engineering and parameter estimation. *Bioinformatics*, **14**: 869–883, 1998.
14. Kyoda KM, Murako M, Kitano H, Construction of a generalized simulator for multi-cellular organisms and its application to SMAD signal transduction. *Pac. Symp. Biocomput.*, **2000**: 317–328, 2000.
15. Nagasaki M, Onami S, Miyano S, Kitano H, Bio-calculus: its concept and molecular interaction. *Genome Inform. Ser. Workshop Genome Inform.*, **10**: 133–143, 1999.
16. Schaff J, Loew LM, The virtual cell. *Pac. Symp. Biocomput.*, **1999**: 228–239, 1999.

17. Mendes P, Kell DB, MEG (model extender for Gepasi): a program for the modelling of complex, heterogeneous, cellular systems. *Bioinformatics,* **17**: 288–289, 2001.

18. Hucka M, Finney A, Sauro HM, Bolouri H, Doyle J, Kitano H, The ERATO Systems Biology Workbench: enabling interaction and exchange between software tools for computational biology. *Pac. Symp. Biocomput.,* **2002**: 450–461, 2002.

19. Hucka M, Finney A, Sauro HM, Bolouri H, Doyle JC, Kitano H, Arkin AP, Bornstein BJ, Bray D, Cornish-Bowden A, Cuellar AA, Dronov S, Gilles ED, Ginkel M, Gor V, Goryanin II, Hedley WJ, Hodgman TC, Hofmeyr JH, Hunter PJ, Juty NS, Kasberger JL, Kremling A, Kummer U, Le Novere N, Loew LM, Lucio D, Mendes P, Minch E, Mjolsness ED, Nakayama Y, Nelson MR, Nielsen PF, Sakurada T, Schaff JC, Shapiro BE, Shimizu TS, Spence HD, Stelling J, Takahashi K, Tomita M, Wagner J, Wang J, SBML Forum. The systems biology markup language (SBML): a medium for representation and exchange of The System Biology Markup Language (SBML): a medium for representation and exchange of biochemical network models. *Bioinformatics,* **19**: 524–531, 2003.

20. Grodins FS, *Control Theory and Biological Systems.* Columbia University Press, New York, 1963.

21. Toates FM, *Control Theory in Biology and Experimental Psychology.* Hutchinson Educational, London, 1975.

22. Edelman GM, Gally JA, Degeneracy and complexity in biological systems, *Proc. Natl. Acad. Sci. USA,* **98**: 13763–13768, 2001.

23. Nowak M A, Boerlijst MC, Cooke J, Maynard Smith J, Evolution of genetic redundancy. *Nature,* **388**: 167–171, 1997.

24. Csete M, Doyle J, Reverse engineering of biological complexity, *Science,* **295**: 1664–1669, 2002.

25. Hartwell L, Hopfield J, Leibler S, Murray A, From molecular to modular cell biology, *Nature,* **402**: C47–C51, 1999.

26. Lauffenburger DA, Cell signaling pathways as control modules: complexity for simplicity, *Proc. Natl. Acad. Sci. USA,* **97**: 5031–5033, 2000.

27. Becskei A, Serrano L, Engineering stability in gene networks by autoregulation. *Nature,* **405**: 590–593, 2000.

28. Hasty J, McMillen D, Collins J, Engineered gene circuits, *Nature,* **420**: 224–230, 2002.

29. Lagally ET, Medintz I, Mathies RA, Single-molecule DNA amplification and analysis in an integrated microfluid device. *Anal. Chem.,* **73**: 565–570, 2001.

30. Simpson P, Roach D, Woolley A, Thorson T, Johnston R, Sensabaugh G, Mathies G, High-throughput genetic analysis using microfabricated 96-sample capillary array electrophoresis microplates. *Proc. Natl. Acad. Sci. USA,* **95**: 2256–2261, 1998.

31. Sulston JE, Schierenberg E, White JG, Thomson JN, The embryonic cell lineage of the nematode *Caenorhabditis elegans. Dev. Biol.,* **100**: 64–199, 1983.

32. Sulston JE, Horvitz HR, Post-embryonic cell lineage of the nematode *Caenorhabditis elegans. Dev. Biol.,* **56**: 110–156, 1997.

33. Onami S, Hamahashi S, Nagasaki M, Miyano S, Kitano H, Automatic acquisition of cell lineage through 4D microscopy and analysis of early *C. elegans* embryogenesis. *Foundations of Systems Biology,* MIT Press, Cambridge, pp. 39–55, 2001.

34. http://www.ncbi.nlm.nih.gov/Genbank/ 2003.

35. Baxevanis AD, The Molecular Biology Database Collection: 2003 update. *Nucleic Acids Res.,* **31**: 1–12, 2003.

36. Ulrich R, Friend SH, Toxicogenomics and drug discovery: will new technologies help us produce better drugs? *Nat. Rev. Drug Discov.,* **1**: 84–88, 2002.

37. von Dassow G, Meir E, Munro EM, Odell GM, The segment polarity network is a robust developmental module. *Nature,* **406**: 188–192, 2000.

38. Csete ME, Doyle JC, Reverse engineering of biological complexity. *Science,* **295**: 1664–1669, 2002.

39. Hasty J, McMillen D, Collins JJ, Engineered gene circuits. *Nature,* **420**: 224–230, 2002.

40. Rao CV, Wolf DM, Arkin AP, Control, exploitation and tolerance of intracellular noise. *Nature,* **420**: 231–237, 2002.

41. Shapiro BE, Levchenko A. Meyerowitz EM, Wold BJ, Mjolsness ED, Cellerator: extending a computer algebra system to include biochemical arrows for signal transduction simulations. *Bioinformatics,* **19**: 677–678, 2003.

42. Kummer U, STODE: automatic stochastic simulation of systems described by differential equations. *Proc. 2nd International Conference Systems Biology* (Yi, Hucka, Morohashi, Kitano, eds.), Omnipress, Madison, USA, 326–333, 2002.

43. Singh K, Prank K, Efficient stochastic simulation of intracellular signalling. *Proc. European Conference Computational Biology* (Oxford University Press), p. 153, 2002.

44. Mendes P, Kell DB, On the analysis of the inverse problem of metabolic pathways using artificial neural networks. *BioSystems,* **38**: 15–28, 1996.

45. Lineweaver H, Burk D, The determination of enzyme dissociation constants. *J. Am. Chem. Soc.,* **56**: 658–666, 1934.

46. Duggleby RG, Progress-curve analysis in enzyme kinetics: numerical solution of integrated rate equations. *Biochem. J.,* **235**: 613–615, 1986.

47. Johnson ML, Why, when, and how biochemists should use least squares. *Anal. Biochem.,* **206**: 215–225, 1992.

48. Levenberg K, A method for the solution of certain nonlinear problems in least squares. *Quart. Appl. Math.* **2**: 164–168, 1944.

49. Marquardt DW, An algorithm for least squares estimation of nonlinear parameters. *SIAM J.,* **11**: 431–441, 1963.

Application of Toxicogenomic: Case Studies

Handbook of Toxicogenomics: Strategies and Applications. Edited by Jürgen Borlak

ISBN: 3-527-30342-1

14
Regulatory Networks of Liver-enriched Transcription Factors in Liver Biology and Disease

Jürgen Borlak, Jürgen Klempnauer, and Harald Schrem

14.1
Introduction

New genomic platform technologies enable the study of complex genomes and proteomes for improved target identification and validation. This leads to high-density datasets, on the order of millions of data points per day. Turning data into knowledge will be one of the biggest challenges of the 21st century. Here we describe concisely the role of liver-enriched transcription factors in regulatory gene networks and focus on liver development function and disease. This knowledge will prove to be indispensable for interpretation of high-density genomic datasets that are being produced in pharmaco- and toxicogenomics.

Numerous studies have established the pivotal role of liver-enriched transcription factors in organ development and cellular function, and there is conclusive evidence for transcription factors acting in concert in liver-specific gene expression. During organ development and in progenitor cells the timely expression of certain transcription factors is necessary for cellular differentiation, and there is overwhelming evidence for hierarchical and cooperative principles in a networked environment of transcription factors. The search for molecular switches that control stem-cell imprinting and liver-specific functions has led to the discovery of many interactions between such different molecules as transcription factors, coactivators, corepressors, enzymes, DNA, and RNA. Many of these interactions either repress or activate liver-specific gene expression. Six families of liver-enriched transcription factors have been characterized so far: HNF-1, HNF-3, HNF-4, HNF-6, C/EBP, and D-binding protein (DBP). The analysis of the tissue distribution of these factors and the determination of their hierarchical relations have led to the hypothesis that cooperation of liver-enriched transcription factors with the ubiquitous trans-activating factors is necessary, and possibly even sufficient, for the maintenance of liver-specific gene transcription. HNFs (hepatocyte nuclear factors) are a heterogeneous class of evolutionarily conserved transcription factors that contain several families of liver-enriched transcription factors (HNF-1, HNF-3, HNF-4, and HNF-6) that are required for hepatocellular differentiation as well as in hepatic carbohydrate, lipid, and pro-

Handbook of Toxicogenomics: Strategies and Applications. Edited by Jürgen Borlak

ISBN: 3-527-30342-1

tein metabolism (Schrem et al., 2002). Major regulatory functions in the liver, including cell cycle control, carcinogenesis, circadian gene regulation, liver regeneration, and apoptosis, are controlled by C/EBPs (CAAT/enhancer binding proteins) (see also Figure 14.2) and DBP (Schrem et al., 2004). In this chapter we highlight striking examples of relevant network interactions of liver-enriched transcription factors with a significant impact on liver biology to further an understanding of the molecular events linked to liver disease and drug-induced toxicity.

14.2
The HNF-1/HNF-4 Network for Liver-specific Gene Expression

Intertypic rat hepatoma–human fibroblast hybrids that show extinction of liver-specific gene expression are deficient in the expression of HNF-4 and HNF-1, and reexpression of liver-specific genes in revertants (or hybrid cell segregants) correlates with the reexpression of both genes (Griffo et al., 1993). Because HNF-4 is an upstream regulator of HNF-1 expression, it was proposed that the HNF-4 gene is the primary target of the pleiotropic extinguisher (Griffo et al., 1993). Dedifferentiated H5 variant cells of a rat hepatoma cell line that show a pleiotropic loss of hepatic functions and fail to express both HNF-1 and HNF-4 (Descharette and Weiss, 1974; Faust et al., 1994) could be directed toward redifferentiation by stable transfection of epitope-tagged HNF-4 cDNA (Späth and Weiss, 1997). The forced expression of only HNF-4 in these H5 variant cells leads to the activation of a subset of liver-specific genes, including alpha1-antitrypsin, fibrinogen, and transthyretin, but not of the endogenous HNF-4 gene. Treatment of the HNF-4tag–expressing cells with dexamethasone increased expression of the transgene 10 fold, resulting in enhanced expression of target genes of both glucocorticoid hormones and HNF-4 (Späth and Weiss, 1997). The set of activated hepatic genes was extended by treatment of cells with the demethylating agent 5-azacytidine followed by selection in dexamethasone-containing glucose-free medium. Some of the colonies that developed reexpressed the entire set of hepatic functions tested (Späth and Weiss, 1997). In dedifferentiated rat hepatoma H5 cells, the effects of HNF-4 expression extend to the reestablishment of differentiated epithelial cell morphology and simple epithelial polarity. The acquisition of epithelial morphology occurs in two steps. First, expression of HNF-4 results in reexpression of cytokeratin proteins and partial reestablishment of E-cadherin production. Only the transfectants are competent to respond to the synthetic glucocorticoid dexamethasone, which induces the second step of morphogenesis, including formation of the junctional complex and expression of a polarized cell phenotype (Späth and Weiss, 1998).

Knockout mice lacking HNF-1alpha fail to thrive and die around weaning after a progressive wasting syndrome with marked liver enlargement. The transcription rate of genes like albumin and alpha1-antitrypsin is reduced, whereas the gene coding for phenylalanine hydroxylase is totally silent, giving rise to phenylketonuria. Mutant mice also suffer from severe Fanconi syndrome caused by renal proximal tubular dysfunction. The resulting massive urinary glucose loss leads to energy and water wasting. HNF1-deficient mice may therefore provide a model for human renal Fanconi syndrome (Pontoglio et al., 1996). Mice deficient in HNF-1alpha develop Laron dwarfism and noninsulin-dependent diabetes mellitus (Lee et al., 1998). Targeted disruption of the HNF-4alpha gene, expressed in visceral endoderm, leads to early embryonic death due to malfunction of the yolk sac and impaired gastrulation in *HNF-4alpha–/–* mouse embryos (Chen et al., 1994; Stoffel and Duncan, 1997; Duncan et al., 1998).

14.2.1
HNF-1 Regulates HNF-4alpha Expression

Liver-specific expression of the mouse HNF-4alpha gene was studied by analyzing the promoter region for required DNA elements. Experiments with reporter constructs in transient transfection assays and in transgenic mice revealed distal enhancer elements at kb –5.5 and –6.5 that were sufficient to drive liver-specific expression of the mouse HNF-4alpha gene in animals (Zhong et al., 1994). An HNF-1-binding site between bp –98 and –68 played an important role in the hepatoma-specific promoter activity of HNF-4 in transient transfection assays but was not sufficient to drive liver-specific expression of a reporter gene in transgenic mice (Zhong et al., 1994).

14.2.2
HNF-1alpha and HNF-4 Regulate HNF-1alpha Expression

The HNF-1 gene contains a relatively short promoter segment located between positions –82 and –40 which directs cell type-specific HNF-1alpha transcription. This region contains a single site for HNF-4alpha (Tian and Schibler, 1991). Transfection experiments revealed that a short region between –118 and –8 is crucial for cell type-specific expression of the HNF-1alpha gene in HepG2 cells. This region contains two positive cis elements called site A, an HNF-4alpha binding site, and site B, an HNF-1alpha binding site. Mutational analyses of these sites and cotransfection assays showed that HNF-4 and HNF-1alpha can trans-activate the HNF-1alpha gene (Miura and Tanaka, 1993). It could be demonstrated that HNF-1alpha negatively regulates its own expression in transient transfection experiments as well as the expression of HNF-4–dependent genes (*ApoCIII* and *ApoAI*) that lack HNF-1alpha binding sites in their promoter region. DNA binding and cell-free transcription experiments failed to demonstrate any direct or indirect interaction of HNF-1alpha with the regulatory regions of *ApoCIII* or *ApoAI*. From these observations it was assumed that HNF-1alpha is able to impede HNF-4 binding or activity. An indirect negative autoregulatory mechanism for HNF-1alpha expression was described, which in turn may affect HNF-4-dependent transcription of other liver-specific genes (Kritis et al., 1993). Later, it could be found that this repression is exerted by a direct interaction of HNF-1alpha with AF-2, the main activation domain of HNF-4. The dual functions of gene activation and repression suggest that HNF-1alpha is a global regulator of the transcriptional network involved in the maintenance of the hepatocyte-specific phenotype (Ktistaki and Talianidis, 1997a). Figure 14.1 depicts an assumed molecular

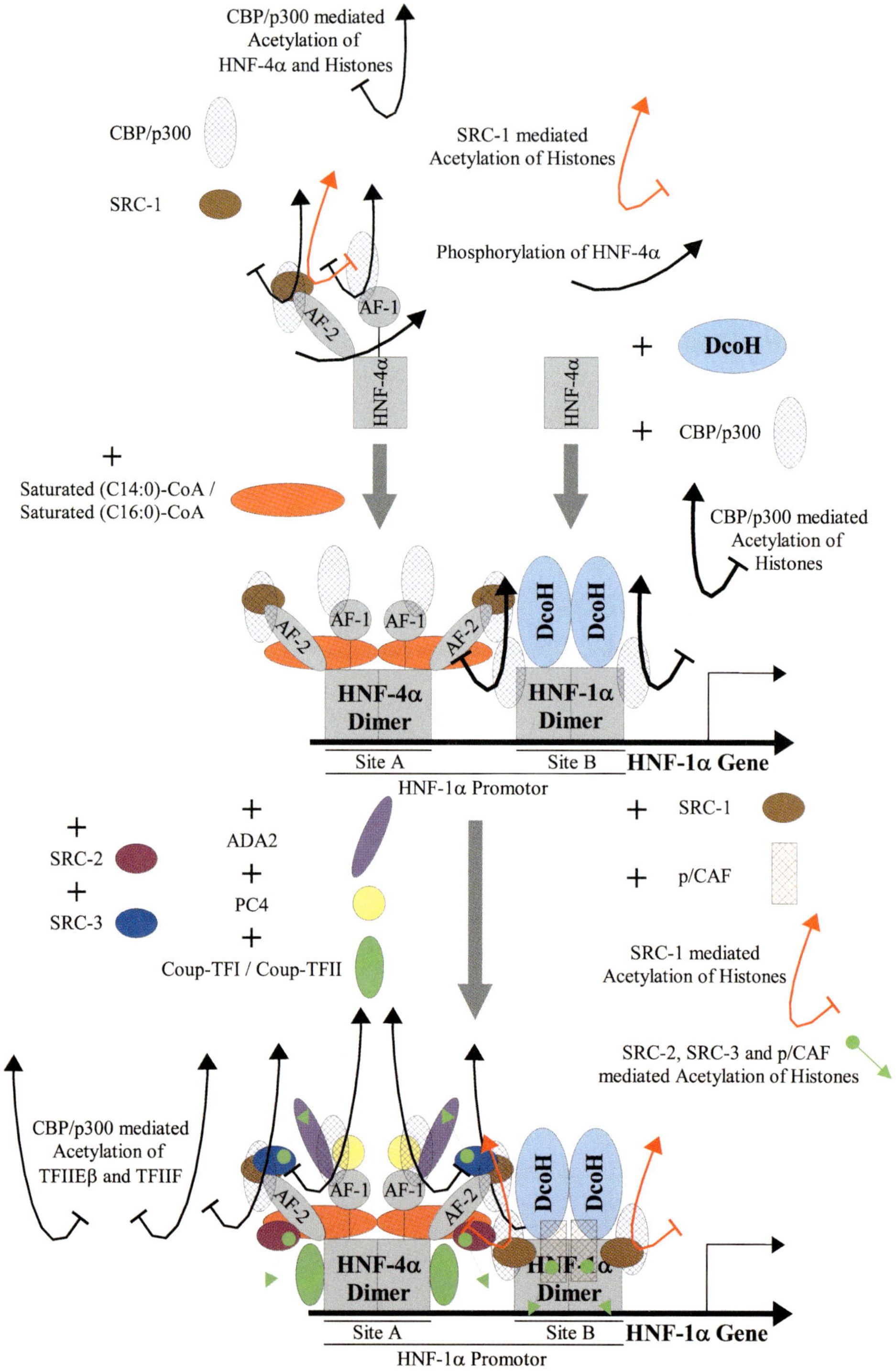
CBP/p300 mediated Acetylation of HNF-4α and Histones
CBP/p300
SRC-1
SRC-1 mediated Acetylation of Histones
Phosphorylation of HNF-4α
AF-2
AF-1
HNF-4α
HNF-4α
+ DcoH
+ CBP/p300
+
Saturated (C14:0)-CoA / Saturated (C16:0)-CoA
CBP/p300 mediated Acetylation of Histones
AF-1
AF-1
AF-2
AF-2
DcoH
DcoH
HNF-4α Dimer
HNF-1α Dimer
Site A
Site B
HNF-1α Gene
HNF-1α Promotor
+ SRC-2
+ SRC-3
+ ADA2
+ PC4
+ Coup-TFI / Coup-TFII
+ SRC-1
+ p/CAF
SRC-1 mediated Acetylation of Histones
SRC-2, SRC-3 and p/CAF mediated Acetylation of Histones
CBP/p300 mediated Acetylation of TFIIEβ and TFIIF
AF-1
AF-1
AF-2
AF-2
DcoH
DcoH
HNF-4α Dimer
HNF-1α Dimer
Site A
Site B
HNF-1α Gene
HNF-1α Promotor

interaction involved in the regulation of the HNF-1alpha gene. Numerous coactivators, as well as the positive HNF-4 ligands, appear to be necessary for optimal HNF-1alpha expression. In this context it is interesting to note that the HNF-4 coactivators p300/CBP, as well as SRC-1 and SRC-3, bind to the activation domain AF-2 of HNF-4. It may well be that HNF-1alpha competes with coactivator binding at the activation domain AF-2 of HNF-4 and thus exerts its indirect negative autoregulation. Additionally, it might be that this hypothetical competition is further modulated by tissue-specific coactivator availability.

14.2.3
Dimerization Cofactor of HNF-1alpha and Liver-specific Gene Expression

Interestingly, HNF-1alpha, but not HNF-1beta, is expressed in the liver. Under physiologic conditions as well as in transfection experiments with HNF-1alpha and HNF-1beta, stable homodimer formation can be found in the liver, whereas in other organs, heterodimers also are detected. From these data it was assumed that the extent of heterodimerization may be regulated in a tissue-specific manner (Mendel et al., 1991 a). A dimerization cofactor of HNF-1alpha (DCoH) could be identified that displays a restricted tissue distribution and does not bind to DNA, but, rather, selectively stabilizes HNF-1alpha homodimers. The formation of a stable tetrameric DCoH–HNF-1alpha complex requires the dimerization domain of HNF-1alpha and does not change the DNA-binding characteristics of HNF-1alpha, but enhances its transcriptional activity. DCoH regulates the formation of transcriptionally active tetrameric complexes and thus may contribute to the developmental and tissue specificity of the complex (Mendel et al., 1991 b). DCoH plays an important role in liver development and liver-specific gene expression, because HNF-1alpha is regarded as an important regulator of the transcriptional network in liver development and liver-specific gene expression.

14.2.4
Agonistic and Antagonistic Ligands for the Orphan Nuclear Receptor HNF-4alpha

In 1998 Hertz and coworkers published the discovery of several ligands for HNF-4 with agonistic and antagonistic effects on HNF-4alpha transcriptional activity. It could be demonstrated that long-chain fatty acids directly modulate the transcriptional activity of HNF-4alpha by binding as their acyl-CoA thioesters to the ligand-binding domain of HNF-4alpha. This binding shifts the oligomer–dimer equili-

◀ **Fig. 14.1** Model of the various interactions occurring at the HNF-1alpha promoter that involve the transcription factors HNF-1alpha, HNF-4alpha, and their respective coactivators, as well as the ligands for HNF-4. Biochemical functions of the coactivators are indicated by arrows of different shapes and colours representing acetylation of various molecules, as indicated. Phosphorylation of HNF-4alpha is also indicated by an arrow. The depicted events and interactions are thought to be necessary for optimal transcription of HNF-1alpha, which plays a major role in the hepatocyte nuclear factor network in liver function and during liver development (for more details and references see the text).

Tab. 14.1 Examples of experimental observations that demonstrate the direct involvement of C/EBPs and HNFs in transcriptional regulation of hepatic cytochrome P450 (*CYP*) genes through interaction with their promoters. TF = transcription factor; IRE-ABP = insulin response element-A binding protein; nts = nucleotides numbered in relation to the start site of transcription within the promoter of the *CYP* gene; agonistic TFs = transcription factors that enhance *CYP* gene expression; antagonistic TFs = transcription factors that inhibit *CYP* gene expression.

CYP gene	*Cell culture*	*Experimental approach*	*Agonistic TF*	*Antagonistic TF*	*C/EBP- or HNF-binding site*	*Reference*
Rat CYP2E1	Primary rat hepatocytes	DNase I footprinting, gel retardation, gel shift competition	HNF-1alpha		nts –127 to –93	Ueno and Gonzalez, 1990
Rat CYP2C12	Human HepG2, COS-1 cells	Direct gel shift	HNF-6alpha, HNF-6beta		nts –53 to –30	Lannoy et al., 1998
Rat CYP2C13	Primary rat hepatocytes	Electrophoretic mobility shift assays (EMSAs) with rat tissue nuclear extracts	HNF-6alpha, HNF-6beta		nts –53 to –41	Samadani and Costa, 1996
Human CYP2B6	Human HepG2 cells	Transfection with Zn-inducible C/EBP-alpha vector to achieve C/EBP-alpha re-expression	C/EBP-alpha			Jover et al., 1998
Human CYP2C9	Human HepG2 cells	Transfection with Zn-inducible C/EBP-alpha vector to achieve C/EBP-alpha re-expression	C/EBP-alpha			Jover et al., 1998
Human CYP2D6	Human HepG2 cells	Transfection with Zn-inducible C/EBP-alpha vector to achieve C/EBP-alpha re-expression	C/EBP-alpha			Jover et al., 1998
Rat CYP2C12 (female-specific)	Primary rat hepatocytes	C/EBP-alpha over-expression in the presence and absence of IRE-ABP, and DNase I footprint analysis, gel mobility shift assays	C/EBP-alpha	IRE-ABP	nts –222 to –204	Buggs et al., 1998
Human CYP3A4	Human HepG2 cells	Cotransfection of C/EBP-alpha and DBP plus promoter deletion experiments with reporter gene assay	C/EBP-alpha		nts –57 to +11	Ourlin et al., 1997
Human CYP3A7	Human HepG2 cells	Cotransfection of C/EBP-alpha and DBP plus promoter deletion experiments with reporter gene assay	C/EBP-alpha		nts –55 to +13	Ourlin et al., 1997

Tab. 14.1 (continued)

CYP gene	*Cell culture*	*Experimental approach*	*Agonistic TF*	*Antagonistic TF*	*C/EBP- or HNF-binding site*	*Reference*
Chicken CYP2H1	Chicken embryo hepatocytes, human HepG2 cells, COS-1 cells	Promoter deletion experiments and DNase I footprint analysis, gel mobility shift assays	rat HNF-1alpha, rat HNF-1beta, rat HNF-3alpha or -beta and chicken C/EBP-alpha	USF (repression, de-repression by phenobarbital through competition at Barbie-box-like sequence)		Dogra and May, 1997
Rat CYP2B1	Human HepG2 cells	Promoter deletion experiments and DNase I footprint analysis, gel mobility shift assays	C/EBP-alpha		nts –64 to –45	Park and Kemper, 1996
Rat CYP2B1	Nuclear extracts from rat livers, primary rat hepatocytes	Promoter deletion experiments and DNase I footprint analysis, gel mobility shift assays, *in vitro* transfection assay	C/EBP-alpha		nts –66 to –42	Luc et al., 1996
Rat CYP2B2	Primary rat hepatocytes	Promoter deletion experiments and DNase I footprint analysis, gel mobility shift assays, *in vitro* transfection assay	C/EBP-alpha		nts –66 to –42	Luc et al., 1996
Rat CYP2C12	Primary rat hepatocytes	Transient transfection of a C/EBP-alpha expression vector plus promoter deletion experiments with reporter gene assay, DNase I footprint analysis, gel mobility supershift assays	C/EBP-alpha		nts –229 to –207	Tollet et al., 1995
Rat CYP2D5	Human HepG2 cells, *Drosophila melanogaster* cells	Transient transfection of a C/EBP-alpha or C/EBP-beta or HNF-1 or a DBP expression vector plus promoter deletion experiments with reporter gene assay, DNase I footprint analysis, gel mobility supershift assays	Sp1, C/EBP-beta forms a ternary complex with a possible agonistic protein–protein interaction Sp1–C/EBP-beta			Lee et al., 1994a

brium of HNF-4alpha, because it could be shown that the binding of saturated (C14 : 0)-CoA to the ligand-binding domain of HNF-4alpha leads to increased HNF-4alpha dimerization and activates binding of the HNF-4alpha dimer to its cognate enhancer element, whereas saturated (C16 : 0)-CoA only activates binding of the HNF-4alpha dimer to its cis-acting element. In contrast, the antagonistic ligands ω-3 and ω-6 polyunsaturated fatty acyl-CoAs, (C18 : 3, w-3)-CoA, and saturated (C18 : 0)-CoA decrease the transcriptional activity of HNF-4alpha. (C18 : 3, w-3)-CoA and saturated (C18 : 0)-CoA were shown to lower the affinity of HNF-4alpha for its cognate enhancer element. Furthermore, it was demonstrated that saturated (C18 : 0)-CoA leads to decreased HNF-4alpha dimerization (Hertz et al., 1998).

14.2.5
Coactivators for HNF-1 and HNF-4 and Their Network Effects in Liver Biology

Multiple coactivators of HNF-1 and HNF-4 have been identified, including CBP, p300, p/CAF, and a series of factors that have been identified biochemically and by expression cloning (Kamei et al., 1996; Torchia et al., 1997; Yoshida et al., 1997; Dell and Hadzopoulou-Cladaras, 1999; Rachez et al., 2000; Soutoglou et al., 2000 a, b). These factors, with a molecular mass around 160 kDa, are members of the p160 protein family and exhibit an intrinsic HAT (histone acetyltransferase activity) (Bannister and Kouzarides, 1996; Ogryzko et al., 1996; Chen et al., 1997; Glass et al., 1997; Spencer et al., 1997). Furthermore, a nuclear receptor coactivator (NCoA) gene family within the p160 protein family has been proposed that includes the homologous factors SRC-1 (also called NCoA-1), SRC-2 (also called NCoA-2, TIF2, GRIP1), and SRC-3 (also called NCoA-3, ACTR, AIB1, p/CIP, TRAM-1, RAC3) (Torchia et al., 1997; Rachez et al., 2000). The NcoA family members SRC-1, SRC-2, and SRC-3 share a conserved N-terminal bHLH, PAS A domain, a serine/threonine-rich region, and a C-terminal glutamine-rich region (Torchia et al., 1997). SRC-1, SRC-3, and CBP all contain several related leucine-rich, charged helical interaction motifs (also termed LCDs) with a consensus core LXXLL sequence motif that is required for the assembly of coactivator complex, which provides receptor-specific mechanisms of gene activation and allows the selective inhibition of distinct signal-transduction pathways. Mutation of this consensus core motif abolishes interaction with nuclear receptors (Torchia et al., 1997). This leads to the inevitable question of whether mutations in these LCD domains may lead to disturbances in liver development or liver function due to reduced HNF-1 and HNF-4 trans-activation potential. Possibly, conformational changes in the CBP holoprotein, perhaps in part contributed by SRC-3 by forming the coactivator complex, modulate interactions with transcription factors and associated regulatory proteins, including protein kinases and histone acetylases (Bannister and Kouzarides, 1996; Ogryzko et al., 1996; Torchia et al., 1997). SRC-1 contains a histone acetylase domain between amino acid residues 1107 and 1216 with intrinsic HAT activity specific for histones H3 and H4 (Spencer et al., 1997). Furthermore, SRC-1 also contains two p/CAF interacting domains between amino acid residues 1207 and 1250 that bind p/CAF, another factor with intrinsic histone acetylase activity (Yang et al., 1996; Spencer et al., 1997). SRC-1 interacts also with

CBP/p300 through a conserved C-terminal domain of CBP/p300 and probably is involved in a three-way interaction with CBP/p300 and an interacting nuclear receptor or transcription factor (Kamei et al., 1996; Yao et al., 1996). SRC-3 and CBP are a functional complex, necessary for the activity of several CBP-dependent transcription factors as well as nuclear receptors (Torchia et al., 1997). Whether SRC-3 is required for trans-activation by HNF-1 or HNF-4 remains to be determined. SRC-3 forms complexes with significant portions of CBP in the cell and is required for transcriptional activity of nuclear receptors and other CBP/p300-dependent transcription factors (Torchia et al., 1997). The major CBP interaction domain of SRC-3 was mapped to amino acid residues 758–1115, with an internal 200-amino acid domain that could still interact, whereas a minimal nuclear receptor interaction domain was mapped N-terminal of the CBP interaction domain to amino acid residues 680–740, which were sufficient for binding a liganded nuclear receptor (Torchia et al., 1997). It could be demonstrated that HNF-1 can physically interact with CBP, p/CAF, SRC-1, and SRC-3 and that these interactions lead to increased HNF-1–dependent transcription in functional assays using a genome-integrated promoter. The transcriptional activation potential of HNF-1 was strictly dependent on the synergistic action of CBP and p/CAF. CBP and p/CAF independently interact with the N-terminal and C-terminal domains of HNF-1, respectively (see also Figure 14.1) (Soutoglou et al., 2000 b). CBP binds to the HNF-4 AF-1 and AF-2 domains with the N terminus and the N and C termini, respectively (Figure 14.1) (Dell and Hadzopoulou-Cladaras, 1999). Interestingly, in contrast to the other nuclear hormone receptors, the interaction between HNF-4 and CBP is ligand-independent and leads to enhanced HNF-4 transcriptional activity for liver-specific apolipoprotein CIII gene expression (Dell and Hadzopoulou-Cladaras, 1999). Recruitment of CBP by HNF-4 results in enhancement of the transcriptional activity of the latter (Yoshida et al., 1997; Dell and Hadzopoulou-Cladaras, 1999). CBP does not activate gene expression in the absence of HNF-4, and dominant negative forms of HNF-4 prevent transcriptional activation by CBP, suggesting that the mere recruitment of CBP by HNF-4 is not sufficient for enhancement of gene expression (Dell and Hadzopoulou-Cladaras, 1999). As expected, it could be demonstrated that p300 acts as a HNF-4 coactivator in a manner similar to that of CBP and that p300 and SRC-1 together can enhance the transcriptional activity of HNF-4 more than SRC-1 or p300 alone (Wang et al., 1998 a, b). The acidic AF-1 domain of the activator HNF-4 interacts specifically with the coactivators CBP, PC4, and ADA2 (Figure 14.1). Green et al. (1998) speculated that AF-1 could affect the preinitiation step through interaction with CBP and/or the ADA2–GCN5 complex by increasing acetylation of histones and rendering the chromatin more accessible to the transcription machinery. Furthermore, AF-1 is hypothesized act also at a post-initiation step, promoting the opening of the DNA double helix through its interaction with PC4 (Brandsen et al., 1997; Green et al., 1998). PC4 and ADA2 are general coactivators that function cooperatively with TBP-associated factors (TAFs) and mediate functional interactions between upstream activators and the general transcriptional machinery (Ge and Roeder, 1994; Barlev et al., 1995). PC4 possesses two ssDNA-binding domains that may be implicated in opening the DNA double helix during gene transcription (Brandsen et al., 1997). Affinity-purified PC2, which lacks independent activity, acts in synergy with the upstream stimulatory activity (USA)-derived coactivator PC4 to mediate the effects of HNF-4 (Malik et al., 2000). ADA2 displays specific interactions with acidic domains of activators such as the HNF-4 AF-1 domain and with the TBP (Barlev et al., 1995). Table 14.1 provides an overview of the HNF-4 coactivators and agonistic ligands, and Figure 14.1 provides a model of protein–protein and protein–DNA interactions including the players HNF-1, HNF-4, and their cofactors at the HNF-1alpha promoter.

14.2.6
The Relevance of HNF-4alpha Splice Variants in Differential Transcriptional Regulation

Further complexity of gene control by HNF-4alpha transcription factors can be anticipated by the differential splicing of the 10 initially identified exons of the HNF-4alpha gene (Nakhei et al., 1998). Thus, so far, seven distinct splice variants have been identified in human and murine cDNA samples. HNF-4alpha1 represents the initially identified transcript, and HNF-4alpha2 through HNF-4alpha7 are the splice variants identified subsequently (Sladek et al., 1990; Hata et al., 1992, 1995; Chartier et al., 1994; Drewes et al., 1996; Kritis et al., 1996; Furuta et al., 1997; Nakhei et al., 1998). In all HNF-4alpha splice variants the DNA-binding domain remains unchanged (Viollet et al., 1997; Nakhei et al., 1998). The impact of these different splice variants on the regulation of downstream target gene regulation remains largely to be determined. The consequences of the existence of different splice variants on the regulation of gene transcription are still not fully understood. Within the 5′-untranslated region of HNF-4alpha, the two splice variants HNF4alpha2 and HNF4alpha3 with additional exons were detected. Both HNF-4alpha splice variants share HNF-4 binding sites with HNF-4alpha1 but have lower DNA binding activities and weaker trans-activation potential than HNF-4alpha1 (Holewa et al., 1997). In cotransfection experiments, evidence was obtained that HNF-4alpha1 is significantly less active than HNF-4alpha2 and that the HNF-4alpha splice variant HNF-4alpha4 has no detectable trans-activation potential. Therefore, the differential expression of distinct HNF-4alpha proteins may play a key role in the differential transcriptional regulation of HNF-4–dependent genes (Drewes et al., 1996).

14.2.7
Activation and Repression by Homo- and Heterodimerization of HNF-4alpha Proteins

Studies with *in vitro* expressed HNF-4alpha protein show that it binds to its recognition site as a dimer (Sladek et al., 1990). It has been proposed that HNF-4alpha forms homodimers, in contrast to other members of the nuclear receptor superfamily that also form heterodimers with other members of the nuclear receptor superfamily like retinoid X receptor alpha (RXR-alpha) (Jiang et al., 1995). Later, it was demonstrated that another 'orphan' member of the nuclear hormone receptor superfamily called SHP (short heterodimers partner), which contains the dimerization and ligand-binding domain found in other family members but lacks the conserved DNA-binding domain (Seol et al., 1996), specifically inhibits trans-activation by

HNF-4 and other hormone receptor superfamily members with which it interacts (Seol et al., 1996; Lee et al., 2000). Therefore, it has been suggested that SHP functions as a negative regulator of receptor-dependent signalling pathways (Seol et al., 1996; Lee et al., 2000). SHP represses nuclear hormone receptor-mediated trans-activation in two separate ways: first by competition with coactivators and second by direct effects of its transcriptional repressor function (Lee et al., 2000).

14.2.8
Posttranscriptional Modification of HNF-4 Function by Phosphorylation and Acetylation

HNF-4 DNA-binding activity is modulated post-translationally by phosphorylation (Ktistaki et al., 1995; Viollet et al., 1997). In cell-free systems and in cultured cells, phosphorylation of tyrosine residue(s) is important for the DNA binding activity of HNF-4 and, consequently, for its trans-activation potential (Ktistaki et al., 1995). Further experiments demonstrated that phosphorylation of HNF-4 by cAMP-dependent protein kinase A at serine residues leads to reduced DNA-binding affinity of HNF-4 *in vitro*. Phosphorylation of HNF-4 by cAMP-dependent protein kinase A at serine residues might be involved in the transcriptional inhibition of liver genes by cAMP inducers (Viollet et al., 1997).

CBP possesses an intrinsic acetyltransferase activity capable of acetylating nucleosomal histones and also several nonhistone proteins. CBP can acetylate HNF-4 at lysine residues within the nuclear localization sequence. CBP-mediated acetylation is crucial for the proper nuclear retention of HNF-4, which is otherwise transported to the cytoplasm by the CRM1 pathway. Acetylation also increases HNF-4 DNA-binding activity and its affinity of interaction with CBP itself and is required for target gene activation (Soutoglou et al., 2000 a).

14.2.9
Cooperation and Competition Between COUP-TF and HNF-4

COUP-TF (chicken ovalbumin upstream promoter-transcription factor) and HNF-4 were both frequently called orphan members of the steroid/thyroid receptor superfamily and exhibit ubiquitous and liver-enriched tissue distribution, respectively (Kimura et al., 1993). COUP-TFs strongly inhibit transcriptional activation mediated by nuclear hormone receptors, including HNF-4. COUP-TFs repress HNF-4–dependent gene expression by competition with HNF-4 for common binding sites found in several regulatory regions (Kimura et al., 1993; Ktistaki and Talianidis, 1997 b). In contrast, promoters such as the HNF-1 promoter, which are recognized by HNF-4 but not by COUP-TFs, are activated by COUP-TFI and COUP-TFII in conjunction with HNF-4 more than 100-fold above basal levels, as opposed to about 8-fold activation by HNF-4 alone (Ktistaki and Talianidis, 1997 b). This enhancement was strictly dependent on an intact HNF-4 E domain. In-vitro and *in vivo* evidence suggests that COUP-TFs enhance HNF-4 activity by a mechanism that involves their physical interaction with the amino acid 227–271 region of HNF-4 (see also Figure 14.1) (Ktistaki and Talianidis, 1997 b). Therefore, in certain promoters, COUP-TFs act as auxiliary cofactors for HNF-4, orienting the HNF-4 activation domain in a more efficient configuration to achieve enhanced transcriptional activity (Kimura et al., 1993; Ktistaki and Talianidis, 1997 b). An example of COUP-TF–associated repression of a liver-specific gene is that of the gene for rat ornithine transcarbamylase, an ornithine cycle enzyme (Kimura et al., 1993). Therefore, COUP-TF plays a dual regulatory role depending on the promoter context. Repression of a tissue-specific promoter by a ubiquitous trans-activator and derepression by a related tissue-enriched trans-activator is potentially an important mechanism for tissue-specific activation of a gene (Kimura et al., 1993; Ktistaki and Talianidis, 1997 b).

14.2.10
The Role of HNFs in CYP Monooxygenase Expression

The foetal liver, the major site of haematopoiesis during embryonic development, acquires additional detoxification functions near birth. The response to xenobiotic exposure with expression of several cytochromes P450 (CYP) monooxygenases and drug efflux transporters is a vital hepatic function. Expression of the genes for these proteins is regulated by nuclear receptors such as the pregnane X receptor (PXR). The expression of several xenobiotic response genes as well as of HNF-4alpha is increased in foetal hepatocytes stimulated by the hepatic maturation factors oncostatin M (OSM) and matrigel. To determine the contribution of HNF-4alpha to xenobiotic responses in the foetal liver, foetal hepatocytes containing floxed HNF-4alpha alleles were cultured, and the HNF-4alpha gene was inactivated by infection with an adenovirus containing the *Cre* gene. As a consequence, expression of CYP3A11 and PXR was suppressed by inactivation of HNF-4alpha. An HNF-4alpha binding site was characterized in the PXR promoter and found to be required for activation of the *PXR* promoter in foetal hepatocytes. It may be assumed that HNF-4alpha is a key transcription factor regulating responses to xenobiotics through activation of the *PXR* gene during foetal liver development (Kamiya et al., 2003). Several putative HNF-3 binding sites have been identified in human CYP2C 5′-flanking regions. Gene reporter experiments with proximal promoters revealed that HNF-3gamma trans-activated CYP2C8, CYP2C9, and CYP2C19 (25-, 4-, and 4-fold, respectively), but it did not trans-activate CYP2C18. However, overexpression of HNF-3gamma in hepatoma cells by means of a recombinant adenovirus induced CYP2C9, CYP2C18, and CYP2C19 mRNAs (4.5-, 20-, and 50-fold, respectively) but did not activate endogenous CYP2C8. The lack of effect of HNF-3gamma on endogenous CYP2C8 could be reversed by treating cells with the deacetylase inhibitor trichostatin A, suggesting the existence of chromatin condensation around functional HNF-3 elements in this gene (Bort et al., 2004). Within the rat CYP2E1 promoter HNF-1alpha binding sites (Ueno and Gonzalez, 1990) and within the chicken CYP2H1 promoter HNF-3alpha, HNF-3beta, and HNF-1alpha binding sites (Dogra and May, 1997) were identified. HNF-6alpha and HNF-6beta binding sites were identified in the promoters of human CYP2C12 and rat CYP2C13 (Lannoy et al., 1998; Samadani and Costa, 1996). Table 14.1 provides examples of experimental findings that demonstrate direct involvement of C/EBPs and HNFs in transcriptional control of hepatic *CYP* genes through interaction with their promoters.

14.3
HNF-6 and HNF-3beta in Liver-specific Transcription Factor Networks

Observations that HNF-6 contributes to control of the expression of transcription factors and is expressed in early stages of liver, pancreas, and neuronal differentiation suggest that HNF-6 participates in several developmental programs (Landry et al., 1997). HNF-6 recognizes the –138 to –126 region of the HNF-3beta promoter. Site--directed mutagenesis of this HNF-6 site diminishes reporter gene expression, suggesting that HNF-6 activates transcription of this promoter and may thus play a role in epithelial cell differentiation of gut endoderm via regulation of HNF-3beta (Samadani and Costa, 1996). Later, it was recognized that HNF-6 is required for HNF-3beta promoter activity and that HNF-6 also recognizes the regulatory region of numerous liver-specific genes (Rausa et al., 1997). In-situ hybridization studies of staged specific embryos demonstrate that HNF-6 and its potential target gene, *HNF-3beta*, are coexpressed in the pancreatic and hepatic diverticulum. More detailed analysis of the developmental expression patterns of HNF-6 and HNF-3beta provides evidence of colocalization in hepatocytes, intestinal epithelial, pancreatic ductal epithelial, and exocrine acinar cells. The expression patterns of these two transcription factors do not overlap in other endoderm-derived tissues or in the neurotube (Rausa et al., 1997).

14.3.1
HNF-6, OC-2, HNF-3beta, and C/EBPs Regulate HNF-3beta Expression

The liver-enriched transcription factor HNF-6 recognizes the –138 to –126 region of the HNF-3beta promoter and is required for HNF-3beta promoter activity (Samadani and Costa, 1996). Similar to HNF-6, another member of the onecut class of transcription factors, called OC-2, with tissue-restricted expression in liver and skin, stimulates transcription of the HNF-3beta gene in transient transfection experiments, suggesting that OC-2 participates in the network of transcription factors required for liver differentiation and metabolism (Jacquemin et al., 1999). Earlier studies showed that promoter activity of HNF-3beta requires –134 bp of HNF-3beta proximal sequences and binds four nuclear proteins, including two ubiquitous factors. One of these promoter sites interacts with a cell-specific factor, LF-H3 beta, whose binding activity correlates with the HNF-3beta tissue expression pattern. Furthermore, there is a binding site for the HNF-3beta protein within its own promoter, suggesting that an autoactivation mechanism is involved in the establishment of HNF-3beta expression. It has been proposed that both the LF-H3 beta and HNF-3 sites play an important role in the cell type-specific expression of the HNF-3beta transcription factor (Pani et al., 1992 b). Later studies demonstrated that members of the C/EBP and proline and acidic amino acid-rich subfamilies of basic region leucine zipper transcription factors bind to the LF-H3 beta site, and cotransfection of HepG2 cells showed that these factors can activate an HNF-3beta promoter reporter construct. The LF-H3 beta-C/EBP binding sequence also confers HNF-3beta promoter stimulation in response to interleukin (IL)-1 and IL-6. Upstream of this HNF-3beta proximal promoter region, an IFN-stimulated response element core sequence (–231 to –210) was found that mediates transcriptional induction by IFN-gamma but not IFN-alpha. Gel mobility supershift assays demonstrated that an IFN-gamma–induced protein–DNA complex is disrupted by an antibody specific for interferon-regulatory-factor-1/interferon-stimulated gene factor-2. Surprisingly, the effect of the three cytokines (IL-1, IL-6, and IFN-gamma) in combination, as assayed by the same model, is not synergistic. HNF-3beta joins the C/EBP family on the list of liver-enriched transcription factors whose expression is modulated by cytokines (Samadani et al., 1995).

14.3.2
Competition and Cooperation Between HNF-3alpha and HNF-3beta

Studies using embryoid bodies in which one or both HNF-3alpha or HNF-3beta genes were inactivated showed that HNF-3beta was necessary for expression of HNF-3alpha. HNF-3beta positively regulated the expression of HNF-4alpha/HNF-1alpha and their downstream targets. In these studies HNF-3alpha acted as a negative regulator of HNF-4alpha/HNF-1alpha, demonstrating that HNF-3alpha and HNF-3beta have antagonistic transcriptional regulatory functions *in vivo*. HNF-3alpha did not appear to act as a classic biochemical repressor but, rather exerted its negative effect by competing for HNF-3 binding sites with the more efficient activator HNF-3beta. In addition, the HNF-3alpha/HNF-3beta ratio was modulated by the presence of insulin, providing evidence that the HNF network may have important roles in mediating the action of insulin (Duncan et al., 1998).

14.4
The Role of C/EBPs in Diverse Physiological Functions

14.4.1
C/EBP-alpha in Energy Metabolism and Detoxification

There is overwhelming evidence that C/EBP-alpha plays a central regulatory role in energy metabolism in the liver (Crosson et al., 1997). High levels of C/EBP-alpha mRNA were observed in tissues known to metabolize lipid and cholesterol-related compounds at uncommonly high rates, which included liver, fat, intestine, lung, adrenal gland, and placenta. C/EBP-alpha is essential for adipogenesis and neonatal gluconeogenesis, as shown by the C/EBP-alpha knockout mouse (Arizmendi et al., 1999). Expression of C/EBP-alpha in the liver is under complex control by both hormonal and metabolic signals, which is consistent with its role as a trans-regulator of genes that play a role in energy metabolism (Crosson et al., 1997) (Figure 14.2). Ammonia produced by amino acid metabolism is detoxified through conversion into urea by the ornithine cycle in the liver, whereas the carbon skeletons of amino acids are converted to glucose by gluconeogenic enzymes. Promoter and enhancer sequences of several genes for ornithine cycle enzymes interact with members of the C/EBP transcription factor family. Disruption of the C/EBP-alpha gene in mice

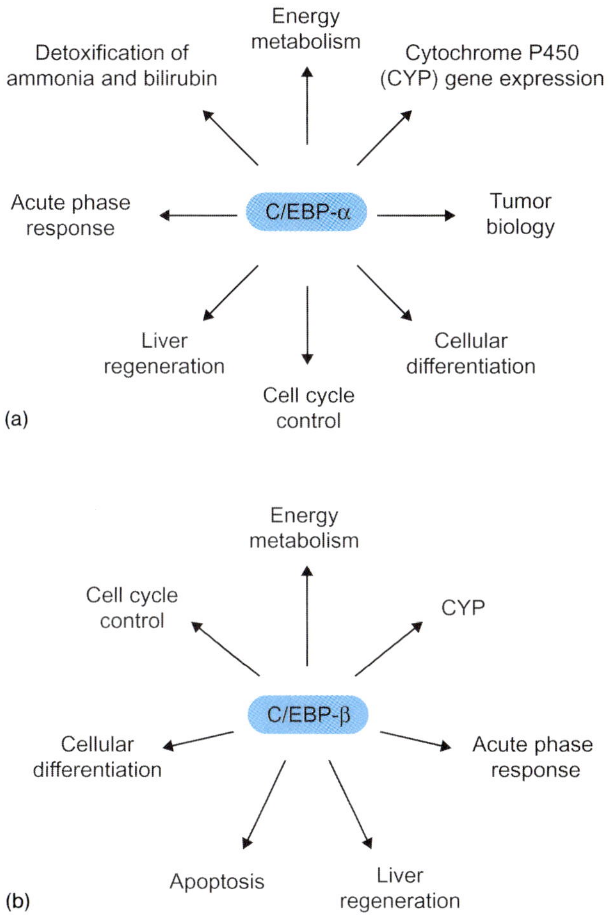

Fig. 14.2 (a) Key Physiological Features of C/EBP-α; (b) Key Physiological Features of C/EBP-β. The involvement of C/EBP-alpha and C/EBP-beta in diverse physiological contexts highlights the important roles of these transcription factors in liver biology. A: the physiological contexts in which C/EBP-alpha plays a major role; B: the same for C/EBP-beta. Interestingly, C/EBP-alpha displays important functional features beyond the functions of a transcription factor, which allow C/EBP-alpha to enable or inhibit proteasomal degradation of important regulatory molecules (e. g., C/EBP-beta, CDK4, and p21) and to engage in inhibitory protein–protein interactions (e. g., disruption of E2F complexes). Details are discussed in the text.

causes hypoglycaemia associated with impaired production of gluconeogenic enzymes. (Kimura et al., 1998) (Figure 14.3). It was previously reported that mice carrying a homozygous null mutation at the *C/EBP-alpha* locus die as neonates due to the absence of hepatic glycogen and the resulting hypoglycaemia. However, the lethal phenotype precluded further analysis of the role of *c/ebp-alpha* in hepatic gene regulation in adult mice. To circumvent this problem, a conditional knockout allele of *c/ebp-alpha* obtained by using the Cre/loxP recombination system was used by Lee

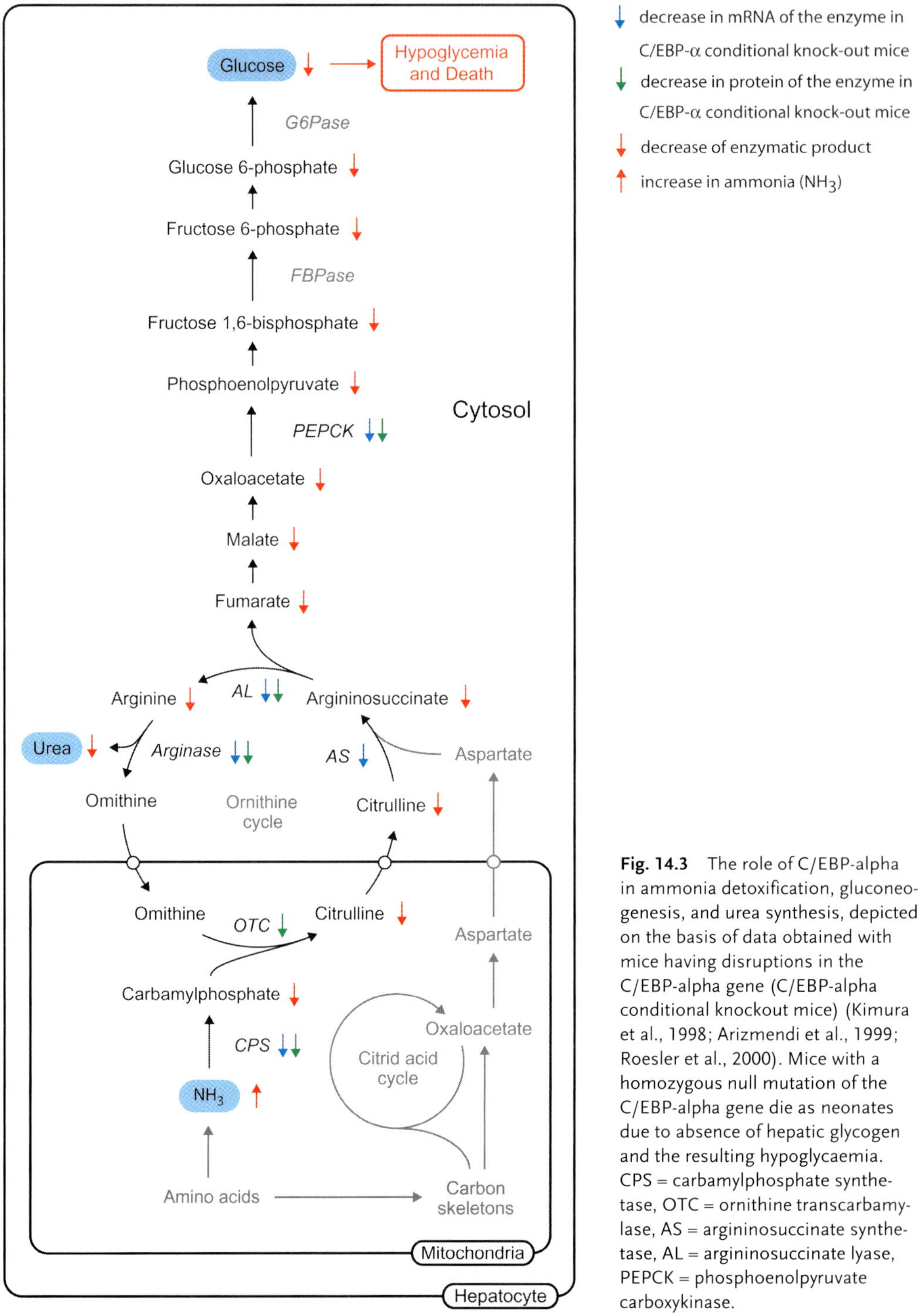

Fig. 14.3 The role of C/EBP-alpha in ammonia detoxification, gluconeogenesis, and urea synthesis, depicted on the basis of data obtained with mice having disruptions in the C/EBP-alpha gene (C/EBP-alpha conditional knockout mice) (Kimura et al., 1998; Arizmendi et al., 1999; Roesler et al., 2000). Mice with a homozygous null mutation of the C/EBP-alpha gene die as neonates due to absence of hepatic glycogen and the resulting hypoglycaemia. CPS = carbamylphosphate synthetase, OTC = ornithine transcarbamylase, AS = argininosuccinate synthetase, AL = argininosuccinate lyase, PEPCK = phosphoenolpyruvate carboxykinase.

et al. (1997 a). This condition resulted in a reduced level of bilirubin UDP-glucuronosyl transferase expression in the liver. After several days, the knockout mice developed severe jaundice due to an increase in unconjugated serum bilirubin. The expression of genes encoding phosphoenolpyruvate carboxykinase, glycogen synthase, and factor IX was also strongly reduced in adult conditional-knockout animals, while the expression of transferrin, apolipoprotein B, and insulin-like growth factor I genes was not affected. These results establish C/EBP-alpha as an essential transcriptional regulator of genes encoding enzymes involved in bilirubin detoxification and gluconeogenesis in the adult mouse liver (Lee et al., 1997 a).

14.4.2
C/EBP-beta in Energy Metabolism

The *C/EBP-beta* gene can be primarily induced by glucocorticoids and by glucagon (Matsuno et al., 1996). C/EBP-beta has been linked to the metabolic and gene regulatory responses to diabetes. C/EBP-beta has also been implicated as an essential factor underlying glucocorticoid-dependent activation of phosphoenolpyruvate carboxykinase (PEPCK) gene transcription *in vivo*. C/EBP-beta binds with high affinity to several sequences of the PEPCK gene promoter, and C/EBP-beta protein is increased 200% in the livers of streptozotocin-diabetic mice, concurrent with increased PEPCK mRNA (Arizmendi et al., 1999). Studies with mice that were heterozygous or homozygous for a null mutation of the gene for C/EBP-beta revealed that C/EBP-beta is not essential to maintaining basal PEPCK mRNA levels (Arizmendi et al., 1999; Roesler, 2000). However, in streptozotocin-diabetic rats C/EBP-beta deletion leads to delayed hyperglycaemia with no increase in free fatty acids in the plasma, limited induction of PEPCK and glucose 6-phosphatase genes, and no increased gluconeogenesis rate. EMSA supershifts of transcription factor C/EBP-alpha, bound to CRE, P3I, and AF-2 sites of the PEPCK promoter, was not increased in diabetic *c/ebpbeta–/–* mouse liver nuclei, suggesting that C/EBP-alpha does not substitute for C/EBP-beta in the diabetic response of liver gene transcription (Arizmendi et al., 1999). Insulin and glucocorticoids reciprocally regulate PEPCK expression primarily at the level of gene transcription. Indeed, it was demonstrated that glucocorticoids promote, whereas insulin disrupts, the association of CREB-binding protein (CBP) and RNA polymerase II with the hepatic PEPCK gene promoter *in vivo*. It was shown that accessory factors, such as the C/EBP-beta isoform LAP, may recruit the coactivator CBP to drive transcription (Ghosh et al., 2001; Duong et al., 2002). Insulin increased protein levels of the C/EBP-beta isoform LIP, an inhibitory form of C/EBP-beta, via phosphatidylinositol-3-kinase–dependent intracellular signal transduction pathways. LIP concomitantly replaced liver-enriched transcriptional activator protein LAP on the PEPCK gene promoter, which can abrogate the recruitment of CBP and polymerase II, culminating in the repression of PEPCK expression and the attenuation of hepatocellular glucose production (Duong et al., 2002).

14.4.3
C/EBPs in the Acute-phase Response

The acute-phase response, an inflammatory process resulting from infection and/or tissue damage, is an early defence mechanism during which striking changes in protein synthesis occur mainly in the liver. The altered expression of many acute-phase protein genes is regulated at the transcriptional level after hepatocyte stimulation by cytokines (e.g., IL-1beta, IL-6, TNF-alpha) and/or lipopolysaccharide (LPS). Some of these acute-phase genes have DNA binding sites for the C/EBP family of transcription factors (for review see Koj, 1996). Figure 14.5 summarizes the events in the hepatocyte during the acute-phase response after stimulation with the cytokines IL-1beta, IL-6, and TNF-alpha.

Lipopolysacharide (LPS)-induced acute-phase response in mouse livers leads to an elevated expression of the low molecular weight C/EBP-beta isoform, liver-enriched transcriptional inhibitory protein (LIP) (Welm et al., 2000) (Figure 14.4). The 5′ region of C/EBP-beta mRNA is involved in the regulation of LIP translation. Binding of cytoplasmic proteins to the 5′ region of C/EBP-beta mRNA is altered in response to LPS administration. One of the major changes is induced binding of a cytoplasmic protein that is immunologically identical to the previously characterized RNA-binding protein CUGBP1 (Timchenko et al., 1999a; Welm et al., 2000). Induction of CUGBP1 binding activity in liver cytoplasm during the acute-phase response is accompanied by elevation of CUGBP1 binding activity to polysomes. CUGBP1 immunoprecipitated from livers of LPS-treated mice, but not from normal animals, is capable of inducing LIP translation in a cell-free translation system. The ability of CUGBP1 to induce LIP translation during the acute-phase response depends on phosphorylation of CUGBP1 (Welm et al., 2000). The elevated LIP translation during the acute-phase response, as well as after partial hepatectomy, leads to increased binding of LIP to the C/EBP consensus site found within the mouse C/EBP-alpha promoter. This binding correlates with the reduction of C/EBP-alpha mRNA levels in both biological situations. Cotransfection experiments showed that full-length C/EBP-beta activates the C/EBP-alpha promoter, while LIP blocks this activation. These data suggest that the dominant negative isoform of C/EBP-beta, LIP, downregulates the C/EBP-alpha promoter in liver and in cultured hepatocytes. Because full-length C/EBP-alpha and C/EBP-beta proteins regulate liver proliferation, this function of LIP may be important in liver growth and differentiation (Welm et al., 2000).

The proinflammatory cytokine TNF-alpha initiates post-transcriptional activation of cytokine-inducible C/EBPs, leading to promotion of the nuclear localization of cytokine-inducible CCAAT-enhancer binding protein isoforms in hepatocytes. This mechanism enables hepatocytes to respond immediately to inflammatory stress (Yin et al., 1996) (Figure 14.5). Interleukin-6 (IL-6) is a pleiotropic cytokine that plays important roles in immunity, hemopoiesis, and inflammation. Both the DNA binding activity and the trans-activating capacity of C/EBP-beta are induced in hepatoma cells by treatment with IL-6 through a posttranslational mechanism, implicating it as a nuclear target of IL-6 and as a mediator of the IL-6–dependent transcriptional activation of liver genes during the acute-phase response (Poli et al., 1990). On the other

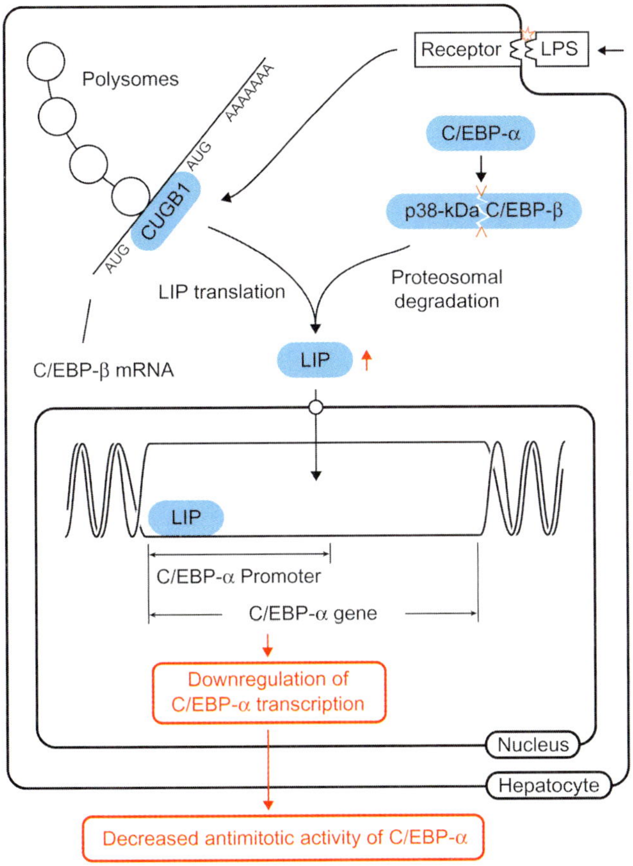

Fig. 14.4 After LPS administration, binding of phosphorylated CUGP1 to the 5′ region of C/EBP-beta mRNA leads to translation of the shorter LIP isoform during the acute-phase response (based on data from Timchenko et al., 1999 a, and Welm et al., 2000). LIP can be produced by two mechanisms: alternative transation, or proteolytic cleavage of full-length C/EBP-beta. In C/EBP-alpha knockout mice (*C/EBPalpha–/–*) the regulation of C/EBP-beta proteasomal degradation is impaired (based on data from Burgess-Beusse et al., 1999 and Welm et al., 1999), whereas the induction of C/EBP-alpha in cultured cells leads to induced cleavage of C/EBP-beta to generate the LIP isoform. Increased LIP levels lead to decreased C/EBP-alpha expression. This mechanism constitutes an alternative indirect autoregulatory loop for regulation of C/EBP-alpha expression. For further details see the text.

hand, C/EBP-beta is involved in activation of the IL-6 promoter in response to IL-1beta and bacterial lipopolysaccharide (LPS). Under some conditions the C/EBP-beta gene is transcriptionally activated by IL-1beta and lipopolysaccharide, whereas in other instances, its binding to cognate DNA sequences is enhanced by cytokines (Akira et al., 1990). IL-6 signalling involves activation of two independent transcription factors: STAT-3 (through phosphorylation by Jak kinases) and C/EBP-beta (through activation of the ras/raf pathway) (Koj, 1996) (Figure 14.5). Experiments

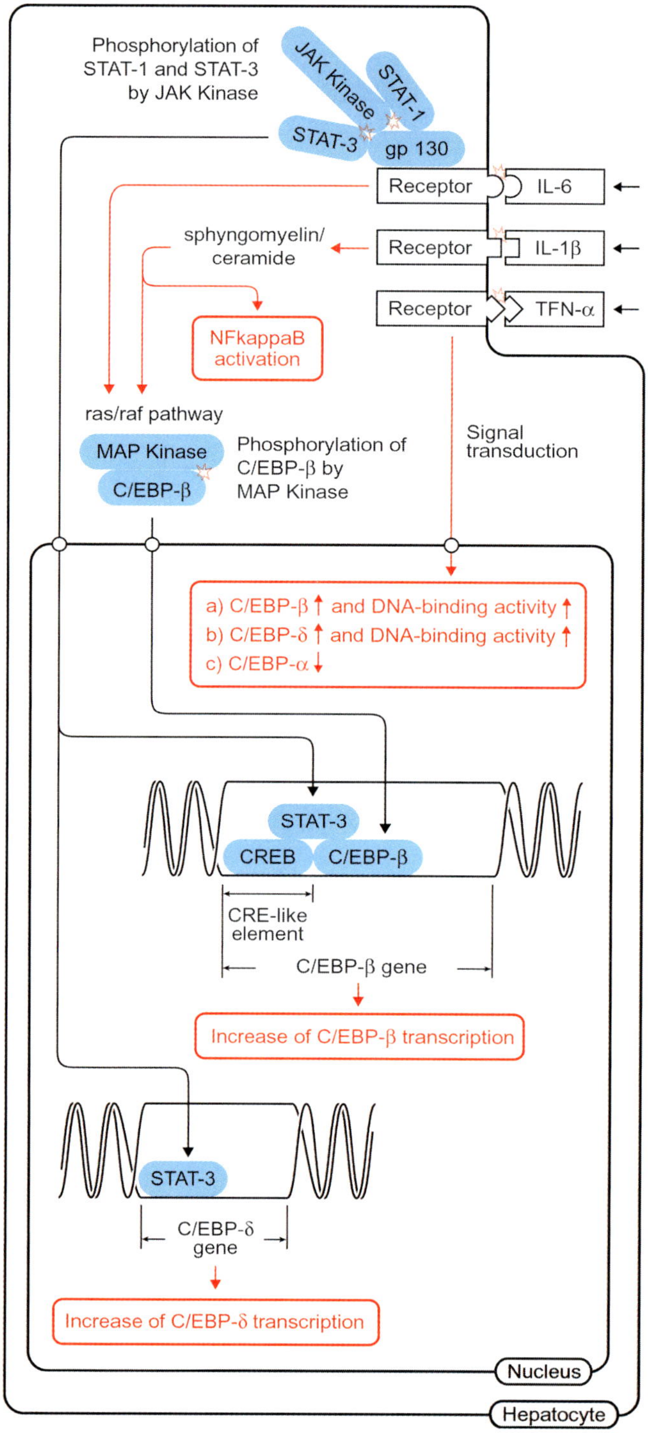

Fig. 14.5 The effects of IL-1beta, IL-6, and TNF-alpha stimulation on hepatocytes during the acute phase response are summarized schematically (for details see the text). Red arrows depict consequences, and black arrows depict actual molecule translocations.

with IL-6–deficient knockout mice demonstrated that IL-6 is essential for the hepatic induction of acute-phase mRNAs like those for alpha1-acid glycoprotein and C-reactive protein (CRP) upon localized tissue damage, but not upon systemically induced inflammation. The defective mRNA induction of acute-phase genes is paralleled by a defective activation of STAT-3, thus suggesting a direct relationship between IL-6 function, STAT-3 activation, and the induction of acute-phase genes. On the other hand, experiments with C/EBP-beta–deficient knockout mice showed that the induction of IL-6 by a variety of stimuli does not necessarily require C/EBP-beta activity *in vivo*. In contrast to the predicted activating role of C/EBP-beta, IL-6 levels are increased in the C/EBP beta-deficient mice, suggesting that C/EBP-beta may act as a modulator of the IL-6 gene *in vivo* (Alonzi et al., 1997). Transfection experiments using promoter constructs with mutated CRE-like elements demonstrated that IL-6 controls C/EBP-beta gene transcription via CRE-like elements in the C/EBP-beta promoter without any STAT-3 DNA binding motifs (Niehof et al., 2001 b) (Figure 14.5). Luciferase reporter gene assays showed that STAT-3 activation through the gp130 signal transducer molecule is involved in mediating IL-6–dependent C/EBP-beta transcription (Niehof et al., 2001 b). It was assumed that protein–protein interactions between STAT-3 and the protein complex at the CRE-like elements of the C/EBP-beta promoter contribute significantly to the regulation of C/EBP-beta transcription.

C/EBP-delta is sharply induced at an early stage of the acute-phase response (Yamada et al., 1997) (Figure 14.5). Treatment of HepG2 cells with IL-6 leads to rapid induction of C/EBP-delta mRNA. Transfection and gel-shift assays led to the identification of a binding site for STAT-3. These findings strongly suggest that C/EBP-delta gene expression is mediated by STAT-3 after IL-6–receptor mediated phosphorylation (Yamada et al., 1997). Several lines of evidence suggest that C/EBP-delta is regulated by phosphorylation and, in conjunction with C/EBP-beta, is one of the major proteins responsible for the increased transcription of the serum amyloid A (SAA) gene in response to inflammatory stimuli (for review see Schrem et al., 2004).

Studies with C/EBP-alpha knockout mice demonstrated that treating neonatal mice with purified bacterial lipopolysaccharide or recombinant IL-1beta resulted in a strong-acute phase response in wild-type mice, but no response in C/EBP-alpha null animals. The C/EBP-alpha knockout and wild-type mice had elevations in C/EBP-beta and -delta mRNA expression and DNA binding as well as increased DNA binding of NF-kappaB, all of which are important in the acute-phase response. Null mice, however, failed to activate STAT-3 binding in response to lipopolysaccharide. A pivotal role for C/EBP-alpha in the induction of the acute-phase response *in vivo* was therefore established (Burgess-Beusse and Darlington, 1998).

14.4.4
Protein–Protein Interactions of C/EBP-beta During the Acute-phase Response

When incubated together, NFkappaB, p65, and C/EBP-beta form a ternary complex by direct protein–protein interaction enabling cross-talk between the transcription factor networks involving NFkappaB and C/EBP-beta, which affects the transcriptional regulation of genes, e. g., during the acute-phase response. Mutational analysis showed that the C-terminal region of the Rel homology domain (RHD) and the C terminus of the activation domain of p65 are important for its interaction with C/EBP-beta (Xia et al., 1997).

NFkappaB and a 140-kDa phosphoprotein named Nopp140 interact with different C/EBP-beta isoforms that are activators for the alpha-1 acid glycoprotein gene. Known inducers of NfkappaB, such as IL-1beta and IL-6, can selectively activate the alpha-1 acid glycoprotein gene via NFkappaB as a coactivator for C/EBP-beta (Lee et al., 1996). In addition to interacting with C/EBP-beta, Nopp140 interacts specifically with TFIIB. Distinct regions of Nopp140 that interact with C/EBP-beta and TFIIB have been characterized, and the sequence of Nopp140 contains several stretches of serine- and acidic amino acid-rich sequences, which are also found in ICP4 of herpes simplex virus type 1, a known transcription factor that interacts with TFIIB. The physical interaction between TFIIB and wild-type Nopp140 or several deletion mutants of Nopp140 correlates well with the ability of Nopp140 to activate the alpha-1 acid glycoprotein gene synergistically with C/EBP-beta. Thus, the molecular mechanism of alpha-1 acid glycoprotein gene activation may involve interaction of C/EBP-beta and TFIIB mediated by the coactivator Nopp140 (Miau et al., 1997).

Physical and functional interactions between C/EBP-beta and heterogeneous nuclear ribonucleoprotein (hnRNP) K result in the repression of C/EBP-beta–dependent trans-activation of the alpha-1 acid glycoprotein gene. Genomic footprinting assays indicate that hnRNP K cannot bind to the promoter region of alpha-1 acid glycoprotein gene or interfere with the binding of C/EBP-beta to its cognate DNA site. Importantly, alpha-1 acid glycoprotein gene activation by the synergistic interaction of Nopp140 and C/EBP-beta is abolished by hnRNP K. The kinetics of appearance of C/EBP-beta–hnRNP K complex in nuclear extracts after initiation of the acute-phase reaction indicates that hnRNP K functions as a negative regulator of C/EBP-beta–mediated activation of the alpha-1 acid glycoprotein gene (Miau et al., 1998).

14.4.5
C/EBPs in Liver Regeneration

Concanavalin A (Con A) injection into mice leads to immune-mediated liver injury. In Con A-induced liver injury, TNF-alpha and IL-6–dependent signalling pathways are activated. TNF-alpha and IL-6 lead to posttranslational activation of C/EBP-beta by phosphorylation and induction of C/EBP-beta transcription via STAT-3, an important regulator of hepatocyte proliferation (Trautwein et al., 1993, 1994 and 1998). Hepatocyte growth factor (HGF) is an inducible cytokine that is essential for the normal growth and development of various tissues, including the liver. HGF confers a major mitogenic stimulus to hepatocytes during liver regeneration (review in Matsumoto and Nakamura, 1992). HGF stimulates the expression of C/EBP-beta and NFkappaB, which are both key transcription factors responsible for the regulation of many genes under stress conditions or during the acute-phase response. Biochemical and functional analyses gave evidence for a HGF-responsive element located in the region –376 to –352 (URE1) of the 5′-upstream regulatory sequence of the gene coding for C/EBP-beta. Activation of NFkappaB by HGF preceded the induction of C/EBP-beta. Further studies indicated that NFkappaB can cooperate with C/EBP-beta or other members of the C/EBP family to activate the C/EBP-beta gene in both a URE1 and a URE2-dependent manner. These results suggest that induction of the C/EBP-beta gene by HGF is mediated at least in part by the activation of NFkappaB. Activated NFkappaB then interacts with C/EBP-beta, resulting in induction of C/EBP-beta (Shen et al., 1997). Additionally, partial hepatectomy, which activates HGF gene expression in the liver, in turn increases C/EBP-beta binding activity to the HGF promoter, with resulting induction of HGF expression, leading to positive feedback during the induction of liver regeneration (Jiang and Zarnegar, 1997). The truncated C/EBP-beta isoform, LIP, is induced in rat livers in response to partial hepatectomy via the alternative translation mechanism (Burgess-Beusse et al., 1999; Welm et al., 1999; Timchenko et al., 1999 a).

Northern blotting was used to examine the expression of C/EBP-alpha mRNA during liver regeneration. C/EBP-alpha mRNA levels decreased to 60% to 80% within 1 to 3 h after partial hepatectomy, as hepatocytes progressed from G0 to G1, and decreased further when cells progressed into S phase. In-vitro transcription analysis was in agreement with the Northern blot data, thus suggesting that C/EBP-alpha is transcriptionally regulated in regenerating liver (Mischoulon et al., 1992).

After two-thirds partial hepatectomy, the liver is able to compensate for the acute loss of mass and maintain serum glucose levels and many of its differentiation-specific functions. Studies of the interplay between differentiation and cell growth during liver regeneration showed that the C/EBP-alpha protein level decreased by more than half during the mid-to-late G1 and S phases (8–24 h after hepatectomy) coordinately with a threefold increase in expression of C/EBP-beta. Renormalization of the levels of these proteins occurred after the major proliferative phase. This inverse regulation of C/EBP-alpha and -beta results in an up to sevenfold increase in the beta/alpha DNA binding ratio between 3 and 24 h after hepatectomy, which may have an important effect on target gene regulation. The persistent expression of C/EBP-alpha and -beta isoforms shows that C/EBP proteins contribute to the function of hepatocytes during physiological growth and that significant amounts of these proteins do not inhibit progression of hepatocytes into S phase of the cell cycle, despite the known antagonist functions of C/EBP-alpha and C/EBP-beta (Greenbaum et al., 1995). The rate of adult rat liver proliferation is normally low and is markedly enhanced during compensatory regeneration. Liver cell proliferation after partial hepatectomy, but not in response to treatment with the antiandrogene cyproterone acetate, is associated with changes in C/EBP-alpha and C/EBP-beta expression. This further supports the notion that changes in expression of transcription factors during liver growth *in vivo* depend on the growth inducer (Skrtic et al., 1997).

14.4.6
C/EBPs and Apoptosis

Apoptotic cell death in the liver in response to activation of the Fas pathway has been implicated in human disease as well as in liver remodelling and tissue repair. Differences in apoptotic cell death in the livers of C/EBP-beta–null mice, assessed by using the Jo-2 agonistic anti-Fas antibody, were investigated. Apoptotic injury was dramatically reduced in *C/EBP-beta –/–* livers, as shown by a nearly 20-fold reduction in apoptotic hepatocytes six hours after Jo-2 treatment in *C/EBPbeta –/–* hepatocytes compared with controls ($P < 0.04$) and also reduced activation of caspase 3. By cleavage occurred in Jo-2–treated *C/EBP-beta –/–* livers, indicating a block of Fas-induced injury distal to the death-inducing signalling complex. The level of the antiapoptotic protein bcl-x(L) was increased greater than tenfold in the mutant animals ($P < 0.04$), which, at least in part, accounts for the protection from Fas-mediated apoptosis. In contrast, bcl-x(L) mRNA levels were unchanged. These observations link C/EBP-beta to Fas-induced hepatocyte apoptosis through a mechanism that likely involves translational or posttranslational regulation of bcl-x(L) (Mukherjee et al., 2001).

14.4.7
C/EBPs in Liver Development

Specific C/EBPs are regulated differentially during the course of postnatal liver development in the rat. During postnatal liver growth, several liver-specific functions emerge, and this coincides with enhanced expression of C/EBP-alpha, -beta, and -delta. Immediately after birth, nuclear expression of the 36-kDa C/EBP-delta protein increases, followed by increased expression of the 38-kDa C/EBP-beta protein and enhanced expression of the 42-kDa C/EBP-alpha protein. Changes in C/EBP–DNA binding activity accompany developmental increases in C/EBP proteins (for review see Diehl et al., 1994 b).

In liver and intestine, C/EBP-alpha mRNA expression is coordinately induced just prior to birth (Birkenmeier et al., 1989). The role of C/EBP-alpha in the developmental expression of a subset of genes governing essential metabolic processes had been elucidated by using a mutant mouse model that lacks C/EBP-alpha. The mutation resulted in the failure of the liver and of white and brown adipose tissue to develop normal metabolic functions in the perinatal period, including hepatic glycogen synthesis and gluconeogenesis and the synthesis and deposition of triglyceride in adipose tissue (for review see Darlington et al., 1995).

14.4.8
The Role of C/EBPs in CYP Monooxygenase Expression During Development

In the human foetal liver, the cytochrome P450 enzyme CYP3A7 is expressed as early as the 13th week of gestation. Its expression continues to the perinatal period but it is sharply repressed immediately after birth. Concomitantly, the expression of CYP3A4, which is not detectable in the foetus, sharply increases in the perinatal period to remain elevated throughout adulthood (review in Hakkola et al., 1998; Hakkola et al., 2001; Williams et al., 2002). CYP3A7 and CYP2A4 respond differently to C/EBP-alpha and DBP, two factors that exhibit a strict proliferation-dependent pattern of expression in the liver (Ourlin et al., 1997). The rat CYP2D5 gene is expressed in liver cells. Its expression commences a few days after birth, and maximal mRNA levels are reached when animals reach puberty. The role of CYP2D5 in developmental programs was therefore studied. Transfection experiments in HepG2 cells using gene fusion constructs of the chloramphenicol acetyltransferase gene and varying portions of the CYP2D5 promoter identified a segment of DNA between nucleotides –55 and –156 that conferred transcriptional activity in HepG2 cells. Activity was markedly increased by cotransfection with a vector expressing C/EBP-beta but was unaffected by vectors producing other liver-enriched transcription factors (C/EBP-alpha, HNF-1alpha, and DBP). DNase I footprinting revealed a region protected by both HepG2 and liver cell nuclear extracts between nucleotides –83 and –112. This region displayed some sequence similarity to the Sp1 consensus sequence and was able to bind the Sp1 protein, as assessed by a gel mobility shift assay. The role of Sp1 in CYP2D5 transcription was confirmed by trans-activation of the 2D5–CAT construct in *D. melanogaster* cells by using an Sp1 expression vector. C/EBP-beta alone was unable to directly bind to the –83 to –112 region of the promoter but was able to produce a ternary complex when combined with HepG2 nuclear extracts or recombinant human Sp1. C/EBP-alpha was unable to substitute for C/EBP-beta in forming this ternary complex. A poor C/EBP binding site is present adjacent to the Sp1 site, and mutagenesis of this site abolished formation of the ternary complex with the CYP2D5 regulatory region. These results established that both factors work in conjunction, possibly by protein–protein interaction, to activate the CYP2D5 gene (Lee et al., 1994) (Table 14.1).

14.4.9
C/EBPs and Their Role in Liver Tumour Biology

p53 is a tumour suppressor and transcription factor that is activated by genotoxic stress and mediates cell cycle arrest and apoptosis. Overexpression of a mutated p53, which is unable to mediate cell cycle arrest and/or apoptosis, is frequently found in undifferentiated hepatocellular carcinomas that typically display a lack of liver-specific gene expression (Tannapfel and Wittekind, 2002). Both wild type p53 and tumour-derived p53 mutant factors repress C/EBP-mediated trans-activation of the albumin promoter via protein–protein interaction. Deletion analysis and domain-swapping experiments showed that repression of C/EBP-beta–mediated trans-activation is dependent on the N-terminal domain of p53 and the trans-activation domain, leucine zipper domain, and inhibitory domain II (amino acids 163–191) of C/EBP-beta (Kubicka et al., 1999).

In an expression profiling study of human hepatocellular carcinoma in Chinese patients, the expression level of C/EBP-alpha was downregulated in the tumour tissues as compared to normal liver tissue from the same patients, whereas hepatocyte nuclear factor 1 (HNF-1), HNF-3beta, HNF-4alpha, and HNF-4gamma were upregulated. These results suggested that liver-enriched transcription factors may play a regulatory role in human hepatocellular carcinoma (Xu et al., 2001). In a study from Japan, comparison of the expression levels of the C/EBP-alpha gene between hepatocellular carcinoma and nontumourous regions in surgical specimens from the same patient revealed also that in 9 out of 13 patients, the expression level in the tumours was decreased compared with that in corresponding nontumourous regions (Tomizawa et al., 2002). Taken together, these data suggest that expression of the C/EBP-alpha gene may be downregulated in the majority of human hepatocellular carcinomas.

The observation that CDP can act as a competitive repressor for C/EBP-alpha–mediated trans-activation (Antes et al., 2000) suggests that CDP may play a significant not-yet-described role in hepatocarcinogenesis, since the negative influence of C/EBP-alpha on cell cycle progression might be abolished when CDP expression is upregulated. Repression by CDP involves competition for binding site occupancy and active repression via the recruitment of a histone deacetylase activity. CDP function is regulated by several post-translational modification events, including phosphorylation, dephosphorylation, and acetylation (for review see Nepveu, 2001).

14.5 Involvement of C/EBP-alpha and C/EBP-beta in Regulation of Cell Cycle Control

14.5.1 C/EBP-alpha Expression and Growth Arrest

In fat and liver tissues, C/EBP-alpha expression is limited to fully differentiated cells (Birkenmeier et al., 1989; Umek et al., 1991). Dedifferentiated cells show decreased levels of C/EBP-alpha expression. Increased C/EBP-alpha expression, e.g., in a stable cell line or in the terminal phase of adipogenesis, is associated with proliferative growth arrest and a specialized cell phenotype (Umek et al., 1991; Runge et al., 1997). Experimental premature expression of C/EBP-alpha in adipoblasts causes direct cessation of mitotic growth (Umek et al., 1991). Mice lacking C/EBP-alpha display hyperproliferation of alveolar type II cells, which implies that C/EBP-alpha has a relevant role in controlled growth arrest of alveolar type II cells (Sugahara et al., 2001). C/EBP-alpha is critically involved in diverse mechanisms of blocking hepatocyte proliferation (see also Schrem et al., 2004), as summarised in Figure 14.6.

14.5.2 Glucocorticoid-induced G1 Cell Cycle Arrest Is Mediated by C/EBP-alpha

The glucocorticoid-stimulated expression of C/EBP-alpha is required for the steroid-mediated G1 cell-cycle arrest of minimal-deviation rat hepatoma cells (Cook et al., 1988). Stimulation of C/EBP-alpha expression is a rapid glucocorticoid receptor-mediated response, associated with G1 cell-cycle arrest (Ramos et al., 1996). Consistent with the role of C/EBP-alpha as a critical intermediate in the growth suppression response, maximal induction of transcription factor mRNA occurs within 2 h of dexamethasone treatment, whereas maximal inhibition of [^{3}H]thymidine incorporation is observed 24 h after steroid treatment (Ramos et al., 1996). As a direct functional approach, abolishment of C/EBP-alpha protein expression and DNA-binding activity by transfection with an antisense C/EBP-alpha expression vector blocked the

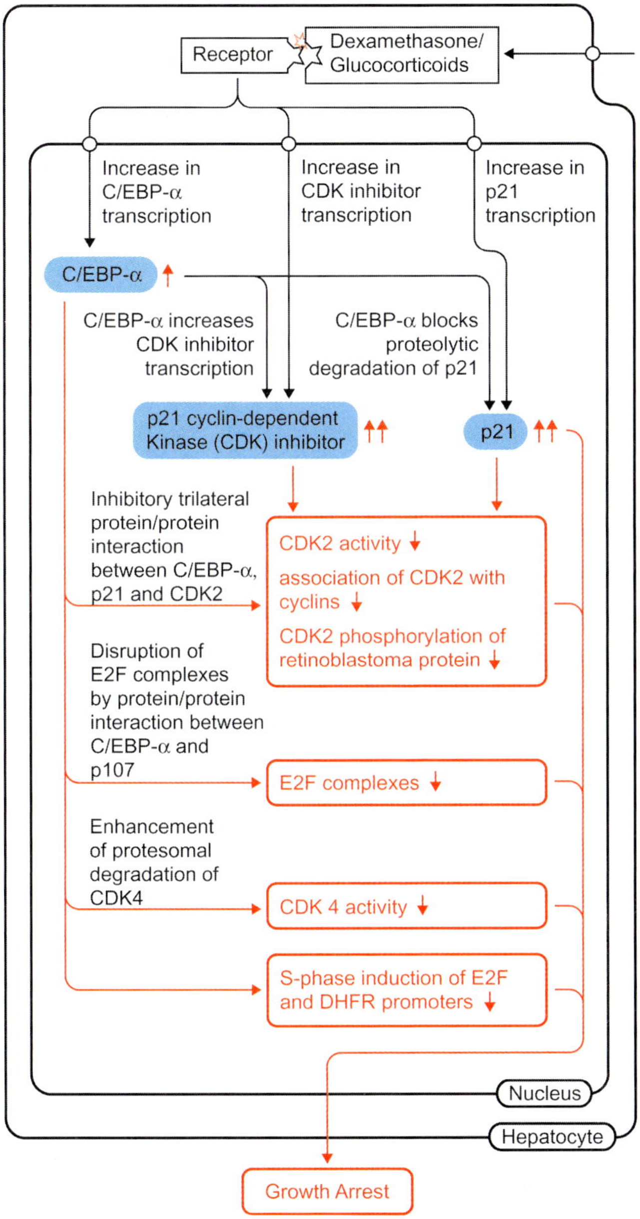

Fig. 14.6 This schematic representation summarizes the findings of Timchenko et al. (1996, 1997, 1998, 1999 a, b), Cha et al. (1998), Cram et al. (1998), Slomiany et al. (2000), Harris et al. (2001), and Wang et al. (2001), who have shown that C/EBP-alpha blocks hepatocyte proliferation via diverse mechanisms. The effects of dexamethasone and glucocorticoid treatment, which lead to growth arrest in hepatocytes, are also shown.

dexamethasone-induced G1 cell-cycle arrest of hepatoma cells but did not alter general glucocorticoid responsiveness. Transforming growth factor beta (TGF-beta) induced a G1 cell-cycle arrest in C/EBP-alpha antisense-transfected minimal-deviation rat hepatoma cells, demonstrating the specific involvement of C/EBP-alpha in the glucocorticoid growth suppression response (Ramos et al., 1996). Numerous experiments have established a functional link between the glucocorticoid receptor signalling pathway that mediates a G1 cell-cycle arrest of rat hepatoma cells and the transcriptional control of p21 by a cascade that requires the steroid-regulated induction of C/EBP-alpha gene expression (Cram et al., 1998; Schrem et al., 2004) (Figure 14.6).

14.5.3 Protein–Protein Interactions Between p21, cdk2, cdk4, and C/EBP-alpha

C/EBP-alpha is expressed at high levels in quiescent (nondividing) hepatocytes. In hepatocytes C/EBP-alpha has a dominant antiproliferative function, but must interact with other factors to regulate hepatocyte-specific gene expression (Diehl et al., 1996). Deletion and cotransfection experiments with human C/EBP-alpha demonstrated that only one of the two intact activation domains AD1 (amino acids 84 to 116) or AD2 (amino acids 154 to 245) is required for antimitotic activity in Hep3B2 cells (hepatoma cell line) (Hendricks-Taylor and Darlington, 1995). In cultured HT1 cells (a mouse preadipocyte cell line that contains the human *C/EBP-alpha* gene under Lac repressor control), C/EBP-alpha inhibits cell proliferation by increasing *p21* gene expression and by post-translational stabilization of p21 protein (also called WAF-1/CIP-1/SDI-1). Furthermore, induction of p21 is responsible for the ability of C/EBP-alpha to inhibit proliferation, because transcription of antisense *p21* mRNA eliminates growth inhibition by C/EBP-alpha (Timchenko et al., 1996) (Figure 14.6). In newborn C/EBP-alpha knockout mice, p21 protein levels are reduced in the liver, and the fraction of hepatocytes synthesizing DNA is increased. More than 30% of the hepatocytes in C/EBP-alpha knockout animals continue to proliferate on day 17 of postnatal life, when cell division in wild-type littermates is low (3%). p21 protein levels are relatively high in wild-type neonates but undetectable in C/EBP-alpha knockout mice (Timchenko et al., 1997). The reduction of p21 protein in the highly proliferating livers that lack C/EBP-alpha suggests that p21 is responsible for C/EBP-alpha–mediated control of liver proliferation in newborn mice (Timchenko et al., 1997). Although C/EBP-alpha controls p21 protein levels, p21 mRNA is not influenced by C/EBP-alpha in the liver. Using coimmunoprecipitation and a mammalian two-hybrid assay system, interaction of C/EBP alpha with p21 protein was demonstrated. Studies of p21 stability in liver nuclear extracts showed that C/EBP-alpha blocks proteolytic degradation of p21. This demonstrates that C/EBP-alpha regulates hepatocyte proliferation in newborn mice and that in the liver the level of p21 protein is under posttranscriptional control, consistent with the hypothesis that protein–protein interaction with C/EBP-alpha determines p21 levels (Timchenko et al., 1997). Two sites within the C/EBP-alpha protein were identified that can interact with p21. One interaction site was localized to the leucine zipper region (amino acids 313–360), whereas the other site was found between amino acids 119 and 226 in activation domain two (AD2) (Harris et al., 2001) (Figure 14.6). CDK2 also interacts with C/EBP-alpha. C/EBP-alpha can cooperate with p21 to inhibit CDK2 activity *in vitro*. Deletion experiments suggested that both the N- and C-terminal p21- and CDK2-binding sites are required for C/EBP-alpha to exert its effects on CDK2 and that a single binding site for p21 or CDK2 is not sufficient to cooperate in inhibiting CDK activity. C/EBP-alpha mutants incapable of inhibiting CDK2 activity *in vitro* do not inhibit proliferation in cultured cells. However, C/EBP-alpha mutants defective in DNA binding inhibit proliferation as effectively as the wild-type protein. These findings show that C/EBP-alpha–mediated growth arrest occurs through protein interactions and is independent of its transcriptional activity (Harris et al., 2001) (Figure 14.6). C/EBP-alpha directly interacts with cdk2 and cdk4 and arrests cell proliferation by inhibiting these kinases. A short growth inhibiting region of C/EBP-alpha has been mapped between amino acids 175 and 187. C/EBP-alpha inhibits cdk2 activity by blocking the association of cdk2 with cyclins. Importantly, the activities of cdk4 and cdk2 are increased in C/EBP-alpha knockout livers, leading to increased proliferation. These data demonstrate that C/EBP-alpha brings about growth arrest through direct inhibition of cdk2 and cdk4 (Wang et al., 2001) (Figure 14.6). C/EBP-alpha enhances proteasome-dependent degradation of cdk4 during growth arrest in the liver of newborn mice and in cultured cells. Overexpression of C/EBP-alpha in several biological systems leads to a decrease in cdk4 protein levels, but not in mRNA levels. Experiments with several tissue culture models revealed that C/EBP-alpha enhances the formation of cdk4–ubiquitin conjugates and induces degradation of cdk4 by a proteasome-dependent pathway. As a result, the half-life of cdk4 is shorter and protein levels of cdk4 are decreased in cells expressing C/EBP-alpha. Gel filtration analysis of cdk4 complexes shows that a chaperone complex cdk4–cdc37–Hsp90, which protects cdk4 from degradation, is abundant in proliferating livers that lack C/EBP-alpha, but this complex is sparse or undetectable in livers expressing C/EBP-alpha. C/EBP-alpha disrupts the cdk4–cdc37–Hsp90 complex by direct interaction with cdk4 and reduces protein levels of cdk4 by increasing proteasome-dependent degradation of cdk4 (Wang et al., 2002) (Figure 14.6).

14.5.4
C/EBP-alpha and p107 Protein–Protein Interaction Disrupts E2F Complexes

C/EBP-alpha controls the composition of E2F complexes through interaction with the retinoblastoma (Rb)-like protein, p107, during prenatal liver development. S-phase–specific E2F complexes containing E2F, DP, cdk2, cyclin A, and p107 were observed in the developing liver. In wild-type animals these complexes disappeared by day 18 of gestation and were no longer present in newborn mice. In the C/EBP-alpha knockout mouse, the S-phase–specific complexes did not diminish and persisted to birth. The elevation of levels of the S-phase–specific E2F–p107 complexes in C/EBP-alpha knockout mice correlated with the increased expression of several E2F-dependent genes, such as those that encode cyclin A, proliferating cell nuclear antigen, and p107. The C/EBP-alpha–mediated regulation of E2F binding is specific, since the deletion of another C/EBP family member, C/EBP-beta, does not change the pattern of E2F binding during prenatal liver development. The addition of bacterially expressed, purified His-C/EBP-alpha to the E2F-binding reaction resulted in disruption of E2F complexes containing p107 in nuclear extracts from C/EBP-alpha knockout mouse livers. Ectopic expression of C/EBP-alpha in cultured cells also led to a decrease in E2F complexes containing Rb family proteins (Timchenko et al., 1999b). Coimmunoprecipitation analyses revealed an interaction of C/EBP-alpha with p107 but none with cdk2, E2F1, or cyclin A. A region of C/EBP-alpha that has sequence similarity to E2F is sufficient for disruption of the E2F–p107 complexes. Despite its role as a DNA binding protein, C/EBP-alpha brings about a change in E2F complex composition through protein–protein interaction. The disruption of E2F–p107 complexes correlates with C/EBP-alpha–mediated growth arrest of hepatocytes in newborn mice (Timchenko et al., 1999b) (Figure 14.6). Using an E2F-DP1–responsive promoter linked to a reporter gene revealed that C/EBP-alpha directly inhibits the induction of this promoter by E2F-DP1 in transient-transfection assays. Furthermore, C/EBP-alpha inhibits the S-phase induction of the E2F and DHFR promoters in permanent cell lines (Slomiany et al., 2000). These findings delineate a straightforward mechanism for C/EBP-alpha–mediated cell growth arrest through repression of E2F-DP–mediated S-phase transcription.

14.5.5 C/EBP-beta Arrests the Cell Cycle Before the G1/S Boundary

During postnatal liver development, C/EBP-beta expression and hepatocyte proliferation are mutually exclusive. In addition to trans-activating liver-specific genes, C/EBP-beta, but not C/EBP-alpha, arrests the cell cycle before the G1–S boundary in HepG2 hepatoma cells. LIP, a liver-inhibitory protein, which is translated from C/EBP-beta mRNA lacking the activation domain of C/EBP-beta, is not only ineffective in blocking hepatoma cell proliferation but also antagonizes the effect of C/EBP-beta on the cell cycle. Deletion analysis indicated that this effect of LIP required only the DNA-binding and leucine zipper domains. In addition, integrity of the C/EBP-beta dimerization and activation domains was indispensable for the arrest of cell proliferation induced by C/EBP-beta (Buck et al., 1994). Thus, hepatocyte differentiation and its characteristic quiescent state may be modulated by the C/EBP-beta LAP/LIP ratio.

14.6 DBP Circadian Gene Regulation in the Liver

In mammals, many physiological processes are subject to circadian regulation. These include sleep–wake cycles, body temperature, heartbeat, blood pressure, endocrine functions, renal activity, and liver metabolism (for review, see Schibler and Lavery, 1999). DBP accumulates in hepatocytes of adult rats according to a strictly controlled circadian rhythm (amplitude approx. 1000-fold). In rat parenchymal hepatocytes, the DBP protein is barely detectable during the morning. At about 2 p.m. DBP levels begin to rise, reach maximal levels at 8 p.m., and decline sharply during the night. This rhythm persists with regard to its amplitude and phase in the absence of external time cues, such as daily dark–light switches (Wuarin and Schibler, 1990; Wuarin et al., 1992). The amplitude of circadian DBP mRNA oscillation can largely account for the daily amplitude in DBP protein oscillation (Fonjallaz et al., 1996). The mRNA accumulation oscillates not only in peripheral tissues such as liver, but also in neurons of the suprachiasmatic nucleus, which are believed to harbour the central circadian pacemaker. According to the currently held model, these oscillators are synchronized via chemical cues by a master pacemaker residing in the suprachiasmatic nucleus of the hypothalamus, which itself is entrained by the photoperiod (Yamazaki et al., 2000).

Although DBP is not essential for embryonic development or survival during adulthood, it is involved in the control of several circadian effects. Mice homozygous for a *DBP* null allele differ from wild-type mice in the period length and the amplitude of circadian locomotor activity, in several electroencephalogram (EEG) parameters of sleeping behaviour (Franken et al., 2000), and in the circadian expression of some liver genes, such as those specifying steroid 15á hydroxylase (CYP2A4) and coumarin 7 hydroxylase (CYP2A5) (Schibler and Lavery; 1999). Run-on experiments with isolated nuclei and physical mapping of nascent RNA chains suggest that circadian transcription plays a pivotal role in rhythmic DBP expression. Since *DBP–/–* mice are still rhythmic and since DBP protein is not required for the circadian expression of its own gene, *DBP* is more likely to be a component of the circadian output pathway than a master gene of the clock (Lopez-Molina et al., 1997).

In the liver, most known genes with rhythmic expression encode enzymes or regulatory proteins involved in food processing and energy homeostasis. These include cholesterol 7alpha hydroxylase (CYP7) (Lavery and Schibler, 1993), the rate-limiting enzyme in the synthesis of bile acids, several cytochrome P450 enzymes involved in detoxification and elimination of food components (e.g., CYP2A5) (Lavery et al., 1999), enzymes involved in carbohydrate metabolism (e.g., PEPCK, glycogen synthase, glycogen phosphorylase), and transcription factors governing fatty acid metabolism (e.g., PPAR and spot 14). At least in the liver, the coordination of physiological needs during the absorptive and postabsorptive phases may be the major function of circadian oscillators. In the liver of nocturnal rats, the phase of the daily DBP mRNA accumulation profile is severely altered when food is offered exclusively during the day (Ogawa et al., 1997). These findings probably have profound implications for the design of animal studies and possibly even for cell culture experiments.

It is believed that the suprachiasmatic nucleus clock entrains the phase of peripheral clocks via chemical cues, such as rhythmically secreted hormones. Temporal feeding restriction under light–dark or dark–dark conditions can change the phase of circadian gene expression in peripheral cell types by up to 12 h while leaving the phase of cyclic gene expression in the suprachiasmatic nucleus unaffected. Therefore, changes in metabolism can lead to an uncoupling of peripheral oscillators from the central pacemaker. Sudden large changes in feeding time, similar to abrupt changes in the photoperiod, reset the phase of rhythmic gene expression gradually and are thus likely to act through a clock-dependent mechanism. Food-induced phase resetting proceeds faster in the liver than in the kidney, heart, or pancreas, but after one week of daytime feeding, the phases of circadian gene expression are similar in all examined peripheral tissues (Damiola et al., 2000).

14.7
Conclusions and Outlook

Considerable evidence stems from the use of knockout and transgenic animal models to demonstrate a pivotal role of HNFs, C/EBPs and DBP in liver biology and key metabolic functions. For example, C/EBP-alpha knockout mice die shortly after birth due to hypoglycaemia. The published evidence points to a complex network of liver-enriched transcription factors and other regulatory proteins to orchestrate the timely and coordinated expression of liver-specific genes, including the proteins necessary for carbohydrate, lipid, and protein metabolism. Other important features include regulatory functions in cell cycle control, carcinogenesis, circadian gene regulation, liver regeneration, and apoptosis.

The importance of C/EBPs in epithelial tumour biology needs to be investigated further to develop a unified understanding of their role in cellular dedifferentiation and malignant transformation. Rescue of high expression levels of C/EBPs may be an important strategy for molecular therapy of liver tumours based on hepatocellular redifferentiation, as observed during liver regeneration.

A fascinating role of DBP lies in the control of circadian gene expression in the liver, which seems to be adapted to and entrained by feeding times. It will therefore be of considerable interest to understand the role of DBP in disease. For instance, rhythmic DBP expression is likely to be altered in unconscious intensive-care patients fed parenterally over prolonged periods of time. The clinically observed deterioration in liver function may be a consequence of desynchronized DBP expression leading to derailed metabolic competence. Likewise, the frequently observed differences in liver gene expression *in vivo* and *in vitro* may be the result of disturbed DBP function.

Proteomics and transcriptomics data on protein changes in human livers in pathologic conditions such as viral hepatitis (e.g., hepatitis B or C), primary sclerosing cholangitis, or primary biliary cirrhosis are still lacking. In the future, proteome analyses using human tumour tissues, which reflect the pathological state of hepatocellular carcinoma or cholangiocellular carcinoma more closely, will be undertaken. This work will complement the gene expression studies of hepatocellular carcinoma, which are already under way. Efforts have also been directed at the proteome analysis of hepatic stellate cells, since these cells play an important role in liver fibrosis. Since liver fibrosis is reversible but cirrhosis is not, it is of considerable importance to identify therapeutic targets that can slow its progression (Seow et al., 2001). Current limitations of the toxicogenomics approach involving speed of throughput are being overcome by increasing automation and the development of new techniques. The isotope-coded affinity tag method appears particularly promising (Kennedy, 2002). Although new associations between proteins and toxicopathological effects are expected to be uncovered by this new technology, limitations include the fact that this methodology offers a new descriptive dimension without any mechanistic insights and an implied temptation to overemphasize epiphenomena. Finally, knowledge of mutations and nucleotide polymorphisms of liver-enriched transcription factors will be invaluable for understanding diseases. In particular, mutations in the single-exon gene C/EBP-alpha might impair growth control and cellular differentiation and thus may play an overwhelming role in liver tumours, as observed in the differentiation block during acute myeloid leukaemia.

The expression of liver-specific genes requires a timely and coordinated expression of different transcription factors from distinct chromosomes. For example, the alpha1-antitrypsin gene contains binding sites for HNF-1, HNF-3, HNF-4, and HNF-6, which interact with the liver-enriched transcription factors HNF-1_, HNF-3_, HNF-4_1, HNF-4_2, HNF-6_, and HNF-6_ (Sladek et al., 1990; De Simone and Cortese, 1991; Samadani and Costa, 1996). Liver-enriched transcription factors that bind to the regulatory sequences of the alpha1-antitrypsin gene have been assigned to human chromosome 12 region q22-qter, chromosome 20q, and chromosome 15 region q21.1–21–2. Furthermore, the transcription factors that bind to the alpha1-antitrypsin regulatory sequence also influence the transcriptional activity of each other. Thus, a considerable challenge for further investigations on the regulation of transcriptional networks will be understanding the molecular basis of the orchestration of transcriptional events that are interdependent and at the same time separated on different chromosomes. It can be expected that the chromatin remodelling complexes, as well as biochemical modifications of chromatin, play pivotal roles in liver development and liver-specific gene expression. In the future, the exact role of higher-order chromatin structure and function in liver development and liver function will need to be determined. Protein–protein interactions between transcription factors and cofactors, as well as between components of multiprotein complexes and transcription factors, are coming more into focus and illustrate the true complexity of gene transcription. In the post-human genome era and with the availability of the human DNA sequence, we find ourselves confronted with a plethora of new challenges ahead that will provide newfound knowledge on the origin of life and the molecular basis of disease. There is optimism that new platform technologies in functional genomics will unveil the secrets of gene regulation and phenotype expression.

Acknowledgments

This work was supported in part by research grants from Novartis Pharma GmbH Germany, BU Transplantation and Immunology, to H.S. and J.K. and from the Lower Saxony Ministry of Science and Culture to J.B. We thank Robert Schrem for producing the excellent figures for this article, as well as for helpful discussions. This article is dedicated to Amanda and Jemima Schrem for their patience with their father during preparation of this article.

References

Akira S, Isshiki H, Sugita T, Tanabe O, Kinoshita S, Nishio Y, Nakajima T, Hirano T, and Kishimoto T (1990) A nuclear factor for IL-6 expression (NF-IL6) is a member of a C/EBP family. EMBO J 9 : 1897–1906.

Alonzi T, Gorgoni B, Screpanti I, Gulino A, and Poli V (1997) Interleukin-6 and CAAT/enhancer binding protein beta-deficient mice act as tools to dissect the IL-6 signalling pathway and IL-6 regulation. Immunobiology 198 : 144–156.

Antes TJ, Chen J, Cooper AD, and Levy-Wilson B (2000) The nuclear matrix protein CDP represses hepatic transcription of the human cholesterol-7alpha hydroxylase gene. J Biol Chem 275 : 26649–26660.

Arizmendi C, Liu S, Croniger C, Poli V, and Friedman JE (1999) The transcription factor CCAAT/enhancer-binding protein alpha regulates gluconeogenesis and phosphoenolpyruvate carboxykinase (GTP) gene transcription during diabetes. J Biol Chem 274 : 13033–13040.

Bannister AJ and Kouzarides T (1996) The CBP co-activator is a histone acetyltransferase. Nature 384 : 641–643.

Barlev NA, Candau R, Wang L, Darpino P, Silverman N, and Berger SL (1995) Characterization of physical interactions of the putative transcriptional adaptor, ADA2, with acidic activation domains and TATA-binding protein. J Biol Chem 33 : 19337–19344.

Birkenmeier EH, Gwynn B, Howard S, Jerry J, Gordon JI, Landschulz WH, and McKnight SL (1989) Tissue-specific expression, developmental regulation and genetic mapping of the gene encoding CCAAT/enhancer binding protein. Genes Dev 3 : 1146–1156.

Bort R, Gomez-Lechon MJ, Castell JV, Jover R (2004). Role of hepatocyte nuclear factor 3 gamma in the expression of human CYP2C genes. Arch Biochem Biophys 426(1) :63–72

Brandsen J, Werten S, van der Vliet PC, Meisterernst M, Kroon J, and Gros P (1997) C-terminal domain of transcription cofactor-PC4 reveals dimeric ssDNA binding site. Nat Struct Biol 4 : 900–903.

Buck M, Turler H, and Chojkier M (1994) LAP (NF-IL-6), a tissue-specific transcriptional activator, is an inhibitor of hepatoma cell proliferation. EMBO J 13 : 851–860.

Buggs C, Nasrin N, Mode A, Tollet P, Zhao HF, Gustafsson JA, and Alexander-Bridges M (1998) IRE-ABP (insulin response element-A binding protein), an SRY-like protein, inhibits C/EBP-alpha (CCAAT/enhancer-binding protein alpha)-stimulated expression of the sex-specific cytochrome P450 2C12 gene. Mol Endocrinol 12 : 1294–1309.

Burgess-Beusse BL, Darlington GJ (1998) C/EBPalpha is critical for the neonatal acute-phase response to inflammation. Mol Cell Biol 18 : 7269–7277.

Burgess-Beusse BL, Timchenko NA, and Darlington GJ (1999) CCAAT/enhancer binding protein alpha (C/EBP-alpha) is an important mediator of mouse C/EBP-beta protein isoform production. Hepatology 29 : 597–601.

Chartier FL, Bossu JP, Laudet V, Fruchart JC, and Laine B (1994) Cloning and sequencing of cDNAs encoding the human hepatocyte nuclear factor 4 indicate the presence of two isoforms in human liver. Gene 147 : 269–272.

Chen HW, Lin RJ, Schlitz D, Chakravarti A, Nash A, Nagy L, Privalsky ML, Nakatani Y, and Evans RM (1997) Nuclear receptor coactivator ACTR is a novel histone acetyltransferase and forms a multimeric activation complex with P/CAF and CBP/p300. Cell 90 : 569–580.

Chen WS, Manova K, Weinstein DC, Duncan SA, Plump AS, Prezioso VR, Bachvarova RF, and Darnell JE, Jr (1994) Disruption of the HNF-4 gene, expressed in visceral endoderm, leads to cell death in embryonic ectoderm and impaired gastrulation of mouse embryos. Genes Dev 8 : 2466–2477.

Cook PW, Swanson KT, Edwards CP, and Firestone GL (1988) Glucocorticoid receptor-dependent inhibition of cellular proliferation in dexamethasone-resistant and hypersensitive rat hepatoma cell variants. Mol Cell Biol 8 : 1449–1459.

Costa RH, Kalinichenko VV, Holterman AX, Wang X (2003) Transcription factors in liver development, differentiation, and regeneration. Hepatology 38 : 1331–1347

Cram EJ, Ramos RA, Wang EC, Cha HH, Nishio Y, and Firestone GL (1998) Role of the CCAAT/enhancer binding protein-alpha transcription factor in the glucocorticoid stimulation of p21waf1/cip1 gene promoter activity in growth-arrested rat hepatoma cells. J Biol Chem 273 : 2008–2014.

Crosson SM, Davies GF, and Roesler WJ (1997) Hepatic expression of CCAAT/enhancer binding protein alpha: hormonal and metabolic regulation in rats. Diabetologia 40 : 1117–1124.

Damiola F, Le Minh N, Preitner N, Kornmann B, Fleury-Olela F, and Schibler U (2000) Restricted feeding uncouples circadian oscillators in peripheral tissues from the central pacemaker in the suprachiasmatic nucleus. Genes Dev 14 : 2950–2961.

Darlington GJ, Wang N, and Hanson RW (1995) C/EBP alpha: a critical regulator of genes governing integrative metabolic processes. Curr Opin Genet Dev 5 : 565–570.

Dell H and Hadzopoulou-Cladaras M (1999) CREB-binding protein is a transcriptional coactivator for hepatocyte nuclear factor-4 and enhances apolipoprotein gene expression. J Biol Chem 274 : 9013–9021.

Descharette J and Weiss MC (1974) Characterization of differentiated and dedifferentiated clones from rat hepatoma. Biochimie 56 : 1603–1611.

Diehl AM, Michaelson P, and Yang SQ (1994) Selective induction of CCAAT/enhancer binding protein isoforms occurs during rat liver development. Gastroenterology 106 : 1625–1637.

Diehl AM, Johns DC, Yang S, Lin H, Yin M, Matelis LA, and Lawrence JH (1996) Adenovirus-mediated transfer of CCAAT/enhancer-binding protein-alpha identifies a dominant antiproliferative role for this isoform in hepatocytes. J Biol Chem 271: 7343–7350.

Dogra SC and May BK (1997) Liver-enriched transcription factors, HNF-1, HNF-3 and C/EBP, are major contributors to the strong activity of the chicken CYP2H1 promoter in chick embryo hepatocytes. DNA Cell Biol 16 : 1407–1418.

Drewes T, Senkel S, Holewa B, and Ryffel GU (1996) Human hepatocyte nuclear factor 4 isoforms are encoded by distinct and differentially expressed genes. Mol Cell Biol 16 : 925–931.

Duncan SA, Navas MA, Dufort D, Rossant J, and Stoffel M (1998) Regulation of a transcription factor network required for differentiation and metabolism. Science 281 : 692–695.

Duong DT, Waltner-Law ME, Sears R, Sealy L, and Granner DK (2002) Insulin inhibits hepatocellular glucose production by utilizing liver-enriched transcriptional inhibitory protein to disrupt the association of CREB-binding protein and RNA polymerase II with the phosphoenolpyruvate carboxykinase gene promoter. J Biol Chem 277 : 32234–32242.

Faust DM, Boshart M, Imaizumi-Scherrer T, Schutz G, and Weiss MC (1994) Constancy of expression of the protein kinase A regulatory subunit R1 alpha in hepatoma cell lines of different phenotypes. Cell Growth Differ 5 : 47–53.

Fonjallaz P, Ossipow V, Wanner G, and Schibler U (1996) The two PAR leucine zipper proteins, TEF and DBP, display similar circadian and tissue-specific expression, but have different target promoter preferences. EMBO J 15 : 351–362.

Franken P, Lopes-Molina L, Marcacci L, Schibler U, and Tafti M (2000) The transcription factor DBP affects circadian sleep consolidation and rhythmic EEG activity. J Neurosci 20 : 617–625.

Furuta H, Iwasaki N, Oda N, Hinokio Y, Horikawa Y, Yamagata K, Yano N, Sugahiro J, Ogata M, Ohgawara H, et al. (1997) Organization and partial sequence of the hepatocyte nuclear factor-4 _/MODY1 gene and identification of a missense mutation, R127W, in a Japanese family with MODY. Diabetes 46: 1652–1657.

Ge H and Roeder RG (1994) Purification, cloning, and characterization of a human coactivator, PC4, that mediates transcriptional activation of class II genes. Cell 78 : 513–523.

Ghosh AK, Lacson R, Liu P, Cichy SB, Danilkovich A, Guo S, and Unterman TG (2001) A nucleoprotein complex containing CCAAT/enhancer-binding protein_ interacts with an insulin response sequence in the insulin-like growth factor binding protein-1 gene and contributes to insulin-regulated gene expression. J Biol Chem 276 : 8507–8515.

Glass CK, Rose DW, and Rosenfeld MG (1997) Nuclear receptor coactivators. Curr Opin Cell Biol 9 : 222–232.

Green VJ, Kokkotou E, and Ladias JA (1998) Critical structural elements and multitarget protein interactions of the transcriptional activator AF-1 of hepatocyte nuclear factor 4. J Biol Chem 273 : 29950–29957.

Greenbaum LE, Cressman DE, Haber BA, and Taub R (1995) Coexistence of C/EBP alpha, beta, growth-induced proteins and DNA synthesis in hepatocytes during liver regeneration. Implications for maintenance of the differentiated state during liver growth. J Clin Invest 96:1351–1365.

Griffo G, Hamon-Benais C, Angrand PO, Fox M, West L, Lecoq O, Povey S, Cassio D, and Weiss M (1993) HNF4 and HNF1 as well as a panel of hepatic functions are extinguished and reexpressed in parallel in chromosomally reduced rat hepatoma–human fibroblast hybrids. J Cell Biol 121:887–898.

Hakkola J, Tanaka E, and Pelkonen O (1998) Developmental expression of cytochrome P450 enzymes in human liver. Pharmacol Toxicol 82:209–217.

Hakkola J, Raunio H, Purkunen R, Saarikoski S, Vahakangas K, Pelkonen O, Edwards RJ, Boobis AR, and Pasanen M (2001) Cytochrome P450 3A expression in the human fetal liver: evidence that CYP3A5 is expressed in only a limited number of fetal livers. Biol Neonate 80:193–201.

Harris TE, Albrecht JH, Nakanishi M, and Darlington GJ (2001) CCAAT/enhancer binding protein-alpha cooperates with p21 to inhibit cyclin-dependent kinase-2 activity and induces growth arrest independent of DNA binding. J Biol Chem 276:29200–29209.

Hata S, Inoue T, Kosuga K, Nakashima T, Tsukamoto T, and Osumi T (1995) Identification of two splice isoforms of mRNA for mouse hepatocyte nuclear factor 4 (HNF-4). Biochim Biophys Acta 1260:55–61.

Hendricks-Taylor LR and Darlington GJ (1995) Inhibition of cell proliferation by C/EBP alpha occurs in many cell types, does not require the presence of p53 or Rb and is not affected by large T-antigen. Nucleic Acids Res 23:4726–4733.

Hertz R, Magenheim J, Berman I, and Bar-Tana J (1998) Fatty acyl-CoA thioesters are ligands of hepatic nuclear factor-4a. Nature 392:512–516.

Holewa B, Zapp D, Drewes T, Senkel S, and Ryffel GU (1997) HNF4alpha, a new gene of the HNF4 family with distinct activation and expression profiles in oogenesis and embryogenesis of Xenopus laevis. Mol Cell Biol 17:687–694.

Jacquemin P, Lannoy VJ, Rousseau GG, and Lemaigre FP (1999) OC-2, a novel mammalian member of the ONECUT class of homeodomain transcription factors whose function in liver partially overlaps with that of hepatocyte nuclear factor-6. J Biol Chem 274:2665–2671.

Jiang G, Nepomuceno L, Hopkins K, and Sladek FM (1995) Exclusive homodimerization of the orphan receptor hepatocyte nuclear factor 4 defines a new subclass of nuclear receptors. Mol Cell Biol 15:5131–5143.

Jiang JG and Zarnegar R (1997) A novel transcriptional regulatory region within the core promoter of the hepatocyte growth factor gene is responsible for its inducibility by cytokines via the C/EBP family of transcription factors. Mol Cell Biol 17:5758–5770.

Jover R, Bort R, Gomez-Lechon MJ, and Castell JV (1998) Re-expression of C/EBP alpha induces CYP2B6, CYP2C9 and CYP2D6 genes in HepG2 cells. FEBS Lett 431: 227–230.

Kamei Y, Xu L, Heinzel T, Torchia J, Kurokawa R, Gloss B, Lin SC, Heyman RA, Rose DW, Glass CK, and Rosenfeld MG (1996) A CBP integrator complex mediates transcriptional activation and AP-1 inhibition by nuclear receptors. Cell 85:403–414.

Kamiya A, Inoue Y, Gonzalez FJ (2003). Role of the hepatocyte nuclear factor 4alpha in control of the pregnane X receptor during fetal liver development. Hepatology 37:1375–1384

Kimura A, Nishiyori A, Murakami T, Tsukamoto T, Hata S, Osumi T, Okamura R, Mori M, and Takiguchi M (1993) Chicken ovalbumin upstream promotertranscription factor (COUP-TF) represses transcription from the promoter of the gene for ornithine transcarbamylase in a manner antagonistic to hepatocyte nuclear factor-4 (HNF-4). J Biol Chem 268:11125–11133.

Kimura T, Christoffels VM, Chowdhury S, Iwase K, Matsuzaki H, Mori M, Lamers WH, Darlington GJ, and Takiguchi M (1998) Hypoglycemia-associated hyperammonemia caused by impaired expression of ornithine cycle enzyme genes in C/EBP-alpha knockout mice. J Biol Chem 273:27505–27510.

Koj A (1996) Initiation of acute phase response and synthesis of cytokines. Biochim Biophys Acta 1317:84–94.

Kritis AA, Ktistaki E, Barda D, Zannis VI, and Talianidis I (1993) An indirect negative autoregulatory mechanism involved in hepatocyte nuclear factor-1 gene expression. Nucleic Acids Res 21:5882–5889.

Kritis AA, Argyrokastritis A, Moschonas NK, Power S, Katrakili N, Zannis VI, Cereghini S, and Talianidis I (1996) Isolation and characterization of a third isoform of human hepatocyte nuclear factor 4. Gene 173 : 275–280.

Ktistaki E and Talianidis I (1997 a) Modulation of hepatic gene expression by hepatocyte nuclear factor 1. Science 277 : 109–112.

Ktistaki E and Talianidis I (1997 b) Chicken ovalbumin upstream promoter transcription factors act as auxiliary cofactors for hepatocyte nuclear factor 4 and enhance hepatic gene expression. Mol Cell Biol 17 : 2790–2797.

Ktistaki E, Ktistakis NT, Papadogeorgaki E, and Talianidis I (1995) Recruitment of hepatocyte nuclear factor 4 into specific intranuclear compartments depends on tyrosine phosphorylation that affects its DNA-binding and transactivation potential. Proc Natl Acad Sci USA 92 : 9876–9880.

Kubicka S, Kuhnel F, Zender L, Rudolph KL, Plumpe J, Manns M, and Trautwein C (1999) p53 represses CAAT enhancer-binding protein (C/EBP)-dependent transcription of the albumin gene. A molecular mechanism involved in viral liver infection with implications for hepatocarcinogenesis. J Biol Chem 274 : 32137–32144.

Landry C, Clotman F, Hioki T, Oda H, Picard JJ, Lemaigre FP, and Rousseau GG (1997) HNF-6 is expressed in endoderm derivatives and nervous system of the mouse embryo and participates to the cross-regulatory network of liver-enriched transcription factors. Dev Biol 192 : 247–257.

Lannoy VJ, Burglin TR, Rousseau GG, Lemaigre FP (1998). Isoforms of hepatocyte nuclear factor-6 differ in DNA-binding properties, contain a bifunctional homeodomain, and define the new ONECUT class of homeodomain proteins. J Biol Chem 273 : 13552–13562

Lavery DJ and Schibler U (1993) Circadian transcription of the cholesterol 7-alpha-hydroxylase gene may involve the liver-enriched bZIP protein DBP. Genes Dev 7 : 1871–1884.

Lavery DJ, Lopez-Molina L, Margueron R, Fleury-Olela F, Conquet F, Schibler U, and Bonfils C (1999) Circadian expression of the steroid 15alpha hydroxylase (cyp2a4) and coumarin 7 hydroxylase (cyp2a5) genes in mouse liver is regulated by the PAR leucine zipper transcription factor DBP. Mol Cell Biol 19 : 6488–6499.

Lee YH, Alberta JA, Gonzalez FJ, and Waxman DJ (1994) Multiple, functional DBP sites on the promoter of the cholesterol-7-alpha-hydroxylase P450 gene, CYP7. Proposed role in diurnal regulation of liver gene expression. J Biol Chem 269 : 14681–14689.

Lee YH, Sauer B, Johnson PF, and Gonzalez FJ (1997) Disruption of the c/ebp alpha gene in adult mouse liver. Mol Cell Biol 17 : 6014–6022.

Lee YH, Sauer B, and Gonzalez FJ (1998) Laron dwarfism and non-insulin dependent diabetes mellitus in the Hnf-1alpha knockout mouse. Mol Cell Biol 18: 3059–3068.

Lee YK, Dell H, Dowhan DH, Hadzopoulou-Cladaras M, and Moore DD (2000) The orphan nuclear receptor SHP inhibits hepatocyte nuclear factor 4 and retinoid X receptor transactivation: two mechanisms for repression. Mol Cell Biol 20 : 187–195.

Lee YM, Miau LH, Chang CJ, and Lee SC (1996) Transcriptional induction of the alpha-1 acid glycoprotein (AGP) gene by synergistic interaction of two alternative activator forms of AGP/enhancer-binding protein (C/EBP beta) and NF-kappaB or Nopp140. Mol Cell Biol 16 : 4257–4263.

Lopez-Molina L, Conquet F, Dubois-Dauphin M, and Schibler U (1997) The DBP gene is expressed according to a circadian rhythm in the suprachiasmatic nucleus and influences circadian behavior. EMBO J 16 : 6762–6771.

Luc PV, Adesnik M, Ganguly S, and Shaw PM (1996) Transcriptional regulation of the CYP2B1 and CYP2B2 genes by C/EBP-related proteins. Biochem Pharmacol 51 : 345–356.

Malik S, Gu W, Wu W, Qin J, and Roeder RG (2000) The USA-derived transcriptional coactivator PC2 is a submodule of TRAP/SMCC and acts synergistically with other PCs. Mol Cell 5 : 753–760.

Matsumoto K and Nakamura T (1992) Hepatocyte growth factor: molecular structure, roles in liver regeneration, and other biological functions. Crit Rev Oncog 3 : 27–54.

Matsuno F, Chowdhury S, Gotoh T, Iwase K, Matsuzaki H, Takatsuki K, Mori M, and Takiguchi M (1996) Induction of the C/EBP beta gene by dexamethasone and glucagon in primary-cultured rat hepatocytes. J Biochem 119 : 524–532.

Mendel DB, Hansen LP, Graves MK, Conley PB, and Crabtree GR (1991 a) HNF-1alpha and HNF-1beta (vHNF-1) share dimerization and homeo domains, but not activation domains, and form heterodimers *in vitro*. Genes Dev 5 : 1042–1056.

Mendel DB, Khavari PA, Conley PB, Graves MK, Hansen LP, Admon A, and Crabtree GR (1991 b) Characterization of a cofactor that regulates dimerization of a mammalian homeodomain protein. Science 254 : 1762–1767.

Miau LH, Chang CJ, Tsai WH, and Lee SC (1997) Identification and characterization of a nucleolar phosphoprotein, Nopp140, as a transcription factor. Mol Cell Biol 17 : 230–239.

Miau LH, Chang CJ, Shen BJ, Tsai WH, and Lee SC (1998) Identification of heterogeneous nuclear ribonucleoprotein K (hnRNP K) as a repressor of C/EBPbeta- mediated gene activation. J Biol Chem 273 : 10784–10791.

Mischoulon D, Rana B, Bucher NL, and Farmer SR (1992) Growth-dependent inhibition of CCAAT enhancer-binding protein (C/EBP alpha) gene expression during hepatocyte proliferation in the regenerating liver and in culture. Mol Cell Biol 12 : 2553–2560.

Miura N and Tanaka K (1993) Analysis of the rat hepatocyte nuclear factor (HNF) 1 gene promoter: synergistic activation by HNF4 and HNF1 proteins. Nucleic Acids Res 21 : 3731–3736.

Mukherjee D, Kaestner KH, Kovalovich KK, and Greenbaum LE (2001) Fas-induced apoptosis in mouse hepatocytes is dependent on C/EBP_. Hepatology 33 : 1166–1172.

Nakhei H, Lingott A, Lemm I, and Ryffel GU (1998) An alternative splice variant of the tissue specific transcription factor HNF4_ predominates in undifferentiated murine cell types. Nucleic Acids Res 26 : 497–504.

Nepveu A (2001) Role of the multifunctional CDP/Cut/Cux homeodomain transcription factor in regulating differentiation, cell growth, and development. Gene 270: 1–15.

Niehof M, Streetz K, Rakemann T, Bischoff SC, Manns MP, Horn F, and Trautwein C (2001) Interleukin-6-induced tethering of STAT3 to the LAP/C/EBP_promoter suggests a new mechanism of transcriptional regulation by STAT3. J Biol Chem 276 : 9016–9027.

Ogawa A, Yano M, Tsujinaka T, Morimoto T, Morita S, Taniguchi M, Shiozaki H, Okamoto K, Sato S, and Monden M (1997) Modulation of circadian expression of D-site binding protein by the schedule of parenteral nutrition in rat liver. Hepatology 26 : 1580–1586.

Ogryzko VV, Schlitz RL, Russanova V, Howard BH, and Nakatani Y (1996) The transcriptional coactivators p300 and CBP are histone acetyltransferases. Cell 87 : 953–959.

Ourlin JC, Jounaidi Y, Maurel P, and Vilarem MJ (1997) Role of the liver-enriched transcription factors C/EBP alpha and DBP in the expression of human CYP3A4 and CYP3A7. J Hepatol 26 Suppl 2 : 54–62.

Pani L, Qian XB, Clevidence D, and Costa RH (1992 b) The restricted promoter activity of the liver transcription factor hepatocyte nuclear factor 3 beta involves a cell-specific factor and positive autoactivation. Mol Cell Biol 12 : 552–562.

Park Y and Kemper B (1996) The CYP2B1 proximal promoter contains a functional C/EBP regulatory element. DNA Cell Biol 5: 693–701.

Poli V, Mancini FP, and Cortese R (1990) IL-6DBP, a nuclear protein involved in interleukin-6 signal transduction, defines a new family of leucine zipper proteins related to C/EBP. Cell 63 : 643–653.

Pontoglio M, Barra J, Hadchouel M, Doyen A, Kress C, Bach JP, Babinet C, and Yaniv M (1996) Hepatocyte nuclear factor 1 inactivation results in hepatic dysfunction, phenylketonuria, and renal Fanconi syndrome. Cell 84 : 575–585.

Rachez C, Gamble M, Chang CPB, Atkins CB, Lazar MA, and Freedman LP (2000) The Drip complex and Src-1/p160 coactivators share similar nuclear receptor binding determinants but constitute functionally distinct complexes. Mol Cell Biol 20 : 2718–2726.

Ramos RA, Nishio Y, Maiyar AC, Simon KE, Ridder CC, Ge Y, and Firestone GL (1996) Glucocorticoid-stimulated CCAAT/enhancer-binding protein alpha expression is required for steroid-induced G1 cell cycle arrest of minimal-deviation rat hepatoma cells. Mol Cell Biol 16 : 5288–5301.

Rausa F, Samadani U, Ye H, Lim L, Fletcher CF, Jenkins NA, Copeland NG, and Costa RH (1997) The cut-homeodomain transcriptional activator HNF-6 is coexpressed with its target gene HNF-3beta in the developing murine liver and pancreas. Dev Biol 192 : 228–246.

Roesler WJ (2000) What is a cAMP response unit? Mol Cell Endocrinol 162 : 1–7.

Runge D, Runge DM, Bowen WC, Locker J, and Michalopoulos GK (1997) Matrix induced re-differentiation of cultured rat hepatocytes and changes of CCAAT/enhancer binding proteins. Biol Chem 378 : 873–881.

Samadani U and Costa RH (1996) The transcriptional activator hepatocyte nuclear factor 6 regulates liver gene expression. Mol Cell Biol 16:6273–6284.

Samadani U, Porcella A, Pani L, Johnson PF, Burch JB, Pine R, and Costa RH (1995) Cytokine regulation of the liver transcription factor hepatocyte nuclear factor-3 beta is mediated by the C/EBP family and interferon regulatory factor 1. Cell Growth Differ 6:879–890.

Schibler U and Lavery DJ (1999) Circadian timing in animals, in: Development: Genetics, Epigenetics and Environmental Regulation (Russo E, Cove D, Edgar L, Jaenisch R, and Salamini F eds.) pp 487–505, Springer-Verlag, Berlin.

Schrem H, Klempnauer J, and Borlak J (2002) Liver-enriched transcription factors in liver function and development. I. The hepatocyte nuclear factor network and liver-specific gene expression. Pharmacol Rev 54:129–158.

Schrem H, Klempnauer J, and Borlak J (2004) Liver-enriched transcription factors in liver function and development. Part II: the C/EBPs and D site-binding protein in cell cycle control, carcinogenesis, circadian gene regulation, liver regeneration, apoptosis, and liver-specific gene regulation. Pharmacol Rev 56:291–330.

Seol W, Choi HS, and Moore DD (1996) An orphan nuclear hormone receptor that lacks a DNA binding domain and heterodimerizes with other receptors. Science 272: 1336–1339.

Shen BJ, Chang CJ, Lee HS, Tsai WH, Miau LH, and Lee SC (1997) Transcriptional induction of the agp/ebp (c/ebp beta) gene by hepatocyte growth factor. DNA Cell Biol 16:703–711.

Skrtic S, Ekberg S, Wallenius V, Enerback S, Hedin L, and Jansson JO (1997) Changes in expression of CCAAT/enhancer binding protein alpha (C/EBP alpha) and C/EBP beta in rat liver after partial hepatectomy but not after treatment with cyproterone acetate. J Hepatol 27:903–911.

Sladek FM, Zhong WM, Lai E, and Darnell JE Jr (1990) Liver-enriched transcription factor HNF-4 is a novel member of the steroid hormone receptor superfamily. Genes Dev 4:2353–2365.

Slomiany BA, D'Arigo KL, Kelly MM, and Kurtz DT (2000) C/EBPalpha inhibits cell growth via direct repression of E2F-DP-mediated transcription. Mol Cell Biol 20: 5986–5997.

Soutoglou E, Katrakili N, and Talianidis I (2000a) Acetylation regulates transcription factor activity at multiple levels. Mol Cell 5: 745–751.

Soutoglou E, Papafotiou G, Katrakili N, and Talianidis I (2000b) Transcriptional activation by hepatocyte nuclear factor-1 requires synergism between multiple coactivator proteins. J Biol Chem 275:12515–12520.

Späth GF and Weiss MC (1997) Hepatocyte nuclear factor 4 expression overcomes repression of the hepatic phenotype in dedifferentiated hepatoma cells. Mol Cell Biol 17: 1913–1922.

Späth GF and Weiss MC (1998) Hepatocyte nuclear factor 4 provokes expression of epithelial marker genes, acting as a morphogen in dedifferentiated hepatoma cells. J Cell Biol 140:935–946.

Spencer TE, Jenster G, Burcin MM, Allis CD, Zhou J, Mizzen CA, McKenna NJ, Onate SA, Tsai SY, Tsai M, and O'Malley BW (1997) Steroid receptor coactivator-1 is a histone acetyltransferase. Nature 389:194–198.

Stoffel M and Duncan SA (1997) The maturity-onset diabetes of the young (MODY1) transcription factor HNF4_ regulates expression of genes required for glucose transport and metabolism. Proc Natl Acad Sci USA 94: 13209–13214.

Sugahara K, Iyama KI, Kimura T, Sano K, Darlington GJ, Akiba T, and Takiguchi M (2001) Mice lacking CCAAT/enhancer-binding protein-alpha show hyperproliferation of alveolar type II cells and increased surfactant protein mRNAs. Cell Tissue Res 306: 57–63.

Tannapfel A and Wittekind C (2002) Genes involved in hepatocellular carcinoma: deregulation in cell cycling and apoptosis. Virchows Arch 440:345–352.

Tian JM and Schibler U (1991) Tissue-specific expression of the gene encoding hepatocyte nuclear factor 1 may involve hepatocyte nuclear factor 4. Genes Dev 5:2225–2234.

Timchenko NA, Wilde M, Nakanishi M, Smith JR, and Darlington GJ (1996) CCAAT/enhancer-binding protein alpha (C/EBP alpha) inhibits cell proliferation through the p21 (WAF-1/CIP-1/SDI-1) protein. Genes Dev 10:804–815.

Timchenko NA, Harris TE, Wilde M, Bilyeu TA, Burgess-Beusse BL, Finegold MJ, and Darlington GJ (1997) CCAAT/enhancer binding protein alpha regulates p21 protein and hepatocyte proliferation in newborn mice. Mol Cell Biol 17:7353–7361.

Timchenko NA, Welm AL, Lu X, and Timchenko LT (1999 a) CUG repeat binding protein (CUGBP1) interacts with the 5′-region of C/EBP-beta mRNA and regulates translation of C/EBP-beta isoforms. Nucleic Acids Res 27:4517–4525.

Timchenko NA, Wilde M, and Darlington GJ (1999 b) C/EBPalpha regulates formation of S-phase–specific E2F–p107 complexes in livers of newborn mice. Mol Cell Biol 19: 2936–2945.

Tollet P, Lahuna O, Ahlgren R, Mode A, and Gustafsson JA (1995) CCAAT/enhancer binding protein-alpha–dependent transactivation of CYP2C12 in rat hepatocytes. Mol Endocrinol 9: 1771–1781.

Tomizawa M, Wang YQ, Ebara M, Saisho H, Watanabe K, Nakagawara A, and Tagawa M (2002) Decreased expression of the CCAAT/enhancer binding protein alpha gene involved in hepatocyte proliferation in human hepatocellular carcinomas. Int J Mol Med 9: 597–600.

Torchia J, Rose DW, Inostroza J, Kamei Y, Westin S, Glass CK, and Rosenfeld MG (1997) The transcriptional co-activator p/CIP binds CBP and mediates nuclear receptor function. Nature 387:677–684.

Trautwein C, Caelles C, van der Geer P, Hunter T, Karin M, and Chojkier M (1993) Transactivation by NF-IL6/LAP is enhanced by phosphorylation of its activation domain. Nature 364:544–547.

Trautwein C, van der Geer P, Karin M, Hunter T, and Chojkier M (1994) Protein kinase A and C site-specific phosphorylations of LAP (NF-IL6) modulate its binding affinity to DNA recognition elements. J Clin Invest 93:2554–2561.

Trautwein C, Rakemann T, Malek NP, Plumpe J, Tiegs G, and Manns MP (1998) Concanavalin A-induced liver injury triggers hepatocyte proliferation. J Clin Invest 101:1960–1969.

Ueno T, Gonzalez FJ (1990). Transcriptional control of the rat hepatic CYP2E1 gene. Mol Cell Biol 10:4495–4505

Umek RM, Friedman AD, and McKnight SL (1991) CCAAT-enhancer binding protein: a component of a differentiation switch. Science 251:288–292.

Viollet B, Kahn A, and Raymondjean M (1997) Protein kinase A-dependent phosphorylation modulates DNA-binding activity of hepatocyte nuclear factor 4. Mol Cell Biol 17: 4208–4219.

Wang H, Iakova P, Wilde M, Welm A, Goode T, Roesler WJ, and Timchenko NA (2001) C/EBPalpha arrests cell proliferation through direct inhibition of Cdk2 and Cdk4. Mol Cell 8:817–828.

Wang H, Goode T, Iakova P, Albrecht JH, and Timchenko NA (2002) C/EBPalpha triggers proteasome-dependent degradation of cdk4 during growth arrest. EMBO J 21:930–941.

Wang JC, Stafford JM, and Granner DK (1998 a) SRC-1 and GRIP1 coactivate transcription with hepatocyte nuclear factor 4. J Biol Chem 273:30847–30850.

Wang L, Liu L, and Berger SL (1998 b) Critical residues for histone acetylation by Gcn5, functioning in Ada and SAGA complexes, are also required for transcriptional function *in vivo*. Genes Dev 12:640–653.

Welm AL, Timchenko NA, and Darlington GJ (1999) C/EBP-alpha regulates generation of C/EBP-beta isoforms through activation of specific proteolytic cleavage. Mol Cell Biol 19: 1695–1704.

Welm AL, Mackey SL, Timchenko LT, Darlington GJ, and Timchenko NA (2000) Translational induction of liver-enriched transcriptional inhibitory protein during acute phase response leads to repression of CCAAT/enhancer binding protein alpha mRNA. J Biol Chem 275:27406–27413.

Williams JA, Ring BJ, Cantrell VE, Jones DR, Eckstein J, Ruterbories K, Hamman MA, Hall SD, and Wrighton SA (2002) Comparative metabolic capabilities of CYP3A4, CYP3A5 and CYP3A7. Drug Metab Dispos 30:883–891.

Wuarin J and Schibler U (1990) Expression of the liver-enriched transcriptional activator protein DBP follows a stringent circadian rhythm. Cell 63:1257–1266.

Wuarin J, Falvey E, Lavery D, Talbot D, Schmidt E, Ossipow V, Fonjallaz P, and Schibler U (1992) The role of the transcriptional activator protein DBP in circadian liver gene expression. J Cell Sci Suppl 16:123–127.

Xia C, Cheshire JK, Patel H, and Woo P (1997) Cross-talk between transcription factors NF-kappaB and C/EBP in the transcriptional regulation of genes. Int J Biochem Cell Biol 29:1525–1539.

Xu L, Hui L, Wang S, Gong J, Jin Y, Wang Y, Ji Y, Wu X, Han Z, and Hu G (2001) Expression profiling suggested a regulatory role of liver-enriched transcription factors in human hepatocellular carcinoma. Cancer Res 61: 3176–3181.

Yamada T, Tobita K, Osada S, Nishihara T, and Imagawa M (1997) CCAAT/enhancer-binding protein delta gene expression is mediated by APRF/STAT3. J Biochem 121: 731–738.

Yamazaki S, Numano R, Abe M, Hida A, Takahashi R, Ueda M, Block GD, Sakaki Y, Menaker M, and Tei H (2000) Resetting central and peripheral circadian oscillators in transgenic rats. Science 288: 682–685.

Yang XJ, Ogryzko VV, Nishikawa JI, Howard BH, and Nakatani Y (1996) A p300/CBP-associated factor that competes with the adenoviral oncoprotein E1A. Nature 382: 319–324.

Yao TP, Ku G, Zhou N, Scully R, Livingston DM (1996) The nuclear hormone receptor coactivator SRC-1 is a specific target of p300. Proc Natl Acad Sci USA 93: 10626–10631.

Yin M, Yang SQ, Lin HZ, Lane MD, Chatterjee S, and Diehl AM (1996) Tumor necrosis factor alpha promotes nuclear localization of cytokine-inducible CCAAT/enhancer binding protein isoforms in hepatocytes. J Biol Chem 271: 17974–17978.

Yoshida E, Aratani S, Itou H, Miyagishi M, Takiguchi M, Osumu T, Murakami K, and Fukamizu A (1997) Functional association between CBP and HNF4 in transactivation. Biochem Biophys Res Commun 241: 664–669.

Zhong W, Mirkovitch J, and Darnell JE Jr (1994) Tissue-specific regulation of mouse hepatocyte nuclear factor 4 expression. Mol Cell Biol 14: 7276–7284.

15
Toxicogenomics Applied to Understanding Cholestasis and Steatosis in the Liver

Timothy W. Gant, Peter Greaves, Andrew G. Smith, and Andreas Gescher

15.1
Introduction

Liver injury can be initiated by a multitude of agents; a few examples are viruses, parasites, and alcohol. Liver injury resulting from these agents takes a number of forms but can be manifest as fatty change, apoptosis, hepatocellular and bile duct damage, cholestasis, inflammation and hepatobiliary regeneration, and fibrosis. Cholestasis of the liver can be associated with liver injury but can also occur as a functional change with little or no associated injury. For instance, it can occur as a reaction to drug treatment or as the phenotypic result of several gene polymorphisms. The latter are a collection of diseases known as progressive familial intrahepatic cholestasis (PFIC), of which three types are linked to three different members of the ATP-binding cassette genes (ABC). These are the phospholipid export pump ABCB4, the bile salt export pump ABCB11, and a third (FIC1) that is presently without known function. The PFIC associated with the FIC1 transporter is known as Byler's disease. In addition to the progressive cholestatic phenotypes, mutations in the genes for the ABC transporters ABCC5/8 and ABCC2 give rise to the conditions of sitosterolemia (a disease characterized by net cholesterol retention) and Dubin–Johnson syndrome, respectively. Dubin–Johnson syndrome is characterized by an inability to transport bilirubin and amphiopathic ions and a persistent jaundice maintained through life. The cholestasis associated with Dubin–Johnson syndrome is not regarded as a true cholestatic phenotype, in comparison with that caused by mutation of the *ABCB4* gene, which is characterized by high serum GGT, portal inflammation, and bile duct proliferation. Patients with mutations in this gene often require liver transplantation. Similarly, Byler's disease is often fatal in the first decade of life without liver transplantation. By comparison, Dubin–Johnson syndrome is rarely fatal. Cholestatic diseases and their associations with transport proteins are reviewed in Trauner and Boyer [1], Trauner et al. [2], and Meier and Stieger [3]. Mutations in genes other than those for the transporter proteins can give rise to hepatobiliary injury with cholestasis. One such gene is the ferrochelatase (*Fech*) gene, which is the focus of two of the four studies presented in this chapter. *Fech* is respon-

Handbook of Toxicogenomics: Strategies and Applications. Edited by Jürgen Borlak

ISBN: 3-527-30342-1

sible for catalysis of the final step in heme biosynthesis, the insertion of the Fe into the protoporphyrin IX ring. Mutations in *Fech* giving rise to insufficiency (about 40 are described in the human population) may result in the deposition of protoporphyrin IX in the liver, which may can bile flow and produce cholestasis. Mutations in *Fech* tend to show differing levels of hepatic penetrance in the human population, suggesting that the full cholestatic phenotype and liver damage depends on the influence of other genes.

15.2
Models of Cholestatsis and Steatosis

15.2.1
The *Fech* Mouse

The ferrochelatase mutant BALB/c mouse (homozygous *Fech*^{m1Pas}/*Fech*^{m1Pas}) is phenotypically characterized by jaundice, hepatomagaly, splenomegaly, bilirubinemia, elevated protoporphyrin levels, and photosensitivity [4]. In this mouse the *Fech* gene carries a T→A transversion within exon 2, which results in a methionine-to-lysine amino acid substitution at position 98 (Figure 15.1) [5]. This mutation arose through random mutagenesis using enthylnitrosourea [4] and is a recessive phenotype inherited in a Mendelian manner. The mutation results in ferrochelatase insufficiency, leading to deposition of protoporphyrin IX in the liver and occlusion of the bile ducts, in turn leading to cholestasis. The level of ferrochelatase activity in the liver in the *Fech*^{m1Pas}/*Fech*^{m1Pas} mouse is approximately 2.7% of normal; the level in the heterozygote (*Fech*^{m1Pas}/*Fech*) is 65% of normal [4]. In addition, the *Fech*^{m1Pas}/*Fech* mouse does not show either deposition of protoporphyrin IX or symptoms of cholestasis, but does show fat deposition in hepatocytes [6]. The *Fech*^{m1Pas}/*Fech*^{m1Pas} mouse is also characterized by severe hepatic steatosis with an associated increase in plasma lipoprotein X and reduced high-density lipids (HDL) [7]. For the study described here, the mice

```
        PagI
           |
gaccgagacctcatgacactt        gaccgagacctcaagacactt
ctggctctggagtactgtgaa        ctggctctggagtactgtgaa
AspArgAspLeuMetThrLeu        AspArgAspLeuLysThrLeu
(a)                          (b)
```

Fig. 15.1 Site of mutation in the ferrochelatase gene in the *Fech* mouse. The T–>A transition is in the second exon and results in a methionine-to-lysine amino acid change (bold type). The wild-type sequence can be cut with restriction enzyme Pag1 (a) and the mutant form cannot (b), which forms the basis of a distinguishing assay. After PCR amplification of a suitable fragment from genomic DNA, cutting at this restriction site gives rise to readily identifiable DNA fragments that identify the three forms, *Fech*/*Fech*, *Fech*/*Fech*^{m1Pas}, and *Fech*^{m1Pas}/*Fech*^{m1Pas}.

were bred with BALB/c mice to give the F_2 generation. Genomic comparison was made of $Fech^{m1Pas}/Fech^{m1Pas}$ and $Fech^{m1Pas}/Fech$ with the wild type ($Fech/Fech$).

15.2.2
Griseofulvin

Griseofulvin has been used topically, primarily too treat fungal infections. When administered to mice, it produces hepatic damage, the chronology of which has been extensively studied [8]. After exposure to griseofulvin, there is an early onset of hepatocyte proliferation that leads to an increase in the liver/bodyweight ratio and an alteration in drug metabolism characteristics, due to enhanced expression of members of the cytochrome P450 family. Griseofulvin is metabolized by cytochrome P450 via a suicide reaction to a metabolite that probably methylates in the haem moiety, giving rise to *N*-methylprotoporphyrin IX which then inhibits ferrochelatase [9]. In this study[10], two strains of mice were subjected to continuous griseofulvin exposure of 1% in the diet. Two strains were utilized to discern if differences in the underlying genetics may affect the response to griseofulvin. There is a previous indication of a difference in response to griseofulvin between mice depending on strain and sex [9].

15.2.3
ET743

Ecteinascidin 743 (ET-743) is a tetrahydroisoquinoline alkaloid, isolated from the marine tunicate *Ecteinascidia turbinata*, which possesses potent antitumour activity [11–13]. Phase I clinical trials showed promising responses, and the drug has now proceeded to Phase II. In the phase II trials, in addition to other side effects, some patients experienced a subclinical hepatic toxicity characterized by elevation of hepatic enzymes and cholangitis (inflammation of the bile ducts), was manifest as elevated alkaline phosphatase and/or bilirubin. A similar toxicity was observed in preclinical studies, where the female rat was identified as a relevant and sensitive model for this toxicity of ET-743. As a direct result of the toxicity seen in the clinical trials and in the rat, a study was performed in our laboratory to investigate the transcriptome changes associated with the development of cholestasis arising from the cholangitis induced by a single i.v. (tail vein) dose of ET743 of 40 $\mu g\ kg^{-1}$ [14].

15.2.4
Alpha-napthylisothiocyanate (ANIT)

ANIT causes cholangitis in the liver of the rat. The mechanism of this toxicity is unclear, but the bile duct damage caused gives rise to a cholestatis [15]. This compound was used as a control for ET743 to enable differentiation of those gene expression effects that were due to the cholangitis from those due to another action of the ET743. Dosing was 100 $mg\ kg^{-1}$ orally once on day zero.

15.3 Pathological and Biochemical Characterization of the Models

15.3.1 Pathological Characterization

A summary of the histopathologically observable liver damage in the above studies is shown in Figure 15.2. In brief, in ANIT-treated animals there was damage and inflammation of the bile ducts (Figure 15.2 f), giving rise to a cholestasis on day two, as shown by an increased level of plasma bilirubin (Figure 15.3 a). By day six, the inflammation had resolved to a chronic inflammatory lesion around the bile ducts, and plasma bilirubin levels had returned to normal. With ET743, three days after dosing an inflammatory process involving the bile ducts appeared (Figure 15.2 g), which gave rise to biochemical evidence of cholestasis, as shown by an increase in plasma bilirubin (Figure 15.3 b). By day 12, the bile duct damage had mainly resolved, but a fibrotic lesion had formed around the portal triad (Figure 15.2 h). A different type of lesion was seen in the mouse models of protoporphyria: in both the griseofulvin-treated and *Fech*^{m1Pas}/*Fech*^{m1Pas} mice, there was deposition of protoporphyrin IX as a result of ferrochelatase insufficiency (Figure 15.2, a–c). Pigment was seen in bile ducts and this was associated with biochemical evidence of cholestasis (Figure 15.3 c). In C57BL/6J griseofulvin-treated mice bile duct inflammation and proliferation occurred by day five, which increased with time and became associated with fibrosis and focal parenchymal necrosis (Figure 15.2 b). A similar lesion was seen only intermittently in the BALB/c griseofulvin-treated mouse and was much less severe (Figure 15.2 e). In the griseofulvin-treated mice, fibrosis was detected by Van Gieson staining in the C57BL/6J mice by day 15 and was extensive by day 22. In contrast, the fibrosis was visible in the BALB/c mice only on day 22 (see Section

Fig. 15.2 Histopathologically observable liver damage in the four cholestasis models used here. (a) Portal zone from a three-month-old *Fech*^{m1Pas}/*Fech*^{m1Pas} mouse, showing bile duct proliferation and a scattering of red-brown pigment located mainly in interstitial cells. Pigment is absent in the interstitial cells (arrowhead). (b) A similar zone from a C57BL/6J mouse administered 1% griseofulvin in the diet for 22 days. Although the pathological changes are similar to those shown in A, they are more florid, as there is more inflammation as well as a focus of overt hepatic necrosis (arrow). (c) and (d) are the same microscopic fields under crossed polarizing filters. Pigment is more abundant in *Fech*^{m1Pas}/*Fech*^{m1Pas} mice, where it is located mainly in the interstitial tissue of the portal tract. (e) Shows a similar view to that in (b), but from a BALB/c mouse treated with griseofulvin for 22 days. The same red-brown pigment is located within the bile ducts, but there is little or no cellular damage or inflammation. (f) Represents a view of the portal zone from a rat two days after treatment with ANIT. There is degeneration of the bile duct epithelium, which is swollen by interstitial tissue and acute inflammatory cells. (g) Shows a similar zone to that in (f), but from a rat treated two days previously with a single dose of 40 μg kg^{-1} i.v. ET743. Although the bile duct epithelium shows degeneration, the surrounding interstitial zone contains fewer inflammatory cells. (h) Represents a similar zone to that seen in (f) and (g), but 12 days after a single dose of ET-743. There is considerable periduct concentric fibrosis around an intact bile duct lined with bile duct cells having variably sized nuclei. All slides were stained with haematoxylin and eosin and are at the same magnification (bar = 140 μm). Original results in Gant et al. [10] and Donald et al. [14]. ▶

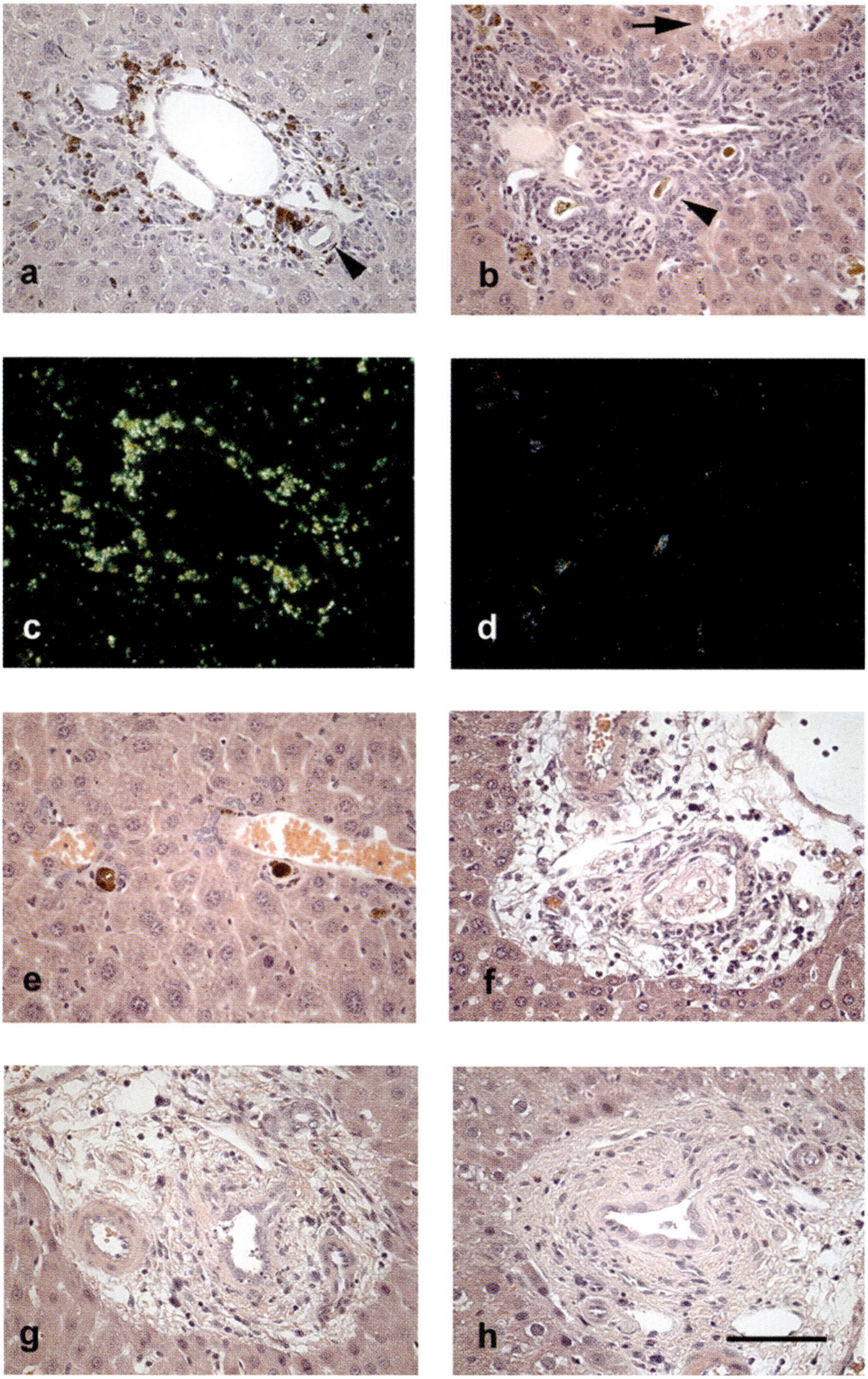
a
b
c
d
e
f
g
h

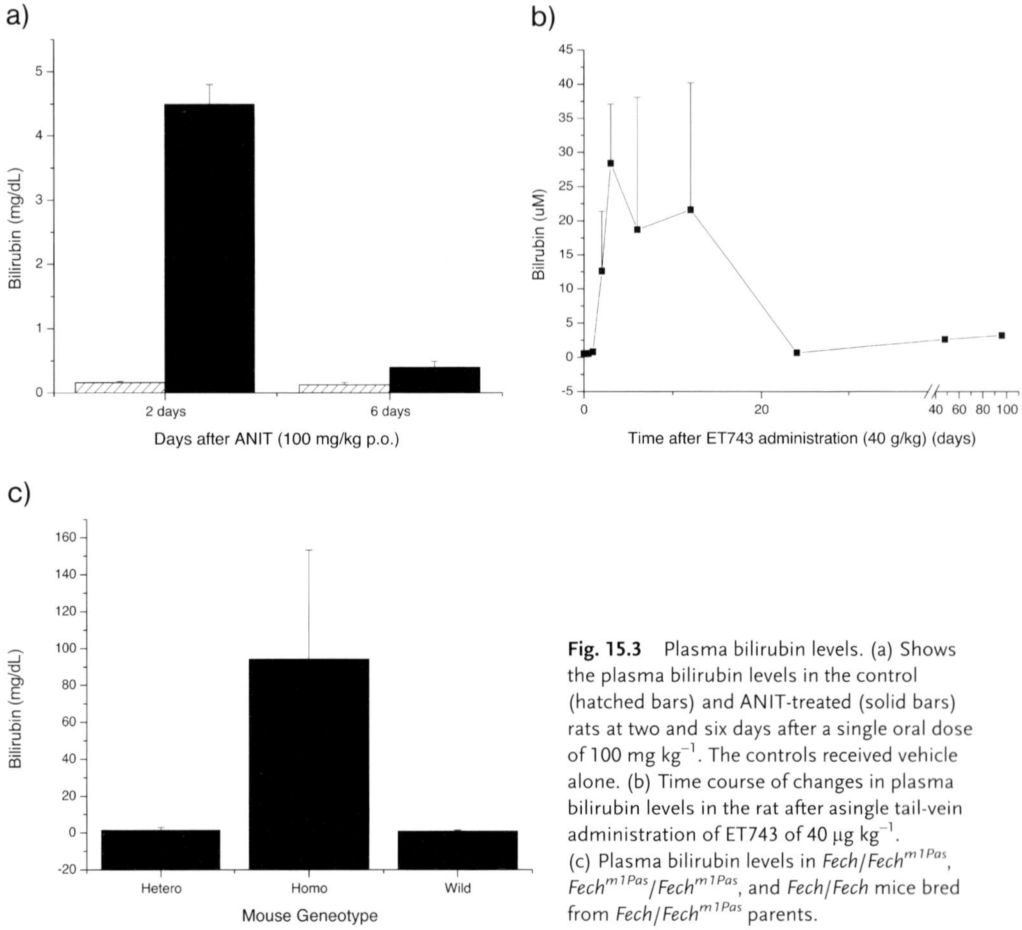

Fig. 15.3 Plasma bilirubin levels. (a) Shows the plasma bilirubin levels in the control (hatched bars) and ANIT-treated (solid bars) rats at two and six days after a single oral dose of 100 mg kg^{-1}. The controls received vehicle alone. (b) Time course of changes in plasma bilirubin levels in the rat after asingle tail-vein administration of ET743 of 40 μg kg^{-1}. (c) Plasma bilirubin levels in *Fech*/*Fech*^{m1Pas}, *Fech*^{m1Pas}/*Fech*^{m1Pas}, and *Fech*/*Fech* mice bred from *Fech*/*Fech*^{m1Pas} parents.

15.6.4 for a discussion of fibrosis in relation to gene expression changes). These changes were associated with an increase in plasma ALT, AST, and AP (Figure 15.4 a, b and c, respectively). In the three-month-old *Fech*^{m1Pas}/*Fech*^{m1Pas} mouse and after 15 and 22 days of griseofulvin treatment in C57BL/6J mice, focal necrosis was seen in the parenchyma, with white cell infiltration (Figure 15.2 a and b, respectively). This pathology was not observed in griseofulvin-treated BALB/c mouse, though the degree of protoporphyrin deposition was similar.

15.3.2
Protoporphyrin IX levels in Models of Ferrochelatase Inhibition

The levels of protoporphyrin IX in both griseofulvin-treated mouse strains at day 22 and in the *Fech*^{m1Pas}/*Fech*^{m1Pas} mouse at two months of age were similar, indicating an equivalent level of ferrochelatase inhibition was being achieved in each (Figure

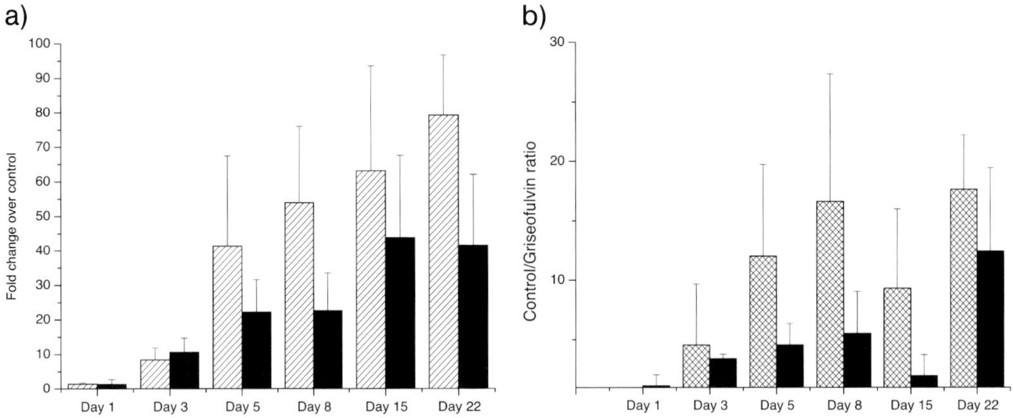

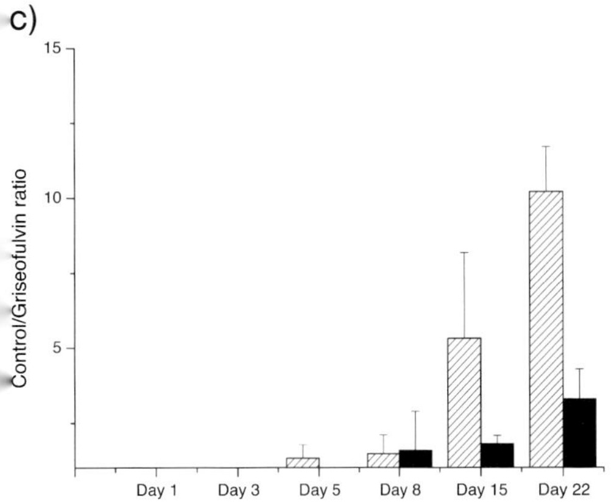

Fig. 15.4 Plasma ALT, AST, and AP levels. (a) Ratio of plasma ALT (to the level in vehicle-treated controls) in C57BL/6J (hatched bars) and BALB/c (solid bars) mice after commencement of a diet containing 1% griseofulvin on day 0; (b) AST; (c) alkaline phosphatase. The experimental details for (b) and (c) are the same as for (a).

15.5). This could be observed histopathologically where a similar level of deposition of brown protoporphyrin IX could be seen in the bile ducts (Figure 15.2 a, b, e).

15.4 Microarray and Bioinformatics Methodology

In our laboratory, we construct our own microarrays using ESTs derived from the IMAGE clone collections [16]. These are printed onto poly-L-lysine slides using a Brown-type arrayer built according to the published details (http://cmgm.stanford.edu/pbrown/mguide/). These microarrays are hybridized in a competitive manner, with both the control and the test samples being hybridized to the same microarray and differentiated by using different fluorescent labels. In this study Cy3 and Cy5 were used. For each time point, time-matched controls were used and four biological

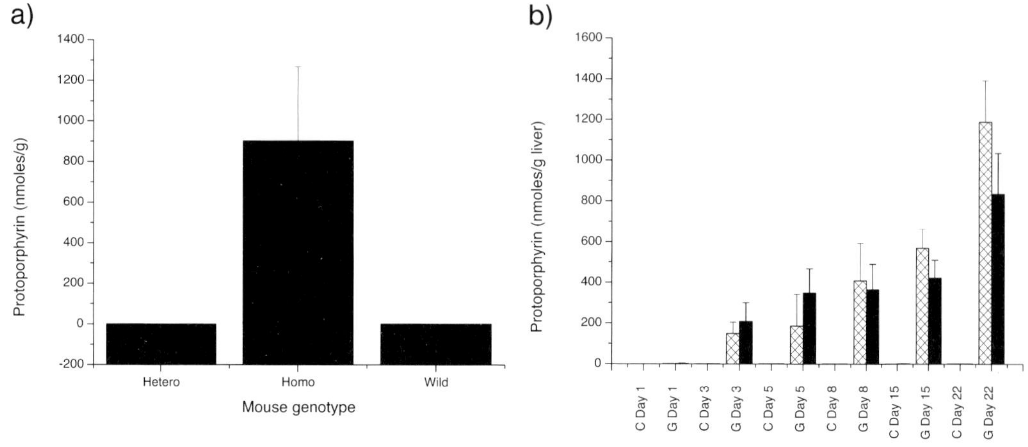

Fig. 15.5 Deposition of protoporphyrin XI in the liver with ferrochelatase insufficiency. (a) Levels of liver protoporphyrin IX in *Fech*/*Fech*^{m1Pas}, *Fech*^{m1Pas}/*Fech*^{m1Pas}, and *Fech*/*Fech* mice bred from *Fech*/*Fech*^{m1Pas} parents. (b) Changes in liver protoporphyrin IX with time in C57BL/6J (hatched bars) and BALB/c (solid bars) mice after commencement of a diet containing 1% griseofulvin on day 0 (g). The controls received diet containing vehicle only (c).

replicates were performed, giving at least three degrees of freedom. At least one of these replicates was reverse-labelled to correct for colour bias. Data were obtained from the image by taking the median value of the pixels within the feature and subtracting the local background. Data was discarded from analysis only if the intensity of fluorescence of the feature for the channel was lower than the local background. The data obtained were normalized by the LOWESS method and the significance was assessed with an unpaired *t* test. Genes were considered significant if the *p* value was less than 0.05. For each of the gene clusters shown in the figures below, the ratio data is shown in two forms: all the data are shown on the left, and statistically significant data points are shown on the right, because the early points in a time course often showed changes in expression that did not achieve significance. Thus, if only the significant points were shown it would appear that the gene expression had gone from nothing to suddenly differentially regulated. By showing all the data, both the transition in the differential gene expression and the achievement of significance are indicated. Software used for the analysis was a mixture of commercial, free, and in-house programs. GenePix (http://www.axon.com/) version 3.06.90 or earlier was used for image capture and analysis. Mapping, mathematical conversion, and statistics were done with our own programs (http://www.le.ac.uk/mrctox/microarray_lab/). Clustering and visualization were done with Cluster3 and TreeView 1.5 (http://rana.lbl.gov/), and principal components analysis was performed with SimcaP10 (http://www.u-metrics. com/). The data were examined in two ways, first by clustering or principal components analysis to look for genes coregulated in expression and second by using specific Gene Ontology (GO) (http://www.geneontology.org/) terms from genes discovered in the above analysis to bring together all the other functionally related genes.

Thus, presentation of the genes is either by coregulated cluster or by GO reference as being in some manner functionally related.

15.5 Liver Gene Expression Altered Directly as a Response to Griseofulvin

One of the most useful aspects of microarray technology in toxicogenomics is to be able to simultaneously determine the expression of all genes in a biochemical pathway after a perturbing event, such as tissue damage or xenobiotic exposure. As this chapter is primarily concerned with the development and consequences of cholestasis, and bilirubin arises from the degradation of heme, differential expression of genes in the heme synthesis pathway was examined. These genes were extracted from the dataset by functionally searching with the GO term 'heme biosynthesis'.

15.5.1 Genes of the Heme Synthesis and Catabolism Pathways

Genes of the heme synthesis and catabolism pathways were selected using the GO search term 'heme biosynthesis' and then hierarchically clustered (Figure 15.6). For genes of the heme synthesis pathway, there were downregulations in gene expression in the mouse cholestatic models of uroporphyrinogen III synthase (*Uros*), uroporphyrinogen III decarboxylase (*Urod*), and erythroid 5-aminolevulinate acid synthase 2 (*Alas2*). These were downregulated in expression through the time course for both the griseofulvin-treated and $Fech^{m1Pas}/Fech^{m1Pas}$ mice against the F_2 *Fech*/*Fech* littermate background. 5-Aminolevulinate acid synthase gene (*Alas1*) expression was induced in the griseofulvin-treated [10] but not $Fech^{m1Pas}/Fech^{m1Pas}$ mice (A. G. Smith, unpublished data).

15.5.1.1 5-Aminolevulinate Acid Synthase 1 and Erythroid 5-Aminolevulinate Acid Synthase 2 (Alas1 and 2)

In both $Fech^{m1Pas}/Fech^{m1Pas}$ and griseofulvin-treated mice there was an unexpected reduction in *Alas2* expression. However, *Alas2* is associated with the synthesis of heme for haemoglobin and not with haemoprotein synthesis in the liver. The downregulation in both $Fech^{m1Pas}/Fech^{m1Pas}$ mice and griseofulvin-treated mice indicates that the downregulation was associated with the loss of the ferrochelatase activity rather than with any direct effect of the griseofulvin. Less clear though is the mechanism by which this occurs. It is apparent this may lead to a loss of haemoglobin in these animals and an associated anaemia, as there is no substitution of *Alas1* for *Alas2* in erythropoiesis [17]. This though would depend on *Alas2* being downregulated in the bone marrow, where it is predominant, and the results above were obtained from liver. It is interesting however to speculate about the control mechanisms that might be regulating the decreased expression in the liver. *Alas2* is controlled both transcriptionally and post-transcriptionally, with posttranscriptional control occurring through a 5′-untranslated iron responsive element (IRE) [17–22] which

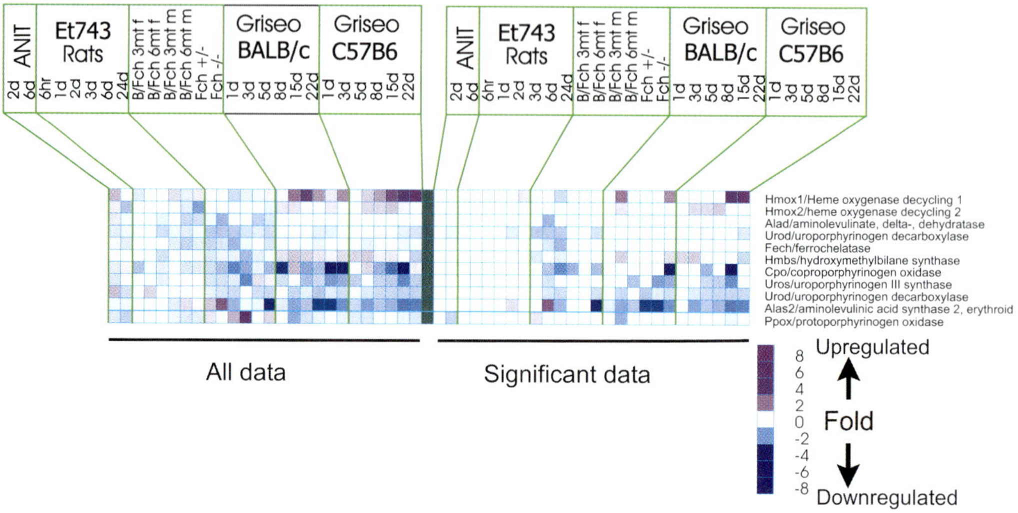

Fig. 15.6 Differential expression of genes involved in the heme synthesis and catabolism cycles in the cholestasis models. The genes were selected by using the GO search term 'heme biosynthesis' and then hierarchically clustered. Each time point or strain comparison is indicated in the legend box above the clustergram. These are, from left to right: ANIT treatment (100 mg kg^{-1} orally) at two and six days compared with a vehicle-treated control. ET743 treatment (40 µg kg^{-1} i.v.) at 6 h and at 1, 2, 3, 6, and 24 days compared with a vehicle-injected control. Ferrochelatase gene expression in $Fech^{m1Pas}/Fech^{m1Pas}$ female (f) mouse at three and six months of age compared with a similarly aged BALB/c mouse; $Fech^{m1Pas}/Fech^{m1Pas}$ male (m) mouse at three and six months compared with a similarly aged BALB/c mouse; male $Fech/Fech^{m1Pas}$ compared with a *Fech/Fech* F_2 mouse bred from heterozygous parents; and a male $Fech^{m1Pas}/Fech^{m1Pas}$ compared with a *Fech/Fech* F_2 mouse bred from heterozygous parents. Griseofulvin-treated BALB/c mice at 1, 3, 5, 8, 15, and 22 days after commencement of a diet containing 1% griseofulvin compared with mice on a diet containing vehicle alone; and C57BL/6J mice at 1, 3, 5, 8, 15, and 22 days treated in the same manner as the BALB/c mice. The left heat map shows all the data, and the right heat map the same data but only the statistically significant data points (two-tailed *t* test, $p<0.05$). The relative changes in gene expression are indicated as a colour gradient from white (not differentially expressed) to magenta (upregulated) or blue (downregulated), as shown in the key. The genes are shown on the right as HUGO gene name/description.

binds to iron regulatory proteins (IRP1 and IRP2) [18, 19] and also possibly ferrochelatase [23]. Under conditions of high iron IRPs are inactivated (IRP1) or degraded (IRP2), allowing translation of the *Alas2* mRNA, but under conditions of low iron, the IRPs bind to the IRE element, leading to repression of translation. *Alas1,* in contrast to *Alas2,* is the gene coding 5-aminolevulinate acid synthase in the haemoprotein biosynthesis pathway of the liver and is transcriptionally regulated by a feedback inhibition loop from heme. Thus, as little heme was being formed in the $Fech^{m1Pas}/Fech^{m1Pas}$ or griseofulvin-treated mice, we might expect that the lack of feedback inhibition to the *Alas1* gene promoter region would result in increased transcriptional activity of the *Alas1* gene. *Alas1* gene expression was determined previously [10], and also by using real-time PCR (data not shown), and the expected result was obtained with both griseofulvin-treated mouse strains, where there was increased transcription of *Alas1*. However, in $Fech^{m1Pas}/Fech^{m1Pas}$ micee the same increase in transcription was not observed (data not shown). The reason for this may be that increased *Alas1* gene transcription in griseofulvin-treated animals was not due to the lack of feedback inhibition from heme but was instead a direct griseofulvin-mediated induction. The *Alas1* gene is inducible by phenobarbital (PB)-like inducers, and griseofulvin is such a compound. *Alas1* is induced through the retinoid X receptor–constitutive active receptor (RXR–CAR) heterodimer, for which it has a binding site [23 a], although CAR per se does not seem to be essential for *Alas1* induction as PB can induce *Alas1* expression in CAR-null mice [24]. Therefore, it is probable that the induction of *Alas1* seen here is not due just to a lack of feedback inhibition from the heme but also to direct induction by griseofulvin. Unlike the *Alas1* gene, *Alas2* is not transcriptionally activated by PB-like compounds [18]. Therefore, one explanation for decreased expression of the *Alas2* gene is that a decreased translation, and probably increased targeted mRNA degradation, occurs as a result of the increased intracellular iron that accumulates due to the failure of ferrochelatase to incorporate it into protoporphryrin IX. In the absence of a PB-like induction from griseofulvin, as occurs for *Alas1*, this effect is manifested as decreased *Alas2* gene expression.

15.5.1.2 Heme Oxygenase 1 and 2 (*Hmox1* and *Hmox2*)

In the griseofulvin-treated mice only, transcription of the *Hmox1* gene increased. This did not occur in $Fech^{m1Pas}/Fech^{m1Pas}$ mice and therefore indicates a mechanism leading to increased transcription that is independent of the inhibition of ferrochelatase. As with *Alas1*, the most likely mechanism is a direct induction by griseofulvin. *Hmox2* is a basally expressed form of heme oxygenase and is responsible for the normal degradation of heme to carbon monoxide and biliverdin. *Hmox1*, by contrast, is an early-response gene induced by stress. In the griseofulvin-treated mice, *Hmox1* gene expression may have been induced as a response to tissue injury or inflammation. However, once again, it is the contrast of two similar models that gives the clue that this is not the correct conclusion. *Hmox1* is not induced significantly in $Fech^{m1Pas}/Fech^{m1Pas}$ mice and increases gradually throughout the time course with griseofulvin in both strains of treated mice. These data suggest a griseofulvin-related induction of transcription. *Hmox1* is induced by both chemical and stress-related stimuli, and induction may occur through the JNK and p38 pathways, possibly through the CRE/AP-1 site. Therefore, griseofulvin may utilize this same mechanism to induce the expression of *Hmox1* [25]. This conclusion is consistent with previous published data both for *Hmox1* and *Alas1* [26]. In the rat there were small changes in the expression of *Hmox1* in response to ANIT and ET743, but these were not statistically significant. These data do, however, indicate the possibility that expression of the *Hmox1* and *Alas1* genes in rat liver also may be altered by ANIT and ET743.

15.5.2
Monooxygenases

In a similar manner to the *Hmox1* and *Alas1* genes, members of the monooxygenase family of genes were induced in the griseofulvin-treated mice only, indicating a direct, chemically mediated induction. The induction of the monooxygenase gene expression was not global, but specific, and limited to members of the *Cyp3a*, *Cyp2b*, and *Cyp2c* gene families (Figure 15.7). Additionally, increased expression of the *Cyp2a5* gene with porphyrinogenic agents in mouse liver has been reported previously [27] and was confirmed here (Figure 15.7). Increased expression of the *Cyp2a5* gene is also reported in preneoplastic and neoplastic liver lesions [28]. Treatment with griseofulvin eventually leads to hepatocarcinogenesis [8], and therefore the increased expression of the *Cyp2a5* gene seen here could be related to this process. Elevated *Cyp2a5* gene expression was also seen in the six- but not the three-month-old *Fech*^{m1Pas}/*Fech*^{m1Pas} mice (Figure 15.7). This *Cyp2a5* expression corresponded to tumour formation, which occurs at about eight months in these mice ([29] and A. G. Smith unpublished data).

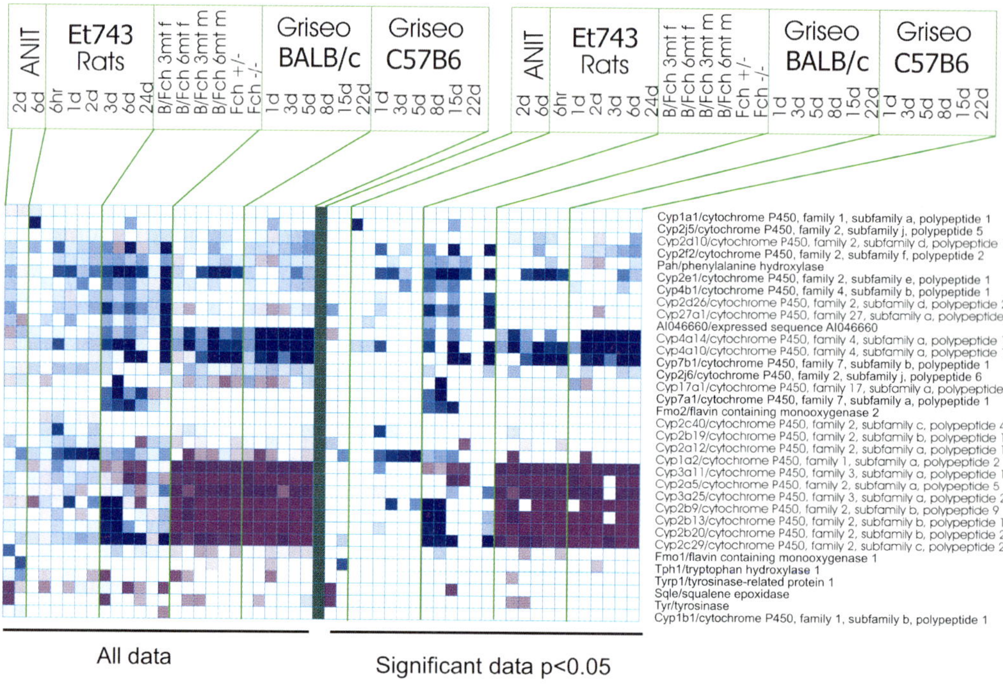

Fig. 15.7 Changes in monooxygenase gene expression across the cholestasis models and at each time point or strain comparison indicated in the legend box above the clustergram. The genes were selected from the full set using the GO search term 'monooxygenase' and then hierarchically clustered. The experimental and figure details are the same as for Figure 15.6. The colour key for the relative changes is shown in Figure 15.6.

The increased expression of members of the *Cyp3a* and *Cyp2c* gene families with PB has previously been characterized and appears due to PB-mediated binding of RXR–CAR heterodimer [30]. Further evidence of the involvement of these receptors is indicated by the decreased ability of PB to induce the *Cyp2b10* and *Cyp3a11* genes in CAR knockout mice [24, 31]. There is also a possibility that some of the monooxygenase gene expression induction seen in this study, in particular that of the *Cyp3a* genes, was mediated through the pregnane X receptor by formation of a heterodimer with RXR in a manner similar to CAR in acting through the same NR1 response element [32]. Figure 15.7 shows not only induction of cytochrome expression but also downregulation, particularly of the *Cyp4a10, Cyp4a14,* and *Cyp4a7b1* genes. The downregulation of the *Cyp7b1* gene is probably related to bile acid biosynthesis from cholesterol, as other genes in the cholesterol and bilirubin biosynthesis pathways are affected (data not shown). Downregulation of the *Cyp4a10* and *Cyp4a14* genes is not a xenobiotic-related phenomenon. as these genes were downregulated in griseofulvin-treated mice, $Fech^{m1Pas}/Fech^{m1Pas}$ mice, and also ET743-treated rats, although only data on *Cyp4a10* gene expression was significant. Downregulation of the *Cyp4a10* and *Cyp4a14* genes occurred prior to liver damage and appeared to be a sensitive indicator of the onset of liver damage. Ueda et al. [24] have shown that PB-mediated induction of the *Cyp4a10* and *Cyp4a14* genes occurs only in CAR-null mice, and so the downregulation of the *Cyp4a10* and *Cyp4a14* genes found here may be related to a transcriptional repression through CAR that is activated in some way by low-level liver damage.

15.6 Gene Expression Changes Associated with Pathological Changes

The ability of genomic profiles to distinguish pathologies and to differentiate closely related pathological subtypes that are not easy to distinguish by other means has been shown particularly well in tumours [33–37]. In toxicogenomics, such gene expression profiling methods are being used to try to distinguish toxicological properties in molecules and to examine pathological change [38–42]. In this section we discuss gene expression profiles associated with pathological change and show how elements of pathological change occurring with cholestasis can be associated with genomic profiles. We also pose the question of what this data adds to a traditional histopathological analysis.

15.6.1 Gene Expression Associated with Inflammation

A set of gene expression subprofiles was evident within the dataset that could be associated with the histopathological change. This gene set primarily included genes associated with inflammation and white cell infiltration, although included amongst them were a subset of the histocompatibility genes (Figure 15.8). The higher levels of increased gene expression were associated with those animals that had the higher levels

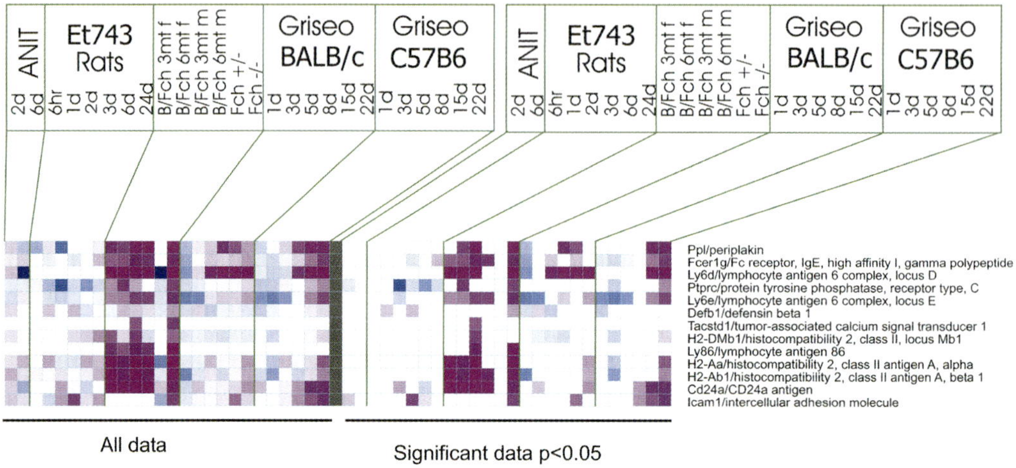

Fig. 15.8 Genes associated with cellular defence, showing increased expression that was closely associated with liver inflammation. This figure shows changes in gene expressions which are a subset (only those that increased in expression) of those on the array sharing the GO term 'defense genes'. The genes were hierarchically clustered after selection. Each time point or strain comparison is indicated in the legend box above the clustergram. The experimental and figure details are the same as for Figure 15.6. The colour key for the relative changes is shown in Figure 15.6.

of liver damage and inflammation, namely the $Fech^{m1Pas}/Fech^{m1Pas}$ and griseofulvin-treated C57BL/6J mice. Most of the genes in the set also show increased expression in the rat models and in the griseofulvin-treated Balb/c mice, but to a much lesser extent which was often not statistically significant. This is in accord with the more localized, reduced levels of damage, seen in the livers of these animals. One exception to this was the *Icam1* (intracellular adhesion molecule) gene, the expression of which correlated closely with the points of maximal inflammation throughout all models. Thus, the most significant expression of this gene was seen two days after ANIT, three days after ET743, in the $Fech^{m1Pas}/Fech^{m1Pas}$ mouse (2 months old), and at 15 and 22 days in the griseofulvin-treated C57BL/6J mice. However, there was little expression in the griseofulvin-treated BALB/c mice, which have considerably less inflammation than the C57BL/6J mice. Of note is that increased *Icam1* expression was not seen when the $Fech^{m1Pas}/Fech^{m1Pas}$ mouse was compared, not to its correct *Fech*/*Fech* littermate, but rather to the BALB/c background. This reflects genetic variation between the strains – the BALB/c background has a higher level of intrinsic expression than the *Fech*/*Fech* F_2 mouse. The above results with *Icam1* gene expression highlight both genetic variability leading to differential gene expression and also the potential for differential toxicity and thus the importance of making sure that the control and treatment groups are matched in toxicogenomics experiments. Both the advantage and disadvantage of genomics experiments is their ability to discern the wider profile of gene expression. The advantage is of course that there are more data, which gives rise to a more accurate and concise gene expression profile reflecting damage and/or phenotype in the tissue. The disadvantage is that small mismatches in the experimental samples, such as different genetic background, circadian rhythm, or cell cycle progression, the have potential to show up very clearly in the genomic profile obtained. It is therefore essential to be able to recognize and understand those gene expression profiles that may arise from controllable variables in the experiment and to distinguish them from those that are caused by the treatment itself.

15.6.2
CD24a

The *Cd24a* gene is expressed in neutrophils and B lymphocytes and has been reported as a marker for breast carcinoma [43]. Its expression here is probably therefore associated with lymphocyte infiltration into inflammatory areas within the liver. Unlike *Icam1*, this gene did not show the same difference in expression with respect to genetic background between $Fech^{m1Pas}/Fech^{m1Pas}$ and griseofulvin-treated BALB/c mice. Significantly increased *Cd24a* gene expression was seen in $Fech^{m1Pas}/Fech^{m1Pas}$ mice, from day eight in griseofulvin-treated C57BL/6J mice, and also, very specifically, on day three after ET743 treatment in rats. These changes in expression very accurately reflected the extent of inflammation, which was maximal in the animals at these time points. Differential expression was also seen in $Fech^{m1Pas}/Fech^{m1Pas}$ and in ANIT treated rats and griseofulvin-treated BALB/c mice, although the difference was not statistically significant. This most probably reflects a very low level of inflammation in these animals and, with the use of more that the four to five replicates used here, might have been significant. As the inflammation at these points was very small, these data indicate the potential utility, sensitivity, and accuracy of a marker such as *CD24a* in reflecting tissue white cell infiltration and inflammation.

15.6.3
Annexins and Liver Damage or Maybe Cholestasis?

Significant expression of annexin genes was seen at all the time points when there was inflammation and damage in the liver, in particular, in the griseofulvin-treated C57BL/6J mice, but also in the griseofulvin-treated BALB/c mice (Figure 15.9). In ET743-treated rats there was increased expression at the three-day time point. There was also expression in the ANIT-treated rats, although it was statistically significant only after the first two-day time point for *Anxa5*. Expression of these genes would therefore also appear to be directly related to and regulated by the inflammatory process.

15.6.4
Fibrosis and Mallory Body Formation

15.6.4.1 Keratin Gene Expression

Common to all models, and closely associated with time points where damage was occurring in the liver, was expression of members of the keratin gene (*Krt*) family, in

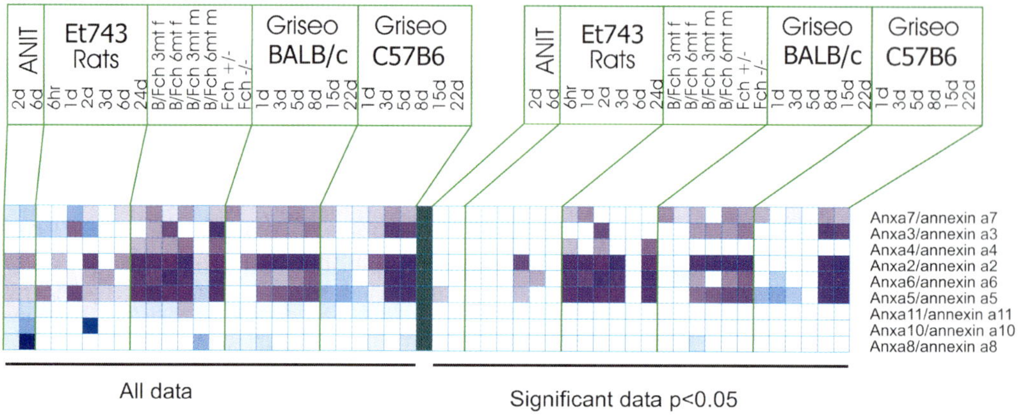

Fig. 15.9 Annexin gene expression in the liver during cholestasis. These genes were abstracted from the full set by searching the gene descriptions for 'annexin' and then hierarchically clustering them. Each time point or strain comparison is indicated in the legend box above the clustergram. The experimental and figure details are the same as for Figure 15.6. The colour key for the relative changes is shown in Figure 15.6.

particular keratins 2–5, 2–6, 2–7, and 2–8 (Figure 15.10). Expression of the *Krt2–8* and *Krt2–18* gene pair was previously observed early in cholestatic disease and leads, if sustained, to aggregates in the hepatocytes and the formation of insoluble deposits called Mallory bodies. The function of Mallory bodies is not entirely clear, but they are a consistent feature of many liver diseases. They may act as a sequestosome for potentially harmful proteins [44]. *Krt2–7* and *Krt2–8* were seen in all models at the points at which maximum liver damage was occurring. An interesting resolution of increased keratin gene expression can be seen for all keratins in the six-day ANIT-treated rats, in which the plasma bilirubin had returned to normal and the bile ducts had reopened. For ET743-treated rats, keratin expression increased from day two as damage was occurring in the liver and remained increased throughout the remainder of the time course. In both the C57BL/6J and BALB/c griseofulvin-treated mice, expression was detectable at three days was statistically significant later in the time course. Interestingly, although the C57BL/6J griseofulvin-treated mice showed a histopathologically increased level of liver damage, keratin expression was higher in the BALB/c mice. This was not a xenobiotic-driven effect, as occurred with monooxygenase gene expression, because the $Fech^{m1Pas}/Fech^{m1Pas}$ mice showed a similarly high level of keratin expression compared with an F_2 *Fech*/*Fech* control. There is however the possibility of transcription being mediated by a component of the bile, as occurs for the *Abcb1* gene (Figure 15.11). The data obtained from the ANIT-treated rats point clearly to this mechanism; their keratin expression resolved at the six-day period when the plasma bilirubin had returned to normal (Figures 15.3 and 15.11). This leads onto some interesting questions on the transcriptional control of the keratin genes. There are no available data detailing transcriptional control of the keratin genes by bile acids. However, the data presented here suggest that there is opportunity for further study.

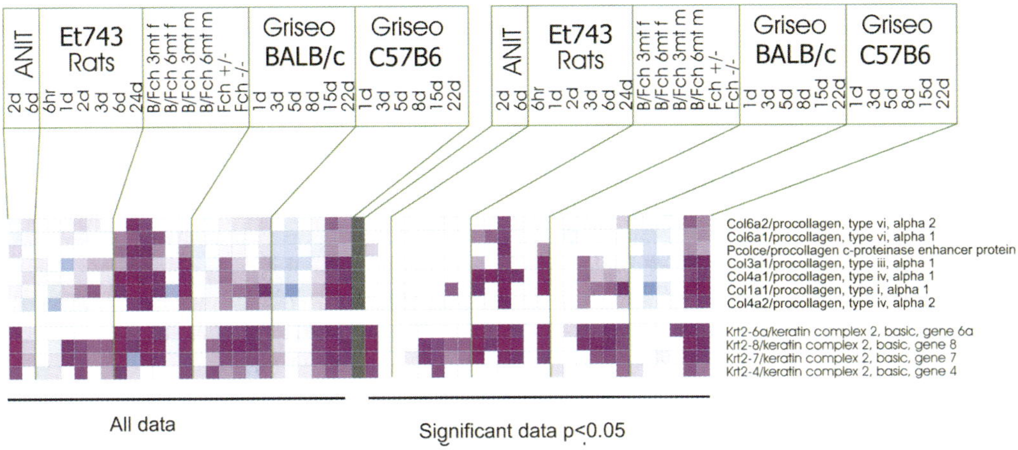

Fig. 15.10 Induced collagen and keratin genes. These genes were abstracted from the full set by a search for the GO terms for 'collagen' (top heat map) or 'keratin' (bottom heat map). These were then hierarchically clustered. Each time point or strain comparison is indicated in the legend box above the heat map. The experimental and figure details are the same as for Figure 15.6. The colour key for the relative changes is shown in Figure 15.6.

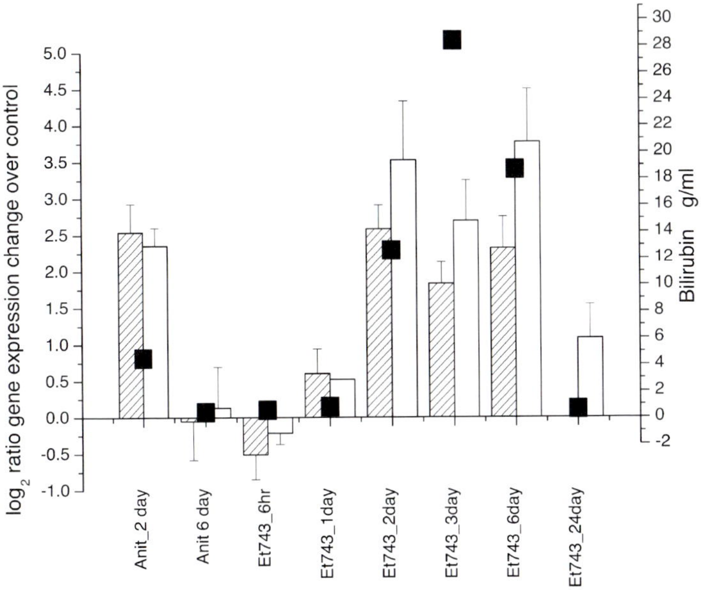

Fig. 15.11 Expression of the *Abcb1* and *Abcb4* genes compared with plasma bilirubin concentration. Liver expression of the *Abcb4* (hatched bars) and *Abcb1* (white bars) genes in the rat cholestasis models and the plasma bilirubin levels (squares) were plotted to indicate the relationship of plasma bilirubin concentration and expression of these two members of the ABC gene family during cholestasis.

15.6.4.2 **Collagen Gene Expression**

Collagen deposition, particularly that of the proteins encoded by *Col1a1* and *Col3a1*, is associated with wound repair and fibrosis. Expression of these collagen genes and additionally the *Col4a1* and *Col4a2* genes was detected in all models, and their expression correlated with the tissue damage and resolution (Figure 15.10). This was particularly true in the C57BL/6J griseofulvin-treated and $Fech^{m1Pas}/Fech^{m1Pas}$ mice, where more extensive damage occurred in the parenchyma. Van Gieson staining showed collagen deposition in damaged areas of the liver commensurate with expression of the collagen genes (Figure 15.12). Interestingly, increased expression of the collagen genes was found in both the BALB/c and C57BL/6J griseofulvin-treated mice, and the increase became statistically significant at an earlier time point in the griseofulvin-treated BALB/c than in the C57BL/6J mice. However, the level of expression finally achieved at the last two time points was higher in the griseofulvin-treated C57BL/6J mouse than in the griseofulvin treated BALB/c mouse. This may reflect a more subacute form of cell damage in the griseofulvin-treated BALB/c mouse, which was less visible histopathologically than that in the C57BL/6J mouse. What is indicated by these data is that assessment of the expression of these genes may be a quantitative means of assessing tissue damage. Combined with the determination of specific gene expressions to assess the degree of inflammation and white cell infiltration, the value of using multiple gene expression determinations in toxicological analysis to both characterize and quantify pathological change can be appreciated.

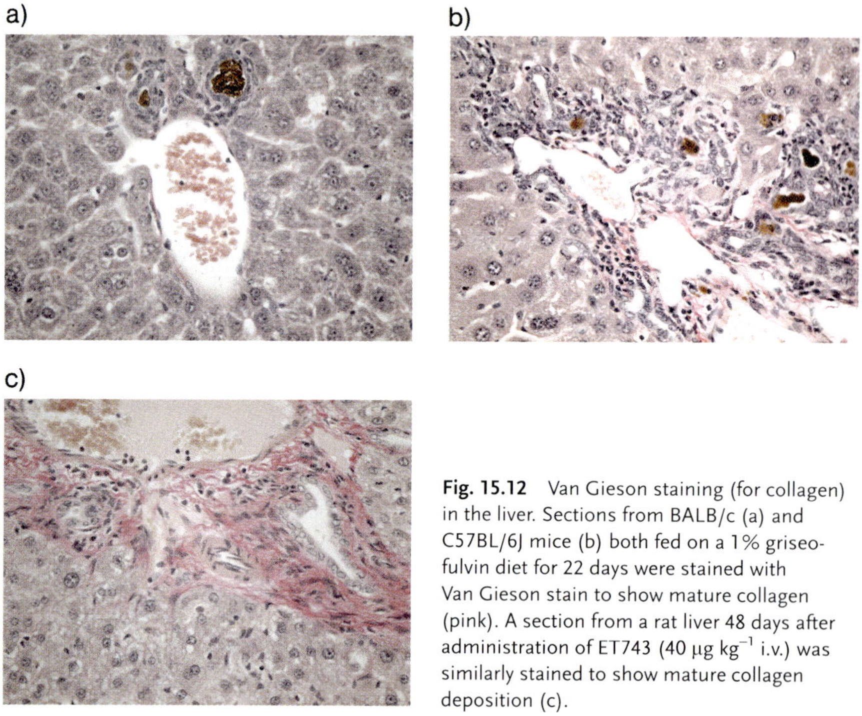

Fig. 15.12 Van Gieson staining (for collagen) in the liver. Sections from BALB/c (a) and C57BL/6J mice (b) both fed on a 1% griseofulvin diet for 22 days were stained with Van Gieson stain to show mature collagen (pink). A section from a rat liver 48 days after administration of ET743 (40 μg kg^{-1} i.v.) was similarly stained to show mature collagen deposition (c).

Gene expression data such as this are therefore useful per se in the absence of histopathological data, but are much more valuable in combination thus adding substantially to the armoury of the pathologist in making toxicological assessments.

15.7 Gleaning New Information on Pathological Changes from Gene Expression Data

Genomic data has the potential to indicate altered pathology both from an analysis of the data as a whole, i.e., taking the whole gene expression profile as one data point, but also from the analysis of individual gene expressions within the profile. The potential of this type of analysis is indicated here by reference to the *Cdc2* gene (mouse homolog of human *Cdc2*) from the cholestasis data sets generated in our laboratory.

A principal components analysis of the data associated with the ET743 study indicated three genes in particular that were able to separate the two- and three-day time points from the rest of the study (Figure 15.13). Two of these were the *Abcb1* and *Abcb4* genes, and the third was the *Cdc2* gene. Increased expression of the *Abcb1* and *Abcb4* genes in the cholestatic ET743-treated rat was not unexpected. Expression of these genes after ANIT administration and bile duct ligation has been described before, and their expression is closely related to plasma bilirubin concentration, suggesting a regulatory control dependent on components of the bile (Figure 15.11) [15]. The expression of *Cdc2* was however unexpected. *Cdc2* is the gene responsible for control of the cell cycle and is normally expressed late in G1, before the protein is required for cell transition from S to G2 and G2 to M [45]. Therefore, expression here indicated the possibility of cell division, although ET743 is an antineoplastic compound. The liver/bodyweight ratio increased during the time period after ET743 administration, and plotting these data along with *Cdc2* gene expression (Figure 15.14 a) indicated that *cdc2* gene expression increased prior to the increase in liver/bodyweight ratio and was possibly the mediating factor behind the increased liver weight. This was further investigated by staining for the S-phase marker Ki67 (Figure 15.14 b), which indicated that the cells in S phase were not in the damaged areas of the liver but rather were hepatocytes in undamaged areas of the parenchyma (Figure 15.14 c); the profile of labelling matched the change in liver/bodyweight ratio. As the *Cdc2* gene controls transition through the cell cycle, it does not appear that the cells are arrested in S phase, since that would give rise to liver hypertrophy. Rather, they are passing though the cell cycle, thus generating liver hyperplasia. These data suggest that *Cdc2* gene expression is therefore induced by ET743 and that the increased expression of *Cdc2* then causes cell-cycle deregulation. Little has been published that either supports or counters this hypothesis, but increased expression of *Cdc2* has been reported in a rat cirrhosis model induced by thioacetamide (TAA) [46]. In the TAA model, increased *Cdc2* gene expression correlated with increased cell division (PCNA staining) and an increase liver/bodyweight ratio. It is possible that the increased expression of the *Cdc2* gene in the TAA model was a response to TAA or cirrhosis. For ET743, the difference in expression between the

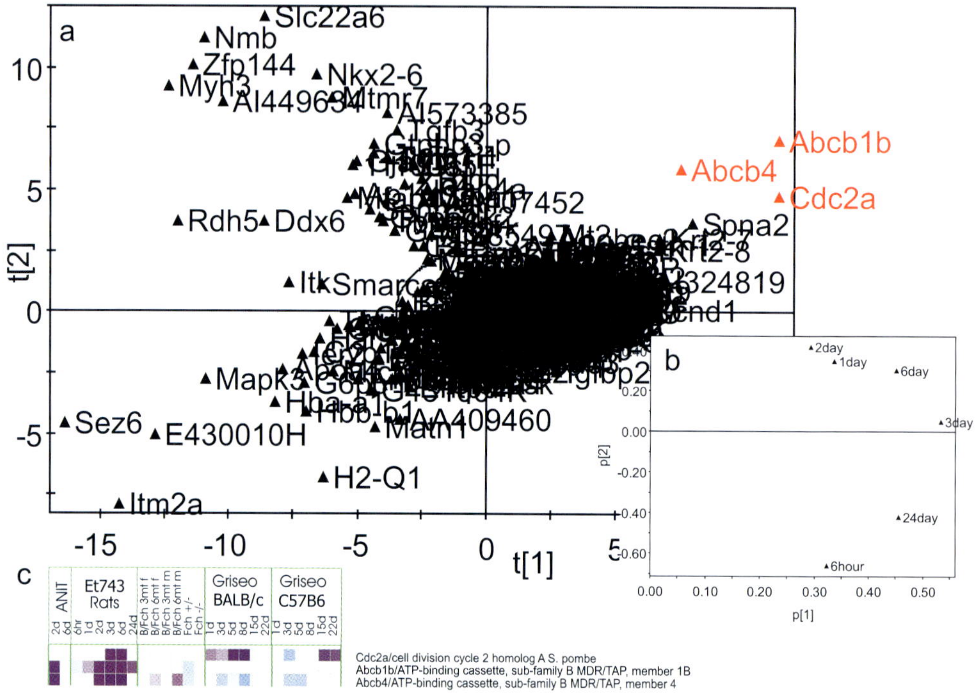

Fig. 15.13 Principal components analysis (PCA) of gene expression data across the time course of cholestasis in the rat after ET743 treatment For this analysis, each set of data obtained at each time point after ET743 injection (40 μg kg^{-1} i.v.) was assessed for similarity by PCA analysis. The similarity is represented in the inset score plot (b). These results show that there is similarity in the gene profiles for the 6 h and 24 day time points, and for the one and two day time points, although these two profiles are very different from the 6 h/24 day set. The three day time point is an outlier; maximal biliary inflammation and damage and the highest level of cholestasis occurred on this day. The gene expressions that contributed most to the separation of the gene expression profile at this time point from the others are shown in the loading plot (a). Shown in red are the major contributing genes *Abcb1*, *Abcb4*, and *Cdc2*. These genes are also shown in the heat map (c), which shows only significant changes in expression of these genes across all models. Each time point or strain comparison is indicated in the legend box above the clustergram. The experimental and figure details are the same as for Figure 15.6. The colour key for the relative changes is shown in Figure 15.6.

models provides clues to support the hypothesis that, with ET743, and quite possibly with TAA, *Cdc2* gene overexpression is mediated by the xenobiotic and is not a pathological change. Significant expression of the *Cdc2* gene was seen not only in the ET743-treated animals but also in the griseofulvin-treated animals, where there was a correlation between expression of the *Cdc2* gene and an increase in the liver/bodyweight ratio (Figure 15.15). However, in the ANIT-treated rats and $Fech^{m1Pas}$/$Fech^{m1Pas}$ mice there was no change in *Cdc2* gene expression even though pathological change and fibrosis occurred. Additionally, in the ANIT-treated rats no change occurred in liver Ki67 labelling (livers from griseofulvin-treated mice has not yet

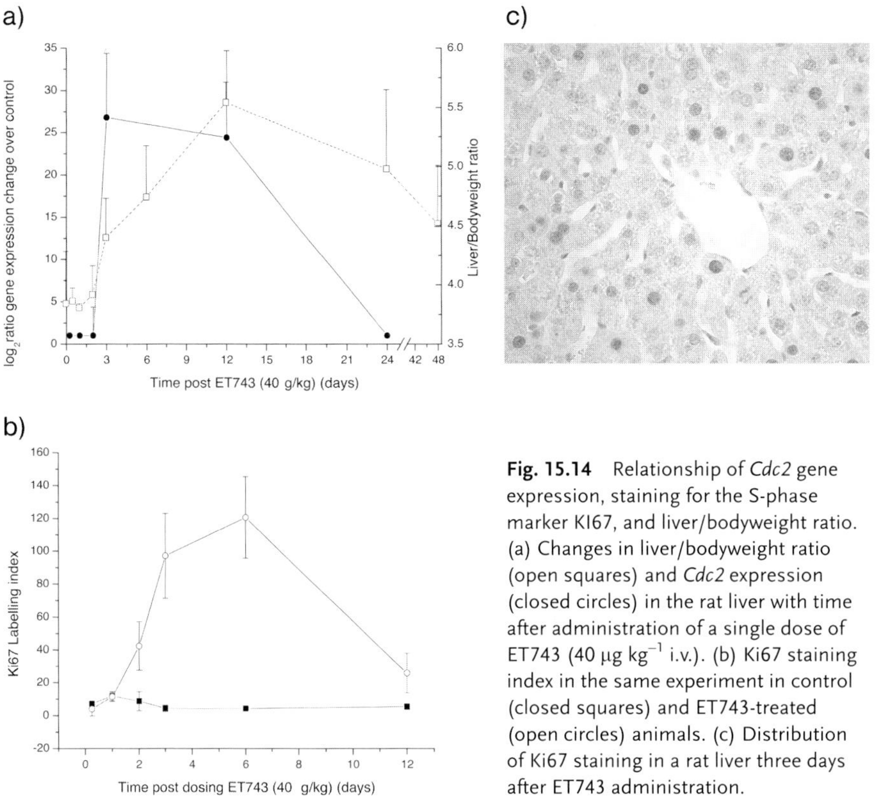

Fig. 15.14 Relationship of *Cdc2* gene expression, staining for the S-phase marker KI67, and liver/bodyweight ratio. (a) Changes in liver/bodyweight ratio (open squares) and *Cdc2* expression (closed circles) in the rat liver with time after administration of a single dose of ET743 (40 μg kg^{-1} i.v.). (b) Ki67 staining index in the same experiment in control (closed squares) and ET743-treated (open circles) animals. (c) Distribution of Ki67 staining in a rat liver three days after ET743 administration.

been assessed by Ki67 labelling; date from ANIT treatment not shown). Therefore the increase in *Cdc2* gene expression was not a response to liver damage but rather appears to be a response to an inductive effect of the xenobiotic. We are therefore left with an interesting scenario in which ET743 and griseofulvin increase *Cdc2* gene transcription in the liver and the aberrant expression of this gene deregulates the hepatocyte cell cycle. This results in hepatocytes entering S phase, causing hyperplasia and increased liver/bodyweight ratio.

15.8 Conclusions

The data presented here are only a fraction of what is available from our toxicogenomic analysis of these models of cholestasis and steatosis, and we also note that this work is still in progress. In particular, we have much information associated with changes in cholesterol synthesis and catabolism, for which there was no room in this chapter. To this end, as more data are generated papers will be submitted to peer-reviewed journals and the data will be made available on the Internet. All of the

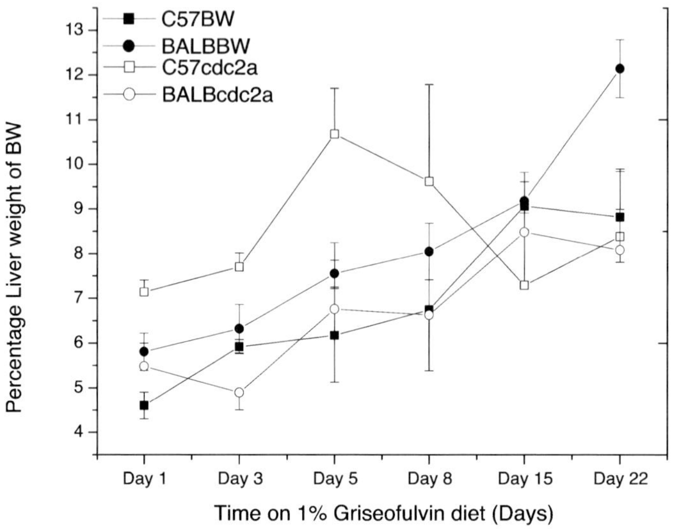

Fig. 15.15 Liver/bodyweight ratio and *Cdc2* expression in C57BL/6J and BALB/c mice fed a diet containing 1% griseofulvin commencing on day zero. Livers were collected on days 1, 3, 5, 8, 15 and 22. Control mice were fed a diet containing vehicle alone. Liver/bodyweight percentages are shown (closed symbols) for the BALB/c (circles) and C57BL/6J (squares) mice, as well as *Cdc2* gene expression, expressed as the $\log_2$ change with respect to the control (open symbols).

data associated with gene profiling of the ET743 and griseofulvin models are already available at http://www.le.ac.uk/mrctox/microarray_lab/.

By using models of cholestasis in rodents, we have tried to illustrate some of the uses and advantages of characterizing toxicity and pathology by using toxicogenomics. Our purpose here was not to suggest that toxicogenomics will replace some of the more traditional toxicological assessments – far from it – but rather that the toxicogenomic approach has much to offer in assessments of toxicity and tissue responses to xenobiotic exposure. Out primary point is that toxicogenomic data should not be assessed in isolation but rather in combination with other measured parameters and histopathology. The question needs to be asked then: if toxicogenomics is not a replacement for traditional methods of toxicity, what does it add to the toxicogenomic assessment that makes it worth undertaking. In the results presented in this chapter on the characterization of inflammation and fibrosis by toxicogenomics, one can see that specific genes can be characterized and used to quantify pathological changes. Moreover, although not presented in detail here, subtle changes occur in the gene expression profiles differentiating the pathological change. Further analysis of the data to find genes making a greater contribution to the individuality of the gene expression profile indicated increased *Cdc2* gene expression in ET743-exposed rat liver. These data in turn led to an analysis of *Ki67* expression analysis and to the derivation of a hypothesis for the mechanism of the liver/bodyweight increase. This example indicates how toxicogenomics can be use to provide a greater understanding of the mechanisms of toxicity and shows that these data may be of use in making risk assessments. The inclusion of the three other phenotypically similar models (defined in narrow terms only as showing a cholestatic phenotype), in which the expression of *Cdc2* was different led to the hypothesis that the increase in *Cdc2* expression was not mediated by liver damage, but rather was a chemically mediated induction, and further, that the aberrant expression of *Cdc2* drove the cell cycle. Similarly, the use of several models enabled us to find that monooxygenase induction was caused by griseofulvin rather than being a response to liver damage. Thus, successful toxicogenomics depends not only on generating reliable genomic data, but also on careful experimental design, cross comparison with other studies, and most importantly, on correlation with other data. The challenge in toxicogenomics is not now the generation of the data, but its analysis.

As a finale the applicability of toxicogenomics to defining the resolution or modulation of toxicity and pathological damage is shown in Figure 15.16. Here the liver damage caused by tail-vein administration of ET743 (40 μg kg^{-1}) was ameliorated by the administration 24 h prior to the ET743 of dexamethasone (10 mg kg^{-1}). This could be observed histopatholgically, but also at the genomic level: all the genes

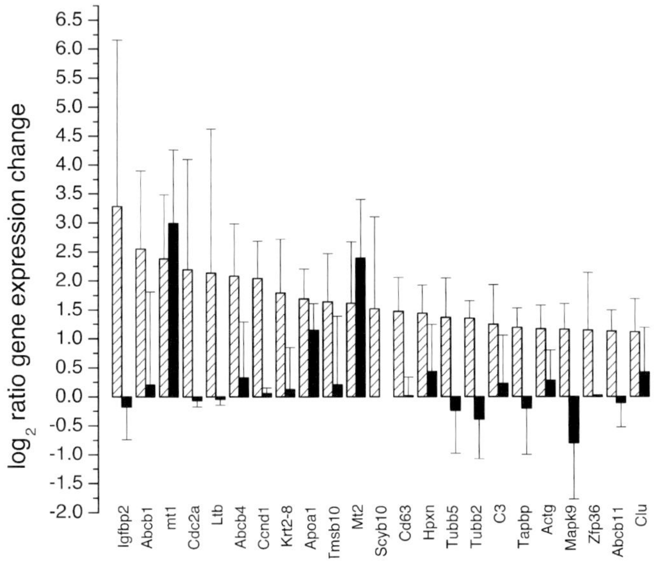

Fig. 15.16 Resolution of ET743-mediated differential gene expression in rat liver by dexamethasone. Shown is the ratio of expression relative to control, of the genes that were maximally differentially expressed in rat liver three days after ET743 injection alone (40 μg kg^{-1} i.v) (hatched bars) and three days after ET743 injection (40 μg kg^{-1} i.v) administered 24 hours after dexamethasone (10 mg kg^{-1}) (black bars). Dexamethasone (10 mg kg^{-1}) administered to rats 24 h prior to i.v. administration of ET743 prevents the liver damage due to ET743. This is reflected in the differential gene expression data: those genes that were maximally differentially expressed after ET743 treatment were unchanged when the ET743 was administered 24 h after dexamethasone, with the exception of the metallothionin genes *Mt1* and *Mt2*.

most induced either as a result of the compound bile duct inflammation and liver damage or the consequent cholestasis were unchanged in expression, with the exception of the metallothionein genes 1 and 2 (*Mt1* and *Mt2*) [47].

Acknowledgements

Many researchers have contributed to the work presented in this chapter and in alphabetical order their contribution is acknowledged here:

Petra Baus, Bruce Clothier, Reginald Davies, Sarah Donald, Jenny Edwards, Richard Edwards, David J. Judah, JinLi Luo, Katie Ridd, Joan Riley, Arenda Shulmann, Colin Travis and the staff of Biomedical Services, Richard Verschoyle, Shu-Dong Zhang.

References

1. Trauner, M. and Boyer, J.L. Bile salt transporters: molecular characterization, function and regulation. Physiol. Rev. 2002, **83**, 633–671.
2. Trauner, M., Meier, P.J. and Boyer, J.L. Molecular pathogenesis of cholestasis. New Engl. J. Med. 1998, **339**, 1217–1227.
3. Meier, P.J. and Stieger, B. Bile salt transporters. Annu. Rev. Physiol. 2002, **64**, 635–661.
4. Tutois, S., Montagutelli, X., Da Silva,V., Jouault, H., Rouyer-Fessard, P., Leroy-Viard, K., Guéne, J.L., Nordmann,Y. and Deybach, J.C. Erythropoietic protoporphyria in the house mouse. J. Clin. Invest. 1991, **88**, 1730–1736.
5. Boulechfar, S., Lamoril, J., Montagutelli, X., Guenet, J.L., Deybach, J.C., Nordmann,Y., Dailey, H., Grandchamp, B. and deVerneuil, H. Ferrochelatase structural mutant ($Fech^{m1Pas}$) in the house mouse. Genomics 1993, **16**, 645–648.
6. Meerman, L., Koopen, N.R., Bloks,V.,Van Goor, H., Havinga, R.,Wolthers, B.G., Kramer,W., Stengelin, S., Muller, M., Kuipers, F. and Jansen, P.L.M. Biliary fibrosis associated with altered bile duct composition in a mouse model of erythropoietic protoporphyria. Gastroenterology 1999, **117**, 696–705.
7. Bloks,V.W., Plosch,T., van Goor, H., Roelofsen, H., Baller, J., Havinga, R., Verkade, H.J., van Tol, A., Jansen, P.L.M. and Kuipers, F. Hyperlipidemia and atherosclerosis associated with liver disease in ferrochelatase-deficient mice. J. Lipid Res. 2001, **42**, 41–50.
8. Knasmuller, S., Parzefall,W., Helma, C., Kassie, F., Ecker, S. and Schulte-Hermann, R. Toxic effects of griseofulvin: disease models, mechanisms and risk assessment. CRC Cr. Rev. Toxicol. 1997, **27**, 495–537.
9. Holley, A., King, L.J., Gibbs, A.H. and De Matteis, F. Strain and sex differences in the response of mice to drugs that induce protoporphyria: role of porphyrin biosynthesis and removal. J. Biochem. Toxicol. 1990, **5**, 175–182.
10. Gant,T.W., Baus, P.R., Clothier, B., Riley, J., Davies, R., Judah, D.J., Edwards, R.E., George, E., Greaves, P. and Smith, A.G. Gene expression profiles associated with inflammation, fibrosis and cholestasis in mouse liver after griseofulvin. EHP Toxicogenomics 2003, **111**, 847–853.
11. Hendricks, H.R., Fiebig, H.H., Giavazzi, R., Langdon, S.P., Jimeno, J.M. and Faircloth, G.T. High antitumor activity of ET-743 against human tumor xenografts from melanoma, non-small cell lung cancer and ovarian cancer. Ann. Oncol. 1999, **10**, 1233–1240.
12. Valoti, G., Nicoletti, M.I., Pellegrino, A., Jimeno, J.M., Hendricks, H., D'Incalci, M., Faircloth, G. and Giavazzi, R. Ecteinascidin-743. Clinical Cancer Research 1999, **4**, 1977–1983.

13. Izbicka, E., Lawrence, R., Raymond, E., Eckhardt, G., Jimeno, J., Clark, G. and VonHoff, D.D. In vitro antitumor activity of the novel marine agent ecteinascidin-743 (ET-743, NSC-648766) against human tumors explanted from patients. Ann. Oncol 1998, **9**, 981–987.
14. Donald, S.,Verschoyle, R.D., Edwards, R., Judah, D.J., Davies, R., Riley, J., Dinsdale, D., Lazaro, L.L., Smith, A.G., Gant, T.W., Greaves, P. and Gescher, A.J. Hepatobiliary damage and changes in hepatic gene expression caused by the antitumor drug ecteinascidin-743 (ET-743) in the female rat. Cancer Res. 2002, **62**, 4256–4262.
15. Schrenk, D., Gant, T.W., Preisegger, K.H., Silverman, J.A., Marino, P.A. and Thorgeirsson, S.S. Induction of multidrug resistance gene expression during cholestasis in rats and nonhuman primates. Hepatology 1993, **17**, 854–860.
16. Turton, N.J., Judah, D.J., Riley, J., Davies, R., Lipson, D., Styles, J.A., Smith, A.G. and Gant, T.W. Gene expression and amplification in breast carcinoma cells with intrinsic and acquired doxorubicin resistance. Oncogene 2001, **20**, 1300–1306.
17. Sadlon, T.J., Dell'Oso, T., Surinya, K.H. and May, B.K. Regulation of erythroid 5-aminolevulinate synthase expression during erythropoiesis. Int. J. Biochem. Cell Biol. 1999, **31**, 1153–1167.
18. Kramer, M.F., Gunaratne, P. and Ferreira, G.C. Transcriptional regulation of the murine erythroid-specific 5-aminolevulinate synthase gene. Gene 2000, **247**, 153–166.
19. Ferreira, G.C. (1999) 5-Aminolevulinate synthase and mammalian heme biosynthesis. In: Iron Metabolism. Inorganic Biochemistry and Regulatory Mechanisms. Eds: Ferreira, G.C., Moura, J.J.G. and Franco, R.) Wiley-VCH,Weinheim, 15–34.
20. Ponka, P. Tissue-specific regulation of iron metabolism and heme synthesis: distinct control mechanisms in arythroid cells. Blood 1997, **89**, 1–25.
21. Cox, T.C., Bawden, M.J., Martin, A. and May, B.K. Human erythroid 5-aminolevulinate synthase: promoter analysis and identification of an iron responsive element in the mRNA. EMBO J. 1991, **7**, 1891–1902.
22. Melefors, O., Goossen, B., Johansson, H.E., Stripecke, R., Gray, N.K. and Hentze, M.W. Translational control of 5-aminolevulinate synthase mRNA by iron-responsive elements in erythroid cells. J. Biol. Chem. 1993, **268**, 5974–5978.
23. Ferreira, G.C. Ferrolchelatase binds the iron responsive element present in the erythroid 5-aminolevulinate synthase mRNA. Biochem. Biophys. Res. Comm. 1995, **214**, 875–878.
23a. Fraser, D.J, Zumsteg, A., and Meyer, U.A. Nuclear receptors constitutive androstane receptor and pregnane X receptor activate a drug-responsive enhancer of the murine 5-aminolevulinic acid synthase gene. J. Biol. Chem. 2003, **278**, 39392–39401.
24. Ueda, A., Hamadeh, H.K.,Webb, H.K., Yamamoto,Y., Sueyoshi,T.L., JM, Afshari, C.A. and Negishi, M. Diverse roles of the nuclear orphan receptor CAR in regulating hepatic genes in response to phenobarbital. Mol. Pharmacol. 2002, **61**, 1–6.
25. Kietzmann, T., Samoylenko, A. and Immenschuh, S. Transcriptional regulation of heme oxygenase-1 gene expression by MAP kinases of the JNK and p38 pathways in primary cultures of rat hepatocytes. J. Biol. Chem. 2003, **278**, 17927–17936.
26. Inafuku, K., Takamiyagi, A., Oshiro, M., Kinjo, T., Nakashima,Y. and Nonaka, S. Alteration of mRNA levels of D-aminolevulinic acid synthase, ferrochelatase and heme oxygenase-1 in griseofulvin induced protoporphyria mice. J. Dermatol. Sci. 1999, **19**, 189–198.
27. Salonpaa, P., Krause, K., Pelkonen, O. and Raunio, H. Up-regulation of CYP2A5 expression by porphrinogenic agents in mouse liver. N-S Arc. Ex. Path. Ph. 1995, **351**, 446–452.
28. Wastl, U.M., Rossmanith,W., Lang, M.A., Camus-Randon, A.M., Grasl-Kraupp, B., Bursch,W. and Schulte-Hermann, R. Expression of cytochrome P450 2A5 in preneoplastic and neoplastic mouse liver lesions. Mol. Carcinogen. 1998, **22**, 229–234.
29. Libbrecht, L., Meerman, L., Kuipers, F., Roskams, T., Desmet,V. and Jansen, P. Liver pathology and hepatocarcinogenesis in a long-term model of erythropoietic protoporphyria. J. Path. 2003, **199**, 191–200.

30. Sueyoshi, T. and Negishi, M. Phenobarbital response elements of cytochrome P450 genes and nuclear receptors. Annu. Rev. Pharmacol. Toxicol. 2001, **41**, 123–143.

31. Zhang, J., Huang, W., Chua, S.S., Wei, P. and Moore, D.D. Modulation of acetaminophen-induced hepatotoxicity by the xenobiotic receptor CAR. Science 2002, **298**, 422–424.

32. Pascussi, J.M., Gerbal-Chaloin, S., Drocourt, L., Maurel, P. and Vilarem, M.J. The expression of *Cyp2b6*, *cyp2c9* and *cyp3a4* genes: a tangle of networks of nuclear and steroid receptors. Biochim. Biophys. Acta 2003, **1619**, 243–253.

33. Alizadeh, A.A., Ross, D.T., Perou, C.M. and van de Rijn, M. Towards a novel classification of human malignancies based on gene expression patterns. J. Path. 2001, **195**, 41–52.

34. Dyrsjot, L., Thykjaer, T., Kruhoffer, M., Jensen, J.L., Marcussen, N., Hamilton-Dutoit, S., Wolf, H. and Orntoft, T.F. Identifying distinct classes of bladder carcinoma using microarrays. Nat. Genet. 2003, **33**, 90–96.

35. Ramaswarmy, S., Ross, K.N., Lander, E.S. and Golub, T.R. A molecular signature of metastasis in primary solid tumours. Nat. Genet. 2003, **33**, 49–54.

36. Alizadeh, A.A., Eisen, M.B., Davis, R.E., Ma, C., Lossos, I.S., Rosenwald, A., Boldrick, J.G., Sabet, H., Tran, T., Yu, X., Powell, J.I., Yang, L.M., Marti, G.E., Moore, T., Hudson, J., Lu, L.S., Lewis, D.B., Tibshirani, R., Sherlock, G., Chan, W.C., Greiner, T.C., Weisenburger, D.D., Armitage, J.O., Warnke, R., Levy, R., Wilson, W., Grever, M.R., Byrd, J.C., Botstein, D., Brown, P.O. and Staudt, L.M. Distinct types of diffuse large B-cell lymphoma identified by gene expression profiling. Nature 2000, **403**, 503–511.

37. Staudt, L.M. Gene expression profiling of lymphoid malignancies. Annu. Rev. Med. 2002, **53**, 303–318.

38. Hamadeh, H.K., Bushel, P.R., Jayadev, S., DiSorbo, O., Bennett, L., Tennant, R., Stoll, R., Barrett, J.C., Paules, R.S., Blanchard, K. and Afshari, C.A. Prediction of compound signature using high density gene expression profiling. Toxicol. Sci. 2002, **67**, 232–240.

39. Hamadeh, H.K., Knight, B.L., Haugen, A.C., Sieber, S., Amin, R.P., Bushel, P.R., Stoll, R., Blanchard, K., Jayadev, S., Tennant, R.W., Cunningham, M.L., Afshari, C.A. and Paules, R.S. Mathapyrilene toxicity: anchorage of pathologic observations to gene expression alterations. Toxicol. Pathol. 2002, **30**, 470–482.

40. Ulrich, R. and Friend, S.H. Toxicogenomics and drug discovery: will new technologies help us produce better drugs? Nat. Rev. Drug Discov. 2002, **1**, 84–88.

41. Waring, J.F., Ciurlionis, R., Jolly, R.A., Heindel, M. and Ulrich, R.G. Microarray analysis of hepatotoxins *in vitro* reveals a correlation between gene expression profiles and mechanisms of toxicity. Toxicol. Lett. 2001, **120**, 359–368.

42. Waring, J.F. and Ulrich, R.G. The impact of genomics-based technologies on drug safety evaluation. Ann. Rev. Pharmacol. Toxicol. 2000, **40**, 335–352.

43. Fogel, M., Friederichs, J., Zeller, Y., Husar, M., Smirnov, A., Roitman, L., Altevogt, P. and Sthoeger, Z.M. CD24 is a marker for human breast carcinoma. Cancer Lett. 1999, **143**, 87–94.

44. Stumptner, C., Fuchsbichler, A., Heid, H., Zatloukal, K. and Denk, H. Mallory body: a disease-associated type of sequestosome. Hepatology 2002, **35**, 1053–1062.

45. Brooks, G., Poolman, R.A. and Li, J.M. Arresting developments in the cardiac myocyte cell cycle: role of cyclin-dependent kinase inhibitors. Cardio. Res. 1998, **39**, 301–311.

46. Jeong, D.-H., Jang, J.-J., Lee, S.-J., Lee, J.-H., Kim, I.-K., Lee, M.-J. and Lee, Y.-S. Expression patterns of cell cycle-related proteins in a rat cirrhotic model induced by CCl_4 or thioacetamide. J. Gastroenterol. 2001, **36**, 24–33.

47. Donald, S., Verschoyle, R.D., Greaves, P., Gant, T.W., Colombo, T., Zaffaroni, M., Frapolli, R., Zucchetti, M., D'Incalci, M., Meco, D., Ricardi, R., Lopez-Lazaro, L., Jimeno, J., and Genscher, A.J. Complete protection by high-dose dexamethasone against the hepatotoxicity of the novel antitumor drug Yondelis (ET-743) in the rat. Cancer Res. 2003, **63**, 5902–5908.

16
Toxicogenomics Applied to Cardiovascular Toxicity

Thomas Thum and Jürgen Borlak

16.1
Introduction

Toxicogenomics is an emerging discipline that uses genomics tools, including gene expression profiling technologies, to address problems of toxicological significance. Initial results are now available from studies in which toxicogenomic approaches have been applied to cardiovascular toxicity resulting from treatment with certain drugs or from environmental pollutants. A variety of drugs were shown to have potential for cardiovascular toxicity. Here, we use a classification based on the phenotype of cardiotoxicity caused by a certain drug and include, whenever available, results from recent toxicogenomic or toxicoproteomic approaches applied to cardiovascular toxicity. We also discuss the impact of environmental pollutants, such as halogenated aromatic hydrocarbons, on the onset of cardiovascular toxicity. Finally, the importance of genetic polymorphisms and tissue-specific metabolism in cardiovascular drug therapy and toxicity is discussed.

16.2
Toxicogenomics Applied to Cardiovascular Toxicity

16.2.1
Drug-induced Cardiac Arrhythmias

Treatment with certain drugs can have both wanted and unwanted electrophysiological effects on the heart. Antiarrhythmics, antihistamines, antidepressants, antimalarial, and other drugs have been associated with arrhythmic events, such as QTc prolongation, torsade-des-pointes arrhythmias, sinus-node disease, atrial and ventricular tachycardias, and sudden cardiac death [1–3].

The paradoxical finding that anti-arrhythmic drugs can cause arrhythmias was shown for the drug quinidine as early as 1918 [4]. In addition, results of the Cardiac Arrhythmia Suppression Trial (CAST) demonstrated an increased mortality in post-

Handbook of Toxicogenomics: Strategies and Applications. Edited by Jürgen Borlak

ISBN: 3-527-30342-1

infarction patients treated with encainide, flecainide, or moricizine [1]. These adverse drug reactions can be, in part, explained by modulation of cardiac ion channels. Indeed, cardiac sodium, calcium, and various potassium channels can be blocked by a variety of drugs. However, the potassium channels, particularly the delayed rectifier K^+ current $K_v11.1$ coded by the human *ether-a-go-go-related* (*HERG*) gene, play the most significant part in drug-induced QT syndromes [5]. Prolonged QT intervals are a risk factor for cardiac sudden death by cardiac arrest [6].

The delayed rectifier K^+ channels are also blocked by the second-generation antihistamines terfenadine and astemizole and the prokinetic $5HT_4$-receptor agonist cisapride [2]. Patients treated with these drugs are also at risk of developing prolonged QT intervals in the ECG and severe arrhythmias [2]. The cardiotoxic effects are pronounced in patients after drug overdosing or who are predisposed to cardiac disease, such as those evincing long-QT syndromes [7]. Cardiac disease is often associated with severe deregulation of ion channels and, in particular, with repression of major potassium channels, as evidenced recently by a knowledge-based genomics study of healthy and diseased human hearts [8]. Because many of the drugs mentioned above are metabolized by the cytochrome P450 isoform CYP3A4, inhibitors of this enzyme system, such as erythromycin or ketoconazole, can lead to enhanced plasma levels and thus to cardiotoxic events [9, 10]. Therefore, proper assessment of the risk profile of the patient must be done before prescribing potential arrhythmic drugs.

An additional group of arrhythmogenic drugs are antidepressants. Indeed, the early use of tricyclic antidepressants (TCA) led to more than 1000 deaths by overdose per year in the late 1970s and early 1980s in the U.S. [11]. In contrast to other drugs, which predominantly affect potassium currents, the observed QTc prolongation under therapy with TCAs is likely due to the blocking of sodium channels during depolarization [12]. Other, older antipsychotic drugs causing cardiotoxicity are the phenothiazines and butyrophenones (e. g., haloperidol), which mainly affect potassium channels but can also block α-adrenergic receptors, thus sometimes leading to unpredictable severe hypotension [13]. In addition, lithium changes the electrical activity of the heart and can lead to sinus-node disease, which is not characterized by QTc prolongation, but most likely is a calcium channel effect on the sinus node [14]. The selective serotonin reuptake inhibitors bupropion and ziprasidone are safer than other antidepressants with respect to cardiac electrophysiology, but single case studies have reported arrhythmic events [15]. A variety of other noncardiac drugs have also been linked to cardiac arrhythmic events, as reviewed recently [16, 17].

In conclusion, patients treated with certain antiarrhythmics, antihistamines, antidepressants, or antimalarials may be at particular risk of suffering from cardiotoxic arrhythmogenic side effects such as QTc prolongation; therefore, drug therapy should monitored with caution.

16.2.2
Drug-induced Myocardial Apoptosis and Necrosis

Apoptosis is a highly regulated, energy-requiring process characterized by cell shrinkage, DNA fragmentation, caspase activation, and membrane blebbing and was first recognized in heart muscle cells in 1994 [18]. Although the rate of apoptosis in diseased hearts is low (<0.5%), it is sufficient for the development of heart failure [19]. Several drugs have been implicated in myocardial apoptosis. Anthracylines, such as doxorubicin, are used in the therapy of leukaemia and cancer, but their use is limited because of their cumulative dose-dependent cardiotoxicity, which was generally attributed to myocardial apoptosis and enhanced production of radical oxygen species (ROS) during cellular metabolism [20]. In addition, studies of catalase-overexpressing transgenic mice demonstrated protection from adriamycin-induced chronic cardiotoxicity [21]. Treatment with anthracylines also enhances expression and secretion of the stress marker atrial natriuretic peptide (ANP) [22] and leads to mitochondrial damage and cytochrome c release [23]. After i.v. administration, the highest tissue-specific concentrations of doxorubicin were found in liver, spleen, kidneys, lung, and heart. Doxorubicin additionally activates a p38 mitogen-activated protein kinase (MAPK), which is critically involved in apoptosis [24] and suppresses the GATA4 transcription factor, an important key regulator of cardiac muscle cells [25]. A complete understanding of the molecular mechanisms leading to anthracyline-induced apoptosis is still lacking, but novel approaches, such as functional genomics, proteomics, and metabonomics will significantly improve our understanding of drug-induced cardiotoxicity. For example, cDNA arrays have been used to gain novel insight into doxorubicin's mode of action. Watts et al. [26] used a human multiple myeloma cell line and identified 29 deregulated genes participating in apoptotic signalling after treatment with doxorubicin. Our group additionally employed a microarray approach to investigate cardiac gene expression after treatment of rats with doxorubicin (4 days, 10 mg kg^{-1}). A major finding was the repression of important transcription factors; in contrast, certain genes coding for cell cycle, extracellular matrix, and metabolism were upregulated [27]. The deregulation of heart-specific transcription factors may provide the rationale for some of the clinical findings observed after treatment with doxorubicin, e.g., metabolic deregulation, apoptosis, and cardiac remodelling. In addition, a proteomics approach was used to investigate the effects of doxorubicin on a cultured human breast cancer cell line (MCF-7). A major finding was that the action of doxorubicin on breast cancer cells may be partly related to deregulation of the heat shock protein 27 [28]. Recent clinical studies have documented high anti-cancer efficacy of trastuzumab, which is a monoclonal antibody used in treatment of HER2 (erbB2/neu)-overexpressing metastatic breast carcinomas. The risk of cardiotoxicity is enhanced when doxorubicin and trastuzumab are administered concomitantly. Treatment of human breast cancer cell lines with trastuzumab enhanced the probability of apoptosis [29] and inhibited expression of fatty acid synthase, which is overexpressed in breast cancer [30]. The observed enhanced cardiotoxicity of combined treatment with doxorubicin and trastuzumab might be due to the loss of erbB2-receptor–dependent myocyte survival pathways [31]. This in turn may create a susceptibility to apoptotic events and may lead to the observed onset of heart failure in certain patients.

In addition to anthracyclines, several other drugs and chemicals also lead to myocardial apoptosis. The α1-adrenoceptor–blocking antihypertensives doxazosin and prazosin have been associated with increased risk of heart failure [32, 33], and it was recently shown in an *in vitro* model of neonatal rat cardiomyocytes that the observed cardiotoxicity was explainable by an enhanced rate of apoptotic events [34]. In addition, zidovudine, a widely used antiviral drug for the treatment of AIDS, results in dilated cardiomyopathy in a selected patient group [35], but the mechanisms leading to cardiotoxicity are still unknown. In addition, the arrhythmogenic potential of antiviral acting α-interferon is potentiated in pathophysiological heart disease [36]. Severe exposure to carbon monoxide can result in myocardial necrosis and cardiomyopathy due to tissue hypoxia [37, 38]. The environmental metals iron, cadmium, cobalt, mercury, and arsenic (also used in the treatment of acute promyelocytic leukaemia) additionally facilitate myocardial apoptosis and lead to ventricular tachycardia and/or cardiomyopathy [39–43].

Whereas some progress in the understanding of anthracycline-induced cardiotoxicity has been made in the past few years, very little is known about other cardiotoxic drugs. Recent findings indicate the presence of cardiac stem cells in the adult heart, which have limited potential for myocyte renewal [44]. It will be interesting to search for toxic effects of drugs on this novel subpopulation of heart cells, because toxic effects on these cells may additionally contribute to the development of chronic heart failure.

16.2.3 Drug-induced Cardiomyopathy and Myocardial Remodelling

Extensive toxic insults persisting for a long time can lead to changes in myocardial morphology. This process is often referred to as 'remodelling'. Myocardial remodelling is first an adaptive response, but is maladaptive in the long term and often leads to cardiac dysfunction and development of cardiomyopathy. Typical molecular responses to cardiotoxic drugs are increases in cell size and protein synthesis [45], upregulation of foetal cardiac genes [46], and induction of immediate–early genes [47]. The observed reprogramming of cardiac gene expression is often correlated with the development of cardiac hypertrophy, which leads to tissue hypoperfusion and, in turn, to the activation of compensatory mechanisms, such as ANP secretion or activation of the renin–angiotensin system [48, 49]. Activation of ANP also triggers myocardial apoptosis [50]. Additional alterations include changes in the extracellular matrix as observed in patients with heart failure [51] and in doxorubicin-treated rats, such as interstitial collagen accumulation [52] or enhanced expression of the fibrillin gene, as observed in a microarray study [27]. Long-term treatment of rats with doxorubicin (1 mg kg^{-1} $week^{-1}$ for 9 weeks) led to significant induction of genes involved in tissue injury and remodelling [53]. Importantly, there is evidence that amifostine or the iron chelator dexrazoxane can reduce myocardial damage when administered concomitantly [54]. Some of the beneficial effects of dexrazoxane could be explained by a microarray approach, where normalization of a variety of doxorubicin-deregulated genes was demonstrated [53].

16.2.4
Drug-induced Myocarditis and Inflammation

Drug-induced toxic myocarditis is rare, but is occasionally seen upon drug treatment with antipsychotics such as amitriptyline or after chronic cocaine abuse [55–57]. For example, signs of severe toxic myocarditis with fibrosis of the heart were shown to be related to treatment with amitriptyline [55]. In addition, 18 instances of myocarditis induced by treatment with clozapine have been reported [58, 59]. These patients showed symptoms such as fever, sinus tachycardia, chest discomfort, and heart failure, and mortality was about 50%. There is also evidence for an association of nonsteroidal antiinflammatory drugs (NSAID) with heart failure [60, 61]. This might be related to selective inhibition of cyclooxygenase-2 and, in turn, impaired renal function, but some reports link treatment with NSAIDs to progressive myocarditis [60]. Nevertheless, further investigations are needed to establish a valid link between myocarditis and the above-mentioned drugs.

16.2.5
Drug-induced Effects on Cardiac Contractility

In general, all drugs that inhibit myocardial contractility can lead to repression of heart function and to severe toxicity when overdosed. In addition, instances have occurred of 'idiopathic' adverse effects after normal dosing, which now can be partly explained by certain genetic polymorphisms with respect to drug-metabolizing enzymes, drug transporters, or receptors (Section 16.3.1) or to drug–drug interactions. The most common adverse effects of β-adrenergic antagonists arise as pharmacological consequences of blocking the beta receptors. Indeed, β-adrenergic blockade can cause or exacerbate heart failure in patients with already-impaired heart function [62]. Nonetheless, the use of β-adrenergic antagonists in the therapy of heart failure in selected patients is very beneficial [63]. This might be due, at least in part, to the normalization of deregulated ion-channel expression or function after treatment of heart failure with β-adrenergic blockers, as suggested recently [8, 64]. In addition, a variety of local or systemic anaesthetics, such as propofol and etomidate, may have negative inotropic effects [65, 66], but the mode of action is still uncertain.

16.2.6
Drug-induced Cardiac Hypertrophy

Cardiac hypertrophy is one end point of chronic myocardial toxicity observed after intake of a variety of drugs and chemicals, including doxorubicin, cocaine, monocrotaline, and anabolics [67–69]. Several underlying molecular events have been identified, including an increase in myocardial radical oxygen species, circulating catecholamines, altered hemodynamics, and enhanced cardiac hypoxia. Characteristic changes in gene expression in cardiac hypertrophy result in elevation of ANP, β-myosin heavy chain, and skeletal α actin, as well as changes in important cardiac transcription factors [48, 70]. These changes have also been observed in drug-induced cardiac hypertrophy with doxorubicin, cocaine, and others [67–69].

Cocaine causes coronary vasoconstriction, increases cardiac sympathetic effects, facilitates arrhythmias, and produces cardiac hypertrophy [68, 71]. The increase in protein content of cardiomyocytes after intake of cocaine has been explained, in part, by protein kinase C–dependent mechanisms [72].

Anabolic drugs (e.g., androstanolon, nandrolon), which are abused for improving athletic performance, have been linked to sudden cardiac death, acute myocardial infarction, and cardiac hypertrophy [69, 73]. Indeed, testosterone influences human left ventricular hypertrophy [74], and modulation of local metabolism of testosterone via certain cytochrome P450 monooxygenases and other steroid-metabolizing enzymes is likely to play a major role in cardiac hypertrophy [48]. In addition, the observed induction of androgen receptor and enhanced production of high-affinity ligands, including dihydrotestosterone, in hypertrophic human hearts, may lead to exaggerated cardiac-specific gene expression [48, 75, 76]. This may accelerate cardiac hypertrophy via an androgen receptor signalling pathway. The latter findings may translate into new concepts in the treatment of cardiac hypertrophy based on modulation of tissue-specific steroid metabolism. Global transcriptome analysis has been used for identifying deregulated genes in both human and experimental cardiac hypertrophy [77, 78] and will be additionally used in the near future for identifying deregulated genes and for generating hypotheses concerning the elucidation of mechanisms leading to drug-induced cardiac hypertrophy.

16.2.7
Drug-induced Vascular Injury

Our understanding of why certain drugs cause vascular injury is limited. Several underlying mechanisms have been discussed, which include (1) biomechanical injury after changes in shear stress, (2) direct toxic effects by pharmacological or chemical perturbation, and (3) immune-mediated injuries.

Drug-induced biomechanical injury was observed after the treatment with drugs that alter local hemodynamics, e.g., the potassium channel opener minoxidil, the selective dopaminergic vasodilator fenoldopam, adenosine agonists, or endothelin receptor antagonists [79–81]. These agents cause profound increases in regional blood flow, thus causing arterial lesions [79]. Allylamine and β-amino-proprionitrile are direct-acting vascular toxicants [82]. In addition, certain drugs can lead to a local activation of the immune system, which can in turn cause vascular injury. There is good evidence that certain hematopoietic growth factors and interferons cause vasculitis [83]. Drugs such as hydralazine, penicillamine, and propyl thiouracil have additionally been associated with vasculitis, but the underlying mechanisms are far from clear [84].

The application of genomic, proteomic, and metabolomic technologies to drug-induced vascular injury is a relatively recent development. To date, most work has focused on phosphodiesterase-4 inhibitor (PDE4)–induced arteriopathy in the rat [85, 86]. Bioinformatics tools such as principal components analysis have enabled a clear discrimination between PDE4-induced vascular injury of rats and healthy controls [86]. Novel technologies can lead to the identification of biomarkers and can provide insight into the mechanisms of drug-induced vascular injury.

16.3 Environmental Pollution and Cardiotoxicity: Effect of Halogenated Aromatic Hydrocarbons

Cardiotoxicity has been linked to air pollution and other environmental insults [87, 88]. Increased exposure to particulate matter contributes to cardiovascular morbidity and mortality [89, 90], which seem to depend on both the composition and the aerodynamic diameter of the particles [89]. Indeed, long-term exposure to fine (< 2.5 μm) particulate air pollution was shown to be an important environmental risk factor for cardiopulmonary mortality [89]. The underlying mechanisms are far from clear; however, initial evidence is now available that immunologic events, such as elevation of the acute-phase response C-reactive protein [91] , as well as direct cardiotoxic effects [92], are of critical importance [20].

Halogenated aromatic hydrocarbons are one of the best known environmental pollutants and have been linked to the development of cardiovascular diseases [93, 94]. The biological risk of these compounds has been correlated with their ability to activate the aryl hydrocarbon receptor (AhR) [95]. This cytosolic receptor is a member of the basic helix–loop–helix/PAS protein family and is bound to a chaperone complex together with two molecules of heat-shock protein 90 (HSP90) and the Ah receptor inhibitory protein [96]. Upon binding of a ligand (e. g., TCDD), AhR translocates into the nucleus and dissociates from its chaperone complex [97]. AhR subsequently dimerizes with its DNA-binding partner, the AhR nuclear translocator (ARNT), and binds to specific dioxin-response elements (DRE) to drive gene transcription of certain genes such as *CYP1A1* and *CYP1A2* (Figure 16.1). AhR plays an important role in HAH-mediated cardiotoxicity, and cardiovascular tissues express a functional AhR, as evidenced by metabolism experiments with 7-ethoxyresorufin, a specific substrate of CYP1A1 (Figure 16.2). Treatment of cardiomyocyte or endothelial cell cultures with Aroclor1254, a mixture of polychlorinated biphenyl (PCB) isomers and congeners, led to significant increases in CYP1A1 gene expression and enzyme activity [98–101]. In addition, PCBs alter the expression of important heart-specific transcription factor genes and downstream target genes, such as the atrial natriuretic peptide (ANP), an established cardiospecific stress marker [102] (Figure 16.1). Also, several groups have reported HAH-mediated cardiotoxic events on the basis of increased heart wet weights in treated chick embryos and development of severe cardiomyopathy [93, 103]. Protein expression of AhR is also increased in human cardiomyopathic left ventricles [104]. Interestingly, complete knockout of AhR in AhR-null mice also leads to cardiac hypertrophy and dysfunction in adult mice [105]. Thus, a delicate balance of AhR seems to be important for normal heart physiology and development. In a recent microarray study with explanted hearts from rats treated with Aroclor1254 (a mixture of PCB congeners and isomers), expression of >30 genes ac-

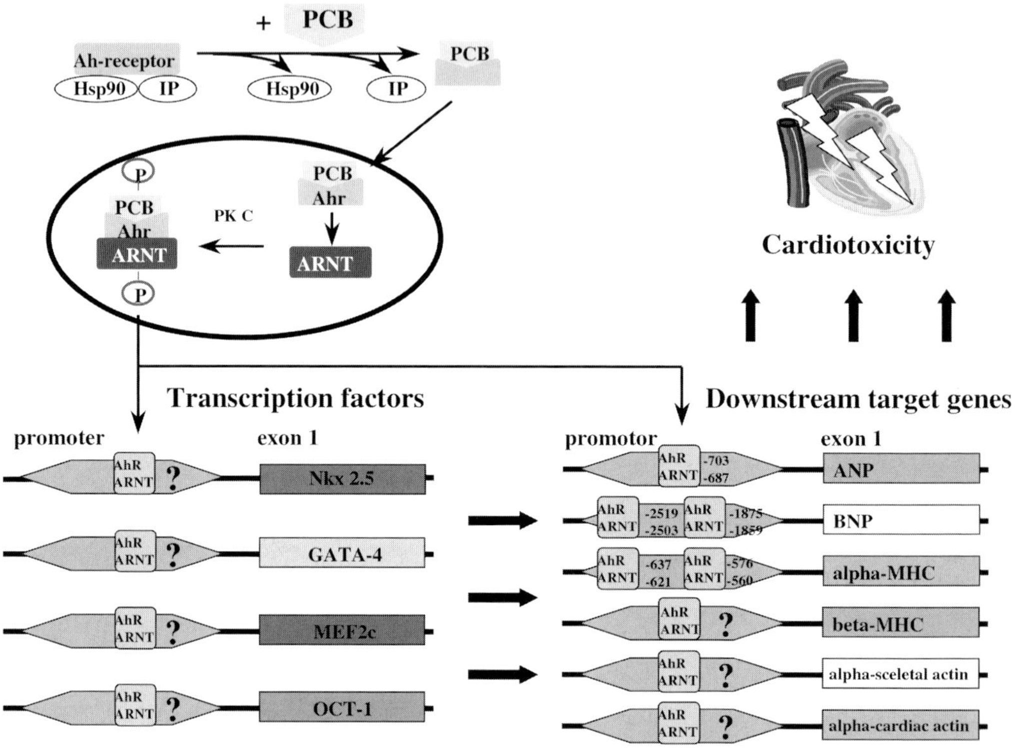

Fig. 16.1 Activation of the aryl-hydrocarbon receptor by polychlorinated biphenyls leads to derailed expression of heart-specific transcription factors and downstream target genes. HSP90, heat-shock protein 90; IP = immunophilin; P = phosphorylated.

tive during metabolism, cellular differentiation, and stress was found to be dramatically altered [106]. These findings may aid our understanding of the observed increase in cardiovascular diseases in polluted areas.

16.4 Importance of Single Nucleotide Polymorphisms (SNPs) and Tissue-specific Drug Metabolism in Cardiovascular Drug Therapy

16.4.1 Single Nucleotide Polymorphisms and Drug Treatment of Cardiovascular Diseases

It is well recognized that different patients respond in different ways to the same medication. Even though differences in the drug response of individuals can result from the effects of age, sex, organ function, concomitant drug therapy, or drug interactions, genetic factors also influence both the efficacy of a drug and the likelihood

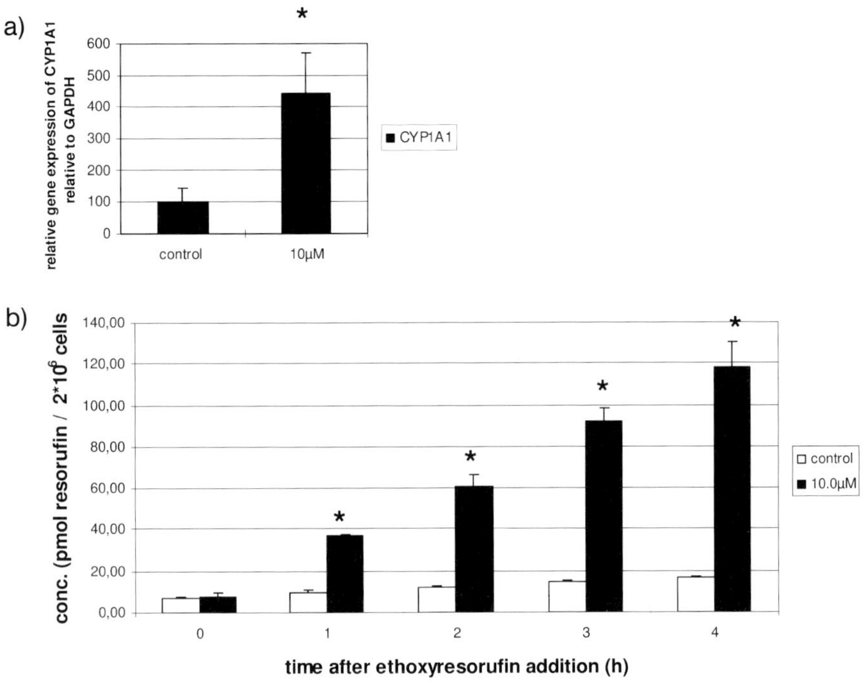

Fig. 16.2 Gene expression (a) and protein activity (b) of CYP1A1 in cultures of adult cardiomyocytes after 24 h treatment with Aroclor 1254 (10 µM). * = $p < 0.05$.

of adverse drug reactions [107]. The initial sequencing of the human genome has identified $>1.4 \times 10^6$ SNPs, of which >60 000 were found in the coding regions of genes [108]. Some of these SNPs have already been linked to substantial changes in the metabolism and efficacy of drugs, and some are also used as predictors of clinical response [109–111]. Genetic polymorphisms in genes coding for proteins involved in drug metabolism or drug transport or for receptors can affect individual responses to cardiovascular agents. It has been known for more than 20 years that approximately 5–10% of Caucasian persons are less able to oxidize the antihypertensive drug debrisoquin or the antiarrhythmic sparteine [112, 113]. These differences could be linked to certain polymorphisms within the cytochrome P450 monooxygenase 2D6 (*CYP2D6*) gene [114]. Further, Rau et al. [115] demonstrated that patients with SNPs in the *CYP2D6* gene have up to 10-times higher plasma concentrations of metoprolol after treatment with this β-adrenoceptor blocking agent. Patients with polymorphisms in drug metabolizing enzymes (DME), which lead to impaired metabolism of drugs, are referred to as 'poor metabolizers'. Indeed, CYP2D6 poor metabolizers are at significantly higher risk for developing adverse effects during metoprolol therapy, due to toxic drug levels after 'normal' dosing [115]. In addition, the antiarrhythmics mexiletine and propafenone are metabolized via CYP2D6, and poor metabolizers had significantly higher plasma concentrations of the respective drug than

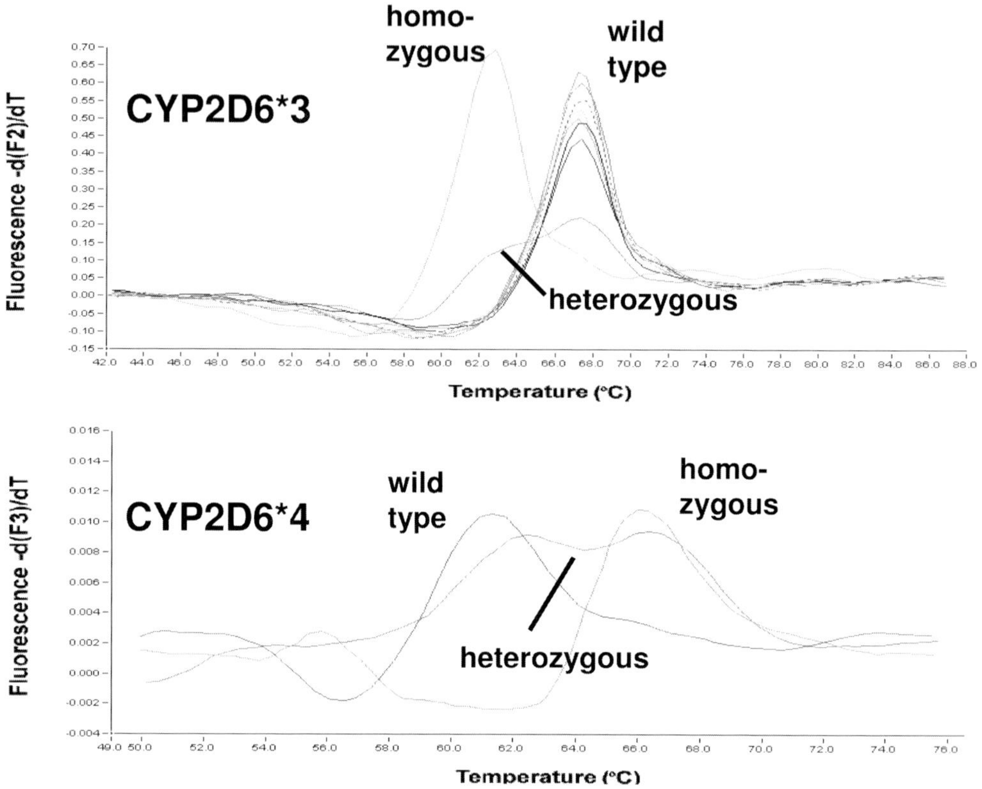

Fig. 16.3 Real-time PCR assay using fluorescence resonance energy transfer hybridization probes for the detection of *CYP2D6* polymorphisms. Melting curves for detection of the wild-type, heterozygous, and homozygous genotypes of the *CYP2D6*3* and *CYP2D6*4* alleles are shown.

did extensive metabolizers [116]. In addition, CYP2C9 and CYP2C19 monooxygenases are responsible for the metabolism of a variety of drugs with cardiotoxic potential, including certain tricyclic antidepressants, barbiturates, β-blockers, and nonsteroidal antiinflamatories [117].

Genetic profiling of important drug-metabolizing enzymes prior to drug therapy will contribute to customized drug therapy and should decrease severe adverse drug reactions [118]. Molecular diagnosis of SNPs can now be easily made for a variety of DME by rapid, cost-effective, accurate methods [111, 119, 120] (Figure 16.3 shows an example in which a method based on fluorescence resonance energy transfer (FRET) revealed various polymorphisms in the *CYP2D6* gene). Future assays will be used to determine more than 10^5 SNPs in a single assay.

16.4.2
Tissue-specific Metabolism in Cardiovascular Tissues

Tissue-specific metabolism of drugs may also affect the efficacy of drug treatment and can lead to striking inter-individual variations in drug response. The vast majority of drug metabolism research has focused on liver tissue, and the metabolic capacity of extrahepatic tissues has long been disregardded. Indeed, several cardiovascular tissues, such as various parts of the heart, arterial coronary, and aortic endothelial cells, as well as smooth muscle cells, express drug-metabolizing enzymes and can metabolize both exogenous and endogenous compounds such as verapamil or testosterone [48, 101, 121–124]. Additionally, endothelial and smooth muscle cells metabolize the drug glyceryl trinitrate to nitric oxide via cytochrome P450s [125]. Although the metabolic competence of cardiovascular tissues is considerably lower than that of liver [123, 124], cellular concentrations of drugs within the target tissue might be affected by local expression of drug-metabolizing enzymes [126]. Underexpression or expression of dysfunctional DMEs due to certain SNPs might then be associated with excessive accumulation and toxic tissue concentrations of a drug, whereas overexpression may lead to impaired drug efficacy or even to the production of toxic metabolites [127].

16.5
Conclusions

Our understanding of cardiovascular toxicity has increased tremendously in recent years. Novel platform technologies, such as global transcriptome analysis, proteomics, and metabonomics, have been integrated in cardiovascular research. As applied to cardiovascular toxicity, toxicogenomics is likely to contribute, at least in part, to a mechanistic understanding, the identification of sensitive and specific biomarkers, and an improved selection of novel compounds for drug development and may also be used for a novel classification of various types of cardiovascular toxicities. Despite the keen interest in the use of proteomics, only a few studies on cardiovascular toxicity using two-dimensional gel electrophoresis and other methods have been done so far [28, 128, 129] – a situation that will soon change. Our understanding of the effects of certain SNPs in the genes for drug-metabolizing enzymes, transporters, and receptors has been considerably improved in the past decade, and pharmacogenetics will further enhance future drug treatment of common cardiovascular diseases.

References

1. Echt DS, Liebson PR, Mitchell LB, Peters RW, Obias-Manno D, Barker AH, Arensberg D, Baker A, Friedman L, Greene HL: Mortality and morbidity in patients receiving encainide, flecainide, or placebo. The Cardiac Arrhythmia Suppression Trial. *N Engl J Med* 1991, 324: 781–788.
2. Paakkari I: Cardiotoxicity of new antihistamines and cisapride. *Toxicol Lett* 2002, 127:279–284.
3. Wesche DL, Schuster BG, Wang WX, Woosley RL: Mechanism of cardiotoxicity of halofantrine. *Clin Pharmacol Ther* 2000, 67:521–529.
4. Frey W: Weitere Erfahrungen mit Chinidin bei absoluter Herzunregelmässigkeit. *Wien Klin Wochenschr* 1918, 55:849–853.
5. Delpon E, Valenzuela C, Tamargo J: Blockade of cardiac potassium and other channels by antihistamines. *Drug Saf* 1999, 21 Suppl 1:11–18.
6. Algra A, Tijssen JG, Roelandt JR, Pool J, Lubsen J: QTc prolongation measured by standard 12-lead electrocardiography is an independent risk factor for sudden death due to cardiac arrest. *Circulation* 1991, 83:1888–1894.
7. Moss AJ: Long QT syndrome. *JAMA* 2003, 289:2041–2044.
8. Borlak J, Thum T: Hallmarks of ion channel gene expression in end-stage heart failure. *FASEB J* 2003, **17**: 1592–1608.
9. Volberg WA, Koci BJ, Su W, Lin J, Zhou J: Blockade of human cardiac potassium channel human *ether-a-go-go-related gene* (HERG) by macrolide antibiotics. *J Pharmacol Exp Ther* 2002, 302:320–327.
10. Monahan BP, Ferguson CL, Killeavy ES, Lloyd BK, Troy J, Cantilena LR Jr.: Torsades de pointes occurring in association with terfenadine use. *JAMA* 1990, 264:2788–2790.
11. Glassman AH: Cardiovascular effects of tricyclic antidepressants. *Annu Rev Med* 1984, 35:503–511.
12. Garson A Jr.: How to measure the QT interval: what is normal? *Am J Cardiol* 1993, 72:14B–16B.
13. Schoenberger JA: Drug-induced orthostatic hypotension. *Drug Saf* 1991, 6: 402–407.
14. Terao T, Abe H, Abe K: Irreversible sinus node dysfunction induced by resumption of lithium therapy. *Acta Psychiatr Scand* 1996, 93:407–408.
15. Biswas AK, Zabrocki LA, Mayes KL, Morris-Kukoski CL: Cardiotoxicity associated with intentional ziprasidone and bupropion overdose. *J Toxicol Clin Toxicol* 2003, 41:101–104.
16. De Ponti F, Poluzzi E, Montanaro N: QT-interval prolongation by non-cardiac drugs: lessons to be learned from recent experience. *Eur J Clin Pharmacol* 2000, 56:1–18.
17. Viskin S, Justo D, Halkin A, Zeltser D: Long QT syndrome caused by noncardiac drugs. *Prog Cardiovasc Dis* 2003, 45: 415–427.
18. Gottlieb RA, Burleson KO, Kloner RA, Babior BM, Engler RL: Reperfusion injury induces apoptosis in rabbit cardiomyocytes. *J Clin Invest* 1994, 94: 1621–1628.
19. Wencker D, Chandra M, Nguyen K, Miao W, Garantziotis S, Factor SM, Shirani J, Armstrong RC, Kitsis RN: A mechanistic role for cardiac myocyte apoptosis in heart failure. *J Clin Invest* 2003, 111:1497.
20. Kang YJ: New understanding in cardiotoxicity. *Curr Opin Drug Discov Dev* 2003, 6:110–116.
21. Kang YJ, Sun X, Chen Y, Zhou Z: Inhibition of doxorubicin chronic toxicity in catalase-overexpressing transgenic mouse hearts. *Chem Res Toxicol* 2002, 15:1–6.
22. Rahman A, Alam M, Rao S, Cai L, Clark LT, Shafiq S, Siddiqui MA: Differential effects of doxorubicin on atrial natriuretic peptide expression *in vivo* and *in vitro*. *Biol Res* 2001, 34: 195–206.
23. Childs AC, Phaneuf SL, Dirks AJ, Phillips T, Leeuwenburgh C: Doxorubicin treatment *in vivo* causes cytochrome c release and cardiomyocyte apoptosis, as well as increased mitochondrial efficiency, superoxide dismu-

tase activity, and Bcl-2:Bax ratio. *Cancer Res* 2002, 62:4592–4598.

24. Kang YJ, Zhou ZX, Wang GW, Buridi A, Klein JB: Suppression by metallothionein of doxorubicin-induced cardiomyocyte apoptosis through inhibition of p38 mitogen-activated protein kinases. *J Biol Chem* 2000, 275: 13690–13698.
25. Kim Y, Ma AG, Kitta K, Fitch SN, Ikeda T, Ihara Y, Simon AR, Evans T, Suzuki YJ: Anthracycline-induced suppression of GATA-4 transcription factor: implication in the regulation of cardiac myocyte apoptosis. *Mol Pharmacol* 2003, 63:368–377.
26. Watts GS, Futscher BW, Isett R, Gleason-Guzman M, Kunkel MW, Salmon SE: cDNA microarray analysis of multidrug resistance: doxorubicin selection produces multiple defects in apoptosis signaling pathways. *J Pharmacol Exp Ther* 2001, 299:434–441.
27. Borlak J, Wagener J, Thum T: Doxorubicin treatment leads to repression of certain transcription factors in rat hearts: a microarray gene expression study in aid of hypothesis generation. [abstract]. *Toxicol Lett* 2003, in press.
28. Chen ST, Pan TL, Tsai YC, Huang CM: Proteomics reveals protein profile changes in doxorubicin-treated MCF-7 human breast cancer cells. *Cancer Lett* 2002, 181:95–107.
29. Lee S, Yang W, Lan KH, Sellappan S, Klos K, Hortobagyi G, Hung MC, Yu D: Enhanced sensitization to taxol-induced apoptosis by herceptin pretreatment in ErbB2-overexpressing breast cancer cells. *Cancer Res* 2002, 62:5703–5710.
30. Kumar-Sinha C, Ignatoski KW, Lippman ME, Ethier SP, Chinnaiyan AM: Transcriptome analysis of HER2 reveals a molecular connection to fatty acid synthesis. *Cancer Res* 2003, 63:132–139.
31. Chien KR: Myocyte survival pathways and cardiomyopathy: implications for trastuzumab cardiotoxicity. *Semin Oncol* 2000, 27:9–14.
32. Messerli FH: Doxazosin and congestive heart failure. *J Am Coll Cardiol* 2001, 38:1295–1296.
33. Sica DA: Doxazosin and congestive heart failure. *Congest Heart Fail* 2002, 8:178–184.
34. Gonzalez-Juanatey JR, Iglesias MJ, Alcaide C, Pineiro R, Lago F: Doxazosin induces apoptosis in cardiomyocytes cultured *in vitro* by a mechanism that is independent of alpha1-adrenergic blockade. *Circulation* 2003, 107: 127–131.
35. Herskowitz A, Willoughby SB, Baughman KL, Schulman SP, Bartlett JD: Cardiomyopathy associated with antiretroviral therapy in patients with HIV infection: a report of six cases. *Ann Intern Med* 1992, 116:311–313.
36. Odashiro K, Hiramatsu S, Yanagi N, Arita T, Maruyama T, Kaji Y, Harada M: Arrhythmogenic and inotropic effects of interferon investigated in perfused and *in vivo* rat hearts: influences of cardiac hypertrophy and isoproterenol. *Circ J* 2002, 66:1161–1167.
37. Marius-Nunez AL: Myocardial infarction with normal coronary arteries after acute exposure to carbon monoxide. *Chest* 1990, 97:491–494.
38. Gandini C, Castoldi AF, Candura SM, Locatelli C, Butera R, Priori S, Manzo L: Carbon monoxide cardiotoxicity. *J Toxicol Clin Toxicol* 2001, 39:35–44.
39. Horwitz LD, Rosenthal EA: Iron-mediated cardiovascular injury. *Vasc Med* 1999, 4:93–99.
40. Suzuki YJ: Stress-induced activation of GATA-4 in cardiac muscle cells. *Free Radical Biol Med* 2003, 34:1589–1598.
41. Limaye DA, Shaikh ZA: Cytotoxicity of cadmium and characteristics of its transport in cardiomyocytes. *Toxicol Appl Pharmacol* 1999, 154:59–66.
42. Centeno JA, Pestaner JP, Mullick FG, Virmani R: An analytical comparison of cobalt cardiomyopathy and idiopathic dilated cardiomyopathy. *Biol Trace Elem Res* 1996, 55:21–30.
43. Li Y, Sun X, Wang L, Zhou Z, Kang YJ: Myocardial toxicity of arsenic trioxide in a mouse model. *Cardiovasc Toxicol* 2002, 2:63–73.
44. Anversa P, Nadal-Ginard B: Myocyte renewal and ventricular remodelling. *Nature* 2002, 415:240–243.

45. Mann DL, Kent RL, Cooper G: Load regulation of the properties of adult feline cardiocytes: growth induction by cellular deformation. *Circ Res* 1989, 64: 1079–1090.
46. Schwartz K, Boheler KR, de la Bastie D, Lompre AM, Mercadier JJ: Switches in cardiac muscle gene expression as a result of pressure and volume overload. *Am J Physiol* 1992, 262:R364–R369.
47. Chien KR, Knowlton KU, Zhu H, Chien S: Regulation of cardiac gene expression during myocardial growth and hypertrophy: molecular studies of an adaptive physiologic response. *FASEB J* 1991, 5: 3037–3046.
48. Thum T, Borlak J: Testosterone, cytochrome P450, and cardiac hypertrophy. *FASEB J* 2002, 16: 1537–1549.
49. Johnston CI, Fabris B, Yoshida K: The cardiac renin–angiotensin system in heart failure. *Am Heart J* 1993, 126: 756–760.
50. Wu CF, Bishopric NH, Pratt RE: Atrial natriuretic peptide induces apoptosis in neonatal rat cardiac myocytes. *J Biol Chem* 1997, 272: 14860–14866.
51. Tan FL, Moravec CS, Li J, Apperson-Hansen C, McCarthy PM, Young JB, Bond M: The gene expression fingerprint of human heart failure. *Proc Natl Acad Sci USA* 2002, 99: 11387.
52. Tokudome T, Mizushige K, Noma T, Manabe K, Murakami K, Tsuji T, Nozaki S, Tomohiro A, Matsuo H: Prevention of doxorubicin (adriamycin)-induced cardiomyopathy by simultaneous administration of angiotensin-converting enzyme inhibitor assessed by acoustic densitometry. *J Cardiovasc Pharmacol* 2000, 36: 361–368.
53. Thompson K, Rosenzweig BA, Pine P, Zhang J, Herman EH, Knapton AD, Honchel R, Shimada B, Kassam S, Finkelstein DB, Lescallet J, Retief JD, Sistare FD: Identification of genes linked to doxorubicin cardiotoxicity and to the cardioprotectant effect of dexrazoxane in rats. *Toxicologist* 2003, 72: 1389.
54. Siveski-Iliskovic N, Hill M, Chow DA, Singal PK: Probucol protects against adriamycin cardiomyopathy without interfering with its antitumor effect. *Circulation* 1995, 91: 10.
55. Ansari A, Maron BJ, Berntson DG: Drug-induced toxic myocarditis. *Tex Heart Inst J* 2003, 30: 76–79.
56. Chokshi SK, Moore R, Pandian NG, Isner JM: Reversible cardiomyopathy associated with cocaine intoxication. *Ann Intern Med* 1989, 111: 1039–1040.
57. Brown J, King A, Francis CK: Cardiovascular effects of alcohol, cocaine, and acquired immune deficiency. *Cardiovasc Clin* 1991, 21: 341–376.
58. Hagg S, Spigset O, Bate A, Soderstrom TG: Myocarditis related to clozapine treatment. *J Clin Psychopharmacol* 2001, 21: 382–388.
59. Idle JR: The heart of psychotropic drug therapy. *Lancet* 2000, 355: 1824–1825.
60. Adachi Y, Yasumizu R, Hashimoto F, Otsuka Y, Okamura A, Kato Y, Oyaizu H, Ikebukuro K, Fukuhara S, Nakai Y, Ikehara S: An autopsy case of giant cell myocarditis probably due to a non-steroidal anti-inflammatory drug. *Pathol Int* 2001, 51: 113–117.
61. Bleumink GS, Van Vliet AC, Van der Tholen A, Stricker BH: Fatal combination of moclobemide overdose and whisky. *Neth J Med* 2003, 61: 88–90.
62. Frishman WH, Furberg CD, Friedewald WT: Beta-adrenergic blockade for survivors of acute myocardial infarction. *N Engl J Med* 1984, 310: 830–837.
63. Hermann DD: Beta-adrenergic blockade 2002: a pharmacologic odyssey in chronic heart failure. *Congest Heart Fail* 2002, 8: 262–269.
64. Reiter MJ, Reiffel JA: Importance of beta blockade in the therapy of serious ventricular arrhythmias. *Am J Cardiol* 1998, 82: 91–191.
65. Fanton JW, Zarr SR, Ewert DL, Woods RW, Koenig SC: Cardiovascular responses to propofol and etomidate in long-term instrumented rhesus monkeys (*Macaca mulatta*). *Comp Med* 2000, 50: 303–308.
66. Mulier JP, Van Aken H: Comparison of eltanolone and propofol on a pressure–volume analysis of the heart. *Anesth Analg* 1996, 83: 233–237.
67. Chen QM, Tu VC, Purdon S, Wood J, Dilley T: Molecular mechanisms of cardiac hypertrophy induced by toxicants. *Cardiovasc Toxicol* 2001, 1: 267–283.

68. Karch SB, Green GS, Young S: Myocardial hypertrophy and coronary artery disease in male cocaine users. *J Forensic Sci* 1995, 40:591–595.
69. Dickerman RD, Schaller F, McConathy WJ: Left ventricular wall thickening does occur in elite power athletes with or without anabolic steroid use. *Cardiology* 1998, 90:145–148.
70. Thum T, Borlak J: Reprogramming of gene expression in cultured cardiomyocytes and in explanted hearts by the myosin ATPase inhibitor butanedione monoxime. *Transplantation* 2001, 71:543–552.
71. Isner JM, Estes NA, III, Thompson PD, Costanzo-Nordin MR, Subramanian R, Miller G, Katsas G, Sweeney K, Sturner WQ: Acute cardiac events temporally related to cocaine abuse. *N Engl J Med* 1986, 315:1438–1443.
72. Henning RJ, Li Y: Cocaine produces cardiac hypertrophy by protein kinase C dependent mechanisms. *J Cardiovasc Pharmacol Ther* 2003, 8:149–160.
73. Fineschi V, Baroldi G, Monciotti F, Paglicci RL, Turillazzi E: Anabolic steroid abuse and cardiac sudden death: a pathologic study. *Arch Pathol Lab Med* 2001, 125:253–255.
74. Hayward CS, Webb CM, Collins P: Effect of sex hormones on cardiac mass. *Lancet* 2001, 357:1354–1356.
75. Morano I, Gerstner J, Ruegg JC, Ganten U, Ganten D, Vosberg HP: Regulation of myosin heavy chain expression in the hearts of hypertensive rats by testosterone. *Circ Res* 1990, 66:1585–1590.
76. Gillardon F, Morano I, Ganten U, Zimmermann M: Regulation of calcitonin gene-related peptide mRNA expression in the hearts of spontaneously hypertensive rats by testosterone. *Neurosci Lett* 1991, 125:77–80.
77. Weinberg EO, Mirotsou M, Gannon J, Dzau VJ, Lee RT, Pratt RE: Sex dependence and temporal dependence of the left ventricular genomic response to pressure overload. *Physiol Genomics* 2003, 12:113.
78. Hwang JJ, Allen PD, Tseng GC, Lam CW, Fananapazir L, Dzau VJ, Liew CC: Microarray gene expression profiles in dilated and hypertrophic cardiomyopathic end-stage heart failure. *Physiol Genomics* 2002, 10:31.
79. Albassam MA, Metz AL, Gragtmans NJ, King LM, Macallum GE, Hallak H, McGuire EJ: Coronary arteriopathy in monkeys following administration of CI-1020, an endothelin A receptor antagonist. *Toxicol Pathol* 1999, 27:156–164.
80. Albassam MA, Smith GS, Macallum GE: Arteriopathy induced by an adenosine agonist-antihypertensive in monkeys. *Toxicol Pathol* 1998, 26:375–380.
81. Louden C, Nambi P, Branch C, Gossett K, Pullen M, Eustis S, Solleveld HA: Coronary arterial lesions in dogs treated with an endothelin receptor antagonist. *J Cardiovasc Pharmacol* 1998, 31 Suppl 1: S384–S385.
82. Boor PJ, Gotlieb AI, Joseph EC, Kerns WD, Roth RA, Tomaszewski KE: Chemical-induced vasculature injury: summary of the symposium presented at the 32nd annual meeting of the Society of Toxicology, New Orleans, Louisiana, March 1993. *Toxicol Appl Pharmacol* 1995, 132:177–195.
83. Merkel PA: Drugs associated with vasculitis. *Curr Opin Rheumatol* 1998, 10:45–50.
84. Norris JH, Leeds J, Jeffrey RF: P-ANCA positive renal vasculitis in association with renal cell carcinoma and prolonged hydralazine therapy. *Ren Fail* 2003, 25:311–314.
85. Slim RM, Robertson DG, Albassam M, Reily MD, Robosky L, Dethloff LA: Effect of dexamethasone on the metabonomics profile associated with phosphodiesterase inhibitor-induced vascular lesions in rats. *Toxicol Appl Pharmacol* 2002, 183:108–109.
86. Robertson DG, Reily MD, Albassam M, Dethloff LA: Metabonomic assessment of vasculitis in rats. *Cardiovasc Toxicol* 2001, 1:7–19.
87. Dockery DW, Pope CA, III, Xu X, Spengler JD, Ware JH, Fay ME, Ferris BG Jr., Speizer FE: An association between air pollution and mortality in six U.S. cities. *N Engl J Med* 1993, 329:1753–1759.

88. Kunzli N, Kaiser R, Medina S, Studnicka M, Chanel O, Filliger P, Herry M, Horak F, Jr., Puybonnieux-Texier V, Quenel P, Schneider J, Seethaler R, Vergnaud JC, Sommer H: Public-health impact of outdoor and traffic-related air pollution: a European assessment. *Lancet* 2000, 356 : 795–801.

89. Pope CA, III, Burnett RT, Thun MJ, Calle EE, Krewski D, Ito K, Thurston GD: Lung cancer, cardiopulmonary mortality, and long-term exposure to fine particulate air pollution. *JAMA* 2002, 287 : 1132–1141.

90. Peters A, Dockery DW, Muller JE, Mittleman MA: Increased particulate air pollution and the triggering of myocardial infarction. *Circulation* 2001, 103 : 2810–2815.

91. Peters A, Frohlich M, Doring A, Immervoll T, Wichmann HE, Hutchinson WL, Pepys MB, Koenig W: Particulate air pollution is associated with an acute phase response in men; results from the MONICA–Augsburg Study. *Eur Heart J* 2001, 22 : 1198–1204.

92. Brook RD, Brook JR, Urch B, Vincent R, Rajagopalan S, Silverman F: Inhalation of fine particulate air pollution and ozone causes acute arterial vasoconstriction in healthy adults. *Circulation* 2002, 105 : 1534–1536.

93. Heid SE, Walker MK, Swanson HI: Correlation of cardiotoxicity mediated by halogenated aromatic hydrocarbons to aryl hydrocarbon receptor activation. *Toxicol Sci* 2001, 61 : 187–196.

94. Toborek M, Barger SW, Mattson MP, Espandiari P, Robertson LW, Hennig B: Exposure to polychlorinated biphenyls causes endothelial cell dysfunction. *J Biochem Toxicol* 1995, 10 : 219–226.

95. Hankinson O: The aryl hydrocarbon receptor complex. *Annu Rev Pharmacol Toxicol* 1995, 35 : 307–340.

96. Chen HS, Perdew GH: Subunit composition of the heteromeric cytosolic aryl hydrocarbon receptor complex. *J Biol Chem* 1994, 269 : 27554–27558.

97. Reyes H, Reisz-Porszasz S, Hankinson O: Identification of the Ah receptor nuclear translocator protein (Arnt) as a component of the DNA binding form of the Ah receptor. *Science* 1992, 256: 1193–1195.

98. Stegeman JJ, Hahn ME, Weisbrod R, Woodin BR, Joy JS, Najibi S, Cohen RA: Induction of cytochrome P450 1A1 by aryl hydrocarbon receptor agonists in porcine aorta endothelial cells in culture and cytochrome P4501A1 activity in intact cells. *Mol Pharmacol* 1995, 47 : 296–306.

99. Schlezinger JJ, Stegeman JJ: Dose- and inducer-dependent induction of cytochrome P450 1A in endothelia of the eel, including in the swim bladder rete mirabile, a model microvascular structure. *Drug Metab Dispos* 2000, 28 : 701–708.

100. Thum T, Haverich A, Borlak J: Cellular dedifferentiation of endothelium is linked to activation and silencing of certain nuclear transcription factors: implications for endothelial dysfunction and vascular biology. *FASEB J* 2000, 14 : 740–751.

101. Thum T, Borlak J: Cytochrome P450 mono-oxygenase gene expression and protein activity in cultures of adult cardiomyocytes of the rat. *Br J Pharmacol* 2000, 130 : 1745–1752.

102. Borlak J, Thum T: PCBs alter gene expression of nuclear transcription factors and other heart-specific genes in cultures of primary cardiomyocytes: possible implications for cardiotoxicity. *Xenobiotica* 2002, 32 : 1173–1183.

103. Walker MK, Catron TF: Characterization of cardiotoxicity induced by 2,3,7,8-tetrachlorodibenzo-*p*-dioxin and related chemicals during early chick embryo development. *Toxicol Appl Pharmacol* 2000, 167 : 210–221.

104. Mehrabi MR, Steiner GE, Dellinger C, Kofler A, Schaufler K, Tamaddon F, Plesch K, Ekmekcioglu C, Maurer G, Glogar HD, Thalhammer T: The arylhydrocarbon receptor (AhR), but not the AhR-nuclear translocator (ARNT), is increased in hearts of patients with cardiomyopathy. *Virchows Arch* 2002, 441 : 481–489.

105. Fernandez-Salguero PM, Ward JM, Sundberg JP, Gonzalez FJ: Lesions of aryl-hydrocarbon receptor-deficient mice. *Vet Pathol* 1997, 34 : 605–614.

106. Thum T, Borlak J: Microarray analysis reveals complex deregulation of gene expression in heart tissue upon Aroclor1254 treatment: implications for cardiotoxicity. *Toxicol Lett.* 2003, **144** (Suppl. 1) S. 93.

107. Evans WE, Relling MV: Pharmacogenomics: translating functional genomics into rational therapeutics. *Science* 1999, 286:487–491.

108. Sachidanandam R, Weissman D, Schmidt SC, Kakol JM, Stein LD, Marth G, Sherry S, Mullikin JC, Mortimore BJ, Willey DL, et al.: A map of human genome sequence variation containing 1.42 million single nucleotide polymorphisms. *Nature* 2001, 409:928–933.

109. McLeod HL, Evans WE: Pharmacogenomics: unlocking the human genome for better drug therapy. *Annu Rev Pharmacol Toxicol* 2001, 41:101–121.

110. Yates CR, Krynetski EY, Loennechen T, Fessing MY, Tai HL, Pui CH, Relling MV, Evans WE: Molecular diagnosis of thiopurine S-methyltransferase deficiency: genetic basis for azathioprine and mercaptopurine intolerance. *Ann Intern Med* 1997, 126:608–614.

111. Borlak J, Hermann R, Erb K, Thum T: A rapid and simple CYP2D6 genotyping assay: case study with the analgesic tramadol. *Metabolism* 2003, **52**: 1439–1443.

112. Mahgoub A, Idle JR, Dring LG, Lancaster R, Smith RL: Polymorphic hydroxylation of debrisoquine in man. *Lancet* 1977, 2:584–586.

113. Eichelbaum M, Spannbrucker N, Dengler HJ: Influence of the defective metabolism of sparteine on its pharmacokinetics. *Eur J Clin Pharmacol* 1979, 16:189–194.

114. Kimura S, Umeno M, Skoda RC, Meyer UA, Gonzalez FJ: The human debrisoquine 4-hydroxylase (*CYP2D*) locus: sequence and identification of the polymorphic *CYP2D6* gene, a related gene, and a pseudogene. *Am J Hum Genet* 1989, 45:889–904.

115. Rau T, Heide R, Bergmann K, Wuttke H, Werner U, Feifel N, Eschenhagen T: Effect of the *CYP2D6* genotype on metoprolol metabolism persists during long-term treatment. *Pharmacogenetics* 2002, 12:465–472.

116. Labbe L, O'Hara G, Lefebvre M, Lessard E, Gilbert M, Adedoyin A, Champagne J, Hamelin B, Turgeon J: Pharmacokinetic and pharmacodynamic interaction between mexiletine and propafenone in human beings. *Clin Pharmacol Ther* 2000, 68:44–57.

117. Goldstein JA, de Morais SM: Biochemistry and molecular biology of the human CYP2C subfamily. *Pharmacogenetics* 1994, 4:285–299.

118. Weinshilboum R: Inheritance and drug response. *N Engl J Med* 2003, 348:529–537.

119. Borlak J, Thum T, Landt O, Erb K, Hermann R: Molecular diagnosis of a familial nonhemolytic hyperbilirubinemia (Gilbert's syndrome) in healthy subjects. *Hepatology* 2000, 32: 792–795.

120. Borlak J, Thum T: Identification of major *CYP2C9* and *CYP2C19* polymorphisms by fluorescence resonance energy transfer analysis. *Clin Chem* 2002, 48:1592–1594.

121. Walles M, Thum T, Levsen K, Borlak J: Verapamil: new insight into the molecular mechanism of drug oxidation in the human heart. *J Chromatogr A* 2002, 970:117–130.

122. Walles M, Thum T, Levsen K, Borlak J: Verapamil metabolism in distinct regions of the heart and in cultures of cardiomyocytes of adult rats. *Drug Metab Dispos* 2001, 29:761–768.

123. Thum T, Borlak J: Gene expression in distinct regions of the heart. *Lancet* 2000, 355:979–983.

124. Borlak J, Walles M, Levsen K, Thum T: Verapamil: Metabolism in cultures of primary human coronary endothelial cells. *Drug Metab Dispos* 2003, 31:888.

125. Salvemini D, Pistelli A, Vane J: Conversion of glyceryl trinitrate to nitric oxide in tolerant and non-tolerant smooth muscle and endothelial cells. *Br J Pharmacol* 1993, 108:162–169.

126. Park BK: Cytochrome P450 enzymes in the heart. *Lancet* 2000, 355: 945–946.

127. Park BK, Pirmohamed M, Kitteringham NR: The role of cytochrome P450 enzymes in hepatic and extrahepatic human drug toxicity. *Pharmacol Ther* 1995, 68 : 385–424.

128. Macri J, Rapundalo ST: Application of proteomics to the study of cardiovascular biology. *Trends Cardiovasc Med* 2001, 11 : 66–75.

129. Arrell DK, Neverova I, Van Eyk JE: Cardiovascular proteomics: evolution and potential. *Circ Res* 2001, 88 : 763–773.

17
Toxicogenomics Applied to Endocrine Disruption

Damian G. Deavall, Jonathan G. Moggs, and George Orphanides

17.1
Introduction

Endocrine disruptors (EDs) have been defined as exogenous substances that alter function(s) of the endocrine system and consequently cause adverse health effects in an intact organism or its progeny or in (sub)populations (World Health Organisation: www.who.int/pcs/emerg_site/edc/edc_descr.html). Since the early 1990s, scientific and media interest in the persistence of such agents in the environment has risen dramatically, as it has been proposed that these compounds may be the cause of a variety of adverse health effects, including cancers and reproductive dysfunction in both humans and wildlife. Consequently, endocrine disruption has become a major international issue that is now the subject of intense research and regulatory initiatives. In this chapter we discuss some of the challenges faced by research into the perceived effects of endocrine disruption and highlight the role toxicogenomics can play in shaping future progress in this area. We focus on how genomics permits a more detailed understanding of the ways in which EDs interact with biological systems and provide a basis for more accurate and realistic safety assessment.

17.1.1
Introduction to Endocrine Disruption

The principle focus of interest in endocrine disruption has been the effects of naturally occurring and industrial synthetic agents on normal physiological control afforded by sex-steroid estrogens and androgens. These hormones, acting via their cognate receptors (estrogen receptor, ER, and androgen receptor, AR), influence many physiological processes and are particularly important in regulating sexual maturation and reproductive function. Thus, if EDs do disrupt normal sex-hormone signalling, they could theoretically represent a challenge to reproductive capacity. Alteration of sex steroid receptor-mediated processes could occur in a number of ways. An agent might alter tissue responsiveness to hormone by modulating receptor levels or affecting normal receptor biology. Changes may occur in the levels of endogenous

Handbook of Toxicogenomics: Strategies and Applications. Edited by Jürgen Borlak

ISBN: 3-527-30342-1

hormone, brought about by effects on synthesis, metabolism, or clearance. Alternatively, a chemical may act directly on the receptor by binding to it and thereby either mimicking or blocking the activity of the endogenous ligand. It has been proposed that increases in a disparate array of adverse human health and environmental effects, for which there had previously been little plausible explanation, are due to endocrine disruptors in the environment which affect normal physiology by one or more of these mechanisms. Particular emphasis has been given to the potential risks to the health of humans and wildlife species posed by exposure to synthetic industrial compounds capable of mimicking the actions of estrogen.

An increasing number of chemicals with estrogenic potential have been identified. Examples include bisphenol A, which is widely used in plastics and resins, organochlorine pesticides such as methoxychlor, a range of pharmaceutical compounds and their metabolites, and constituents of some personal-care products. The increased use of these agents and the resulting potential for accumulation in the environment (particularly in water supplies) has been proposed as the underlying cause of the increased incidence of breast cancer [1], feminisation of aquatic wildlife species [2, 3], and a reduction in reproductive fitness associated with the alleged decrease in human sperm counts over the past five decades [4]. The evidence for some of these assertions is stronger than for others. For example, it is acknowledged that fish living in waterways containing high levels of estrogens do undergo a feminisation progression [5, 6]. Conversely, although some studies have positively associated concentrations of organochlorines with increased risk of breast cancer [7], others have failed to demonstrate this link [8], and a review of the epidemiological data regarding this association has found no conclusive link between organochlorine exposure and breast cancer risk. Thus, the debate continues as to the significance of EDs, particularly with regard to human health, as much of the data associating EDs with increased occurrence of adverse effects has been questioned. So far it has not been possible to eliminate a role for other environmental factors.

Although interest in endocrine disruption has risen dramatically in the past 10 years, it is not a new phenomenon, and some widely accepted effects of EDs have been reported since the 1950s. For example, the synthetic estrogen diethylstilbestrol (DES) was implicated in abnormal breast development in men consuming meat from animals treated with this compound as a growth promoter. Some years later, the use of DES in the clinic to prevent miscarriages was discontinued when offspring of the women using this drug were found to be at higher risk of reproductive and immunological abnormalities [9]. Also in the 1950s, a range of natural plant estrogens was discovered. These phytoestrogens were implicated in sheep sterility, observed in flocks grazing on clover-rich land. There have been many reports of abnormalities in the reproductive organs of laboratory animals resulting from exposure to endocrine-disrupting chemicals. Superficially, these data appear to correlate with the findings of a small number of epidemiologic studies reporting subfertility and reproductive organ dysfunction after occupational exposure to solvents and pesticides. However, epidemiological studies have failed to reveal a link between exposure and pathology, as such data are extremely difficult to collect and correctly interpret. Nevertheless, concern over the potential for adverse health effects has triggered research and regulatory activity, and the U.S. Environmental Protection Agency (EPA) and the Organization for Economic Cooperation and Development (OECD) are now involved in dictating testing requirements for EDs.

In contrast to concern over levels of synthetic estrogens in the environment, a more positive role in human health has been assigned to naturally occurring estrogenic compounds. These include flavonoids, phytosterols, lignans, and microbial products, for example zearalenones. Soy-based foods are particularly rich in phytoestrogens such as genistein, and an association has been made between diets rich in soy products and low incidence of breast cancer, particularly in the Japanese population. It is interesting to note that such observations have led to a perception that synthetic estrogens might adversely affect health whilst natural estrogens are thought to promote it. There is little evidence for such broad assertions, and both classes of compound mimic estrogens to cause similar outcomes in animal studies. Indeed, synthetic estrogenic and anti-estrogenic compounds are now successfully being used in the clinic to treat a variety of disease states (see Section 17.1.2)

There is intense debate, research, and regulatory activity into endocrine disruption, as illustrated by issues surrounding exposure to xenoestrogens. High-quality research allows a much more detailed appreciation of the way in which EDs interact with biological systems, and this will facilitate a clearer view of how human health may be affected, beneficially or adversely, by exposure. Powerful research tools, such as toxicogenomics platforms, are required in addition to existing approaches (see Section 17.3). Regulatory pressures will necessarily demand a precautionary approach aimed at reducing exposure to existing EDs and limiting potential for exposure to new compounds with such profiles. Progress in understanding ED action will translate into improved paradigms for safety assessment.

17.1.2 Therapeutic Endocrine Modulators

In addition to the potential adverse effects of endocrine disruption previously described, pharmacological use of endocrine modulators represents an important therapeutic area. Regarding modulators of estrogen function, estrogen receptor agonists and antagonists are now widely used to treat a number of diverse pathophysiological conditions, including hormone-dependent breast cancer and osteoporosis.

Approximately 70–80% of all breast tumours express ERα (ER+), and expression is both an important prognostic factor and an indictor of the most likely beneficial therapeutic approach [10]. The use of selective estrogen receptor modulators (SERMs) is currently a widespread approach to successfully treating ER+ breast tumours and to prophylactically reducing the risk of developing ER+ breast cancers in woman defined as high-risk for the disease.

SERMs may be broadly subdivided into two categories, determined by their mode of action. First-generation SERMs such as tamoxifen and raloxifene disrupt ligand–receptor interaction of ER with endogenous estradiol, thus preventing ER from acting as a ligand-activated transcription factor (see Section 17.2.1). However, first-generation SERMs display mixed agonist/antagonist properties, such that tamoxifen treatment may be associated with an increased risk of uterine cancer due to agonist activity in this tissue. More recently ER 'destroyers' have been developed (fulvestrant/faslodex/ICI 182,780), which bind to ER and subsequently decrease the abundance of transcriptionally competent receptor in the nucleus. This again prevents estrogen receptor acting as a transcription modulator. It is hoped that treatment with compounds such as faslodex will be associated with fewer adverse effects than tamoxifen treatment. The use of both classes of compound leads to tumour regression, a decrease in the number of cells in S phase, and an induction of apoptosis markers, and hence this type of endocrine modulation represents a beneficial use of synthetic estrogenic compounds.

In addition to the use of SERMs in oncology, they may also be beneficial in the treatment of other diseases known to be associated with the action of sex hormones. One example is osteoporosis [11]. Bone mass loss in post-menopausal women is increasing in incidence in ageing Western populations. Among current treatments, sex-steroid hormone replacement therapy (HRT) is favoured, but estrogen replacement therapy (ERT) is reported to have undesirable effects on reproductive tissues, as it may increase the risk of breast and uterine cancer [12, 13]. Thus, selective estrogen receptor modulators (SERMs) have been proposed as candidate treatments for osteoporosis, as the ideal SERM would have the beneficial effects of estrogen in bone without the undesirable effects in breast and uterus. The current gold-standard SERM for use in this area is raloxifene, which has been shown to prevent bone loss and reduce the occurrence of fractures in short-term trials [14].

Among the uses of estrogens as pharmaceutically active compounds, the most widespread in Western society is as a contraceptive agent. It has been estimated that the dose of estrogens in the birth control pill, based on its *in vitro* potency relative to endogenous estradiol, equates to approximately 17 000 µg per day, compared to approximately 100 µg from estrogen flavonoids (depending on diet) and 2.5 pg from organochlorine pesticides [15]. Ironically, the widespread use of estrogenic pharmaceutically active compounds is potentially a major contributor of estrogens to water supplies in which feminisation of aquatic species has been demonstrated.

What is clear is that the targeted endocrine disruption described here can be advantageous to human health. The use and further development of endocrine modulators such as SERMs requires continued research as we continue to elucidate the mechanisms by which these compounds bring about both desirable endpoints and unwanted side effects. Toxicogenomics is a valuable tool for evaluating the modes of action of these therapies by providing a readout of their transcriptional effects. This may aid future research and development strategies for pharmaceutical compounds of this type.

17.2
Molecular Mechanisms of Estrogen Signalling

To appreciate the contribution of toxicogenomics to endocrine disruption research, it is necessary to be familiar with the current state of scientific research underlying the mechanistic action of EDs. The emphasis in our laboratories has been on the biology of ER action, as this will allow us to appreciate the cellular processes that may be altered by estrogenic endocrine disruptors. With this is mind, a brief outline of the molecular mechanisms by which estrogens act will help to clarify the role of toxicogenomics in furthering our understanding of these processes.

17.2.1 Introduction to Estrogen Receptor Action

The cellular effects of estrogenic compounds are mediated by two subtypes of estrogen receptor: ERα and ERβ. These receptors belong to a superfamily of nuclear receptors that act as ligand-activated transcription factors and show tissue-specific distribution patterns, with both ER subtypes being expressed in uterus, mammary gland, ovary, prostate, epdidymus, testis, pituitary, kidney, thymus, bone, and central nervous system. ER is activated upon estrogen binding to the ligand-binding domain. This results in homodimerisation, DNA binding at an estrogen response element (ERE) within a target gene, and a conformational change that facilitates interaction of the receptor with chromatin remodelling proteins [16].

ER modulates gene expression in the nucleus by forming protein complexes with cofactors [17, 18]. These ER-associated cofactors facilitate and augment the recruitment of the basal transcriptional machinery by remodelling the repressive chromatin environment in which genes are constrained, and thus they mediate ER-dependent transcription. The tissue-specific expression of these cofactor proteins may provide another level at which specificity in the effects of estrogens in different tissues can be achieved [19]. In addition to ERE-bound ER forming complexes with cofactors, ER may itself be capable of exhibiting cofactor activity, as it has been shown to interact with DNA-bound AP-1 transcription factor and to determine transcriptional responses in a manner that does not depend on its own direct interaction with DNA [20].

17.2.2 Extranuclear Action of Estrogen Receptors Signalling Through Kinase Cascades to Pleiotropic Transcriptional Effects

In the classical model of estrogen receptor action, estrogenic compounds diffuse into the cell and bind to ER, inducing the receptor to dimerise and bind to specific EREs in the promoter regions of target genes to regulate gene expression. However, it is now established that the mode of action of ER is much more complex than this classical model.

Both ER subtypes possess two distinct transactivation domains, termed AF-1 and AF-2. In addition to ligand-dependent activation via the AF-2 region, ER may influence gene expression in a ligand-independent manner via the AF-1 domain. Activation of AF-1 is due, at least in part, to phosphorylation of conserved serine residues. As AF-1 and AF-2 may interact in a synergistic fashion to influence promoter activity [21], there is considerable potential for interplay between ER ligand binding and the activation of kinase signalling cascades to influence gene expression.

In addition to the nuclear activity of ER, rapid extranuclear actions have been demonstrated, including activation of mitogen-activated protein kinases that have pleiotropic cellular effects at both genomic and nongenomic levels [22]. The realisation that ERs employ diverse molecular mechanisms for regulating gene transcription has generated a need for more holistic studies of alterations in gene expression in response to estrogenic chemicals. Although a relatively small number of genes have been described as being directly ER-responsive, estrogens may yet influence the expression of many more genes via the activation of alternative signalling cascades. This is of particular relevance to the field of endocrine disruption, as the ability of ER to respond to widespread, diverse signals may alter the way in which compounds are classified as EDs, since compounds that act via estrogen receptor to bring about genomic effects may do so in the absence of direct interaction with the receptor itself.

17.3
Current Methods for Assessing Endocrine-disrupting Potential

Given the potential of EDs to alter normal physiology, it has been necessary to develop techniques to evaluate the potential of a compound to act as an endocrine disruptors. The approaches currently widely used in assessment may be subdivided into those that examine a surrogate physiological endpoint for altered steroid-like activity and those that directly establish the ability of a putative ED to bind to and/or activate a given hormone receptor. In this section, we discuss some of these techniques and their limitations, to highlight the potential benefits of genomic analysis. Our emphasis is on assays for sex-steroid EDs, and we discuss the relevance of surrogate molecular markers for estrogenicity.

17.3.1
Nuclear Receptor Binding Assays and Yeast Transactivation Assays

One of the principle mechanisms by which EDs bring about changes in sex-steroid–mediated homeostasis is via direct interaction between receptor and chemical. Thus, use of receptor binding and transactivation assays as early screens to detect ligand–receptor interaction is widespread. *In vitro* ligand-binding assays are well established and have been rigorously validated as a method of determining direct ligand–receptor interactions [23]. Such techniques have undergone many refinements, yet are based on a common principle of competitive displacement, whereby the test substance displaces a receptor-bound probe molecule, which is typically radiolabelled, from a crude receptor preparation of cell line or tissue origin. Since the conception of this assay, modifications have addressed technical shortcomings, such as the time-consuming nature of such assays and their reliance on radioactive chemicals. The use of solid-phase immobilisation of the receptor, fluorescence polarization techniques, and immunoassay protocols has resulted in a robust and straightforward system [24, 25]. However, this approach still cannot assay the effect of ligand on ER function, does not provide any indication of physiological outcome in response to receptor–ligand interaction (as *in vivo* assays can, see Section 17.3.2), and depends on a direct interaction between the test compound and the receptor.

The issue of effects on receptor functionality has been successfully addressed, at least in part, by yeast hybrid assays in which mammalian steroid receptors introduced into *Saccharomyces cerevisiae* can function as steroid-dependent activators of transcription [26, 27]. Such assays employ a reporter-based approach in which yeast are transformed with a receptor expression plasmid and a reporter comprising a response element motif upstream of a gene encoding a readily measurable enzyme, which is incorporated into the yeast genome. Such assays are successfully used for both androgenicity and estrogenicity screens and serve as a useful tool to examine transactivation function in isolation from other signalling events. Similar reporter assays have also been developed in mammalian cell lines [28]. Like the ligand-binding assay, yeast hybrid systems represent an easily manipulated, rapid, relatively inexpensive method to pre-screen large numbers of potential EDs. However, both approaches are essentially simplistic in the parameters they seek to examine, as they both assay binding of test compounds to receptors. As such, they are not capable of assessing the effects EDs may elicit through indirect action on steroid receptors. Furthermore, they cannot be used to determine systemic effects of EDs or progression to pathology in response to EDs. Consequently, this pre-screening has typically been followed up with more informative bioassays that examine surrogate endpoints for the physiological effects of endocrine disruption. The surrogate *in vivo* assay also has its limitations, and the power of current techniques will be greatly magnified by the use of toxicogenomics as a predictive tool for identification of EDs, a tool for determining mode of action, and a method of predicating likely physiological changes induced by genomic effects.

17.3.2
End-point *in vivo* Assays for Potential Endocrine Disruptors

In addition to assays for ligand–receptor interaction, a number of approaches have been developed to look at biological endpoints induced by ED action. These assays have been performed in cell culture and *in vivo*, typically in rodent models. Of the cell culture assays, the most widespread has been the E-SCREEN, which relies on use of the estrogen-sensitive mammary tumour cell line MCF-7 [29, 30]. In this cell type, estrogen exposure correlates with increased proliferation, and thus a readily measurable endpoint exists to compare the effects of ED exposure to those observed with a reference estrogen (17β-estradiol).

Two *in vivo* assays are widely performed to assess potential EDs for estrogenicity or androgenicity: the rodent uterotrophic assay [23] and the rat Hershberger assay [31], respectively. The uterotrophic assay relies on the observation that the uterine weight of sexually immature or ovariectomised rodents increases in response to estrogen administration. Thus, uterine wet weight can be employed as an endpoint to measure estrogenicity of a test compound. This assay can be used in conjunction with measurements of sensitive morphological and biochemical endpoints in the uterus, such as uterine epithelial cell height increases and induction of the estrogen-responsive proteins lactotransferrin and progesterone receptor [32, 33]. Although a positive response in the uterotrophic assay may be accompanied by adverse effects, such as carcinogenesis [34], the increase in uterine weight itself is not an adverse endpoint. Consequently, the results of multigenerational rodent studies looking at long-term effects of exposure to EDs may not correlate with positive uterotrophic data [35, 36]. This assay has now undergone extensive evaluation and validation under OECD direction [37].

Also undergoing OECD validation is the Hershberger castrated male rat androgen assay [38]. Surgically or chemically castrated sexually mature male rats are subject to a regression of tissues maintained by androgens, such as the prostate and seminal vesicles, and this can be at least partly restored by the addition of androgen. A potential anti-androgen ED can be assayed according to its ability to block this restoration upon its administration. As with the uterotrophic assay, one of the key problems with this gravimetric endpoint determination is that it may represent a relatively insensitive measure of changes occurring in response to EDs.

Although it is clear that physiological endpoints such as these are valuable in evaluating ED action, they can no doubt be greatly augmented by the concomitant evaluation of precursor genomic changes underlying ED activity. Genome screening platforms provide an exquisitely sensitive method of determining the transcriptional events underlying not only the increases in organ growth seen in the uterotrophic and Hershberger assays, but also the changes underlying other phenotypic alterations that cannot be tested by these methods. As these *in vivo* assays are surrogates for physiological perturbation in response to EDs, it is of enormous potential benefit to use them in conjunction with other techniques that can provide a far greater wealth of data, particularly the molecular mechanistic data provided by genomics.

17.4 Value of Toxicogenomic Platforms to ED Toxicology

17.4.1 Genome-scale Microarray Experiments Facilitate a Global View of Gene Expression

Transcriptional regulation is one of the key mechanisms a cell utilises to respond to a changing external environment. Consequently, environmental influences impinging upon a cell are typically accompanied by alterations in gene expression. Thus, the effects of EDs (as with a variety of toxicological stimuli) may be assessed on the basis of their effects at the genomic level. Previously, measurement of transcriptional effects has been limited by the necessity to examine each gene individually. So, although it has been possible to measure, for example, mRNA abundance by Northern blot analysis of a known estrogen-responsive gene (such as that encoding the trefoil factor protein TFF1/pS2) in a defined estrogen-responsive system (such as MCF-7 cells) in response to estrogenic compounds, it has been impractical to use such systems to examine multiple transcript profiles. However, with the development of genome-wide transcript profiling techniques, it has become feasible to simultaneously and rapidly measure the expression levels of thousands of genes. The adoption of this technology by toxicologists has led to the development and validation of toxicogenomics platforms that can be successfully employed to address key issues in the field of endocrine disruption. Thus, as discussed, genomic analysis techniques can vastly increase the scope of data on potential EDs, their modes of action, and their likely biological effects.

Of particular interest among the genomic technologies applicable to endocrine disruption research are microarray platforms for gene expression analysis. These arrays may be broad in coverage, enabling profiling of numerous cellular functions or pathways, or may be application-targeted, allowing assay of a subset of genes known to be involved in a particular process. These platforms have undergone extensive technological development in recent years. Earlier formats consisted of cDNA fragments from a few hundred genes immobilised on a nylon membrane. These membranes can easily be hybridised with radiolabelled cDNA synthesised from the RNA pool extracted from a tissue or cell type under investigation. In addition to being widely available commercially, this format is readily customised. Consequently, it is possible to generate focused arrays containing genes relevant to the researcher's particular area of interest. For example, our laboratory has developed a series of microarrays (ToxBlots) that facilitate the transcriptional analysis of biological processes related to general mechanisms of toxicity [39] and gene expression events underlying specific toxic endpoints involved in, for example, oxidative stress. Technological development of microarrays has resulted in improvements in ease of handling, reduction of variability, and increases in gene number represented on the matrix. Currently, there is a shift to the use of microarrays printed on glass slides, possessing surface chemistry that increases the efficiency and uniformity of hybridisation, using fluorescent labelled (rather than radioactive) probes. With this approach, in contrast to the nylon filters, it is possible to hybridise two samples (for example, control and treated samples) simultaneously on the same slide by labelling each with a different fluorescent marker, thus decreasing the inherent variability present between arrays.

In addition to the use of cDNA microarrays, current leading-edge technology favours the use of oligonucleotides on the array surface, rather than cDNA sequences. This is advantageous as short oligonucleotides provide higher specificity. Arrays in this format have now been developed to allow entire-genome–scale transcriptional analysis. These array chips are hybridised with samples that have been first reverse-transcribed to produce cDNA that is then *in vitro* transcribed to produce cRNA. To generate these arrays, multiple oligonucleotide probes (typically 11–16) are designed for each gene to be represented on the array. Complementary probes are accompanied by single base mismatch sequences for each oligonucleotide to allow quantification of nonspecific cross hybridisation. The inclusion in this array format of multiple probe sets for each gene and internal probe hybridisation controls produces a high degree of reproducibility between arrays, which it has been difficult to demonstrate with, for example, custom nylon arrays. Consequently, this technology is being adopted as the gold-standard method of generating reliable array data.

Microarray techniques such as these may be used to predict the mode of action of toxicants based on the transcription signature they produce. This 'fingerprinting' relies on correlating gene changes with biological responses and functions primarily to facilitate comparison of toxicants with each other and with reference toxicants. Alternatively, molecular mechanisms affected by a toxicant can be assayed, and these can be related to a known endpoint. Both of these contexts are equally applicable to ED research, and toxicogenomics platforms may be used to predict whether or not a compound is a potential ED, and if so, how it might act to alter normal cellular physiology. The potential of a compound to act as an ED can be evaluated by comparison of the gene expression changes it produces with those of a reference compound (for example 17β-estradiol). Furthermore, the molecular mechanisms underlying a reference physiological change known to be associated with endocrine disruption, such as surrogate end-point changes to uterine weight in response to estrogen exposure, can be determined. This latter approach may facilitate the identification of robust, novel molecular markers of endocrine disruption that may increase the sensitivity of a surrogate end-point assay, or in some instances, provide an alternative to it.

The facility to examine genome-wide gene expression changes is the key advantage of microarray technology, particularly with regard to its use in endocrine disruption research. Although focused arrays can be used to examine molecular changes known to underlie a defined endpoint, genome-scale analysis is not biased toward predefined gene changes. As previously discussed, a variety of physiological processes may potentially be subject to endocrine disruption (see Section 17.1), and thus a global, holistic view of transcriptional changes in response to ED challenge would be more desirable, in order to establish a comprehensive view of alterations in cell function. The identification of robust classifying signatures to 'fingerprint' ED action also initially relies on the use of a genome-scale platform. For screening putative EDs based on a comparison of gene expression changes in relation to those of a reference compound, it would be possible to use one of the cell line or rodent models currently used to identify potential EDs, for example, the MCF-7 cell line used in the E-SCREEN or rodent uterine tissue. As we discuss in Section 17.4.2, the use of 'conventional' ED assays in parallel with toxicogenomics is a powerful approach for identifying endocrine disrupting potential. However, the scope of microarray use in this area of toxicology extends beyond its use as a screening method.

One of the key concerns of ED exposure is biological challenge due to long-term environmental exposure to doses of EDs that may fall below the no-effect level observed in surrogate end-point assays such as the uterotrophic assay. Toxicogenomics tools can be used to evaluate gene expression changes that may occur in response to low-dose long-term exposure, as such changes necessarily precede any physiological endpoint. It may also be possible to correlate genomic effects preceding phenotypic changes, such as carcinogenesis, that would not be detectable over the time scale of the surrogate endpoint assay. This again allows microarrays to be used in a predictive mode, in an attempt to clarify the strength of association between progression to adverse phenotypes and ED exposure. In a similar fashion, toxicogenomics can be used to investigate the potential side effects of pharmaceutical endocrine modulators such as SERMs, as the pattern of gene expression changes in tissues other than the desired target tissue could be used to predict likely undesirable phenotypic changes.

Data are now being published from studies validating the use of microarrays to examine large-scale gene expression changes in response to ED exposure. For example, studies have examined the possibility of using microarrays in risk assessment to evaluate the endocrine disruption potential of compounds, based on their transcriptional signature in steroid hormone sensitive cell lines [40], uterine tissue from ovariectomised mice [41, 42], and testicular tissue from neonate mice [43]. Studies from our laboratory and others have also successfully coupled the use of surrogate endpoint assays and microarray platforms [44], which has increased understanding of the molecular mechanisms underlying the increase in uterine weight in response to estrogen. Such studies may, in time, be able to sufficiently validate transcript profiling such that measurement of gene expression markers in response to endocrine disruption will itself form the basis of accurate assays for ED potential and mode-of-action studies. In addition to publications on the use of microarrays in animal and cell-line models, work has been published which suggests that toxicogenomics can be successfully used to assess the effects of ED exposure on human development, by examining gene expression in umbilical tissue [45]. The developmental stage at which ED exposure occurs may be a primary determinant of the subsequent progression to adverse changes in normal physiology. Approaches that can address this will increase our understanding of the significance of endocrine disruption to human health and environmental change. Toxicogenomics is uniquely positioned to address such issues if it is possible to fingerprint transcriptional changes that are associated with progression to a future pathology.

Microarray data have the potential to revolutionise ED research, but the use of these platforms is, predictably, not without limitations, and their use will no doubt be augmented by the concomitant use of alternative genomics platforms. Reverse-transcription polymerase chain reaction (RT–PCR) has been successfully used to correlate individual gene expression changes with ED exposure in mammalian and aquatic species [46–48]. The use of real-time fluorescence RT–PCR enables quantitative determination of gene expression changes in response to EDs to be readily achieved. Thus, RT–PCR follow-up studies can be successfully used to track expression levels of biomarkers identified by genome-scale analysis. However, although real-time PCR methods permit the analysis of thousands of samples in a day with high sensitivity, it is limited by the number of genes it is possible to study in one reaction, due to the necessity for multiple fluorescent probes. Although microarrays successfully address the need to analyse many genes simultaneously, the technology can be prohibitively expensive. In addition to the cost of either commercial gene-chip systems or in-house array-printing facilities, analytical instruments and software represent a further capital outlay. Thus, there is demand for a low-cost, high-speed method of measuring the expression of multiple genes, and this need may, in part, be met by the use of bead-based expression bioassays such as the BADGE assay [49], recently developed for gene expression analysis in food crops. This system, which is equally applicable to endocrine disruption research in mammalian systems, utilises oligonucleotide capture probes that are linked to commercially available colour-coded beads. To assay gene expression, biotin-labelled cRNA samples are synthesised and hybridised to the beads, which are then passed through a counting device to record the bead identification and the intensity of reporter fluorescence associated with it. Commercially, sets of up to 100 distinct microspheres are available (Luminex^{TM}), and thus it is possible to measure the expression levels of 100 genes in a single assay. Although this represents a far smaller gene set than those represented by genome-scale microarrays, it would be possible to use this technology to identify the effect of EDs on gene expression in a transcriptional fingerprint of up to 100 genes previously identified using microarrays. Given its considerable cost and time benefits, this technology is well positioned to replace focused arrays representing very limited gene sets.

In conclusion, therefore, the impact of toxicogenomics platforms on endocrine disruption research is considerable. Continued validation of current technologies and development of new, more efficient, or powerful platforms will aid in this revolution. However, such technological advances will prove to be of value only if the experiments in which they are used are well designed and the data they produce are interpreted in a meaningful way. We now give some consideration to these points.

17.4.2
Experimental Design

17.4.2.1 Coupling *in vivo* Assays and Genomic Analysis

The key to realising the potential of toxicogenomics in ED research is appropriate experimental design, which necessitates the use of an appropriate model in which to investigate genomic effects. Initial observations would seek to correlate transcriptional changes and phenotypic changes, and it is likely that the concomitant use of conventional ED assays (such as uterotrophic and multigenerational *in vivo* assays and also cell line models such as MCF-7) and toxicogenomics platforms will be the most beneficial approach. Genomics applications will enhance the sensitivity of such assays, as it will be possible to observe transcriptional events that precede and determine the phenotypic changes observed. Although a number of molecular markers for estrogenicity are successfully studied at the gene-expression level by techniques such as RT–PCR (for example, lactoferrin [34] and progesterone receptor [50]), they are not currently used as replacements for endpoint observations, as there is uncertainty about the significance of precursor molecular events that have been observed in the absence of phenotypic change, such as an increase in uterine weight [51]. However, the possibility of identifying more molecular signatures, not only of (for example) estrogenicity, but also of adverse effects resulting from ED exposure, will help to validate new markers as alternative surrogates, which, when used with endpoint assays, will no doubt increase sensitivity. However, it is important to note that validation of molecular markers must be multifaceted. One must consider the specificity of changes observed in expression of a single marker gene, the significance of the kinetics and magnitude of change, and the correlation with phenotypic alteration.

Endpoints such as prostate size and uterine weight increase are not in themselves adverse effects. To appreciate how EDs might affect physiology, it is necessary to examine the gene expression changes that underlie progression to an observable adverse biological effect in the tissue in which this change is seen. Toxicogenomics can be used to establish transcription signatures in any target tissue, and these expression changes can then be correlated with the appearance of adverse phenotypic effects. The capacity to observe early gene expression changes and effects in multiple tissues will facilitate the formulation of predictive hypotheses on the transcriptional programmes underlying ED action. These can be related to endpoint changes currently used as markers of ED potential.

17.4.2.2 Transgenic Animals and Cell Lines

Understanding the molecular mechanisms by which exposure to endocrine disruptors affects physiology can be facilitated by the use of genomics technologies. As discussed, the use of appropriate models is the key to realising the potential of such approaches. The power of genomics in elucidating the mechanisms by which toxicants act can be increased by the use of biological systems in which key components have been disrupted, for example, transgenic animals and genetically modified cell lines. This is applicable to endocrine disruption research. For example, when investigating the effects of compounds that may alter sex-steroid function, it would be valuable to study gene expression changes in animals devoid of the steroid receptor targeted by the test agent. Thus, it would be possible to establish whether gene expression changes seen in wild-type animals depend on the receptor in question, or alternatively, are due to another mode of action of the compound. Hormone receptor knockout mice, such as the estrogen receptor alpha knockout ERKO [52] and the androgen receptor knockout AR KO [53] have been developed to investigate molecular mechanisms of estrogen and androgen action, respectively, and could be used to further our understanding of the contribution these receptors have to the effects of ED exposure.

Cell lines are highly suitable for mechanistic studies. The relative ease of genetically modifying cell lines compared to animals facilitates the construction of models in which signalling pathways and receptor expression can be manipulated. Thus, the effects of ED exposure on transcriptional programmes in the presence or absence of altered production of a given protein can be assessed. Manipulation of intracellular pathways in this way allows their contribution to the response to EDs to be readily determined. For example, in our laboratory we are using cell line models to assess the differential effects of estrogen-induced gene expression via ERα versus ERβ [54]. Given the requirement to understand molecular mechanisms associated with ED-induced gene expression, cell lines and the genetic modification of cell lines will have increasing importance in the application of toxicogenomics to endocrine disruption research.

17.5 Data Interpretation

17.5.1 The Use of Hierarchical Gene Clustering to Fingerprint ED Modes of Action Will Allow Mechanistic Determination

Genomics platforms, such as the high-density microarrays described in Section 17.4.1, are capable of producing extremely large datasets of gene expression changes. Given the complexity of this information it is essential that it be interpreted in a meaningful manner. The raw output of microarray experiments is a list of gene or expressed sequence tag (EST) identities and a measure of their relative abundance in the transcript pool. Thus, raw data are of little use unless one correlates expression levels with gene function. For genes of known identity, functional information is obtained through database searches. With the information arising from genome sequencing initiatives, it is increasingly possible (and indeed essential) to functionally annotate a greater proportion of the elements represented on a gene array. This can be done in-house for custom arrays (although such hand-annotation takes considerable time) or by reference to gene identification material available from the providers of commercial arrays (for example, the Affymetrix NetAffx™ Analysis Center [55]).

One of the most successful ways of interpreting expression data is to use analysis software capable of grouping, and hence classifying, observed gene expression changes based on functional annotations. Gene clustering allows patterns of expression of functionally related genes to be determined and hence allows inferences to be made as to the potential cellular effects of differential regulation of specific cellular pathways. Selection of the appropriate clustering criteria is determined by the nature of information required from the experiment, again illustrating the need not only to plan the experimental model and protocol, but also to consider the goals for the output of the experiment. Depending on the type of data required, it may be an advantage to combine clustering approaches to elucidate biological pathways [56]. For example, we have studied the effects of 17β-estradiol on gene expression in the mouse uterus. Initial unsupervised (hierarchical) clustering was used to divide genes into temporally coregulated groups. A subsequent supervised clustering approach, using universal gene ontology descriptions, allowed us to identify gene functions that predominate in a cluster. By combining clustering tools in this way, we have revealed how 17β-estradiol induces uterine growth and maturation by regulating the activities of different biological pathways successively (Figure 17.1).

The acquisition of an appropriate gene cluster fingerprint obtained for a putative ED compound can potentially be used in a predictive manner to make inferences as to the likely cellular effects of exposure. Furthermore, this fingerprint could be used in a comparative manner to assay the effects of multiple test compounds in comparison to the effects observed with an appropriate reference compound [57]. In this laboratory, we have used gene clustering based on functional annotation to understand, at the molecular level, the gene changes associated with estrogen exposure and how these relate to the physiological changes seen in the uterus with estrogen treatment (unpublished data, J.G.M., H. Tinwell, T. Spurway, A. Soames, I. Kimber, J. Ashby, G.O.). Similar protocols could be use to investigate gene expression changes associated not only with other surrogate endpoints, but also with adverse health effects seen in longer-term end-point studies, such as progression to carcinogenesis.

17.5.2
Pathway Analysis of ED Action

The key to understanding the mode of action of putative endocrine-disrupting compounds is to understand which cellular pathways they modulate and how such path-

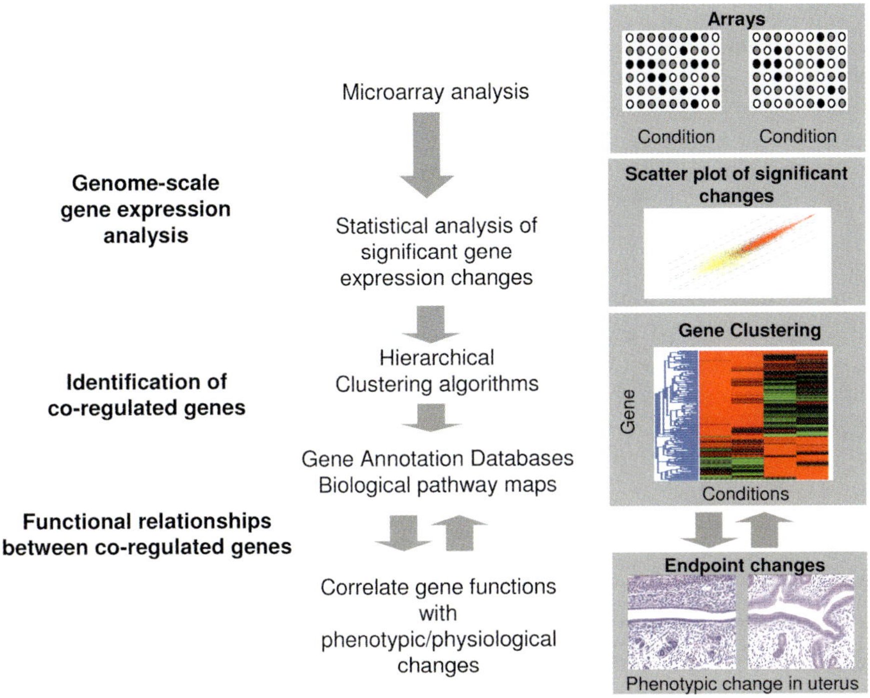

Fig. 17.1 Bioinformatic analysis of gene expression data. Interpretation of microarray data requires the use of advanced bioinformatics tools. For example, statistical analysis, gene clustering based on functional annotation, and superimposition of data onto biological pathway maps can all be utilised to understand the functional relationships of coregulated genes and how these may bring about physiological changes. The schematic shown here illustrates the approaches we have used to correlate gene expression changes with physiological changes in the uterus in response to estrogens.

ways ordinarily control cellular physiology. This is equally important in appreciating how environmental EDs may bring about adverse health and environmental effects and in appreciating the desirable and undesirable effects of pharmaceutical endocrine modulators. Consequently, as well as an understanding the identity and function of a given gene, when assessing the biological relevance of an expression change it is necessary to appreciate the interplay of numerous genes in cell physiology pathways. This requires considerable biological knowledge to support data interpretation and will be aided by the continued development of bioinformatics tools that allow data to be overlaid onto knowledge-based pathway analysis maps [58].

Bioinformatics resources have been developed to describe intracellular pathways associated with a range of biological processes. For example, the Kyoto Encyclopaedia of Genes and Genomes (KEGG; http://www.genome.ad.jp/kegg) is a resource for understanding the molecular mechanisms involved in many cellular processes, including apoptosis, mitogen-activated kinase-mediated signal transduction, membrane transport, and circadian rhythm. By collating available experimental evidence it has been possible to identify gene products involved in these processes. Consequently, gene expression data from transcript profiling can be analysed by superimposing data on these maps and identifying gene changes occurring in a given pathway of interest. By analysing gene expression changes in terms of their relevance to given pathways, it will be possible to interpret their likely biological significance. With this issue of biological relevance in mind, microarray analysis software (for example GeneSpring™ software, Silicon Genetics, Redwood City, CA) is being continually updated to allow transcriptional changes to be interpreted in terms of the pathways they might affect.

An important and rapidly evolving area of toxicogenomics is the bioinformatic analysis of gene regulatory sequences associated with coregulated genes that have been identified through transcript-profiling experiments. Elucidating key regulatory sequences in the promoters of ED-responsive genes represents a powerful approach for predicting the molecular mechanisms by which EDs signal their target genes. The recent completion of the human and rodent genome sequences [59, 60] and the development of new mammalian promoter analysis tools [61] will greatly facilitate this approach.

17.5.3
Predictive Testing of ED Potential Based on Transcript Profiling

A well designed and appropriately interpreted genomics experiment provides a molecular signature of transcriptional effects in response to toxicant exposure. For endocrine disruption research, this can be used to establish transcriptional changes underlying an observed physiological/pathophysiological change and also to aid in the identification and classification of future test compounds in a comparative approach. Classification could be based on assigning agents to subsets based on their transcript profile and would be applicable to both environmental agents and pharmaceutically active compounds.

The use of transcript profiling to test potential EDs has several advantages not offered by current investigative methods. For example, detailed mode-of-action studies are critical in evaluating the potential for ED exposure to produce an adverse phenotypic change. By describing molecular events underlying such changes for an appropriately wide variety of potential EDs, it would be possible to describe future test compounds based on the similarity of the transcript profile produced to a reference library of results. This will enable assessments of the likely outcome of compound exposure to be made based on the correlation between exposure-induced gene expression changes and the biological outcome of such exposure. A reference database such as this would increase confidence in predicting the outcome of ED exposure, which would be of great benefit in the current climate of regulatory pressure. Proof-of-concept for this predictive mode of toxicogenomics has been provided in studies of liver toxicant mode of action [62]. Predictive mode-of-action testing will also be useful in the ongoing search for therapeutic endocrine modulators. As discussed, toxicogenomics platforms help to determine the mechanistic basis of the therapeutic benefits of such compounds and also the basis of unwanted side effects. If sufficient correlation exists between structure and effects, molecular signatures can form the basis for advanced-stage compound characterisation, with the aim of reducing the number of unpredicted adverse effects seen when these treatments are used in the clinic. This approach may be useful in directing development initiatives intended to uncover new modes of action that maintain a therapeutic benefit with fewer associated adverse effects than current treatments.

Clearly, in addition to studying the effects of known EDs and endocrine modulators, toxicogenomics is highly valuable as a tool to predict the mode of action of new test compounds. As the technology for such studies becomes more accessible, it is likely that predictive testing will increasingly rely on genomics tools to supplement existing techniques.

17.6 Summary

Clarifying the existence of a link between endocrine disruptors and adverse health effects in humans and wildlife species is a challenge for toxicology. Given the perception of likely harm of hormonal perturbation, and in particular disruption of estrogen- and androgen-driven processes, this issue is subject to intensive investigation and pressure from regulatory bodies. Toxicogenomics platforms have the potential to substantially advance research into not only endocrine disruption, but also pharmaceutically active endocrine modulators. The key benefit of genomics is the depth of knowledge it is possible to obtain with a global approach examining gene expression changes. The power of this technology is enhanced by continued development of databases and data-analysis software that facilitates knowledge-based interpretation of genomics data. The adoption of toxicogenomics allows detailed mechanistic profiles to be constructed for putative ED/endocrine modulator compounds, based on transcriptional effects in suitable biological models. This is turn will facilitate the validation of new molecular markers for use in ED screening. Approaches such as those highlighted here allow toxicologists to address a number of key questions. For example, what is the molecular basis for tissue/species specificity of EDs, and do different classes of estrogenic compounds induce their effects through different mechanisms?

In addition to the use of gene expression profiling, the application of other technologies to endocrine disruption research will further increase our understanding. Gene transcription represents a primary mechanism by which a cell attempts to adapt to environmental changes, as this alters the intracellular protein composition. Post-translational modification of proteins, including those that control gene transcription, may be subject to alteration by EDs. To investigate the effects of EDs on protein modification, it will be necessary to adopt sensitive proteomics technologies, such as electrophoretic or chromatographic separation of proteins coupled to mass spectrometry. A combination of proteomic and genomic approaches will provide a more complete picture of the cellular response to EDs. Concomitant use of tools of the genomic era, together with existing methods, will facilitate a more detailed appreciation of the mechanisms by which health and environmental factors might be subjected to change by endocrine disruption.

Acknowledgments

The authors thank Drs. John Ashby and Ian Kimber for critical evaluation of the manuscript.

References

1. Dewailly, E., Dodin, S., Verreault, R., Ayotte, P., Sauve, L., Morin, J. and Brisson, J.: High organochlorine body burden in women with estrogen receptor positive breast cancer. *Journal of the National Cancer Institute* 1994, **86** 232–234
2. Colborn, T., vom Saal, F. and Soto, A.: Developmental effects of endocrine-disrupting chemicals in wildlife and humans. *Environmental Health Perspectives* 1993, **101**, 378–384
3. Guillette, L., Gross, T., Masson, G., Matter, J., Percival, H. and Woodward, A.: Developmental abnormalities of the gonad and abnormal sex hormone concentrations in juvenile alligators from contaminated and control lakes in Florida. *Environmental Health Perspectives* 1994, **102**, 680–688
4. Sharpe, R. and Skakkebaek, N.: Are estrogens involved in falling sperm counts and disorders of the male reproductive tract? *Lancet* 1993, **341**, 1392–1395
5. Sumpter, J.: Feminized responses in fish to environmental estrogens. *Toxicology Letters* 1995, **82**, 737–742
6. Segner, H., Caroll, K., Fenske, M., Janssen, C., Maack, G., Pascoe, D., Scafers, C., Vandenbergh, G., Watts, M. and Wenzel, A.: Identification of endocrine-disrupting effects in aquatic vertebrates and invertebrates: report from the European IDEA project. *Ecotoxicology and Environmental Safety* 2003, **54**, 302–314
7. Hoyer, A., Grandjean, P., Jorgensen, T., Brock, J. and Hartig, H.: Organochlorine exposure and risk of breast cancer. *Lancet* 1998, **352**, 1816–1820
8. Hunter, D., Hanksinson, S., Laden, F., Colditz, G., Mason, J., Willet, W., Speizer, F. and Woeff, M.: Plasma organochlorine levels and the risk of breast cancer. *New England Journal of Medicine* 1997, **33**, 1253–1258
9. Giusti, R., Iwamoto, K. and Hatch, E.: Diethylstilbestrol revisited: a review of the long-term health effects. *Annals of Internal Medicine* 1995, **122**, 778–788
10. Keen, J. and Davidson, N.: The biology of breast carcinoma. *Cancer* 2003, **97**, 825–833
11. Moggs, J., Deavall, D. and Orphanides, G.: Sex steroids, ANGELS and osteoporosis. *BioEssays* 2003, **25**, 195–199
12. Cauley, J., Lucas, F., Kuller, L., Stone, K., Browner, W. and Cummings, S.: Elevated serum estradiol and testosterone concentrations are associated with a high risk of breast cancer: study of osteoporotic fractures research group. *Annals of Internal Medicine* 1999, **130**, 270–277
13. Vesey, M.: Exogenous hormones in the etiology of cancer in women. *Journal of the Royal Society of Medicine* 1984, **77**, 542–549
14. Boyack, M., Lookinland, S. and Chasson, S.: Efficacy of raloxifene for treatment of menopause: a systematic review. *Journal of the American Academy of Nurse Practitioners* 2002, **14**, 150–165
15. Amaral Mendes, J.: The endocrine disrupters: a major medical challenge. *Food and Chemical Toxicology* 2002, **40**, 781–788

16. Moggs, J. and Orphanides, G.: Estrogen receptors: orchestrators of pleiotropic cellular responses. *EMBO Reports* 2001, **2**, 775–781
17. Shang, Y., Hu, X., DiRenzo, J., Lazar, M. and Brown, M.: Cofactor dynamics and sufficiency in estrogen receptor-regulated transcription. *Cell* 2000, **103**, 843–852
18. McKenna, N. and O'Malley, B.: Combinatorial control of gene expression by nuclear receptors and coregulators. *Cell* 2002, **108**, 465–474
19. Shang, Y. and Brown, M.: Molecular determinants for the tissue specificity of SERMs. *Science* 2002, **295**, 2465–2468
20. Gaub, M., Bellard, M., Scheuer, I., Chambon, P. and Sassone-Corsi, P.: Activation of the ovalbumin gene by the estrogen receptor involves the fos–jun complex. *Cell* 1990, **63**, 1267–1276
21. Metivier, R., Penot, G., Flouriot, G. and Pakdel, F.: Synergism between ERalpha transactivation function 1 (AF-1) and AF-2 mediated by steroid receptor coactivator protein-1: requirement for the AF-1 alpha-helical core and for a direct interaction between the N- and C-terminal domains. *Molecular Endocrinology* 2001, **15**, 1953–1970
22. Falkenstein, E., Tillmann, H., Christ, M., Feuring, M. and Wehling, M.: Multiple actions of steroid hormones: a focus on rapid, non-genomic effects. *Pharmacological Reviews* 2000, **52**, 513–556
23. Shelby, M., Newbold, R., Tully, D., Chae, K. and Davis, V.: Assessing environmental chemicals for estrogenicity using a combination of *in vivo* and *in vitro* assays. *Environmental Health Perspectives* 1996, **104**, 1296–1300
24. Garrett, S., Lee, H. and Morgan, M.: A nonisotopic estrogen receptor-based assay to detect estrogenic compounds. *Nature Biotechnology* 1999, **17**, 1219–1222
25. Bolger, R., Weise, T., Ervin, K., Nestich, S. and Checovich, W.: Rapid screening of environmental chemicals for estrogen receptor binding capacity. *Environmental Health Perspectives* 1998, **106**, 551–557
26. Gaido, K. W., Leonard, L. S., Lovell, S., J.C, G., Babai, D., Portier, C. J. and McDonnell, D. P.: Evaluation of chemicals with endocrine modulating activity in a yeast-based steroid hormone receptor gene transcription assay. *Toxicology and Applied Pharmacology* 1997, **143**, 205–212
27. Metzger, D., White, J. and Chambon, P.: The human estrogen receptor functions in yeast. *Nature* 1988, **334**, 31–36
28. Pennie, W., Aldridge, T. and Brooks, A.: Differential activation by xenoestrogens of ER alpha and ER beta when linked to different response elements. *Journal of Endocrinology* 1998, **158**, R11–14
29. Villalobos, M., Olea, N., Brotons, J., Olea-Serrano, M., Ruiz de Almodovar, J. and Pedraza, V.: The E-Screen assay: a comparison of different MCF-7 cell stocks. *Environmental Health Perspectives* 1995, **103**, 844–850
30. Soto, A., Lin, T., Justicia, H., Silvia, R. and Sonnenschein, C. An 'in culture' bioassay to assess the estrogenicity of xenobiotics (E-screen). In: Colborn, T., and Clement, C. (eds.). *Chemically Induced Alterations in Sexual and Functional Development: The Wildlife/Human Connection.* Princeton Scientific Publishing, Princeton, NJ, 1992, 295–309
31. Hershberger, L., Shipley, E. and Meyer, R.: Myotrophic activity of 19-nortestosterone and other steroids determined by modified levator ani muscle method. *Proceedings of the Society of Experimental Biology and Medicine* 1953, **83**, 175–180
32. Jefferson, W., Padilla-Banks, E., Clark, G. and Newbold, R.: Assessing estrogenic activity of phytochemicals using transcriptional activation and immature mouse uterotrophic responses. *Journal of Chromatography B* 2002, **777**, 179–189
33. Diel, P., Schulz, T., Smolnikar, K., Strunck, E., Vollmer, G. and Michna, H.: Ability of xeno- and phytoestrogens to modulate expression of estrogen-sensitive genes in rat uterus: estrogenicity profiles and uterotrophic activity. *Journal of Steroid Biochemistry and Molecular Biology* 2000, **73**, 1–10
34. Newbold, R., Banks, E., Bullock, B. and Jefferson, W.: Uterine adenocarcinoma in mice treated neonatally with genestein. *Cancer Research* 2001, **61**, 4325–4328

35. Tyl, R., Myers, R., Marr, M., Thomas, B., Keimowitz, A., Brine, D., Veselica, M., Fail, P., Chang, T., Seely, J., Joiner, R., Butala, J., Dimond, S., Cagen, S., Shiotsuka, R., Stropp, G. and Waechter, J.: Three-generation reproductive toxicity study of dietary bisphenol A in CD Sprague–Dawley rats. *Toxicological Sciences* 2002, **68**, 121–146
36. Ashby, J. and Tinwell, H.: Uterotrophic activity of bisphenol A in the immature rat. *Environmental Health Perspectives* 1998, **106**, 719–720
37. Ashby, J. and Owens, J.: Critical review and evaluation of the uterotrophic bioassay for the identification of possible estrogen agonists and antagonists: in support of the validation of the OECD uterotrophic protocols for the laboratory rodent. Organisation for Economic Co-operation and Development. *Critical Reviews in Toxicology* 2002, **32**, 445–520
38. Ashby, J. and Lefevre, P. A.: Preliminary evaluation of the major protocol variables for the Hershberger castrated male rat assay. *Regulatory Toxicology and Pharmacology* 2000, **31**, 92–105
39. Pennie, W., Woodyatt, N., Aldridge, T. and Orphanides, G.: Application of genomics to the definition of the molecular basis for toxicity. *Toxicology Letters* 2001, **120**, 353–358
40. Inoue, A., Yoshida, N., Omoto, Y., Oguchi, S., Yamori, T., Kiyama, R. and Hayashi, S.: Development of cDNA microarray for expression profiling of estrogen-responsive genes. *Journal of Molecular Endocrinology* 2002, **29**, 175–192
41. Watanabe, H., Suzuki, A., Kobayashi, M., Takahashi, E., Itamoto, M., Lubahn, D., Handa, H. and Iguchi, T.: Analysis of temporal changes in the expression of estrogen-regulated genes in the uterus. *Journal of Molecular Endocrinology* 2003, **30**, 347–358
42. Watanabe, H., Suzuki, A., Mizutani, T., Handa, H. and Iguchi, T. Large-scale gene expression analysis for evaluation of endocrine disruptors. In: Inoue, T., and Pennie, W. (eds.). *Toxicogenomics*. Springer-Verlag, Tokyo, 2003, 149–155
43. Komiyama, A., Ono, Y., Koh, K., Sakurai, K., Shibayama, T., Kato, M., Yoshikawa, T., Seki, N., Iguchi, T. and Mori, C.: Toxicogenomic effects of neonatal exposure to diethylstilbestrol on mouse testicular gene expression in the long term: a study using cDNA microarray analysis. *Molecular Reproduction and Development* 2002, **36**, 17–23
44. Naciff, J., Overmann, G., Torontali, S., Carr, G., Tiesman, J., Richardson, B. and Daston, G.: Gene expression profile induced by 17 alpha-ethynyl estradiol in the prepubertal female reproductive system of the rat. *Toxicological Sciences* 2003, **72**, 314–330
45. Mori, C., Komiyama, A., Adachi, T., Sakurai, K., Takashima, K. and Todaka, E.: Application of toxicogenomic analysis to risk assessment of delayed long-term effects of multiple chemicals, including endocrine disruptors in human fetuses. *Environmental Health Perspectives* 2003, **111**, 803–809
46. Kawai, M., Swan, K., Green, A., Edwards, D., Anderson, M. and Henson, M.: Placental endocrine disruption induced by cadmium: effects on P450 cholesterol side-chain cleavage and 3beta-hydroxysteroid dehydrogenase enzymes in cultured human trophoblasts. *Biology of Reproductive* 2002, **67**, 178–183
47. Halm, S., Pounds, N., Maddix, S., Rand-Weaver, M., Sumpter, J., Hutchinson, T. and Tyler, C.: Exposure to exogenous 17beta-oestradiol disrupts p450aromB mRNA expression in the brain and gonad of adult fathead minnows (*Pimephales promelas*). *Aquatic Toxicology* 2002, **60**, 285–299
48. Takeyoshi, M., Anai, S. and Shinoda, K.: Hepatic alpha(2u)-globulin mRNA levels and diethylstilbestrol-associated testicular atrophy in rats. *Reproductive Toxicology* 2000, **14**, 355–357
49. Yang, L., Tran, D. and Wang, X.: BADGE, BeadsArray for the detection of gene expression, a high-throughput diagnostic bioassay. *Genome Research* 2001, **11**, 1888–1898
50. Waters, K., Safe, S. and Gaido, K.: Differential gene expression in response to methoxychlor and estradiol through ERalpha, ERbeta, and AR in reproductive

tissues of female mice. *Toxicological Sciences* 2001, **63**, 47–56

51. Ashby, J.: The leading role and responsibility of the international scientific community in test development. *Toxicology Letters* 2003, **140–401**, 37–42

52. Couse, J., Curtis, S., Washburn, T., Lindzey, J., Golding, T., Lubahn, D., Smithies, O. and Korach, K.: Analysis of transcription and estrogen insensitivity in the female mouse after targeted disruption of the estrogen receptor gene. *Molecular Endocrinology* 1995, **9**, 1441–1454

53. Kato, S.: Androgen structure and function from knock-out mouse. *Clinical Pediatric Endocrinology* 2002, **11**, 1–7

54. Murphy, T. and Orphanides, G.: Characterisation of the molecular responses to xenoestrogens using gene expression profiling. *Phytochemistry Reviews* 2002, **1**, 199–208

55. Lui, G., Loraine, A., Shigeta, R., Cline, M., Cheng, J., Chervitz, S., Kulp, D. and Siani-Rose, M. NetAffx: Affymetrix probesets and annotations. *Nucleic Acids Research* 2003, **31**(1), 82–86

56. Quackenbush, J.: Microarray data normalisation and transformation. *Nature Genetics* 2002, **32**, 496–501

57. Larkin, P., Folmar, L., Hemmer, M., Poston, A. and Denslow, N.: Expression profiling of estrogenic compounds using a sheepshead minnow cDNA macroarray. *Environmental Health Perspectives* 2003, **111**, 839–846

58. Slonim, D.: From patterns to pathways: gene expression data analysis comes of age. *Nature Genetics* 2002, **32**, 502–508

59. International Human Genome Sequencing Consortium: Initial sequencing and analysis of the human genome. *Nature* 2001, **409**, 860–921

60. Mouse Genome Sequencing Consortium: Initial sequencing and analysis of the mouse genome. *Nature* 2003, **420**, 520–562

61. Aerts, S., Thijs, G., Coessens, B., Staes, M., Moreau, Y. and De Moor, B.: Toucan: Deciphering the cis-regulatory logic of coregulated genes. *Nucleic Acids Research* 2003, **31**, 1753–1764

62. Waring, J., Cavet, G., Jolly, R., McDowell, J., Dai, H., Ciurlionis, R., Zhang, C., Stoughton, R., Lum, P., Ferguson, A., Roberts, C. and Ulrich, R.: Development of a DNA microarray for toxicology based on hepatotoxin-regulated sequences. *Environmental Health Perspectives* 2003, 111, 863–870

18
Toxicogenomics Applied to Teratogenicity Studies

Philip G. Hewitt, Peter-J. Kramer, and Jürgen Borlak

18.1
Introduction

Teratology is the study of birth defects – structural or functional abnormalities that are present at birth. In humans, most of the observed birth defects are caused by random genetic errors; however, some are caused by environmental factors. For a chemical to be labelled a teratogen it must significantly increase the occurrence of structural or functional abnormalities in offspring at a dose that does not cause severe toxicity in the mother. Adverse effects on development under these conditions maybe secondary to the stress on the maternal system. The malformations are dependent on two major factors; namely, exposure level and timing of exposure. It is also a common finding that foetuses react differently within the same womb. This is probably due to certain foetuses being exposed to higher concentrations of toxicant or to genetic variations in susceptibility.

Teratology, the study of 'monsters' (terata), was based originally only on observations and had perceived supernatural implications. The acceptance of the basic genetics concepts in the early 20th century provided a scientific basis for the cause of congenital defects. Very early in the 20th century scientists began to link environmental insults to birth defects [for example, ionising radiation (Hipple and Pagenstrecher, 1907), sex hormones (Lillie, 1917), and chemicals (Gillman et al., 1948)]. The supposed safety of the human foetus was refuted as far back as 1941, after thousands of children exposed to German measles were born with cataracts, deafness, and congenital heart disease (Greg, 1941). This was confirmed by the thalidomide disaster in the late 1950s and early 1960s, which involved at least 12 000 children in 46 countries (McBride, 1961; Lenz, 1962; Colborn et al., 1996). This instance, in particular, prompted government intervention to assure appropriate testing of drugs and other xenobiotics in pregnant mammals. More recently (June 2000) it was reported that approximately 50 % of all pregnancies in the U.S.A. result in prenatal or postnatal death or an otherwise less than healthy baby.

The term 'teratogenicity' has been largely replaced by the more general term developmental toxicology, to allow for more adverse developmental problems – and to take

Handbook of Toxicogenomics: Strategies and Applications. Edited by Jürgen Borlak

ISBN: 3-527-30342-1

into account species differences. Developmental toxicity can be described as any structural or functional alteration, reversible or irreversible, caused by environmental insults, which interferes with homeostasis, normal growth, differentiation, development, and/or behaviour. The potential targets include the fertilized egg or zygote (prior to implantation and prior to formation of the three primary germ layers), the embryo during major organ development (organogenesis), the foetus in the post-embryonic period, and the neonate or postnatal offspring. In the developing foetus there is the necessity for very precise temporal and spatial sequencing of specific cell numbers and types for normal differentiation, including programmed cell death. In most animals, cells communicate via signalling pathways, which are repeatedly used in various combinations at different times and locations in the embryo and foetus. Chemical disruption of these pathways clearly leads to abnormal development of the foetus.

Teratogenicity testing is traditionally performed in test animals, which may respond differently from humans. Susceptibility to teratogenic effects shows extreme variability between different species, including responses to ACE inhibitors, aspirin, vitamin A, and thalidomide, which are negative in certain animal species (especially the rat) but which have been shown to be teratogenic in humans (Table 18.1). A comprehensive list of drugs and chemicals that are teratogenic are referenced in Schardein (1985). As a result of this discrepancy between animals and humans, there is a strong need for good (better) testing strategies. A better testing strategy is required, as a positive teratogenicity result in an animal model alone should not be a reason for halting drug development or lead to removal of the drug from the market. In other words, teratogenicity can be controlled in humans (i.e., do not prescribe to pregnant women) or be safely prescribed (for example, vitamin A and aspirin), as a low but pharmacologically active dose of such a compound may have beneficial effects but no teratogenicity at all.

The sedative thalidomide has become the most notorious teratogenic agent known to man. The type of defect observed in children was positively correlated to the time of treatment. When taken by women in the first three months of pregnancy (specifically, weeks 7–8), rare birth defects were observed in thousands of children, that is, phocomelia (severe shortening of the limbs) and amelia (lack of limbs). Weeks 7–8 were subsequently shown to be the critical time for limb development in the foetus. Although the mechanism of teratogenesis and determinants of risk remain unclear, it is known that thalidomide is bioactivated by embryonic prostaglandin H synthase (PHS) to a free-radical intermediate. This produces reactive oxygen species (ROS), which cause oxidative damage to DNA and other cellular macromolecules. Similarly, thalidomide is bioactivated by horseradish peroxidase and oxidizes DNA and glutathione, indicating free radical-mediated oxidative stress. Furthermore, thalidomide teratogenicity in rabbits is reduced by the PHS inhibitor acetylsalicylic acid, indicating PHS-catalysed bioactivation. This oxidative stress modulates intracellular glutathione (GSH) and redox status, which can perturb redox-sensitive processes, such as transcription factor activation and/or binding. Nuclear factor-kappa B (NF-κB), a redox-sensitive transcription factor involved in limb outgrowth, may be modulated by thalidomide-induced redox shifts. NF-κB and regulatory genes that initiate and maintain limb outgrowth and development, such as *Twist* and *Fgf-10*, are selectively expressed in the progress zone

Tab. 18.1 Summary of birth defects, types and incidence, caused by well known drugs and chemicals that are positive human teratogens.

Chemical/drug	*Most common abnormality*	*Test species*								
		Mouse	*Rat*	*Guinea pig*	*Hamster*	*Rabbit*	*Dog*	*Cat*	*Pig*	*Monkey*
Alcohol	craniofacial, limb, CV defects	Y	+	+		–	Y			
Aminopterin	skeletal defects	–	Y				+	–	+	–
Analapril	renal, CV effects	Y								
Antithyroid compounds	hyperthyroidism	Y	Y	Y		Y				
6-Azauridine		+	+			+				
Busulfan	multiple renal and CNS defects	+	+							
Coumarin anticoagulants	nose and skeletal defects	–	–			–			–	
Cyclo-phosphamide	digit effects	Y	Y			+				+
Cytarabine	limb and ear defects	+	Y							
Diethyl-stilbestrol	uterine lesions	Y	Y		–	–				+
5-Fluorouracil	multiple	Y	Y	Y		+				+
Procarbazine	limb and ear defects	+	Y			Y				Y
Methotrexate	skeletal defects	+	+		–	Y	–	Y		+
Methyl mercury	microcephaly, neurological deficit	Y	Y		+	–	–	Y	–	–
Streptomycin	inner ear	–	Y	–		–				
Thalidomide	limb defects	+	+	–	+	Y	+	+	+	Y
Trimethadione	limb facial anomalies. mental retardation	+	–							+
Vitamin A	CNS, heart, ear	+	+		+	–				+

Y = teratogenic, similar effects in humans; + teratogenic; – not teratogenic.

of the developing limb bud (which is important in the proximo-distal patterning of the limbs). Hansen et al. (2002) showed by in situ hybridization a preferential decrease in *Twist*, *Fgf-8*, and *Fgf-10* expression after thalidomide treatment (400 mg kg^{-1} day^{-1}) in rabbit embryos, whereas expression in rat embryos was not affected. This could help to explain the difference in sensitivities to thalidomide between these two species.

However, it is clear that thalidomide is still an excellent pharmaceutical and, under today's regulations, may not have been withdrawn. In fact, thalidomide is starting to make a resurgence, especially in the areas of leprosy, skin diseases, and cancer therapy (Nasca et al., 2003; Matthews and McCoy, 2003).

Retinoic acid (RA) is essential for both embryonic and adult growth, activating gene transcription via specific nuclear receptors. It is generated, via a retinaldehyde intermediate, from retinol (vitamin A). When RA concentrations deviate from their normal range in either direction, abnormal growth and development occur. RA has been described as a universal teratogen and, as such, is routinely used as a positive control (as seen in the studies reported later in this chapter). Hypervitaminosis A induces multiple abnormalities, but typical reactions include exencephaly in rats (Cohlan, 1953), facial and digit malformations in rabbits (Giroud and Martinet, 1958), and behavioural changes in rats at subteratogenic doses. High concentrations of RA result in abnormal development of cerebellum and hindbrain nuclei. The latter parallels the malformations seen in the human embryo exposed to RA due to treatment of the mother with the anti-acne drug Accutane (13-cis RA) and, when the child survives beyond birth, a particular set of behavioural anomalies has been described (McCaffery et al., 2003).

18.1.1
Current Testing Strategies: Established Procedures

Before the thalidomide incident in the 1960s there was no legislation covering reproduction toxicity. There was also little knowledge of the molecular mechanisms of teratogenicity (no molecular biology, no toxicogenomics, no developmental biology). Therefore, one important consequence of the thalidomide disaster was that nearly every country introduced legal requirements for the testing of potential new drugs. Therefore, detailed reproductive tests were included as part of the testing battery. Both the FDA and OECD have established guidelines for evaluating reproductive and developmental toxicity. In 1993, new guidelines for the testing of drugs were implemented internationally (ICH, 1993), whereby strategies followed in the U.S.A., Europe, and Japan were harmonised. The major theme of these new guidelines is scientific flexibility. Factors specified as relevant included anticipated drug use in relation to reproduction; the form and routes of administration intended for humans; and existing data on toxicity, pharmacodynamics, kinetics, and similarity to other compounds in structure/activity. To be able to detect immediate and delayed affects, it is recommended that exposure should be throughout one complete life cycle. Section II of these guidelines covers teratogenicity. The current guidelines call for the use of a rodent and a nonrodent species. Usually rat (several strains are available, for example, Wistar, Sprague–Dawley, and Fischer 344) and the rabbit (usually the New Zealand While albino or Dutch Belted black and white) are used. In fact, the use of the rabbit is more historical, as thalidomide was positive in this species. An overview of the new requirements is given in Table 18.2. When using laboratory animals for teratogenicity, testing numerous factors must be considered. Because of interspecies differences in developmental pathways, xenobiotic metabolism, and pharmacokinetics, the choice of species is critical. It is strongly recommended that early pharmacokinetic studies be performed prior to the main reproduction toxicity study, as the results may indicate the need for alternative species, study design, or dosing schedule. There should also be a comparison between pregnant and nonpregnant animals, as the pharmacokinetics may be very different. The route of administration

Tab. 18.2 Developmental toxicity testing requirements.

Parameter	*Requirement*
Maternal endpoints	
Assignment of dose group	By a body-weight–dependent random procedure
Definition of high-dose group	Should induce developmental and/or maternal toxicity, but no more than 10% maternal deaths
Test substance administration: period of dosing	Dose from implantation through termination (days 6–20 or 21 in rats, 6–17 or 18 in mice and 6–29 or 30 in rabbits); option to start at GD 0
Test substance administration: dose adjustment	Dosage adjusted periodically throughout the period of administration by body weight
Number of pregnant animals at termination	Rodents and rabbits: 20 per group
Maternal post-mortem data: corpora lutea counts	Data required for all species (including mice)
Foetal endpoints	
Rodents: assignment of foetuses for evaluation	Half of each litter assigned for skeletal evaluation, the remainder for visceral evaluation
Rabbits: coronal section	Required (50% coronal section, 50% serial sections)
Ossified and cartilaginous skeletal evaluation	Both ossified and cartilaginous skeletal examination required

chosen should be the same as that intended for human use. Exposure should continue throughout the length of the gestation period, especially during organogenesis (which is obviously different from species to species). There are also practical considerations when choosing the species. For example, availability (need a large number of animals born at the same time), size, cost, gestation length (as short as possible), mothering ability, and litter size (to help with statistics). Scientific considerations include metabolism, reproduction physiology, embryology, maturation post partum (short), species and strain sensitivity, and as much background data as possible.

18.1.2
Calcium Signalling and Foetal Development

The integrated communications control system within an embryo requires short-range (subcellular) and long-range (pan-embryonic) abilities; it has to be flexible and, at the same time, robust enough to operate in a dynamically changing environment without information being lost or misinterpreted. Although many signalling elements appear, disappear, and sometimes reappear during embryo/foetal development, it is becoming clear that embryos also depend on a ubiquitous, persistent, and highly versatile signalling system that is based around a single messenger, namely,

Ca^{2+} (Webb and Miller, 2003). Features of Ca^{2+} signalling pathways that have been described previously in mature cells and tissues are now being described during embryogenesis. The elementary Ca^{2+} events that constitute intracellular signalling during fertilization and early zygotic developmental stages are thought to drive many, if not all, of the subsequent intracellular and intercellular signalling events that occur as development proceeds. The increase in embryonic cell number is accompanied by a reduction in cell size, with the result that individual cells become surrounded by an increasing number of neighbouring cells. This increase in complexity is accompanied by developmental events being initiated that require coordinated activity and, as a consequence, there is an initiation of localized intercellular Ca^{2+} signalling. During the extensive cellular rearrangements that occur during gastrulation, germ-layer formation, and establishment of the body axes, there is an increasing requirement for coordination on a broader scale. This is reflected in the intercellular Ca^{2+} signalling events that begin to display a more extensive global nature. Once the germ layers and major body axes have been established, there is a return to more localized intercellular signalling events, which are associated with the generation of specific embryonic organs, such as the brain and heart, and a reappearance of intracellular signalling events from single cells. Efforts to identify the downstream targets and overall function of these Ca^{2+} signals in specific developmental events are now a very active part of developmental biological research.

It is therefore of great toxicological significance if a substance causes imbalances in the calcium signalling pathways during any of these steps of embryogenesis.

18.1.3
Effect of Dose on Embryo Development

Pregnancy itself may actually increase uptake of possible toxicants, as well as increasing the uptake into target tissues (due to a decrease in circulating plasma albumin). The placenta itself provides little in the way of restricting molecules entering the foetus.

Three general dose–response patterns have been identified: (1) cause malformations of the entire litter at exposure levels not causing embryo lethality (rare); (2) combination of embryo lethality, malformation, growth retardation, and apparently normal foetuses [the latter response pattern is more common and results from agents that cause cytotoxicity to replicating cells via alterations in replication, transcription, translation, or cell division (Ritter, 1977)]; and (3) growth retardation and embryo lethality without malformation. Compounds producing this effect are considered to be embryotoxic and not teratogenic and usually act on fundamental cellular processes, such as glycolysis, mitochondrial function, and membrane integrity (Bass et al., 1978). We should also note that, due to the size of the embryo, there could be a much higher equimolar concentration due to the size/volume ratio, compared to the mother.

18.1.4
Effect of Time on Embryo Development

The timing of exposure to a teratogen is critical in determining the potential effects. Exposure very early, before implantation, usually causes death; exposure during middle stages of development (organogenesis) leads to structural defects; and, finally, in late stages of development, exposure is most likely to cause growth retardation. Exposure to a teratogen during a critical period for a particular organ system may lead to malformations in that system. One example that highlights the importance of time of exposure is that of thalidomide.

Exposure of the stem cells (in either the female or the male) during gametogenesis can lead to mutations and hence the transfer of somatic mutations to the offspring. Potentially toxic substances can affect this maturation process in many different ways. For example, chronic cocaine exposure is known to reduce testicular expression levels of the nuclear factor cAMP response element modulator, and this maybe one of the mechanisms responsible for disruption or impairment of spermatogenesis in the testes (Li et al., 2003).

The post-fertilization period of susceptibility differs from exposures of gametes, the latter producing excessive pre- and peri-implantational death and low rates of foetal anomalies predominated by growth retardation. Retinoic acid administered prior to gastrulation produces novel malformation syndromes indicative of specific gene expression modification. The rates and types of defects from retinoic acid treatment of both gametes and the early conceptus contrast with those resulting from embryonic treatment during organogenesis, and their mechanisms are likely to differ. The pregastrulation period has not been explored to the extent reported during gametogenesis or organogenesis. Pregastrulation teratology is a new area of investigation with relevance both to reproductive toxicology and to mammalian developmental biology (Rutledge, 1997).

18.1.5
Issues Linked to the Placenta as a Barrier

The term 'placental barrier' is a misnomer, since the placenta allows the transfer of most xenobiotics from the mother to the foetus. However, chemicals with a molecular weight of over 1000 do not pass through so easily (Morgan, 1997). Species differences in placenta structure may also influence the transplacental transfer of chemicals. For example, the placental thickness depends upon the number of foetal and maternal cell layers. The rat and the rabbit have a single layer of cells, primates and humans have three layers of cells, and pigs and horses have six. In general, the more complex multilayered placenta of higher animals makes it more difficult for xenobiotics to reach the foetus. The role of active transport is believed to be limited, and the major mechanism of transfer is diffusion (simple or facilitated). The placenta is known to have both phase 1 and phase 2 metabolising enzyme systems and as such may still protect the developing foetus from potentially toxic agents (for example, high butyrylcholinesterase activity metabolises cocaine and therefore acts as a metabolic barrier to protect the foetus (Sastry, 1995)). Xenobiotic-metabolising enzymes may also activate certain compounds. For example, oxon metabolites of organophosphorus insecticides and epoxides of cyclodiene chlorinated hydrocarbons have a greater potential for foetotoxicity/teratogenicity than the mother substrates.

18.1.6
Effect of Xenobiotic and Endogenous Metabolism

Xenobiotic metabolism of toxicants is thought to occur mostly in maternal tissues or the placenta. This is due to the very low levels of both phase I and II xenobiotic drug-metabolising enzymes in the developing foetus. Monooxygenase activity has been reported to be absent from the foetus (rat) but shortly before birth (gestation day (GD) 20), there is a burst of activity (Borlakoglu et al. 1993 a, b). Specific isoforms of cytochrome P450 have been shown to be present. The greatest interest appears to be in P450s 1A1, 1B1, 2E1, and 3A7, each of which has been reported to be expressed at toxicologically significant levels or at least at potentially toxicologically significant levels during organogenesis (Juchau et al., 1998). However, activities of phase II enzymes, such as UDP-glucuronyltransferase, glutathione S-transferase, and epoxide hydrolase, were measurable as early as GD 10. Wells and Winn (1996) stated that teratological susceptibility is determined by the ability of the embryo to metabolise compounds and to subsequently repair any damage caused by reactive intermediates. If detoxification and repair mechanisms are immature (or completely lacking) in the embryo, then these embryos have increased susceptibility to teratogenic compounds.

The cytochrome P450s also play a crucial role in the metabolism of endogenous substrates, such as steroids, fatty acids, prostaglandins, and RA. Otto et al. (2003) demonstrated that the cytochrome P450 system (including cytochrome P450 reductase, *cpr*) plays a key role in early embryonic development. The process appears to be, at least in part, controlled by regional concentrations of RA and has profound effects on blood vessel formation. Knockout mice were bred with a double deletion of the *cpr* gene, and 70% of the animals showed many defects, which included an open neural tube, lack of branchial arches and limb buds, enlarged heart, reduced number of somites, and shortening of the anteroposterior axis. These defects were prevented when mothers were fed a vitamin A-deficient diet.

In the developing human foetus, the liver plays another essential role, that of haematopoietic stem cells derivation, up until the time of birth, when the bone marrow takes over. Perturbations of foetal erythropoiesis, such as by the well known teratogen, 5-fluorouracil, have obvious effects on the ability of the developing foetus to initiate an immune response. 5-Fluorouracil has been shown to produces foetal anaemia on GD 16–17, as evidenced by dose-dependent decreases in the cell counts, haematocrit, and haemoglobin content of foetal blood obtained by cardiac puncture (Zucker et al., 1995). These data suggest that 5-fluorouracil inhibits both erythroid cell proliferation and RNA synthesis reversibly, resulting in an anaemia that triggers compensatory release of immature reticulocytes.

18.1.7
Mechanisms of Teratogenicity

The biochemical mechanisms of action of many teratogens are unknown; however, it is obvious that any chemical that interferes with cell division is likely to damage developing organisms. One form of malformation for which much mechanistic information is available is the cleft palate. Cleft palate occurs when there is a disruption in the growth and fusion of the maxillary and palatine process, involving cell division, migration, apoptosis, and other complex processes. For example, TCDD binds to specific proteins in the cytosol blocking apoptosis and subsequently causing cleft palate. High levels of glucocorticoids also cause cleft palate, by interacting with the glucocorticoid receptors in the maxillary cells and inhibiting cell growth.

Neurological effects on the foetus are common, as there is increased permeability of the foetal blood–brain barrier, allowing greater access to teratogens. There are also many very specialised steps in neurological development that can be potentially disrupted.

Thalidomide has been hypothesised to directly damage developing limb tissue or to interfere with communication between that tissue and surrounding tissue (Stine and Brown, 1996). Cocaine potentiates the effects of norepinepherine by blocking reuptake. Norepinepherine stimulates blood vessel contraction, causing a decrease in blood flow to the foetus and resulting in hypoxia.

It is well documented that these affects are not rare but, in fact, fairly common. This is illustrated by the case study presented here, namely the teratogenicity of the drug EMD 82571, which was developed by Merck, Darmstadt. This drug was halted during clinical development, primarily due to positive developmental toxicity data.

18.2
Alternative Methods

18.2.1
Embryonic Stem Cells

Blastocyte-derived pluripotent embryonic stem cells can be induced to differentiate into a variety of cell types and have been used to try to predict teratogenicity, although with limited success to date. As far back as 1991, Laschinski et al. reported an early teratogenicity screening test based on cytotoxicity testing in mouse embryonic stem cells. This test has been improved to look specifically at stem cell derived cardiomyocytes (Scholz et al, 1999). ECVAM (EU Centre for Validation of Alternative Methods) has since validated these techniques (Genschow et al., 2002; Spielmann and Liebsch, 2002). The same ECVAM validation procedure was also used to validate the micromasses test, the whole embryo culture test, and the mouse embryonic stem cell test (Spielmann and Liebsch, 2001).

Permanent embryonic germ cell lines have also been employed as an *in vitro* alternative to *in vivo* germ cell mutagenicity tests (BALB/cJ mice; Klemm et al., 2001).

This test system was proven to be a sensitive and highly predictive germ cell mutagenicity method.

18.2.2 Micromasses and Other Cell Culture Systems

Cell culture systems have certain advantages when one is looking at specific toxicity endpoints. For example, Uyeki et al. (1996), Hwang et al. (1988), and Thal et al. (1986) have reported the use of mesenchymal cells from chick limb buds, which were cultured as micromasses, where they differentiated into chondrocytes. Similarly, De Bari et al. (2001) cultured adult human periosteum-derived cells as micromasses for use in the repair of joint surface defects.

Some nonmammalian cell culture systems have also been previously used. These include cells derived from *Drosophila* eggs, hydra cells, and *Xenopus* embryos (Stine and Brown, 1996).

18.2.3 Whole-embryo Culture

Young rat or mouse embryos have been maintained in culture, exposed to potential teratogens, and then observed for changes in normal development in response to the drug treatment. The whole-embryo culture technique has been shown, on numerous occasions, to support normal embryonic growth and development during early organogenesis (New, 1978). Studies using whole-embryo cultures allow assessment of the direct effect of a toxicant on the embryo and precise control of the variables of interest. For example, Tabacova et al. (1996) reported the use of ICR and CD1 mouse embryos to study the effect of inorganic arsenic toxicity (oxidation state, time, dose, and gestational age dependence). The malformation pattern produced *in vitro* closely corresponded to that observed after maternal administration at the same gestational stage. This showed that use of such a system was predictive, at least for inorganic arsenic. Other examples include studies by Mirkes and Greenaway (1982), Greenaway et al. (1985), Hunter et al. (1996), and Winn and Wells (2002). However, these embryo cultures have not been widely used, especially in the pharmaceutical industry. Safety studies still rely wholly on *in vivo* developmental studies, because it is estimated that these *in vitro* methods show a concordance of only approximately 60% with *in vivo* data (Report from Reprotox Arbeitskreis, 2002). Therefore, decisions on a new drug's safety are still made on the basis of *in vivo* studies.

Other types of embryo cultures have also been developed more recently, for example, chick embryos in ovo. Whitsel et al. (2002) reported the use of such a system to try to elucidate the teratogenic mechanism of an anticonvulsant drug, valproic acid (VPA). Chicken embryos exposed to VPA in ovo showed increased mortality, growth delay, and abnormalities similar to those previously reported in humans (neural tube, cardiovascular, craniofacial, limb, and skeletal abnormalities). Pax-2 and Pax-6 protein expression was qualitatively diminished in the eye. Localized exposure of the wing bud to VPA caused structural abnormalities in the developing wing in the absence of other anomalies in the embryos. These wing defects were similar to those observed after topical whole-embryo VPA application. These authors determined that at least one mechanism of VPA teratogenicity involved its direct action on the developing tissue. Fuller et al. (2002) proposed altered neural crest cell migration and proliferation as mechanisms of teratogenicity. Neural tube segments from chick embryos were cultured with VPA and showed markedly decreased proportions of cells migrating individually, promoting migration as epithelial sheets. Immunostaining of VPA-exposed explants revealed N-cadherin–positive cell boundaries, but independent neural crest cells did not stain. F-actin staining was reduced in independent neural crest cells. The data suggest a mechanism involving interference with epithelial–mesenchymal transition.

18.2.4 Gene Expression Profiling

Very limited data are available on the use of global gene expression profiling for prediction or elucidation of the mechanism of teratogenicity. However, more and more research is being published on the role of specific genes in teratogenicity (see Section 18.3.1).

18.2.5 In Silico Studies

Knudsen recently reported (2003) the use of functional genomics and computational biology to try to elucidate specific teratogenic mechanisms, by using global gene expression changes relating to specific teratogens. A comprehensive gene expression matrix that captures the biological complexity of the embryonic transcriptome and its regulation can be used to predict the state of the embryo during a toxic insult.

18.3 Molecular Aspects of Teratogenicity

18.3.1 Genes Responsible for Causing Birth Defects

The reproductive cycle comprises a wide range of complex interactions at the molecular, cellular, and structural level within a very specific chronological sequence. These events are different in different animal species. The complexity of this system makes it vulnerable to multiple toxic interferences, meaning that many traditional tests would be required to identify all the possible effects. Therefore, it makes sense to try to develop better screening assays to try to accurately predict what will occur in humans, using quicker and cheaper test systems that can monitor multiple pathways. These new testing strategies will have to rely on knowledge of molecular mechanisms involved in the processes of teratogenicity. It is evident from current literature that more and more information is becoming available that shows the involvement of specific genes and transcription factors (Table 18.3).

Numerous studies have established the pivotal role of transcription factors in organ development and cellular function, and there is conclusive evidence that transcription factors act in concert in liver-specific gene expression. During organ development and in progenitor cells, the timely expression of certain transcription factors is necessary for cellular differentiation. There is overwhelming evidence for hierarchical and cooperative principles in a networked environment of transcription factors. The search for molecular switches that control stem-cell imprinting and liver-specific functions has led to the discovery of many interactions between markedly

Tab. 18.3 Known transcription factors involved in teratogenic responses.

Transcription factor	***Affected by or altered in***	***Function***	***Reference***
NF-κB	thalidomide	inflammatory response	Meierhofer and Wiedermann, 2003
Pax 1	valproic acid	organogenesis	Barnes et al., 1996
Pax 2	valproic acid	organogenesis	Whitsel at el., 2002
Pax 3	valproic acid	organogenesis	Whitsel at el., 2002
Scleraxis	5-azadeoxycytidine	early tendon morphogenesis	Rosen and Chernoff, 2002
PPAR-delta	valproic acid	adipogenic mechanisms	Lampen et al., 2001
Activating protein-2	valproic acid	organogenesis	Werling et al., 2001
Goosecoid	retinoic acid	*homeobox* gene, RXR dependent	Zhu et al., 1999
BMP-2	retinoic acid	bone development	Zhu et al., 1999
BMP-4	retinoic acid	bone development	Zhu et al., 1999
TBX5	thalidomide, Holt–Oram syndrome	limb development	Guenzler, 1999
E2F-1		cell cycle promoting	Henry et al., 2003
Aryl hydrocarbon receptor	TCDD	xenobiotic metabolising enzymes	Peters et al., 1999
RARalpha, RXR heterodimer	retinoic acid	neural tube closure	Aaku-Saraste et al., 1997 Dreyer et al., 1996
Sonic hedgehog	retinoic acid	limb development	Smith et al., 2003
Lis1	neuronal migration disorder	neuronal migration	Assadi et al., 2003
SALL4	Holt–Oram syndrome; Okihiro syndrome		Kohlhase et al., 2003
Sp1	thalidomide	DNA mismatch repair	Drucker et al., 2003; Gazzoli and Kolodner, 2003

different molecules, such as transcription factors, coactivators, corepressors, enzymes, DNA, and RNA. Thus, specific mutational changes in liver-enriched transcription factors can be demonstrated to lead to altered intermolecular interactions, with the consequence of human disease (Schrem et al., 2002). With the advent of gene expression arrays, it may be possible in the future to monitor these gene expression changes (toxicogenomics) in an embryo (in culture, stem cells, etc.) so as to indicate specific birth defects. The promise of genomics (and proteomics) is not only to perform screening tests, but also to allow the elucidation of the underlying mechanism(s) that cause specific cellular responses that mediate or are responsible for teratogenic effects.

A new revolution in reproduction toxicology is approaching, and toxicogenomics will be at the forefront. Gene expression profiling will help to bridge the gap between traditional toxicology and the molecular biology of the developing foetus. Not only will these technologies aid in elucidation of toxic mechanisms in the foetus (and mother) but will also lead to a greater understanding of organogenesis (stem cell biology).

Modulation of gene expression is of paramount importance in the mechanisms of drug-induced toxicity, and major efforts are being made to determine the relevance of gene expression in response to drug exposure. DNA arrays offer the unique opportunity to explore the simultaneous gene expression of literally thousands of genes, but its cost-effective use requires rational gene selection. In conjunction with other molecular endpoints, reliable predictions of drug safety becomes feasible at early stages of drug development.

18.3.2
Specific Genes Involved in Birth Defects

Endothelins are known to play a role in foetal development. Treinen et al. (1999) showed that malformations in both rats and mice are produced after treatment with two endothelin receptor antagonists. These malformations were consistent with the pattern of endothelin-1 gene expression in mouse embryonic pharyngeal arches and heart and with the craniofacial and cardiovascular malformations observed in endothelin-1–deficient mice.

Bennett et al. (2000) investigated the effect of VPA on the expression of specific genes within developing foetuses (specifically during neurulation). Several genes were identified that were significantly increased during VPA treatment, with alterations in the transcriptional activities of critical neurotrophic and growth factor genes – including *tgfα*, *tgfβ*, *ngf*, *bdnf*, and *bfgf*. VPA treatment has also been reported to not simply disrupt development in a nonspecific manner, but to act by specifically altering *HOX* gene expression (Faiella et al., 2000).

It was also recently reported that thalidomide teratogenicity is due to transcriptional control of the inflammatory response via NF-κ (Meierhofer and Wiedermann, 2003). NF-κB is also an integral part of the apoptosis mechanism and is very important in normal foetal development.

Apoptosis has been reported to be responsible for the deleterious effects of several compounds on the foetal system:

- 2,3,7,8-Tetrachlorodibenzo-*p*-dioxin (TCDD) causes cardiovascular toxicity, culminating in death of mammalian embryos. A chick embryo model was used by Ivnitski et al. (2001) to determine whether TCDD alters coronary artery development and whether this alteration is associated with apoptosis and/or changes in myocyte proliferation. They showed that a TCDD-induced increase in apoptosis occurs early in embryo development and therefore may contribute to changes in myocyte proliferation, coronary development, and cardiac structural malformations.
- 2,4-Dichlorophenoxyacetic acid (2,4-D) and its derivatives are herbicides and have been associated with a range of adverse effects in humans and various animal species, from embryotoxicity and teratogenicity to neurotoxicity. It has been demonstrated that 2,4-D induces apoptosis in cerebellar granule cells in culture, apparently by a direct effect on mitochondria, leading to cytochrome c release and consequent activation of caspase-3, thereby triggering events that may cause apoptosis (DeMoliner et al., 2002).
- Ethylnitrosourea (ENU), a well known DNA alkylating agent, induces anomalies in the central nervous system, craniofacial tissues, limbs, and male reproductive organs. Katayama et al. (2000) reported that excess cell death caused by apoptosis occurs in these organs and tissues of rat foetuses from dams treated with ENU on day 13 of gestation (GD 13). In addition, a high incidence of microencephaly, ectrodactyly, and curved caudal vertebrae was observed in the offspring from dams treated with ENU at GD 13. It was strongly suggested that ENU-induced apoptosis in rat foetal tissues might play an important role in the induction of anomalies in the corresponding tissues.

Bone morphogenic proteins (e. g., BMP-4 is repressed by retinoic acid treatment in mice) also play a crucial role in teratogenicity (Zhu et al., 1999). Regulation of cranial fusion can also be affected by antagonists of BMPs, such as noggin, which has been shown to prevent cranial closure (Warren et al., 2003).

Disruption of the *c-ski* proto-oncogene causes changes in morphogenesis of craniofacial structures (as seen after EMD 82571 treatment), skeletal muscle development, and the central nervous system. Mice that lack this gene present with defects caused by failed closure of the cranial neural tube (Berk et al., 1997).

18.4
Case Study: Elucidation of Mechanisms of Teratogenic Toxicity of the Developmental Drug EMD 82571

18.4.1
Properties of EMD 57033 and EMD 82571

EMD 57033 has been characterised as a calcium sensitizer and was developed to treat coronary heart disease. Calcium ions play a pivotal role in control of myocardial contractility, and an increase in contraction force can be elicited by increasing the transient free Ca^{2+} concentration and/or by augmenting the myofibrillar sensitivity to Ca^{2+}. Traditionally, drugs have been developed which increase the force of contraction by strengthening the myocardial contractility, ultimately by raising the Ca^{2+} concentration. For example, β-sympathomimetics, phosphodiesterase III (PDE_{III}) inhibitors, and cardiac glycosides.

EMD 82571, a pro-drug of EMD 57033, was the first drug developed which was shown to increase contraction primarily via calcium sensitisation. It also has PDE_{III} inhibitory properties, contributing to its overall cardiovascular profile. The compound acts through downstream mechanisms at the level of the actin–myosin cross-bridges, by increasing the contribution of each cross-bridge to the contractile force (Merck internal report).

The acute toxicity of EMD 82571 in rodents was shown to be low. Female rats were considerably more sensitive, due to large differences observed in the first pass metabolism. Bioavailability of the active drug was only 9% in male rats but 60% in the female rat. Repeat dose studies showed a no-observable-effect level of 10 mg kg^{-1} in both rats and dogs. At higher doses, mild toxicity was observed, with the principle target organ being the liver, which increased in weight and demonstrated centrilobular hypertrophy associated with increases in liver enzymes. Histologically, perivasculitis and vacuolation of the centrilobular hepatocytes was observed. The Ames test (±S9), the rat micronucleus test, and the mouse lymphoma cell assay (+S9) were all negative. Mutation frequencies were slightly increased in the absence of S9 activation in the mouse lymphoma cell assay.

Embryo–foetal toxicity of EMD 82571, EMD 57033, and the ester group (*N*-methylpiperidinol) was studied in rats. Administration was oral and from gestation days 6 to 17. All the high-dose (150 mg kg^{-1}) foetuses were malformed after EMD 82571 treatment. The most common abnormalities were exencephaly, micrognathia, and palatoschisis (Figure 18.1). Treatment with EMD 57033 or *N*-methylpiperidinol did not cause an increase in the frequency of malformations, even at concentrations of 300 mg kg^{-1} (Merck internal report).

To elucidate the teratogenic mechanism of EMD 82571, two different approaches were taken, both involving gene expression profiling. The first was to concentrate on specific, relevant genes (hypothesis-based) and the second was based on global gene expression analysis (Affymetrix rat 230A array).

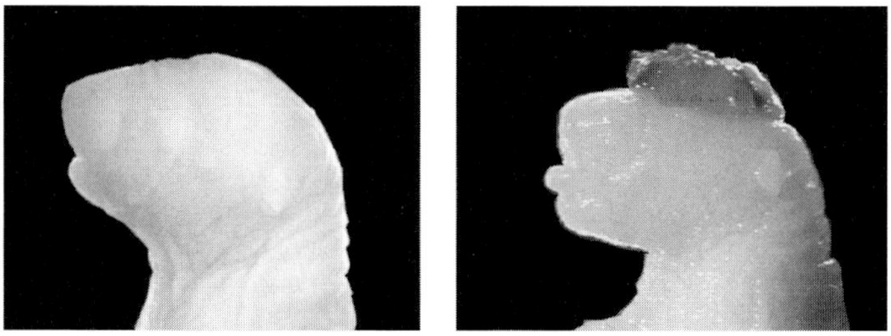

Fig. 18.1 Foetal malformations caused by treatment with EMD 82571 and retinoic acid.

18.4.2 Hypothesis-driven Gene Expression Array

18.4.2.1 Gene Selection

Genes (246) were selected based on specific genes reported to be involved in teratogenic processes and foetal development. Additional genes were also selected, based on their putative role in EMD 82571's mode of action and its toxicological profile (Table 18.4).

Tab. 18.4 Rational for selecting genes for focused cDNA array.

Area of activity	*Proteins encoded*
Developmental regulators	BMPs, WNTs, HNFs, Hoxs, PAXs, RXRs, RASs, CEBP, CREB, etc.
Extracellular matrix/cytoskeleton structural proteins, matrix metalloproteinases, adhesion molecules	Collagens, lamanins, integrins, fibrillins, micrifibrillar proteins, bone specific proteins, calcium handling proteins, MMPs, TIMPs, endonucleases, cartilage, osteopoetin, microfibullar proteins, aggrecan core proteins
Cell cycle	DNA polymerase, topoisomerase, E2F1, CDKs, replication factors, ribosomal proteins, GADDs, etc.
Growth factors/nuclear factors	Connective tissue growth factors, granulocyte colony-stimulating factor, TGF, TGFRs, IGF, IGFR, PDGFs, VEGFs, CAR, CXR, PXR, PPAR, etc.
Acute phase response/heat shock response	Heat shock proteins, ubiquitin, α1-AT, CRP, α2-macroglobulin, etc.
Detoxification	CYPS, UGTs, STs, steroid metabolism, FMOs, HPRT, etc.
Metabolism	Protein, lipid, carbohydrate

18.4.2.2 Study Design

In Vivo Embryotoxicity Study

Pregnant female Wistar rats were dosed daily with either EMD 82571 (50 mg kg^{-1} or 150 mg kg^{-1}) or RA (12 mg kg^{-1} or 20 mg kg^{-1}) on gestational days 6–17 (Table 18.5). RA was chosen as a positive control because of its very well documented effects on developing foetuses – including similar malformations as observed for EMD 82571 (Sakai and Langille, 1992; Cunningham et al., 1994; Mulder et al., 2000).

On gestational days 12 and 20, the female was killed and the foetuses were removed (visible malformations were noted; Table 18.6). The maternal liver, whole embryo (day 12), foetal liver (day 20), or foetal bone (cranium, mandibular bone) were removed from all animals in the study and immediately snap-frozen in liquid nitrogen.

Tab. 18.5 In-vivo developmental study details: treatment.

Treatment	*Days of treatment*	*Day of section*	*Number of animals*
Control	6–11	12	5
50 mg kg^{-1} EMD 82571	6–11	12	5
150 mg kg^{-1} EMD 82571	6–11	12	5
Control	6–11	20	5
50 mg kg^{-1} EMD 82571	6–11	20	5
150 mg kg^{-1} EMD 82571	6–11	20	5
Retinoic acid[a)]	6–17	20	5

a) Dose chosen according to Emmanouil-Nikoloussi et al. (2000).

Tab. 18.6 Malformations caused by high-dose EMD 82571.

		Individual external observation (# foetuses)				
Female No.	*Number of foetuses*	*Exencephaly*	*Exencephaly, micrognathia/ agnathia*	*Exencephaly, facial cleft*	*Exencephaly, micrognathia/ agnathia, facial cleft*	*Within normal limits*
1	6	3	1	1	–	1
2	11	–	6	–	5	–
3	10	–	–	–	–	10
4	10	–	2	–	1	7
5	13	6	–	4	–	3

18.4.2.3 Gene Expression Experimental Design

- *cDNA Array Production*: Defined 200–400-bp fragments of the 246 selected cDNAs derived from rat liver tissue were cloned, amplified, purified, and checked for size and purity on agarose gel. Amplified inserts were gridded on treated glass slides (Memorec) using an ink-jet micro arrayer (Luigs and Neumann, Ratingen and Memorec).
- *Sample Labelling and Hybridization*: Total RNA was extracted, and 40 µg of total RNA was used for each hybridisation. Control samples were labelled with Cy3, treated samples with Cy5. Hybridisation was carried according to the protocol described by Borlak et al. (2003).
- *Data Analysis and Normalization:* Arrays were read using ScanArray3000 (GSI Lumonics). Signal intensities of Cy3 and Cy5 samples were normalized to the median of the housekeeping gene signals and were determined with standard procedures in the laboratory of Prof. Borlak (Borlak et al., 2003).

18.4.2.4 Results and Discussion

Genes (246) were selected based on their putative role in EMD 82571's mode of action and their importance in known teratogenic pathways and were analysed using a custom-made BioChip. Induction and suppression of many genes clearly occurred after treatment with EMD 82571 and RA in both maternal liver and the various embryonic tissues taken. These could be grouped into compound-specific gene changes and common gene changes (Table 18.7).

Specific changes caused by EMD 82571 included (1) induction of HSC 73 (heat shock cognate 73–kd protein), Fen 1 (Flap endonuclease 1), HSP105, collagen 2A1, bone morphogenic protein 7 (Bmp 7), and connective tissue growth factor precursor (CTGF); (2) suppression of epithelial–cadherin precursor (Cdh-1) and alpha-1-antitrypsin precursor (AT1).

Genes that were commonly induced by both EMD 82571 and RA included those for hypoxanthine-guanine phosphoribosyltransferase (HPRT), GAPDH, glucuronosyltransferase 2B2 (UGT2B2), cytochrome P450 2E1, cytochrome P450 7A1, and insulin-like growth factor II (IGFII).

It is clear that both EMD 82571 and RA caused significant changes in gene expression in both the maternal liver and the target tissue. These changes can be specifically linked to general cellular stress (e. g., Hsc 73, Hsc 105, DNA topoisomerase IIb, Fen1), but more importantly, to specific changes during foetal development: Bmp7, collagen 2A1, and Ctgf. The induction of HPRT could explain the significant ($P<0.05$) reduction in serum urea levels observed during previous *in vivo* toxicity studies (internal report, Merck). It is also known that HPRT oxidase inhibitors also cause an increase in HPRT activity, leading to teratogenic effects similar to those seen in these studies.

The metabolic modulation observed might lead to changes in bile acid synthesis. This would lead to high levels of circulating bile acids (such as deoxycholic acid), which have been reported to cause foetal resorption, as well as significant increases in foetal malformations (Zimber and Zusman, 1990). These effects have also been reported in humans. The Zellweger (or cerebro-hepato-renal) syndrome is a congeni-

Tab. 18.7 Number of genes affected (by class) in embryo liver and bone tissue after treatment with retinoic acid (RA) or EMD 82571.

Pathway	*RA-induced*	*RA-suppressed*	*EMD-induced*	*EMD-suppressed*	*Commonly induced*	*Commonly suppressed*
Signal transduction	2	1	1	0	1	0
Protooncogenes	0	0	0	1	0	1
ECM, cytoskeleton	7	0	2	2	0	0
Metabolism	1	1	6	0	4	0
Protein turnover	2	1	4	1	1	0
Miscellaneous	1	0	0	0	1	2

tal disorder characterized by cerebral dysfunction, craniofacial dysmorphic features, transient cholestasis, and renal cysts. Patients fail to thrive and usually die in their first year of life. Several biochemical abnormalities have been observed, including elevated levels of coprostanic acids and the C-29 dicarboxylic bile acid (Eyessen et al., 1985). Therefore, it was postulated that EMD 82571 acts directly on the maternal liver, subsequently causing the teratogenic effects observed.

Many congenital malformations are produced during the gastrulation and neurulation stages of embryogenesis. Altered maternal metabolism in rats has been reported to have a direct impact on the embryo or an indirect effect via disruption of the nutritive function of the yolk sac. It is essential to remember that the metabolic status of the embryo is rapidly changing and that the embryo responds differently at different times of gestation. If the mother is compromised in any way, this has a consequent effect on the foetuses.

Interestingly, both EMD 82571 and RA induced the expression of GAPDH; the responsible gene is commonly considered as a housekeeping gene. This suggests that such simple normalisation procedures will not be adequate for large gene expression studies.

We need to attempt to discern from the literature which genes are the most relevant for the application. The microarray approach is a completely closed system that provides results only for strictly predetermined genes, which may already be well characterised. This selection will not be representative of the entire genome. The advantage of smaller size and reduced complexity is that it facilitates the task of making a high specificity, high quality microarray for quantitative use. This is useful for focusing on mechanisms of action, when they are known (Bartosiewicz et al., 2001; Gerhold et al., 2001). Other advantages of using such a hypothesis-driven microarray include costs, manpower, ease of use, and ease of data interpretation. However, the major disadvantage is the limited number of genes chosen. No amount of forethought can really predict all the important gene expression changes that may occur. In addition, the rat genome has yet to be completely sequenced and, as a consequence, annotation is difficult. At the moment, one of the most advanced rat array systems available is that from Affymetrix (the A chip has 15 900 annotated genes and the B chip an additional 13 000 ESTs).

Therefore, to further test the hypothesis suggested from the smaller focused array, that of bile acid teratogenicity, a global expression analysis study using the same tissue samples was initiated.

18.4.3
Global Expression Array (Affymetrix)

18.4.3.1 Chip Design

Rat sequences (15 900) were chosen from the GenBank, bdEST, and RefSeq databases. Oligonucleotide probes complementary to each corresponding sequence were synthesised in situ on the arrays, and 11 pairs of probes were used for each gene (Murphy, 2002).

18.4.3.2 Experimental Design

The same bone (20-d embryo), liver (maternal and 20-d embryos), and total embryo (12-d) RNA samples as from the previous experiment were taken, pooled, and processed for global expression profiling.

Sample Labelling and Hybridisation

cRNA was prepared according to the manufacturer's recommendation. Briefly, double-stranded cDNA was synthesized from 10 μg total RNA by using Superscript II RT (Invitrogen) and an oligo dT_{24}-T7 promoter primer (GenSet). The obtained cDNA was first cleaned using Phase Lock Gel (Eppendorf) – phenol/chloroform extraction, followed by ethanol precipitation. The cleaned-up cDNA was used as a template for *in vitro* transcription using the Megascript kit and biotinylated nucleotides (Bio-11-CTP and Bio-16-UTP) to produce biotin-labelled cRNA (Enzo^{R} BioArray High Yield RNA Transcription Labelling Kit, Affymetrix). The purified material was then assessed for yield, purity, and integrity by spectrophotometric and Bioanalyzer analyses. Fragmented (35–200 bases) *in vitro* transcripts (cRNAs) were purified with Rn.easy spin columns (Qiagen) before hybridising (10 μg) overnight onto the Affymetrix GeneChip Rat Expression 230A array (16 h at 60 rpm in a 45 °C GeneChip hybridisation oven 640). The hybridised samples were stained with streptavidin-R/phycoerythrin (SAPE, Molecular Probes), and the signal was amplified with a biotinylated goat antistreptavidin antibody (Vector Laboratories), followed by a final staining with SAP. Washing, staining, and amplification were carried out using the Affymetrix GeneChip Fluidics station 400. The arrays were also scanned using the GeneArray scanner from Agilent.

Data Analysis and Normalization

The rat 230A array includes a set of rat maintenance genes to facilitate normalisation and scaling of gene expression experiments. These normalisation genes show consistent levels of expression over defined sample sets. The raw data obtained was first quality-checked using Expressionist Refiner software (GeneData) before further analysis using Expressionist Analyst (GeneData). The RMA algorithm, by which treated and control groups can be compared, was used for normalisation. Default parameters provided in Expressionist software were used for all analysis. A threshold value of a two-fold change was applied to the data to aid in interpretation of the limited dataset.

18.4.4 Results and Discussion

Hierarchical cluster analysis using all genes expressed showed a good separation of each tissue studied (embryo day 12, embryo bone day 20, embryo liver day 20, and maternal liver) (Figure 18.2). However, any indication of compound effects on gene expression was not possible from this analysis. It is also suggestive that the largest influence on overall gene expression came from the individual tissues themselves.

Figure 18.3 shows the number of genes differentially expressed for all tissues tested. It is clear that many more genes were differentially regulated in the target or-

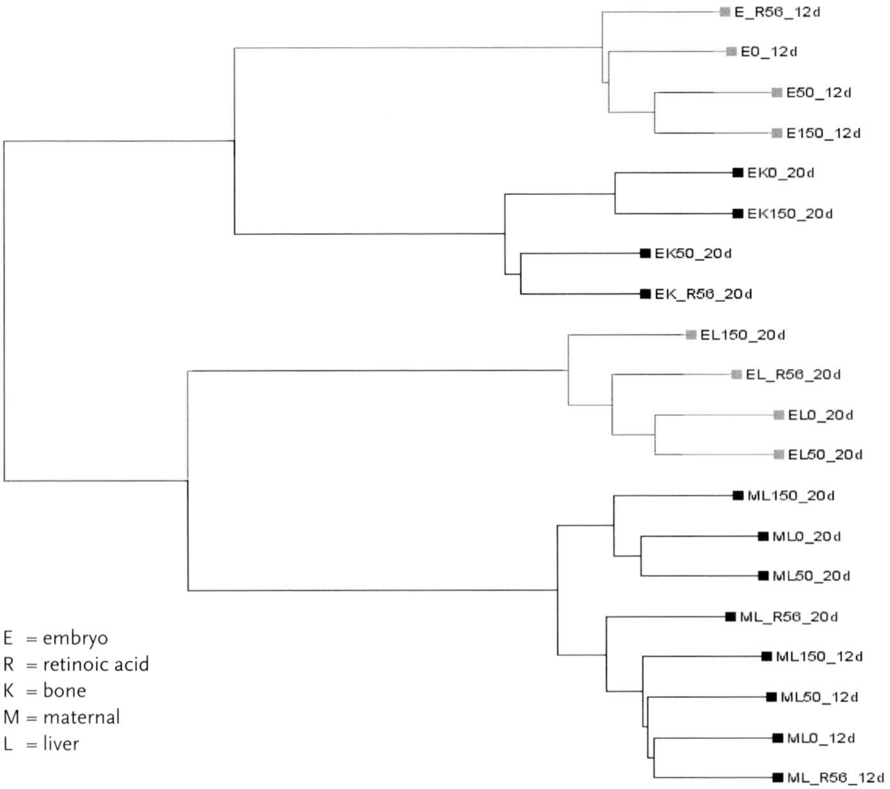

Fig. 18.2 Effects of EMD 82571 and retinoic acid on embryo liver and bone tissue gene expression.

gan in the foetus, namely the bone. Surprisingly, many more genes were regulated after low-dose EMD 82571 treatment than after high-dose treatment. The model compound, retinoic acid, which is a powerful teratogen, had a serious affect on most of the tissues tested, with many more genes upregulated than after EMD 82571 exposure.

These data show that very little gene expression deregulation occurred in the maternal liver after 12 days gestation, and only retinoic acid had a significant effect after 20 days. Of those genes that were up- or down-regulated, none matched those reported for the hypothesis-driven array presented above.

Table 18.8 gives a summary of the relevant genes that were deregulated in the foetal tissue, irrespective of time and tissue. Several very important pathways were clearly affected by both EMD 82571 and retinoic acid treatment, with many of these genes being involved in differentiation/development, calcium-regulated signalling pathways, ion-channel activity, and the extracellular matrix. These common mechanisms appear to have been affected by all three treatments and can be linked directly to the developing foetus (and hence deregulation leading to birth defects).

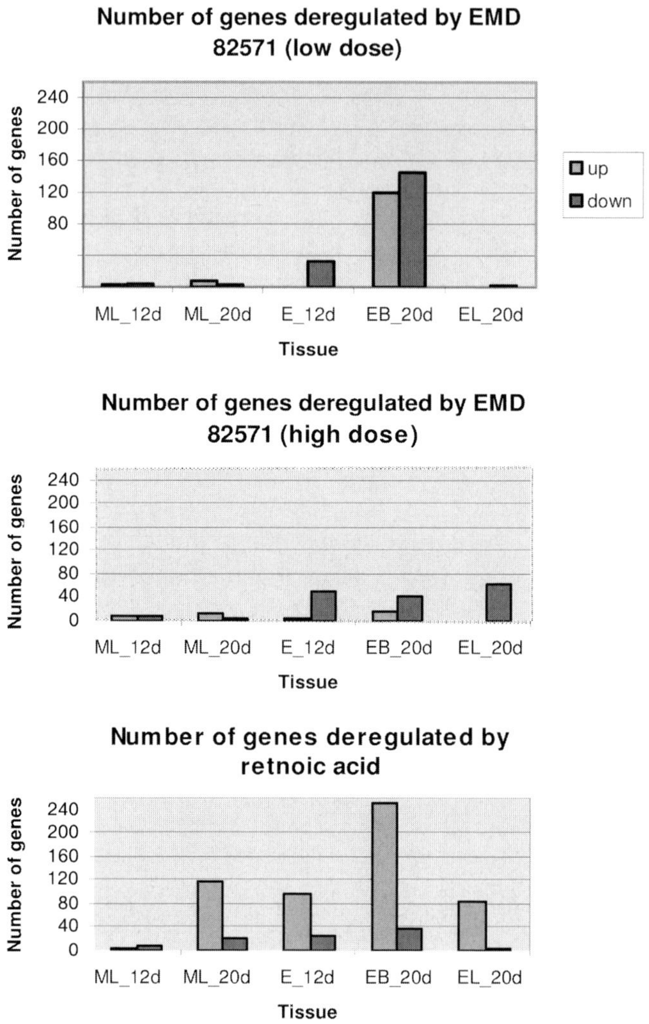

Fig. 18.3 Variation in the number of differentially expressed genes in different tissues after treatment with either EMD 82571 or retinoic acid (B = bone).

18.4.4.1 **Calcium Homeostasis**

As discussed in the introduction, it is clear that embryos depend on a ubiquitous, persistent, and highly versatile signalling system that is based around calcium, especially during the cellular rearrangements that occur during gastrulation, germ-layer formation, and establishment of the body axis. It is therefore no surprise that a substance designed to modulate calcium sensitivity has a profound effect on a developing embryo, as occurs with EMD 82571. Calcium channel blockers have been shown to pose no major teratogenic risk to humans (Magee et al., 1996). As already stated,

Tab. 18.8 Summary of highly up and down regulated/relevant genes by EMD 82571 and retinoic acid

Gene	*Gene description*	*Gene symbol*	*Function*	*Fold change*
Calcium homeostasis				
Low Dose EMD 82571				
1387137_at	Cartilage oligomeric matrix protein	Comp	calcium ion binding	2.36
1369621_s_at	FK506 binding protein 2	Fkbp2	modulation of calcium flux properties/histone chaperone	2.19
1387081_at	reticulocalbin 2	Rcn2	calcium ion binding	2.04
1370198_at	triadin 1	Trdn	calcium handling	2.15
1367797_at	Multiple endocrine neoplasia 1	Men1	calcium homeostasis	0.45
1369142_at	bone gamma-carboxy-glutamate protein	Bglap	calcium ion binding	0.49
1368339_at	calbindin 3	Calb3	calcium ion binding	0.33
High Dose EMD 82571				
1368044_at	secretogranin 2	Scg2	calcium ion binding	2.05
1369142_at	bone gamma-carboxy-glutamate protein	Bglap	calcium ion binding	0.32
Retinoic acid				
1367614_at	annexin 1	Anxa1	calcium-dependent phospholipid binding, calcium ion binding	2.03
1368955_at	calcium/calmodulin-dependent serine protein kinase	Cask	protein kinase activity, intracellular signaling cascade	2.07
1387401_at	calsequestrin 2	Casq2	calcium ion storage activity	2.74
1368988_at	calsequestrin 2	Casq2	calcium ion storage activity	2.77
1367846_at	S100 calcium-binding protein A4	S100a4	calcium ion binding	2.06
1387455_a_at	Very low density lipoprotein receptor	Vldlr	calcium ion binding	2.22
1367562_at	Secreted acidic cystein-rich glycoprotein (osteonectin)	Sparc	basement membrane, calcium ion binding	2.11
Bone Specific				
Low Dose EMD 82571				
1371052_at	Noggin	Nog	Inhibitor of BMP's, inhibition of bone formation	3.08
1368161_a_at	alpha-2-HS-glycoprotein	Ahsg	cysteine protease inhibitor activity, ossification	0.14
1367581_a_at	secreted phosphoprotein 1	Spp1	ossification, cell adhesion molecule activity	0.47
1369142_at	bone gamma-carboxy-glutamate protein	Bglap	calcium ion binding	0.49
1369175_a_at	Ameloblastin	Ambn	tooth enamel development	0.26

Tab. 18.8 (continued)

Gene	*Gene description*	*Gene symbol*	*Function*	*Fold change*
1388007_x_at	Amelogenin	Amel	bone development	0.50
1390398_at	BMP receptor 1A	Bmpr1a	bone development	0.50
High Dose EMD 82571				
1368161_a_at	alpha-2-HS-glycoprotein	Ahsg	cysteine protease inhibitor activity, ossification	0.15
1369142_at	bone gamma-carboxy-glutamate protein	Bglap	calcium ion binding	0.32
1369773_at	Bone morphogenic protein 3	BMP3	bone development	0.47
1300734_a_at	Dentin sailophospho-protein	dspp	tooth development	0.48
1388007_x_at	Amelogenin	Amel	bone development	0.32
1370582_a_at	Amelogenin	Amel	bone development	0.31
1369589_x_at	Amelogenin	Amel	bone development	0.33
1387634_a_at	Amelogenin	Amel	bone development	0.18
Ion-channels and transporters				
Low Dose EMD 82571				
1370407_at	chloride ion pump-associated 55 kDa protein	Clp55	ion channel/transport	2.08
1370973_at	sodium channel, voltage-gated, type 6, alpha	Scn6a	ion channel/transport	2.30
1368082_at	solute carrier family 4, member 2	Slc4a2	inorganic anion exchanger activity	0.37
1369625_at	aquaporin 1	Aqp1	water channel activity	0.28
1387651_at	aquaporin 1	Aqp1	water channel activity	0.41
1369074_at	amino acid transport system A3	Ata3	amino acid transport	0.39
1368335_at	apolipoprotein A-I	Apoa1	lipid transport, steroid biosynthesis	0.27
1369727_at	apolipoprotein A-II	Apoa2	lipid transport	0.29
1370862_at	apolipoprotein E	Apoe	lipid transport	0.40
1370228_at	Transferrin	Tf	iron ion transporter activity	0.29
1367758_at	alpha-fetoprotein	Afp	beta-glucuronidase activity, transport, carrier activity	0.06
1370228_at	Transferrin	Tf	iron ion transporter activity	0.18
1369319_at	glutamate transporter EAAC1 interacting protein	Gtrap 3-18	neuronal, cholesterol	0.44
1369929_at	prosaposin	Psap	glycosphingolipid catabolic pathways and glycolipid transport	0.41
High Dose EMD 82571				
1368335_at	apolipoprotein A-I	Apoa1	lipid transport, steroid biosynthesis	0.14

Tab. 18.8 (continued)

Gene	*Gene description*	*Gene symbol*	*Function*	*Fold change*
1369074_at	amino acid transport system A3	Ata3	amino acid transport	0.37
1370862_at	apolipoprotein E	Apoe	lipid transport	0.29
1370228_at	transferrin	Tf	iron ion transporter activity	0.23
1386909_a_at	voltage-dependent anion channel 1	Vdac1	ion channel	0.43
Retinoic acid				
1367989_at	solute carrier family 2, member 4	Slc2a4	glucose transporter activity	2.23
1383080_at	transferrin	Tf	iron ion transporter activity	2.32
1370069_at	solute carrier family 12, member 5	Slc12a5	potassium-chloride transporter	0.44
1368057_at	ATP-binding cassette, sub-family D (ALD), member 3	Abcd3	ATP-binding cassette (ABC) transporter activity	0.42
Differentiation and Development				
Low Dose EMD 82571				
1373812_at	cyclin-dependent kinase inhibitor 1B	Cdkn1b	cell cycle arrest, negative regulation of cell proliferation	2.51
1373499_at	growth arrest specific 5	Gas5	cell cycle arrest, negative regulation of cell proliferation	2.29
1369735_at	growth arrest specific 6	Gas6	cell cycle arrest, negative regulation of cell proliferation	2.23
1369679_a_at	nuclear factor I/A	Nfia	transcription factor activity DNA replication	2.98
1387349_at	short stature homeobox 2	Shox2	transcription factor activity	2.10
1367703_at	crystallin, gamma D	Crygd	sensory organ development, structural constituent of eye lens	0.40
1368821_at	follistatin-like	Fstl	FSTL3 is a local regulator of activin action in gonadal development and gametogenesis	0.28
1368822_at	follistatin-like	Fstl	FSTL3 is a local regulator of activin action in gonadal development and gametogenesis	0.47
1387919_at	mitofusin 2	Mfn2	mitochondrial fusion is essential for embryonic development	0.49
1369793_a_at	l-gicerin	Mcam	immunoglobulin (Ig) super-family expression only observed in developmental stage when neurons extend neurites and migrate	0.20
1367570_at	transgelin (smooth muscle 22 protein)	Tagln	muscle development	0.38
1398823_at	translin-associated factor X	Tsnax	essential for normal cell proliferation	0.36

Tab. 18.8 (continued)

Gene	*Gene description*	*Gene symbol*	*Function*	*Fold change*
1388101_at	collapsin	Crmp4	regulation of axonal growth and branching	0.48
1369244_at	aryl hydrocarbon receptor nuclear translocator 1	Arnt1	transcription factor, developmental signalling	0.23
High Dose EMD 82571				
1387634_a_at	amelogenin	Amel	tooth development	0.18
1370582_a_at	amelogenin	Amel	tooth development	0.31
1388007_x_at	amelogenin	Amel	tooth development	0.32
1369589_x_at	amelogenin	Amel	tooth development	0.33
Retinoic acid				
1388206_a_at	eukaryotic initiation factor 5 (eIF-5)	Eif5	differentiation	2.53
1367713_at	eukaryotic translation initiation factor 2, subunit 1 (alpha)	Eif2s1	differentiation	2.39
1398799_at	eukaryotic translation initiation factor 4E	Eif4e	differentiation	2.59
1369679_a_at	nuclear factor I/A	Nfia	transcription factor activity, DNA replication	2.04
1372143_at	ubiquitin-conjugating enzyme E2 variant 2	Ube2v2	protein degradation	2.71
1369617_at	ubiquitin-conjugating enzyme E2N	Ube2n	protein degradation	2.15
1399143_at	ubiquitin-conjugating enzyme E2N	Ube2n	protein degradation	2.55
1368632_at	forkhead box O1	Foxo1	transcription factor activity	0.21
1368867_at	GERp95	Gerp95	development + differentiation; stem cell differentiation	0.26
1368866_at	GERp95	Gerp95	development + differentiation; stem cell differentiation	0.41
Extracellular Matrix				
Low Dose EMD 82571				
1367845_at	neurofilament 3, medium	Nef3	intermediate filament	2.67
1370059_at	neurofilament, light polypeptide	Nfl	intermediate filament	2.81
1368028_at	peripherin 1	Prph1	intermediate filament	4.44
1370944_at	procollagen, type X, alpha 1	Col10a1	structural	4.37
1374353_x_at	actin alpha cardiac 1	Actc1	cytoskeleton	0.30
1374352_at	actin alpha cardiac 1	Actc1	cytoskeleton	0.34
1370086_at	fibrinogen, gamma polypeptide	Fgg	cytoskeleton	0.41

Tab. 18.8 (continued)

Gene	*Gene description*	*Gene symbol*	*Function*	*Fold change*
1371530_at	keratin 8	Krt8	cytoskeleton	0.29
1388155_at	keratin complex 1, acidic, gene 18	Krt1-18	cytoskeleton	0.29
1388433_at	keratin complex 1, acidic, gene 19	Krt1-19	cytoskeleton	0.37
1369166_at	matrix metalloproteinase 9 (type IV collagenase)	Mmp9	tissue repair/collagen degradation	0.31
1371053_at	myosin, heavy polypeptide 8, skeletal muscle	Myh8	cytoskeleton	0.35
1398321_a_at	procollagen, type XII, alpha 1	Col12a1	extracellular matrix structural constituent, cell adhesion	0.35
1370288_a_at	tropomyosin 1, alpha	Tpm1	structural constituent of cytoskeleton, muscle thin filament tropomyosin	0.21
1371239_s_at	tropomyosin 3, gamma	Tpm3	structural constituent of cytoskeleton, muscle thin filament tropomyosin	0.23
1367964_at	troponin 1, type 2	Tnni2	actin binding, muscle development, structural constituent of cytoskeleton	0.46
1371618_s_at	tubulin, beta 3	Tubb3	cytoskeleton	0.20
1387892_at	tubulin, beta 5	Tubb5	cytoskeleton	0.45
High Dose EMD 82571				
1367845_at	neurofilament 3, medium	Nef3	intermediate filament	2.15
1370059_at	neurofilament, light polypeptide	Nfl	intermediate filament	2.06
1368028_at	peripherin 1	Prph1	intermediate filament	3.45
1388204_at	matrix metalloproteinase 13	Mmp13	tissue repair/collagen degradation. Osteoblastic development	0.47
1398275_at	matrix metalloproteinase 9 (IV collagenase)	Mmp9	tissue repair/collagen degradation	0.32
1398866_at	scaffolding protein SLIPR	Slipr	structural constituent of cytoskeleton	0.45
1387854_at	procollagen, type I, alpha 2	Col1a2	cytoskeleton	0.48
1370155_at	procollagen, type I, alpha 2	Col1a2	cytoskeleton	0.45
1388155_at	keratin complex 1, acidic, gene 18	Krt1–18	cytoskeleton	0.22
1371530_at	keratin 8	Krt8	cytoskeleton	0.25
1388433_at	keratin complex 1, acidic, gene 19	Krt1-19	cytoskeleton	0.31
1367592_at	troponin T2	Tnnt2	structural constituent of cytoskeleton, muscle development	0.35

Tab. 18.8 (continued)

Gene	*Gene description*	*Gene symbol*	*Function*	*Fold change*
Retinoic acid				
1367562_at	secreted acidic cystein-rich glycoprotein (osteonectin)	Sparc	basement membrane, calcium ion binding	2.23
1367749_at	lumican	Lum	collagen-binding leucine-rich proteoglycans, distributed in interstitial connective tissues	2.00
1370854_at	nexilin	LOC 246172	actin filament-binding protein localized at cell-matrix adherens junction	2.13
1370697_a_at	nexilin	LOC 246172	actin filament-binding protein localized at cell-matrix adherens junction	2.65
1388204_at	matrix metallo-proteinase 13	Mmp13	tissue repair/collagen degradation	2.78
1370944_at	procollagen, type X, alpha 1	Col10a1	structural	2.48
1371530_at	keratin 8	Krt8	cytoskeleton	0.48
1388155_at	keratin complex 1, acidic, gene 18	Krt1-18	cytoskeleton	0.42
1388433_at	keratin complex 1, acidic, gene 19	Krt1-19	cytoskeleton	0.49
1368411_a_at	microtubule-associated protein 2	Mtap2	cytoskeleton	0.47
1375469_at	SWI/SNF related, actin dependent regulator of chromatin, a4	Smarca4	cytoskeleton	0.48
1387226_at	internexin, alpha	Inexa	intermediate filament	0.50
1367572_at	myosin light chain 3, alkali, cardiac ventricles	Myl3	cytoskeleton, muscle development	0.48
1371618_s_at	tubulin, beta 3	Tubb3	cytoskeleton	0.21

voltage-sensitive calcium channels are essential for correct bone formation (Li et al., 2002), and therefore any substance that may change levels of calcium in the developing foetus will have profound effects on bone development.

18.4.4.2 **Bone Formation**

The major target organ is the foetal bone, and many important genes responsible for bone development were down regulated, for example, BMP3, which is important for cartilage formation (Tsumaki et al., 2002). In addition, noggin was upregulated and is known to be an inhibitor of bone morphogenic proteins (and therefore inhibits bone development – membranous ossification) (Aspenberg et al, 2001; Devlin et al., 2003). In fact, introduction of noggin into developing chick embryos causes facial abnormalities (Lee et al., 2001). Several of these deregulated genes are also calcium sensitive and therefore could have been regulated due to the calcium-sensitizing effects of EMD 82571. Not only bone-specific genes were altered, but several genes important in tooth development were also down-regulated.

18.4.4.3 Ion Channels and Transporters

Several important ion channels were regulated (Table 18.8), and their function in foetal development is not clear. However, changes in pH can affect bone and tooth development (Sui et al., 2003). Verapomil was also shown recently to mediate bone formation via voltage-sensitive calcium channels (Li et al., 2003).

18.4.4.4 Differentiation and Development

Francis-West et al. (2003) recently published data on the molecular cascades that control craniofacial development. Their studies emphasize how unique the head actually is, with each individual part governed by a distinct set of cellular signalling interactions/cascades. The processes that control neural tube closure, together with correct development of the skull and differentiation of the facial primordia and the branchial arches, is extremely complex, and defects in these processes result in several syndromes, such as exencephaly.

18.4.4.5 Extracellular Matrix

The complex and largely obscure regulatory processes that underlie ossification and fusion of the sutures during skull morphogenesis depend on the conditions of the extracellular microenvironment (Carinci et al., 2000). Distribution and sites of synthesis of a cartilage extracellular matrix protein, cartilage oligomeric matrix protein (COMP), and of a bone extracellular matrix protein, bone sialoprotein (BSP), are all important in femoral head development in the rat (Shen et al., 1995). Longitudinal growth of the skeleton is a result of the endochondral ossification that occurs at the growth plate. Through a sequential process of cell proliferation, extracellular matrix synthesis, cellular hypertrophy, matrix mineralization, vascular invasion, and eventually apoptosis, cartilage is continually replaced by bone as bone length increases (Ballock and O'Keefe, 2003). There is a well known relationship between the insoluble matrix and soluble factors during limb patterning, usually involving interactions with BMPs (Arteaga-Solis et al., 2001). Therefore, it is not surprising that a compound that causes such severe limb and cranial defects in the developing rat regulates genes for many different extracellular matrix proteins.

It is well known that gene expression is not a static process and that expression levels of genes are not stable with time. The differences observed in these studies between gestation days 12 and 20 could be due to responses to the administered compound or to effects caused earlier by the compounds. However, it is also possible that gene expression is inherently different in a developing foetus than in a maternal animal that is on the verge of giving birth.

In conclusion, pronounced gene expression changes were seen under most conditions tested, and these patterns of gene expression changes were indicative of a specific phenotype. From the possible metabolic deregulation in the maternal liver to the specific alterations of foetal bone development, a specific gene expression pattern will be produced. Numerous genes that are involved in numerous different pathways, such as bile acid production, calcium homeostasis, transport proteins, ion channel activity, extracellular matrix, etc., are regulated. These studies are preliminary but give us an excellent springboard for further research.

18.5 Importance of Surrogate Markers for Prediction of Teratogenicity

The studies described in the chapter have relied on the use of tissue from control and malformed foetuses. It is of little benefit to use such a system to identify possible teratogens during drug testing – as the malformations will already be evident. Therefore, the search for surrogate markers is essential. From the studies performed here, in which liver tissue was studied and compared to *in vitro* hepatocyte cultures (data not shown, and Borlak et al, 2002) it was clear that there were very significant differences in the *in vivo* and *in vitro* changes in gene expression and that using this system would not enable the finding a surrogate marker(s).

18.6 Summary and Future of Gene Expression Profiling for Teratogenicity Studies

From both experimental approaches, it is clear that significant changes are occurring at the gene expression level in both the maternal animal and the offspring. There is a definite effect on calcium signalling, resulting in perturbations of numerous genes that are known to be involved in differentiation of bone tissue and teeth, these being the two major malformations observed in foetuses after EMD 82571 treatment. This should not be too surprising, considering the mode of action of this developmental drug. However, not all foetuses were malformed and, of those that were, not all were similarly altered. In addition, some litters were completely unaffected by treatment. This leads to the question of the metabolic disturbance suggested by the knowledge-based array, where it is suggested that an increase in circulating bile acids could cause the birth defects observed. Follow-up studies on pregnant rats showed that EMD 82571 does indeed increase the levels of circulating bile acids (e.g., cholic acid, taurocholic acid; data not shown). But the effect that these bile acids may have in the developing embryo remains speculative. Additional support for this 'indirect' teratogenic effect comes form the pharmacokinetics data for EMD 82571, which clearly show that no pro-drug is circulating in the adult rat and that the active drug (EMD 57033) does not cause any significant increase in birth defects. Therefore, it is possible that the alterations caused by the calcium sensitizer itself (changes in calcium homeostasis, ion channel function, cellular signalling, etc.) cause certain developing foetuses to be more susceptible to these increased levels of circulating foetotoxic bile acids.

It is apparent that too little is known about the adaptive, homeostatic, and repair factors in the early embryo. Increased efforts should be undertaken to model and quantify those processes that determine the amount of chemical that reaches the site of toxicity (molecular dose) and how these teratogenic effects are propagated. The use of traditional developmental procedures does not help in this understanding. A more molecular approach is therefore essential, and the use of toxicogenomics to try to elucidate mechanisms of toxicity and to try to predict teratogenicity is the way forward in the future.

Acknowledgements

I would like to thank Prof. Jürgen Borlak for his patience with the writing of this chapter. Also to Dr. Anja von Heydebreck and Suse Beyer for their bioinformatics support of the affymetrix data.

References

Aaku-Saraste E, Oback B, Hellwig A, and Huttner WB (1997). Neuroepithelial cells downregulate their plasma membrane polarity prior to neural tube closure and neurogenesis. *Mech. Dev.*, **69(1–2)**, 71–81.

Arteaga-Solis E, Gayraud B, Lee SY, Shum L, Sakai L, and Ramirez F (2001). Regulation of limb patterning by extracellular microfibrils. *J. Cell Biol.*, **154(2)**, 275–281.

Aspenberg P, Jeppsson C, and Economides AN (2001). The bone morphogenetic proteins antagonist Noggin inhibits membranous ossification. *J. Bone Miner. Res.*, **16(3)**, 497–500.

Assadi AH, Zhang G, Beffert U, McNeil RS, Renfro AL, Niu S, Quattrocchi CC, Antalffy BA, Sheldon M, Armstrong DD, Wynshaw-Boris A, Herz J, D'Arcangelo G, and Clark GD (2003). Interaction of reelin signaling and Lis1 in brain development. *Nat. Genet.*, **35(3)**, 270–276.

Ballock RT, and O'Keefe RJ (2003). Physiology and pathophysiology of the growth plate. *Birth Defects Res. Part C Embryo Today*, **69(2)**, 123–143.

Barnes GL, Mariani BD, and Tuan RS (1996). Valproic acid-induced somite teratogenesis in the chick embryo: relationship with Pax-1 gene expression. *Teratology*, **54(2)**, 93–102.

Bartosiewicz M, Penn S, and Buckpitt A (2001). Applications of gene arrays in environmental toxicology: fingerprints of gene regulation associated with cadmium chloride, benzo(a)pyrene, and trichloroethylene. *Environ. Health Perspect.*, **109(1)**, 71–74.

Bass R, Oerter D, Krowke R and Speilmann H (1978). Embryonic development and mitochondrial function. III. Inhibition of respiration and ATP generation in rat embryos by thiamphenicol. *Teratology*, **18**, 93–102.

Bennett GD, Wlodarczyk B, Calvin JA, Craig JC, and Finnell RH (2000). Valproic acid-induced alterations in growth and neurotrophic factor. *Reproductive Toxicology*, **14**, 1–11.

Berk M, Desai SY, Heyman HC, and Colmenares C (1997). Mice lacking the *ski* proto-oncogene have defects in neurulation, craniofacial patterning, and skeletal muscle development. *Genes and Development*, **11**, 2029–2039.

Borlak J, Bosio A, Kramer, P-J, and Hewitt PG (2002). A knowledge based toxicogenomic approach to predict teratogenicity of new drug candidates. Poster presentation, Toxicology Letters 135, 583.

Borlak J, Drewes J, Hofmann K and Bosio A (2004). Toxicogenomics applied to *in vitro* toxicology: an array based gene expression and protein activity study in human hepatocyte cultures upon treatment with Aroclor 1254. *Xenobiotica*, submitted

Borlakoglu JT, Scott A, Henderson CJ, and Wolf CR (1993 a). Alterations in rat hepatic drug metabolism during pregnancy and lactation. *Biochemical Pharmacology*, **46(1)**, 29–36.

Borlakoglu JT, Scott A, Henderson CJ, Jenke HJ, Wolf CR (1993 b). Transplacental transfer of polychlorinated biphenyls induces simultaneously the expression of P450 isoenzymes and the protooncogenes c-Ha-ras and c-raf. *Biochemical Pharmacology*, **45(7)**, 1373–1386.

Buchenau P, Saumweber H, and Arndt-Jovin DJ (1993). Consequences of topoisomerase II inhibition in early embryogenesis of *Drosophila* revealed by *in vivo* confocal laser scanning microscopy. *J Cell Sci.*, **104**, 1175–1185.

Carinci P, Becchetti E, and Bodo M (2000). Role of the extracellular matrix and growth factors in skull morphogenesis and in the pathogenesis of craniosynostosis. *Int. J. Dev. Biol.*, **44(6)**, 715–723.

Cohlan SQ (1953). Excessive intake of vitamin A as a cause of congenital anomalies in the rat. *Science*, **117(3046)**, 535–536.

Colborn T, Smolen M, and Rolland R (1996). Taking a lead from wildlife. *Neurotoxicol. Teratol.*, **18(3)**, 235–7.

Cunningham ML, Mac Auley A, and Mirkes PE (1994). From gestation to neurulation: transition in retinoic acid sensitive identifies distinct stages of neural patterning in the rat. *Dev. Dyn.*, **200**, 227–241.

De Bari C, Dell'Accio F, and Luyten FP (2001). Human periosteum-derived cells maintain phenotypic stability and chondrogenic potential throughout expansion regardless of donor age. *Arthritis Rheum.*, **44(1)**, 85–95.

De Moliner KL, Evangelista de Duffard AM, Soto E, Duffard R, and Adamo AM (2002). Induction of apoptosis in cerebellar granule cells by 2,4-dichlorophenoxyacetic acid. *Neurochem. Res.*, **27(11)**, 1439–1446.

Devlin RD, Du Z, Pereira RC, Kimble RB, Economides AN, Jorgetti V, and Canalis E (2003). Skeletal overexpression of noggin results in osteopenia and reduced bone formation. *Endocrinology*, **144(5)**,1972–1978.

Dreyer C, and Ellinger-Ziegelbauer H (1996). Retinoic acid receptors and nuclear orphan receptors in the development of Xenopus laevis. *Int. J. Dev. Biol.*, **40(1)**, 255–262.

Drucker L, Uziel O, Tohami T, Shapiro H, Radnay J, Yarkoni S, Lahav M, and Lishner M (2003). Thalidomide down-regulates transcript levels of GC-rich promoter genes in multiple myeloma. *Mol. Pharmacol.*, **64(2)**, 415–420.

Emmanouil-Nikoloussi EN, Goret-Nicaise M, Foroglou P, Kerameos-Foroglou C, Persaud TV, Thliveris JA, and Dhem A (2000). Histological observations of palatal malformations in rat embryos induced by retinoic acid treatment. *Exp. Toxicol. Pathol.*, **52**, 437–444.

Faiella A, Wernig M, Consalez GG, Hostick U, Hofmann C, Hustert E, Boncinelli E, Balling R, and Nadeau JH (2000). A mouse model for valproate teratogenicity: parental effects, homeotic transformations, and altered *HOX* expression. *Human Molecular Genetics*, **9**, 227–236.

Francis-West PH, Robson L, and Evans DJ (2003). Craniofacial development: the tissue and molecular interactions that control development of the head. *Adv. Anat. Embryol. Cell Biol.*, **169(III-VI)**, 1–138.

Fuller LC, Cornelius SK, Murphy CW, and Wiens DJ (2002). Neural crest cell motility in valproic acid. *Reprod. Toxicol.*, **16(6)**, 825–839.

Gazzoli I, and Kolodner RD (2003). Regulation of the human MSH6 gene by the Sp1 transcription factor and alteration of promoter activity and expression by polymorphisms. *Mol. Cell. Biol.*, **23(22)**, 7992–8007.

Genschow E, Spielmann H, Scholz G, Seiler A, Brown N, Piersma A, Brady M, Clemann N, Huuskonen H, Pailard F, Bremer S, and Becker K (2002). The ECVAM international validation study on *in vitro* embryotoxicity tests: results of the definitive phase and evaluation of prediction models. European Centre for the Validation of Alternative Methods. *Altern. Lab. Anim.*, **30(2)**, 151–176.

Gerhold D, Lu M, Xu J, Austin C, Caskey CT, and Rushmore T (2001). Monitoring expression of genes involved in drug metabolism and toxicology using DNA microarrays. *Physiol. Genomics*, **5(4)**, 161–170.

Gillman J, Gilbert C, Gillman T, and Sence I (1948). A preliminary report on hydrocephalus, spina bifida, and other congenital anomalies in the rat produced by trypan blue. *S. African J. Med. Sci.*, **13**, 47.

Giroud A, and Martinet M (1958). Consequences of hypervitaminosis A in the rabbit embryo. *C. R. Seances Soc. Biol. Fil.*, **152(6)**, 931–932.

Greenaway JC, Mirkes PE, Walker EA, Juchau MR, Shepard TH, and Fantel AG (1985). The effect of oxygen concentration on the teratogenicity of salicylate, niridazole, cyclophosphamide, and phosphormide mustard in rat embryos *in vitro*. *Teratology*, **32**, 287–295.

GREGG NM (1941). Congenital cataract following German measles in the mother. *Trans. Ophthalmol. Sco. Aust.*, **3**, 35–46.

GUENZLER V (1999). Mechanisms of thalidomide teratogenicity. *Nat. Med.*, **5(8)**, 853.

HIPPLE V, and PAGENSTRECHER H (1907). Über den Einfluss des Cholins und der Röntgenstrahlen auf den Ablauf der Gravidität. *Münch. Med. Wochenschr.*, **54**, 452–456.

HUNTER, ES III, ROGERS EH, SCHMID JE, and RICHARD A (1996). Comparative effects of haloacetic acids in whole embryo cultures. *Teratology*, **54**, 57–64.

HWANG PM, BYRNE DH, and KITOS PA (1988). Effects of molecular oxygen on chick limb bud chondrogenesis. *Differentiation*, **37**, 14–19.

IVNITSKI I, ELMAOUED R, and WALKER MK (2001). 2,3,7,8-tetrachlorodibenzo-p-dioxin (TCDD) inhibition of coronary development is preceded by a decrease in myocyte proliferation and an increase in cardiac apoptosis. *Teratology*, **64(4)**, 201–212.

JUCHAU MR, BOUTELET-BOCHAN H, and HUANG Y (1998). Cytochrome-P450-dependent biotransformation of xenobiotics in human and rodent embryonic tissues. *Drug. Metab. Rev.*, **30(3)**, 541–568.

KATAYAMA K, ISHIGAMI N, UETSUKA K, NAKAYAMA H, and DOI K (2000). Ethylnitrosourea (ENU)-induced apoptosis in the rat fetal tissues. *Histol. Histopathol.*, **15(3)**, 707–711.

KLEMM M, GENSCHOW E, POHL, I, BARRABAS C, LIEBSCH M, and SPIELMANN H (2001). Permanent embryonic germ cell lines of BALB/cJ mice – an *in vitro* alternative for *in vivo* germ cell mutagenicity tests. *Toxicology In Vitro*, **15**, 447–453.

KNUDSEN ST, FOSS CH, POULSEN PL, BEK T, LEDET T, MOGENSEN CE, and RASMUSSEN LM (2003). E-selectin-inducing activity in plasma from type 2 diabetic patients with maculopathy. *Am. J. Physiol. Endocrinol. Metab.*, **284(1)**, E1–6.

KOHLHASE J, SCHUBERT L, LIEBERS M, RAUCH A, BECKER K, MOHAMMED SN, NEWBURY-ECOB R, and REARDON W (2003). Mutations at the SALL4 locus on chromosome 20 result in a range of clinically overlapping phenotypes, including Okihiro syndrome, Holt-Oram syndrome, acro-renal-ocular syndrome, and patients previously reported to represent thalidomide embryopathy. *J. Med. Genet.*, **40(7)**, 473–478.

LAMPEN A, GOTTLICHER M, and NAU H (2001). Prediction of embryotoxic effects of valproic acid-derivatives with molecular *in vitro* methods. *ALTEX*, **18(2)**, 123–126.

LASCHINSKI G,VOGEL R and SPIELMAN H (1991). Cytotoxicity test using blastocyte-derived euploid embryonal stem cells: a new approach to *in vitro* teratogenesis screening. *Reprod. Toxicol.*, **5**, 57–64.

LEE SH, FU KK, HUI JN, and RICHMAN JM (2001). Noggin and retinoic acid transform the identity of avian facial prominences. *Nature*, **414(6866)**, 909–912.

LENZ W. VON and KNAPP K (1962). Die thalidomid-embryopathie. *Deutsche medizinische Wochenschrift*, Stuttgart, **87(24)**, 1232–1242.

LI H, DUNBAR JC, and DHABUWALA CB (2003). Expression of cAMP-responsive element modulator (CREM) in rat testes following chronic cocaine administration. *J. Environ. Pathol. Toxicol. Oncol.*, **22(2)**, 111–116.

LI J, DUNCAN RL, BURR DB, and TURNER CH (2002). L-type calcium channels mediate mechanically induced bone formation *in vivo*. *J. Bone Miner. Res.*, **17(10)**, 1795–8000.

LILLIE FR (1917). The free-martin: A study in the action of sex hormones in the fetal life of cattle. *J. Exp. Zool.*, **23**, 371–452.

MAGEE LA, SCHICK B, DONNENFELD AE, SAGE SR, CONOVER B, COOK L, MCELHATTON P, SCHMIDT MA, AND KOREN G (1996). The safety of calcium channel blockers in human pregnancy: a prospective, multicenter cohort study. *Am. J. Obstet. Gynecol.*, **174**, 823–828.

MATTHEWS SJ, and MCCOY C (2003). Thalidomide: a review of approved and investigational uses. *Clin. Ther.*, **25(2)**, 342–395.

MCBRIDE WG (1961). Thalidomide and congenital abnormalities. *The Lancet*, **2**, 1358.

MCCAFFERY PJ, ADAMS J, MADEN M, and ROSA-MOLINAR E (2003). Too much of a good thing: retinoic acid as an endogenous regulator of neural differentiation and exogenous teratogen. *Eur. J. Neurosci.*, **18(3)**, 457–472.

MEIERHOFER C, and WIEDERMANN CJ (2003). New insights into the pharmacological and toxicological effects of thalidomide. *Current Opinions in Drug Discovery Development*, **6**, 92–99.

MIRKES, PE, and GREENAWAY, JC (1982). Teratogenicity of chlorambucil in rat embryos in vitro. *Teratology*, **26**, 135–143.

Morgan DJ (1997). Drug disposition in mother and foetus. *Clin. Exp. Pharmacol. Physiol.*, **24(11)**, 869–873.

Mulder GB, Manley N, Grant J, Schmidt K, Zeng W, Eckhoff C, and Maggio-Price L (2000). Effects of excess vitamin A on development of cranial neural crest-derived structures: a neonatal and embryonic study. *Teratology*, **62**, 214–226.

Murphy D (2002). Gene expression studies using microarrays: principles, problems, and prospects. *Advances in Physiology Education*, **26(4)**, 256–270.

Nasca MR, Micali G, Cheigh NH, West LE, and West DP (2003). Dermatologic and non-dermatologic uses of thalidomide. *Ann Pharmacother.*, **37(9)**,1307–1320.

New DAT (1978). Whole embryo culture and the study of mammalian embryos during organogenesis. *Biol. Rev.*, **53**, 81–122.

Otto DM, Henderson CJ, Carrie D, Davey M, Gundersen TE, Blomhoff R, Adams RH, Tickle C, and Wolf CR (2003). Identification of novel roles of the cytochrome p450 system in early embryogenesis: effects on vasculogenesis and retinoic acid homeostasis. *Mol. Cell. Biol.*, **23(17)**, 6103–6116.

Peters JM, Narotsky MG, Elizondo G, Fernandez-Salguero PM, Gonzalez FJ, and Abbott BD (1999). Amelioration of TCDD-induced teratogenesis in aryl hydrocarbon receptor (AhR)-null mice. *Toxicol. Sci.*, **47(1)**, 86–92.

Principles of Toxicology, eds KE Stine, TM Brown. Chapter 6, pp 83, 85 CRC Press, Boca Raton, FL 1983.

Ritter EJ (1977). Altered biosynthesis. *Handbook of Teratology: Mechanisms and Pathogenesis*, Vol 2, JG Wilson, FC Fraser (ed.), pp. 99–116. Plenum, New York.

Rosen MB, and Chernoff N (2002). 5-Aza-2′-deoxycytidine-induced cytotoxicity and limb reduction defects in the mouse. *Teratology*, **65(4)**, 180–190.

Rutledge JC (1997). Developmental toxicity induced during early stages of mammalian embryogenesis. *Mutat. Res.*, **396(1–2)**, 113–127.

Sakai A, and Langille RM (1992). Differential and stage dependent effects of retinoic acid on chondrogenesis and synthesis of extracellular matrix macromolecules in chick craniofacial mesenchyme *in vitro*. *Differentiation*, **52**, 19–32.

Sastry BV (1995). Neuropharmacology of nicotine: effects on the autoregulation of acetylcholine release by substance P and methionine enkephalin in rodent cerebral slices and toxicological implications. *Clin. Exp. Pharmacol. Physiol.*, **22(4)**, 288–290.

Schardein JL (1985). Current status of drugs as teratogens in man. *Prog. Clin. Biol. Res.*, **163C**, 181–190.

Scholz G, Pohl I, Genschow E, Klemm M, and Spielmann H (1999). Embryotoxicity screening using embyonic stem cells *in vitro*: correlation to *in vivo* teratogenicity. *Cells Tissues Organs*, **165(3–4)**, 203–211.

Schrem H, Klempnauer J, and Borlak J (2002). Liver-enriched transcription factors in liver function and development. Part I: the hepatocyte nuclear factor network and liver-specific gene expression. *Pharmacol. Rev.*, **54(1)**, 129–158.

Shen Z, Heinegard D, and Sommarin Y (1995). Distribution and expression of cartilage oligomeric matrix protein and bone sialoprotein show marked changes during rat femoral head development. *Matrix Biol.*, **14(9)**, 773–781.

Smith DG, Wilburn C, and McCarthy RA (2003). Methoprene photolytic compounds disrupt zebrafish development, producing phenocopies of mutants in the sonic hedgehog signaling pathway. *Mar. Biotechnol. (NY)*, **5(2)**, 201–212.

Spielmann H, and Liebsch M (2001). Lessons learned from validation of *in vitro* toxicity test: from failure to acceptance into regulatory practice. *Toxicology In Vitro*, **15**, 585–590.

Spielmann H, and Liebsch M (2002). Validation success: chemicals. *Altern. Lab. Anim.*, **30 Suppl. 2**, 33–40.

Sui W, Boyd C, and Wright JT (2003). Altered pH regulation during enamel development in the cystic fibrosis mouse incisor. *J. Dent. Res.*, **82(5)**, 388–392.

Tabacova S, Hunter ES III, and Gladen BC (1996). Developmental toxicity of inorganic arsenic in whole embryo culture: oxidation state, dose, time, and gestational age dependence. *Toxicology and Applied Pharmacology*, **138**, 298–307.

Thal G, Sasse J, Holtzer H, and Pacifici M (1986). Differential survival of cartilage and muscle cells in chick limb-bud co-cultures maintained in chemically defined and serum-free media. *Differentiation*, **31**, 20–28.

Treinen KA, Louden C, Dennis, MJ, and Wier PJ (1999). Developmental toxicity and toxicokinetics of two endothelin receptor antagonists in rats and rabbits. *Teratology*, **59**, 51–59.

Tsumaki N, Nakase T, Miyaji T, Kakiuchi M, Kimura T, Ochi T, and Yoshikawa H (2002). Bone morphogenetic protein signals are required for cartilage formation and differently regulate joint development during skeletogenesis. *J. Bone Miner. Res.*, **17(5)**, 898–906.

Ujeki EM, Nakanashi S, and Fremming L (1986). Chromium effects on chondrocytic differentiation *in vitro*. *Journal of Toxicology and Environmental Health*, **19**, 137–145.

Warren SM, Brunet LJ, Harland RM, Economides AN, and Longaker MT (2003). The BMP antagonist noggin regulates cranial suture fusion. *Nature*, **422**, 625–629.

Webb SE, and Miller AL (2003). Calcium signalling during embryonic development. *Nat. Rev. Mol. Cell. Biol.*, **4(7)**, 539–551.

Wells PG, and Winn LM (1996). Biochemical toxicology of chemical teratogenesis. *Crit. Rev. Biochem. Mol. Biol.*, **31**, 1–40.

Werling U, Siehler S, Litfin M, Nau H, and Gottlicher M (2001). Induction of differentiation in F9 cells and activation of peroxisome proliferator-activated receptor delta by valproic acid and its teratogenic derivatives. *Mol. Pharmacol.*, **59(5)**, 1269–1276.

Whitsel AI, Johnson CB, and Forehand CJ (2002). An in ovo chicken model to study the systemic and localised teratogenic effects of valproic acid. *Teratology*, **66**, 153–163.

Winn LM, and Wells PG (2002). Evidence for Ras-dependent signal transduction in phenytoin teratogenicity. *Toxicology and Applied Pharmacology*, **184**, 144–152.

Zhu CC, Yamada G, and Blum M (1999). Retinoic acid teratogenicity: the role of goosecoid and BMP-4. *Cell Mol. Biol.*, **45**, 617–629.

Zimber A, and Zusman I (1990). Effects of secondary bile acids on the intrauterine development in rats. *Teratology*, **42**, 215–224.

Zucker RM, Elstein KH, Shuey DL, and Rogers JM (1995). Flow cytometric detection of abnormal fetal erythropoiesis: application to 5-fluorouracil-induced anemia. *Teratology*, **51(1)**, 37–44.

19
Toxicogenomics Applied to Nephrotoxicity

Anke Lühe and Heinz Hildebrand

19.1
Brief Survey of Nephrotoxicity

19.1.1
Relevance and Occurrence of Nephrotoxic Effects

The kidneys are frequent targets of drug- or chemical-induced organ toxicity. The anticancer drug cisplatin, for example, causes renal failure in up to 25% of patients after a single-dose treatment [1]. Aminoglycoside antibiotics are known to induce nephrotoxicity in 10–20% of all therapeutic courses [2], and the incidence of renal syndromes related to the NSAID ibuprofen is believed to reach 18% [3].

This high vulnerability of the kidney can be ascribed to several kidney-specific characteristics. A vast amount of xenobiotics as well as many chemical compounds are renally excreted from the organism. These compounds reach concentrations during their passage through the nephron (Figure 19.1) that are far beyond those other organs are exposed to. This is due to the high kidney blood flow (which amounts to 25% of the resting cardiac output) and a high rate of accumulation of compounds in the kidney.

Accumulation of toxicants in the kidney can occur through different mechanisms. One of the main kidney functions is water recovery, which results in concentration of solutes in the tubular lumen. This can lead to crystallisation of compounds with low solubility and finally to obstruction of the kidney.

Additionally, the kidney possesses several active and passive transport systems, which are not only able to recover or secrete ions, amino acids, and carbohydrates, but are also responsible for the uptake or secretion of most of the renally eliminated xenobiotics and chemicals. Mercuric ion, for example, binds to sulfhydryl groups of brush border membrane proteins and is finally internalised [4], and aminoglycosides are supposed to be taken up via specific binding to anionic phospholipids in the brush border membrane and subsequent pinocytosis [5]. Additionally, aminoglycosides are supposed to be reabsorbed actively via binding to the megalin receptor [6]. Finally, beta-lactam antibiotics are known to concentrate in proximal tubular cells due to uptake by the renal organic anion transport system [7].

Handbook of Toxicogenomics: Strategies and Applications. Edited by Jürgen Borlak

ISBN: 3-527-30342-1

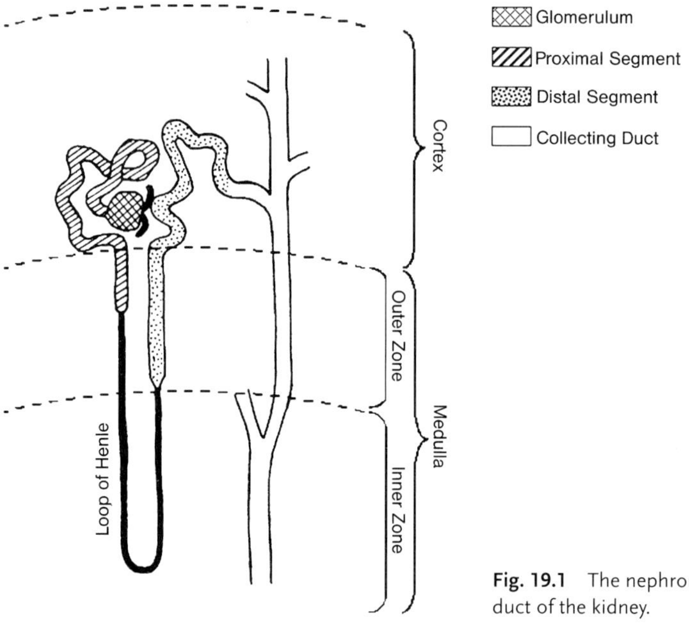

Fig. 19.1 The nephron and the collecting duct of the kidney.

Most of the reabsorption processes in the kidney, if not energy-dependent themselves, depend on ATP-consuming Na^+ uptake as a driving force. Thus, the kidney is especially vulnerable to ischemic insults that can lead to depletion of ATP and consequently inhibit the formation of a sodium gradient across the membranes [6].

Another characteristic that makes the kidney particularly vulnerable to toxins is the fact that the kidney expresses a variety of metabolic enzymes, such as kidney-specific cytochrome P450-dependent monooxygenases, glutathione-S-transferases, gamma-glutamyl transferase, and sulfotransferases. Many compounds, although harmless at first, are eventually bioactivated by these enzymes to toxic metabolites. For example, hexachlorobutadiene is conjugated with glutathione in the liver and further bioactivated by kidney-specific cysteine-conjugate beta-lyase to a toxic metabolite [8]. The carcinogen vinylidene chloride is bioactivated in the kidney by an androgen-dependent member of the cytochrome P450 family, which in mice, is exclusively expressed in the proximal tubule of males [9].

19.1.2
Different Modes of Nephrotoxicity

Nephrotoxicants can exert their effects on the kidney through one specific mechanism or through different mechanisms simultaneously. Several approaches have been made to group nephrotoxic events according to the place of action of the nephrotoxicant [10] or according to the generic toxic effect of the compound [5]. In the following we focus on the most predominant events related to nephrotoxicity.

19.1.2.1 Acute Renal Failure

Acute renal failure (ARF) is characterised by a rapid decrease in all renal functions and occurs as a consequence of several other events induced by nephrotoxic compounds. The underlying mechanisms include acute tubular necrosis, acute interstitial nephritis, intratubular obstruction, decreased renal perfusion, and thrombotic insults leading to haemolytic uremic syndrome.

Acute tubular necrosis is usually due to direct tubular injury resulting from site-specific accumulation and/or uptake of the toxin which can lead to alterations in mitochondrial functions and hence in energy metabolism (example toxins: mercuric ion, cisplatin), inhibition of phospholipid metabolism and changes in intracellular calcium levels (aminoglycosides), impairment of transport activities (CCl_4), and increase of membrane permeability (amphotericin B).

Acute interstitial nephritis is characterised by an inflammatory reaction of the interstitium and its infiltration with lymphocytes, monocytes, and plasma cells. It is typically induced by penicillins, cephalosporins, sulphonamides, nonsteroidal anti-inflammatory drugs (NSAIDs), allopurinol, and some Chinese herbs.

Decreased renal perfusion can result after application of hyperosmolar radiocontrast media [10] or can occur due to a combination of preexisting renal ischemia and prolonged use of NSAIDs. Ischemia leads to vasoconstriction mediated by induction of angiotensin II and vasopressin. This effect is enhanced by NSAIDs, which inhibit the synthesis of vasodilatating prostaglandins and thus support vasoconstriction [11].

19.1.2.2 Chronic Renal Failure

Chronic renal failure (CRF) is considered a tubulointerstitial disease, which can develop from several kidney diseases such as ARF, primary glomerulopathy, nephrosclerosis, and stenosis of the renal artery when they are accompanied by interstitial fibrosis [12]. Cyclosporin, for example, is known to induce tubulointerstitial lesions and as a consequence leads to CRF [13]. Long-term consumption of Ochratoxin A–contaminated food leads to marked interstitial fibrosis and tubular atrophy. This clinical presentation is associated with chronic nephropathy in pigs as well as with endemic Balkan nephropathy in humans [14]. Primary glomerulopathy can occur after treatment with D-penicillamine or captopril, which exert damage through binding to glomerular structures via their sulfhydrylgroups and thus lead to changes in the filtration capacity of the glomerulum [10]. Chronic abuse of NSAIDs can also lead to the development of CFR, due to primary glomerulopathy, interstitial nephritis, and/or papillary necrosis [13].

19.1.2.3 Toxic Insults Leading to Altered Fluid and Electrolyte Balance

One of the main functions of the kidney is the maintenance of water and electrolyte homeostasis of the organism. Some nephrotoxicants can disrupt the highly vulnerable processes of urine concentration and electrolyte or solute reabsorption and hence lead to increased excretion. Lithium, for example, is responsible for the development of nephrogenic diabetes insipidus in 20–70% of all treated patients, due to its direct interference with the actions of antidiuretic hormone in the distal tubule and collecting duct [15]. Changes in potassium handling are induced by cyclosporin, which is supposed to suppress plasma renin activity and to cause tubular insensitivity to aldosterone [16].

19.1.2.4 Renal Carcinogenesis

In several laboratory studies, as well as in various carcinogenicity assays, a sizeable number of compounds have been demonstrated to cause the development of renal cancers [17]. A variety of mechanisms have been reported to be involved in renal carcinogenesis, such as formation of DNA adducts by nitrosamines or Ochratoxin A [18], oxidative damage of DNA mediated by potassium bromate [19], and increased stimulation of cell proliferation by D-limonene or perchloroethylene due to lysosomal accumulation of alpha-2-microglobulin, specifically in male rats [20, 21].

19.1.3 Actual Situation in Diagnosis and Mechanistic Investigation

Early diagnosis of toxin-induced renal diseases is of outstanding importance, because many acute nephrotoxic effects can be almost completely reversed, or development of a chronic status can be prevented, by discontinuation of exposure to the toxicant. Gaining knowledge about the mechanistic mode of action of a toxicant helps to select new drugs with low nephrotoxic potential from a group of candidates. It may also serve to counteract the nephrotoxicity of substances by coapplication of compounds with attenuating effects, such as cotreatment with pentoxifylline, which has preventive effects on cyclosporine-induced renal failure [22], or mitigation of adriamycin nephrotoxicity by curcumin administration [23].

So far, toxic renal events have been investigated with various methods, including *in vivo* as well as a broad spectrum of *in vitro* technologies. Traditionally, the changes in excretion of urinary enzymes such as N-acetyl-beta-D-glucosaminidase, alkaline phosphatase, alanine aminopeptidase, and beta2-microglobulin have been assayed and are still in use as indicators of nephrotoxic insults [24]. Measurements of serum creatinine levels and blood urea nitrogen (BUN) have also been widely used. Development of techniques such as proton nuclear magnetic resonance (proton NMR) spectroscopic examination of urinary protein content offers the opportunity to analyze the whole protein content of urine samples in one experiment and facilitates the identification of biomarkers for nephrotoxicity [25]. Proteomic approaches also promise to be suitable for identification of biomarkers involved in the development of nephrotoxicity. Two-dimensional gel electrophoresis followed by mass spectrometric identification of altered proteins has already been used in several studies to define biomarkers involved in renal diseases [26, 27].

Changes in the release or activity of marker enzymes can also be evaluated in several *in vitro* models. Available *in vitro* models for testing of nephrotoxicity range from isolated perfused whole kidneys or nephron segments from rat or rabbit to renal tissue slices, freshly isolated tubular fragments or renal cells, and several permanent renal cell culture models. Although perfused kidneys or nephron segments offer the opportunity to study functional characteristics of certain nephron segments under maintenance of tubulovascular tissue integrity, they are not widely used because of their short life span of only a few hours.

In contrast, renal tissue slices are still frequently employed for study of transport and toxicity. The major disadvantage of tissue slices is that surfaces may be severely damaged during cutting.

Primary cell cultures of proximal tubule cells, collecting duct cells, or freshly isolated glomeruli are suitable models for assessing cell-type–specific toxic effects, but they fail to reveal nephrotoxic effects that are due to damage of cell types other than the one investigated, and their isolation and handling is usually difficult and time-consuming.

Permanent cell lines such as LLC-PK1 (pig proximal tubule cells), OK (opossum proximal tubule cells), NRK (rat proximal tubule cells), and MDCK (dog collecting duct cells) offer the advantage of easy cultivation and unlimited life span. However, they have lost several kidney-specific characteristics, such as some metabolic and transport activities [28–30], and therefore results obtained with permanent cell lines from studies addressing the nephrotoxic potential of compounds have to be evaluated carefully.

One major problem in the investigation of kidney toxicity, which occurs with almost all of the mentioned test methods, is the fact that very early toxic effects are usually not detectable. After being injured by a toxic compound, the kidney reacts almost immediately with counter-regulatory mechanisms to maintain normal kidney function for as long as possible. This so-called 'functional reserve' is capable of masking the first symptoms of an early nephrotoxic insult, which might not be noticeable until 70–80% of the renal epithelial mass has been injured [31]. Thus, early detection of renal damage is almost impossible until the functional reserve has been used up.

19.1.4 New Perspectives Offered by Toxicogenomics

Toxicogenomic approaches offer the opportunity to investigate genome-wide transcriptional changes after the occurrence of a toxic insult. Differential display methods and especially microarrays containing hundreds or thousands of cDNAs or oligonucleotides are widely used to investigate toxicologically altered gene expression. Quantitative PCR is usually employed to verify selected expression data derived from toxicogenomic experiments. Differential display techniques are suitable for discovering new genes and biochemical pathways involved in disease, whereas microarrays allow the assignment of biochemical functions to known genes and ESTs (expressed sequence tags) [32].

With regard to investigation of nephrotoxic events, toxicogenomics offers very early insight into toxin-induced lesions in the kidney, even before clinical or histopathological changes may be visible. Activation of the functional reserve of the kidney may be accompanied by transcriptional changes, which can be detected on the mRNA level, even if changes in urinary volume, protein content, or glomerular filtration rate are not yet observable.

Mechanistic analysis of gene expression patterns derived from toxin-treated samples provide considerable insight into the mode of action of different groups of nephrotoxicants and may be suitable for ranking compounds with similar toxic mechanisms so as to find the least toxic one.

Comparison of gene expression profiles from samples treated with several nephrotoxicants known to involve similar pathways of nephrotoxicity can help to select toxicity-related genes, which might serve as markers for predicting the nephrotoxic potential of unknown compounds. On the diagnostic level, toxicogenomic analysis of single nucleotide polymorphisms (SNPs) may help to identify individuals with high risk of developing nephrotoxic symptoms after treatment with certain compounds.

19.2 Toxicogenomic Approaches in Prediction of Toxicity and Mechanistic Studies (Case Studies)

19.2.1 Prediction of Toxicity: Toxicogenomics Aimed at the Identification of Markers of Renal Toxicity ('Fingerprinting')

Gene expression profiling in renal toxicity can be exploited as a predictive tool by adressing three different issues:

- prediction of an individual's susceptibility to develop renal disorders,
- identification of key genes involved in the progression of nephrotoxic lesions,
- prediction of the toxic potential of a compound.

The first topic involves the identification of marker genes, whose nonabundance/abundance or mutation can indicate an individual's predisposition to developing renal diseases or cancers. This approach has already been used successfully. For example, Guay-Woodford and colleagues [33] reviewed renal diseases with a known or supposed genetic cause and described disease-susceptible genes for more than 20 monogenic renal disorders. Diagnostic analysis of SNPs affecting these genes may facilitate a more reliable risk assessment in the area of renal diseases with genetic origin.

Knowledge of key transcripts involved in the progression of various renal disorders might be of great benefit in future diagnosis and treatment of these diseases. Several recent research projects, which focussed at the identification of such predictive markers, have been rather successful. For example, one research group investigated gene expression changes during renal ischemia–reperfusion in the rat to select subsets of genes that are indicative of different stages of acute renal failure [34]. Katsuma and colleagues [35] reported 173 differentially expressed genes that were involved in the progression of nephrolithiasis. Skubitz and Skubitz [36] identified several genes that were differentially expressed in clear-cell renal cell carcinoma, normal kidneys, and nonmalignant diseased kidneys and which thus could facilitate early cancer diagnosis. Another relevant work by Scherer and colleagues [37] describes the identification of 10 genes that proved suitable for predicting the occurence or nonoccurence of renal chronic allograft rejection after transplantation.

Furthermore, predictive toxicogenomics especially aims at the identification of marker genes that could be used to predict the nephrotoxic potential of compounds, but little work has been carried out in this area so far. Major advantages would be the possibility to monitor candidate drugs for their likelihood to induce toxic lesions in the kidney so that high-risk compounds could be withdrawn from the pipeline at an early stage of drug development. Treatments with drugs that are already in use and known to induce nephrotoxic lesions may be more easily adjusted with respect to dose and duration so as to permit a nontoxic treatment course.

The difficulty in identification of marker genes that are suitable for predicting the nephrotoxic potential of a compound becomes evident upon consideration of the following points:

- Nephrotoxicity is manifested in a vast number of different clinical outcomes, which all involve different toxic mechanisms. As a consequence, it is very likely that there are various sets of genes, which could serve as markers for the different modes of nephrotoxicity.
- To extract consistent marker genes, it is necessary to conduct a considerable amount of toxicogenomic studies with well known compounds that mediate their toxicity through different modes.
- Definition of the appropriate application dose of the compound, as well as the optimum timepoint for sample preparation, appear to be very critical in toxicogenomic studies, especially with completely unknown candidate drugs.
- The huge amount of data arising from this mass of toxicogenomic studies will have to be analyzed and stored in a database.

As far as the liver is concerned, the first steps have been made in the direction of exploiting array-derived transcriptional datasets for prediction of certain toxicological presentations, but lack of standardized study designs still limits their predictive capacity [38].

Burczynski et al. [39], for example, performed toxicogenomic studies of two different classes of hepatotoxicants, representing both cytotoxic anti-inflammatory drugs on the one hand and DNA-damaging agents on the other hand. They were able to select a subset of genes, which proved to have discriminating capacity for this learning set of compounds. Cluster analyses, applying this subset of genes to a database containing ~100 compounds of various hepatotoxic mechanisms, demonstrated the highly predictive value of this gene subset.

To our knowledge, comparable approaches aimed at the generation of a database of kidney-derived array data have not been reported so far.

Although a database for marker genes for use in predicting the nephrotoxic potential of compounds is not available yet, the advantages of predictive toxicology have already been exploited to a certain extend. For example, analysis of gene expression changes in the kidney cortex of paraquat-treated rats revealed 157 differentially ex-

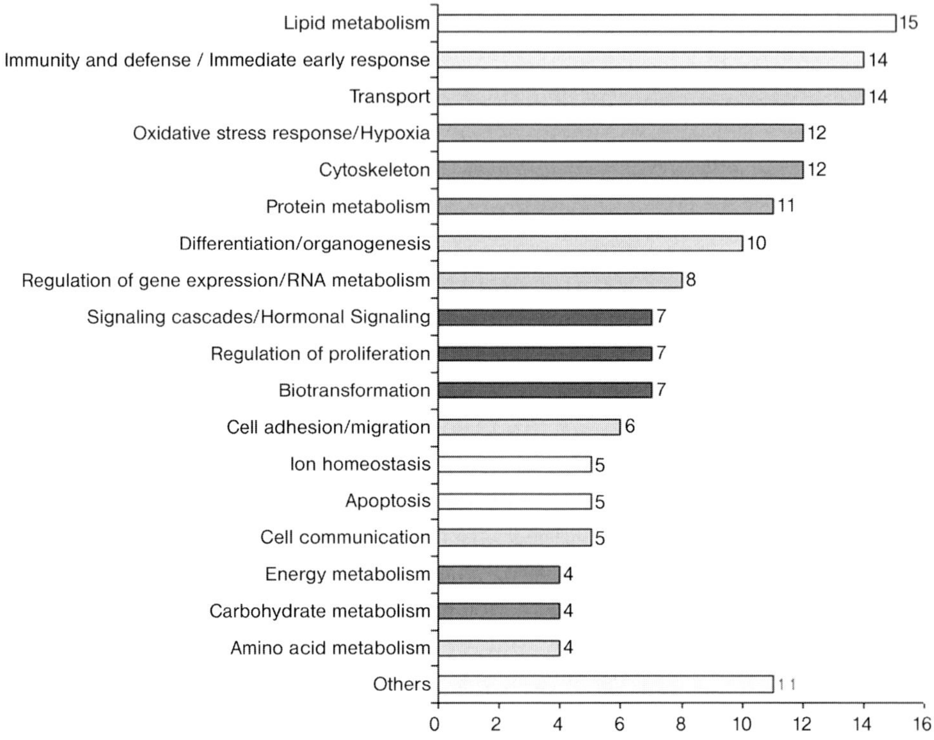

Fig. 19.2 Ranking of biochemical pathways affected in rat kidney cortex after paraquat treatment. The number of genes belonging to each pathway is shown next to the bars.

pressed genes after seven days of consecutive application [40]. The regulated genes were mainly associated with the development of oxidative stress, the enhancement of lipid degradation, and the occurence of early inflammatory responses (Figure 19.2), which represents an early state of the toxic insult known to be induced by paraquat [41]. Interestingly, after seven days of treatment, no histopathological lesions were yet detectable. This example may illustrate the capacity of toxicogenomic studies for predicting a toxic outcome at early stages of intoxication, even without evidence of visible changes in tissue morphology.

19.2.2
Mechanistic Studies: Toxicogenomics Aimed at Elucidating the Mode of Nephrotoxic Action

Mechanistic investigation of the mode of action of toxicants may also be a promising application of toxicogenomics. With regard to the kidney, only a few approaches have so far been aimed at better understanding of the mechanisms underlying the nephrotoxic effects of compounds. Below we discuss selected research projects indicating the suitability of toxicogenomics for detection of mechanistic networks involved in nephrotoxicity.

19.2.2.1 Mechanistic Characterization of Nephrotoxicants: Applicability of *in vitro* Models and Correlation with *in vivo* Data

To investigate the suitability of a rat proximal tubule cell culture model (PTC) for mechanistic characterization of Ochratoxin A (OTA) nephrotoxicity, gene expression data derived from kidney cortices of Wistar rats treated with a low dose (1 mg kg^{-1}) and a high dose (10 mg kg^{-1}) of OTA for 24 h and 72 h, respectively, and gene expression data derived from PTC also treated with a low (5 μM) and a high (12.5 μM) concentration of OTA for 24 h and 72 h, respectively, were compared [42].

In vivo experiments were carried out by daily gavage with vehicle control (corn oil) or OTA (1 mg kg^{-1} or 10 mg kg^{-1}) of three animals per dose group, which were analyzed separately after exsanguination and extraction of total RNA from kidney cortex on cDNA microarrays containing 700 toxicologically relevant gene sequences. *In vitro* experiments were carried out in duplicate for each dose group, and samples were hybridized on cDNA microarrays following the same protocol as with *in vivo* samples.

Analysis of differentially regulated genes from *in vitro* and *in vivo* experiments revealed 254 genes that showed significant up- or down-regulation (more than two-fold) in comparison to controls. With regard to assessment of the mode of action underlying OTA nephrotoxicity, genes with different expression profiles *in vivo* and *in vitro* were excluded from mechanistic analyses. Instead, these so-called discriminator genes were clustered by a hierarchical clustering method, and it was possible to identify three groups of genes (Figure 19.3), which behaved differently *in vivo* and *in vitro* after treatment with OTA, indicating that their regulation might be due to model-specific handling of OTA intoxication.

Genes that were grouped together in the first cluster included those encoding 60S ribosomal protein L6 and activin receptor II, whose expression was up-regulated *in vivo* but barely changed *in vitro*. Genes in cluster two showed significant down-regulation *in vitro*, but their expression was barely changed *in vivo* (e.g., alpha prothymosin and ID-1). 60S ribosomal protein L6 and activin receptor II are known to be positive regulators of tissue repair after injury [43], whereas alpha prothymosin and ID-1 are reported to negatively influence regeneration processes [44, 45]. Hence, these results suggest that tissue regeneration is mediated, at least in part, differently *in vivo* and *in vitro*.

The third cluster comprised genes whose expression was down-regulated *in vivo* but barely changed *in vitro*. Most of the genes in this group produce proteins that function in metabolism and/or biotransformation, such as cytochrome P450 2D18, D-dopachrome tautomerase, and gamma-glutamyl-transpeptidase, or proteins that play a role in the transport system of the kidney, such as organic anion transporter K1, organic cation transporter 2, and renal organic anion transporter. These results are in agreement with knowledge about the limited capacity of primary cells in culture to maintain metabolic and transport activities [46].

Returning to the mechanistic analysis of OTA toxicity in PTC and kidney cortex *in vivo*, the remaining 215 'common genes' were analysed with respect to dose- and

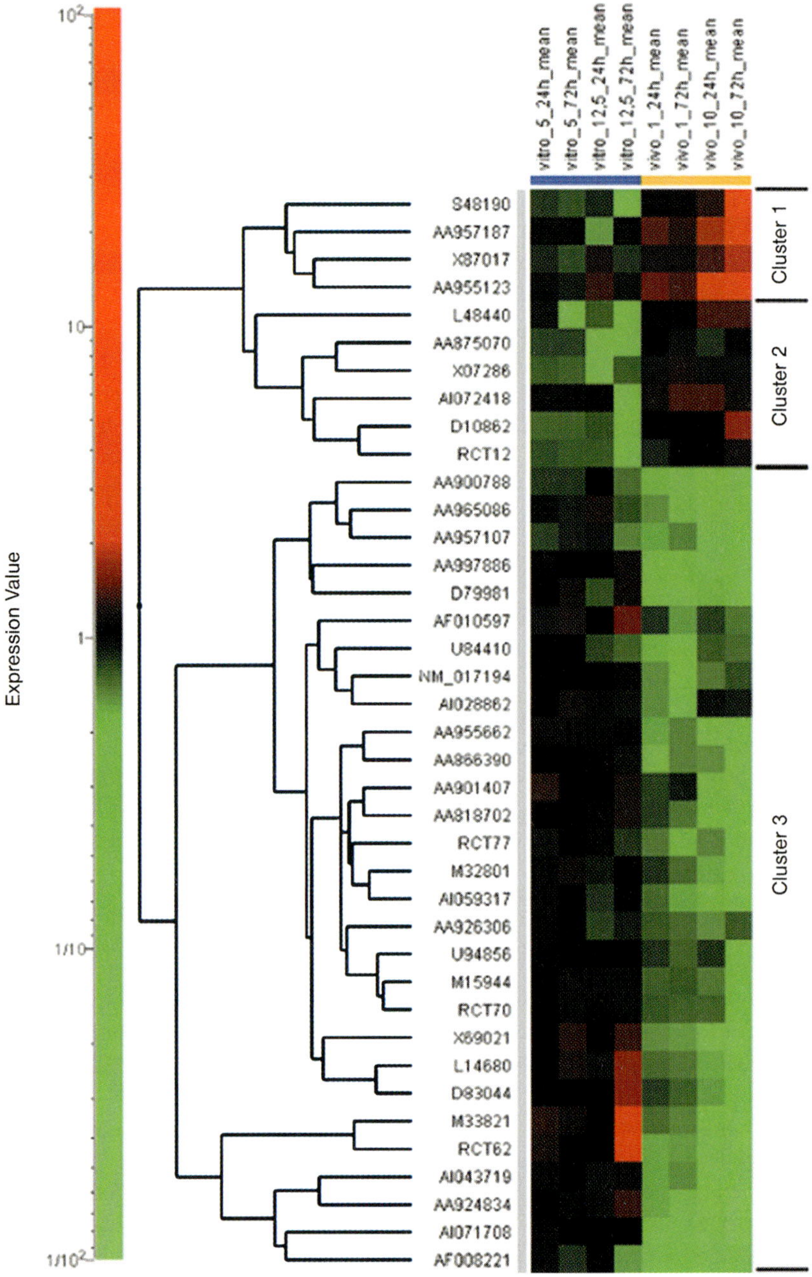

Fig. 19.3 Hierarchical clustering of 39 genes that are differentially regulated *in vivo* and *in vitro* after treatment with Ochratoxin A. There are three groups of genes exhibiting different expression profiles. The scale on the left represents the colour code according to the relative changes of gene expressions in each experiment (from [42]).

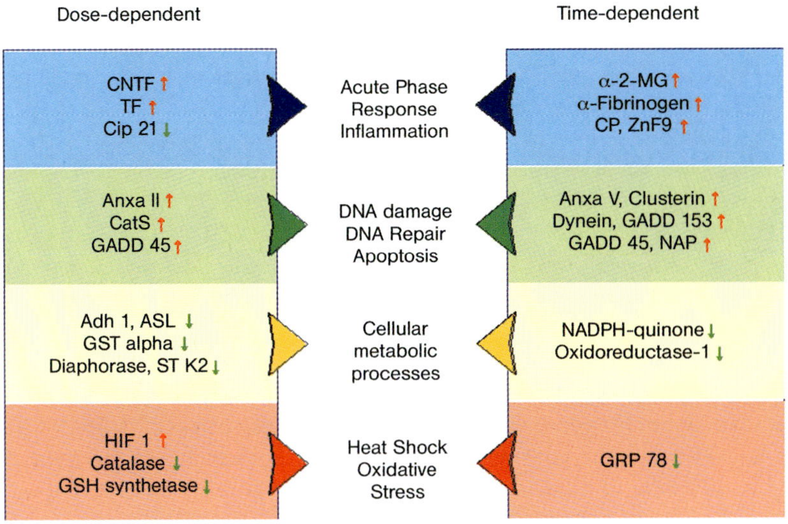

Fig. 19.4 Grouping of genes that are differentially regulated in rat kidney cortex and rat proximal tubule cell culture in a dose- or time-dependent manner after treatment with Ochratoxin A. Red arrows indicate upregulation, green arrows indicate downregulation.

time-dependent changes in gene expression after exposure to OTA. According to the biological function of the encoded proteins, these genes were clustered into four different groups (Figure 19.4):

- acute-phase response and inflammation,
- DNA damage, DNA repair, and apoptosis,
- cellular metabolic processes,
- heat-shock and oxidative-stress response.

Interestingly, changes in cellular metabolism and oxidative stress appeared to be more dose-dependent, but inflammation and acute-phase responses, as well as responses to DNA damage, predominantly occurred in a time-dependent manner.

In these studies most of the literature-described effects of OTA, such as DNA damage possibly mediated by oxidative stress, were confirmed on the transcriptional level. Furthermore, there is much evidence for acute-phase responses, for severe tissue lesions, and for massive deterioration of cellular metabolism. Transcriptional changes and gene expression networks such as up-regulation of the genes for calpactin I heavy chain, annexin V, Gadd153, clusterin, and hypoxia-inducible factor I have been detected, which were not described before as being involved in mediation of OTA-induced nephrotoxicity. Summarizing the above, toxicogenomics proved to be a suitable method for investigation of Ochratoxin A–induced nephrotoxicity.

19.2.2.2 Mechanistic Characterization of Nephrotoxicants Acting on the Tubular System: Cisplatin and Mercuric Chloride

So far, little work has been published on assessment of the mode of action of nephrotoxicants that act on the tubular system [42, 48].

The toxic mechanisms by which atypically elevated levels of physiological compounds like angiotensin II can affect gene transcription in the renal medulla were recently investigated by Yuan et al. [47]. Intravenous application of angiotensin II to Sprague–Dawley rats followed by microarray analysis of induced alterations in gene expression revealed several differentially regulated genes with known functions in the development of oxidative stress and interstitial fibrosis in the outer medulla.

Huang et al. [48] assessed the transcriptional changes that occurred after treatment of rats with two doses of cisplatin (0.5 mg kg^{-1} d^{-1} and 1 mg kg^{-1} d^{-1}) in comparison to saline-glucose–treated controls, using cDNA microarrays containing 250 toxicologically relevant rat genes. Use of the anticancer drug cisplatin is limited by its severe side effects on the proximal tubules of the kidney, which take the form of significant impairment of tubular reabsorption; decrease in mitochondrial respiratory function, enzymatic activity in the respiratory chain, and glutathione peroxidase; and possible interference with the control of cellular calcium homeostasis [49].

After statistical analysis of the cisplatin-treated samples, Huang et al. [48] identified 22 genes that exhibited significant alterations (>2-fold) in their expression after 7-days of treatment with cisplatin. They assigned these 22 genes to eight categories of different biochemical functions, which were in agreement with the literature-described toxic mode of action of cisplatin. Significantly regulated genes were found to be associated with apoptosis and/or necrosis (clusterin, Waf-1, CD44), tubular transport (down-regulation of genes for the organic anion transporters K1, P1, and 3), oxidative stress (catalase gene), inflammatory responses (genes for ceruloplasmin and IP-10), maintenance of Ca^{2+} homeostasis (senescence marker protein-30), and tissue regeneration (insulin-like growth factor binding protein-1, tissue inhibitor of metalloproteinases-1), but the most predominant changes were observed for multi-drug-resistance gene-1 (MDR1) and the gene for P-glycoprotein (P-gp), which indicate the beginning of cisplatin resistance.

Another study was carried out on the mechanism of mercuric chloride nephrotoxicity [40]. Mercuric chloride is well known as a serious environmental pollutant, which mainly causes toxicity in the proximal tubules of the kidney. Suggested mechanisms of tubular injury include reaction with sulfhydryl groups of tubular membrane proteins, alteration of membrane permeability, generation of reactive oxygen species, impairment of mitochondrial function, interference with Ca^{2+} homeostasis, and induction of autoimmune responses [50–52].

After treatment of male Wistar rats with two doses of mercuric chloride (1.8 mg kg^{-1} d^{-1} and 18 mg kg^{-1} d^{-1}) for one or three days, respectively, the gene expression changes in kidney cortex were analyzed on Affymetrix RG U34A microarrays containing approximately 8800 probe sets of about 5000 rat genes. According to *t*-test comparison of mercuric chloride-treated samples with vehicle-treated control samples ($P = 0.001$, >2-fold change), 385 significantly regulated probe sets corresponding to 311 different genes were identified. These differentially expressed genes were assigned to 18 biochemical pathways.

The most pronounced transcriptional changes induced by mercuric chloride seemed to be associated with protein metabolism; responses of the immune system; interference with cell signalling, biotransformation, and transport processes; and induction of changes affecting the cytoskeleton and cell adhesion, which corresponded well with literature-based knowledge.

Toxicogenomic approaches addressing the transcriptional mechanisms underlying compound-induced nephrotoxicity have not been at the centre of researchers' interest so far, despite the fact that much work has already been performed on the field of hepatotoxicity. Nevertheless, as evidenced by the studies described above, toxicogenomics will be of outstanding importance in future research elucidating the mechanisms through which renal toxicity is mediated.

19.3 Perspectives

Future directions in toxicology research will more and more require miniaturizable, automatable, high-throughput technologies, which allow researchers to cope with the increasing need for early, reliable toxicological information about unknown compounds and drug candidates. Toxicogenomics has proven to be a suitable tool for various toxicological applications, and research has already been successful in minimizing current limitations, such as high costs and the requirement for large amounts of RNA.

Building up a database for nephrotoxic compounds, as well as further characterization of existing *in vitro* models for application in toxicogenomic studies, will provide time- and cost-saving tools for investigation of the toxic properties of candidate compounds at an early stage of development.

Toxicogenomics-derived knowledge about the transcriptional changes occurring in response to nephrotoxicant exposure can be combined with histopathological findings and results gained from toxicoproteomic and toxicometabolomic analyses of urine samples. Such comprehensive approaches may provide almost exhaustive information about the circumstances involved in renal toxicity and will address both the transcriptional and translational levels.

References

1. Madias N.E., Harrington J.T.: Platinum nephrotoxicity. *Am J Med.* 1978 **65**: 307–314
2. Swan S.K.: Aminoglycoside nephrotoxicity. *Semin Nephrol* 1997 **17**: 27–33
3. Murray M.D., Brater D.C., Tierney W.M., Hui S.L., McDonald C.J.: Ibuprofen-associated renal impairment in a large general internal medicine practice. *Am J Med Sci* 1990 **299**: 222–229
4. Diamond G.L., Zalups R.K.: Understanding renal toxicity of heavy metals. *Toxicol Pathol* 1998, **26**: 92–103
5. Werner M., Costa M.J., Mitchell L.G., Nayar R.: Nephrotoxicity of xenobiotics. *Clin Chim Acta* 1995, **237**: 107–154
6. Fanos V., Cataldi L.: Renal transport of antibiotics and nephrotoxicity: a review. *J Chemother* 2001, **13**: 461–472
7. Kaloyanides G.J.: Antibiotic-related nephrotoxicity. *Nephrol Dial Transplant* 1994, **9 Suppl 4**: 130–134
8. Dekant W., Vamvakas S.: Biotransformation and membrane transport in nephrotoxicity. *Crit Rev Toxicol* 1996, **26**: 309–334
9. Dekant W.: Biotransformation and renal processing of nephrotoxic agents. *Arch Toxicol Suppl* 1996, **18**: 163–172
10. Koren G.: The nephrotoxic potential of drugs and chemicals: pharmacological basis and clinical relevance. *Med Toxicol Adverse Drug Exp* 1989, **4**: 59–72
11. Bennett W.M., Porter G.A.: Nephrotoxicity of common drugs used by urologists. *Urol Clin North Am* 199, **17**: 145–156
12. Bohle A., Kressel G., Muller C.A., Muller G.A.: The pathogenesis of chronic renal failure. *Pathol Res Pract* 1989, **185**: 421–440
13. Paller M.S.: Drug-induced nephropathies. *Med Clin North Am* 1990, **74**: 909–917
14. Stefanovic V., Polenakovic M.H.: Balkan nephropathy: kidney disease beyond the Balkans? *Am J Nephrol* 1991, **11**: 1–11
15. Gabutti L., Gugger M., Marti H.P.: Impaired kidney function in lithium therapy. *Ther Umsch* 1998, **55**: 562–564
16. Bantle J.P., Nath K.A., Sutherland D.E., Najarian J.S., Ferris T.F.: Effects of cyclosporine on the renin–angiotensin–aldosterone system and potassium excretion in renal transplant recipients. *Arch Intern Med* 1985, **145**: 505–508.
17. Huff J.: Chemicals associated with tumours of the kidney, urinary bladder and thyroid gland in laboratory rodents from 2000 U.S. National Toxicology Program/National Cancer Institute bioassays for carcinogenicity. *IARC Sci Publ* 1999, **147**: 211–225
18. Obrecht-Pflumio S., Dirheimer G.: In vitro DNA and dGMP adducts formation caused by Ochratoxin A. *Chem Biol Interact* 2000, **127**: 29–44
19. Umemura T., Takagi A., Sai K., Hasegawa R., Kurokawa Y.: Oxidative DNA damage and cell proliferation in kidneys of male and female rats during 13-weeks exposure to potassium bromate ($KBrO_3$). *Arch Toxicol* 1998, **72**: 264–269
20. Dietrich D.R., Swenberg J.A.: The presence of alpha 2u-globulin is necessary for D-limonene promotion of male rat kidney tumors. *Cancer Res* 1991, **51**: 3512–3521
21. Goldsworthy T.L., Lyght O., Burnett V.L., Popp J.A.: Potential role of alpha-2 mu-globulin, protein droplet accumulation, and cell replication in the renal carcinogenicity of rats exposed to trichloroethylene, perchloroethylene, and pentachloroethane. *Toxicol Appl Pharmacol* 1988, **96**: 367–379
22. Kaputlu I., Sadan G., Karayalcin B., Boz A.: Beneficial effects of pentoxifylline on cyclosporine-induced nephrotoxicity. *Clin Exp Pharmacol Physiol* 1997, **24**: 365–369
23. Venkatesan N., Punithavathi D., Arumugam V.: Curcumin prevents adriamycin nephrotoxicity in rats. *Br J Pharmacol* 2000, **129**: 231–234
24. Kunin C.M., Chesney R.W., Craig W.A., England A.C., DeAngelis C.: Enzymuria as a marker of renal injury and disease: studies of N-acetyl-beta-glucosaminidase in the general population and in patients with renal disease. *Pediatrics* 1978, **62**: 751–760
25. Holmes E., Bonner F.W., Sweatman B.C., Lindon J.C., Beddell C.R., Rahr E., Nicholson J.K.: Nuclear magnetic resonance spectroscopy and pattern recognition analysis of the biochemical processes

associated with the progression of and recovery from nephrotoxic lesions in the rat induced by mercury(II) chloride and 2-bromoethanamine. *Mol Pharmacol* 1992, **42**: 922–930

26. Rasmussen H.H., Orntoft T.F., Wolf H., Celis J.E.: Towards a comprehensive database of proteins from the urine of patients with bladder cancer. *J Urol* 1996, **155**: 2113–2119
27. Pang J.X., Ginanni N., Dongre A.R., Hefta S.A., Opitek G.J.: Biomarker discovery in urine by proteomics. *J Proteome Res* 2002, **1**: 161–169
28. Courjault-Gautier F., Chevalier J., Abbou C.C., Chopin D.K., Toutain H.J.: Consecutive use of hormonally defined serum-free media to establish highly differentiated human renal proximal tubule cells in primary culture. *J Am Soc Nephrol* 1995, **5**: 1949–1963
29. Gstraunthaler G.J.: Epithelial cells in tissue culture. *Ren Physiol Biochem* 1988, **11**: 1–42
30. Aleo M.D., Taub M.L., Nickerson P.A., Kostyniak P.J.: Primary cultures of rabbit renal proximal tubule cells: I. Growth and biochemical characteristics. *In Vitro Cell Dev Biol* 1989, **25**: 776–783
31. Pfaller W., Gstraunthaler G.: Nephrotoxicity testing *in vitro*: what we know and what we need to know. *Environ Health Perspect* 1998, **106 Suppl 2**: 559–69
32. Alcorta D.A., Prakash K., Waga I., Sasai H., Munger W., Jennette J.C., Falk R.J.: Future molecular approaches to the diagnosis and treatment of glomerular disease. *Semin Nephrol* 2000, **20**: 20–31
33. Guay-Woodford L.M.: Overview: the genetics of renal disease. *Semin Nephrol* 1999, **19**: 312–318
34. Yoshida T., Kurella M., Beato F., Min H., Ingelfinger J.R., Stears R.L., Swinford R.D., Gullans S.R., Tang S.S.: Monitoring changes in gene expression in renal ischemia–reperfusion in the rat. *Kidney Int* 2002, **61**: 1646–1654
35. Katsuma S., Shiojima S., Hirasawa A., Takagaki K., Kaminishi Y., Koba M., Hagidai Y., Murai M., Ohgi T., Yano J., Tsujimoto G.: Global analysis of differentially expressed genes during progression of calcium oxalate nephrolithiasis. *Biochem Biophys Res Commun* 2002, **296**: 544–552
36. Skubitz K.M., Skubitz A.P.: Differential gene expression in renal-cell cancer. *J Lab Clin Med* 2002, **140**: 52–64
37. Scherer A., Krause A., Walker J.R., Korn A., Niese D., Raulf F.: Early prognosis of the development of renal chronic allograft rejection by gene expression profiling of human protocol biopsies. *Transplantation* 2003, **75**: 1323–1330
38. Storck T., von Brevern M.C., Behrens C.K., Scheel J., Bach A.: Transcriptomics in predictive toxicology. *Curr Opin Drug Discov Dev* 2002, **5**: 90–97
39. Burczynski M.E., McMillian M., Ciervo J., Li L., Parker J.B., Dunn R.T. II, Hicken S., Farr S., Johnson M.D.: Toxicogenomics-based discrimination of toxic mechanism in HepG2 human hepatoma cells. *Toxicol Sci* 2000, **58**: 399–415
40. Lühe A.: Toxicogenomics applied to the kidney: gene expression analysis *in vitro* and *in vivo* after treatment with nephrotoxicants. 2003, PhD thesis, Johann-Wolfgang-Goethe-University, Frankfurt/Main, Germany.
41. Adachi J., Tomita M., Yamakawa S., Asano M., Naito T., Ueno Y.: 7-Hydroperoxycholesterol as a marker of oxidative stress in rat kidney induced by paraquat. *Free Radic Res* 2000, **33**: 321–327
42. Lühe A., Hildebrand H., Bach U., Dingermann T., Ahr H.J.: A new approach to studying Ochratoxin A (OTA)-induced nephrotoxicity: expression profiling *in vivo* and *in vitro* employing cDNA microarrays. *Toxicol Sci* 2003, **73**: 315–328
43. Maeshima, A., Zhang, Y., Nojima, Y., Naruse, T., Kojima, I.: Involvement of the activin–follistatin system in tubular regeneration after renal ischemia in rats. *J. Am. Soc. Nephrol* 2001, **12**: 1685–1695
44. Rodriguez, P., Vinuela, J.E., Alvarez-Fernandez, L., Buceta, M., Vidal, A., Dominguez, F., Gomez-Marquez, J.: Overexpression of prothymosin alpha accelerates proliferation and retards differentiation in HL-60 cells. *Biochem J* 1998, **331**: 753–761
45. Matejka, G.L., Thornemo, M., Kernholt, A., Lindahl, A.: Expression of Id-1 mRNA and protein in the post-ischemic regenerating rat kidney. *Exp Nephrol* 1998, **6**: 253–264

46. Dickmann K.G., and Mandel L.J.: Glycolytic and oxidative metabolism in primary renal proximal tubule cultures. *Am J Physiol* 1989, **257**, C333–340
47. Yuan B., Liang M., Yang Z., Rute E., Taylor N., Olivier M., Cowley A.W. Jr.: Gene expression reveals vulnerability to oxidative stress and interstitial fibrosis of renal outer medulla to nonhypertensive elevations of ANG II. *Am J Physiol Regul Integr Comp Physiol* 2003, **284**: R1219–1230
48. Huang Q., Dunn R.T. 2nd, Jayadev S., DiSorbo O., Pack F.D., Farr S.B., Stoll R.E., Blanchard K.T.: Assessment of cisplatin-induced nephrotoxicity by microarray technology. *Toxicol Sci* 2001. **63**: 196–207
49. Anand A.J., Bashey B.: Newer insights into cisplatin nephrotoxicity. *Ann Pharmacother* 1993, **27**: 1519–1525
50. Werner M., Costa M.J., Mitchell L.G., Nayar R.: Nephrotoxicity of xenobiotics. *Clin Chim Acta* 1995, **237**: 107–154
51. Nath K.A., Croatt A.J., Likely S., Behrens T.W., Warden D.: Renal oxidant injury and oxidant response induced by mercury. *Kidney Int* 1996, **50**: 1032–1043
52. Moszczynski P.: Mercury compounds and the immune system: a review. *Int J Occup Med Environ Health* 1997, **10**: 247–258

20
Toxicogenomic Analysis of Human Umbilical Cords to Establish a New Risk Assessment of Human Foetal Exposure to Multiple Chemicals

Masatoshi Komiyama and Chisato Mori

20.1
Introduction

Low-level but constant exposure to multiple chemicals occurs throughout our lives from air, water, soil, food, and household products [1]. Chemical exposure has been suggested as a cause of human health disorders [2–7]. Human foetuses and infants are significantly more sensitive to a variety of environmental toxicants than adults [1, 7, 8]. In fact, they are especially vulnerable to the toxic effects of environmental tobacco smoke, pesticides, polychlorinated biphenyls (PCBs), and metals [9–15]. Also in animal experiments, it has been shown that adverse effects of chemicals such as endocrine disrupters appear in the reproductive and nervous systems, particularly when exposure occurs during foetal or neonatal periods [3, 16–18].

Our previous studies using umbilical cords have shown that human foetuses are exposed to multiple chemicals in Japan [19, 20]. There is anxiety that these multiple chemical exposures may cause delayed long-term effects after the foetuses are born and grow up. However, the current risk-assessment strategy, established in 1983 by the U.S. National Research Council, is based on the risk of only single chemicals and does not consider the risk of complex mixtures of chemicals [21]. Further, it focuses on adverse health effects on adults, not on children or foetuses. Therefore, in addition to the current risk assessment, it is urgently necessary to establish a new method of evaluating health risks of exposure to multiple chemicals during the foetal period.

Toxicogenomics is a new scientific subdiscipline derived from a combination of the fields of toxicology and genomics. It is the study of genes and their products that are important in adaptive response to toxic exposure, for identifying potential human and environmental toxicants and for determining their putative mechanisms of action through the use of genomics resources [22, 23]. One such resource is DNA microarrays, which allow high-throughput analysis of gene expression. Alteration of gene expression precedes histopathological changes in organs upon exposure to toxicants. Changes in expression occur in some genes even if histopathological changes are not obvious and continue in the long term [24–27]. Thus, gene expression changes should be sensitive predictive biomarkers of adverse effects of chemical ex-

Handbook of Toxicogenomics: Strategies and Applications. Edited by Jürgen Borlak

ISBN: 3-527-30342-1

posures. If gene expression profiles are linked to adverse effects of chemicals, they will be useful for predictive evaluation of health risks derived from exposure to multiple chemicals.

This chapter reviews our recent studies on the application of toxicogenomics to develop a new method of evaluating health risks derived from foetal exposure to multiple chemicals, together with some additional results from further analyses. It covers the following topics: strategy for establishment of a new risk assessment, concentration of chemicals in human umbilical cords, gene expression in the umbilical cords, and toxicogenomic analysis of the umbilical cords.

20.2 Strategy for Establishment of a New Risk-assessment Method for Human Foetal Exposure to Multiple Chemicals

We have recently started using toxicogenomic analyses based on DNA microarrays to develop a new risk-assessment method to evaluate the effects of foetal exposure to multiple chemicals using human umbilical cords (Figure 20.1) [28]. Umbilical cord is a tissue that is purely derived from the foetus, unlike the placenta, which is a mixture of foetal and maternal tissues. This characteristic of the umbilical cord allows the response to chemicals of only the foetus to be monitored by analyzing its gene expression profile. In addition, it is technically and socially easy to collect umbilical cords. Therefore, the use of umbilical cords seems to be ideal for risk assessment of chemical effects on foetuses.

In the framework, toxicogenomic analysis of umbilical cords consists of four steps (Figure 20.1):

1. Step 1 is global gene expression analysis of umbilical cords using DNA microarrays.

2. Step 2 is a combined analysis of the data from Step 1 and exposure assessment data in each umbilical cord. This analysis will clarify the relationship between a global gene expression profile and chemical exposure levels.

3. Step 3 analysis consists of *in vitro* experiments using human umbilical cord-derived cells (HUCCs). Here, the change in gene expression in HUCCs is analyzed by DNA microarrays after experimental exposures to chemicals, and we can determine how HUCCs genes respond to various chemicals at various concentrations. For this purpose, cultured human umbilical vein endothelial cells (HUVEC) are one of the candidates, as we found that HUVEC genes change their expression after chemical exposure (unpublished data). Although HUVEC can be used in this step, other cells from umbilical cords also may be applicable.

4. Step 4 is an integrated comparative analysis of data from Step 2 and Step 3. In this integrated analysis, biological reactions at the molecular level caused by exposure to multiple chemicals in foetuses can be detected by comparing data from Step 2 with those of Step 3 that are the results of exposure to known chemicals at known concentrations.

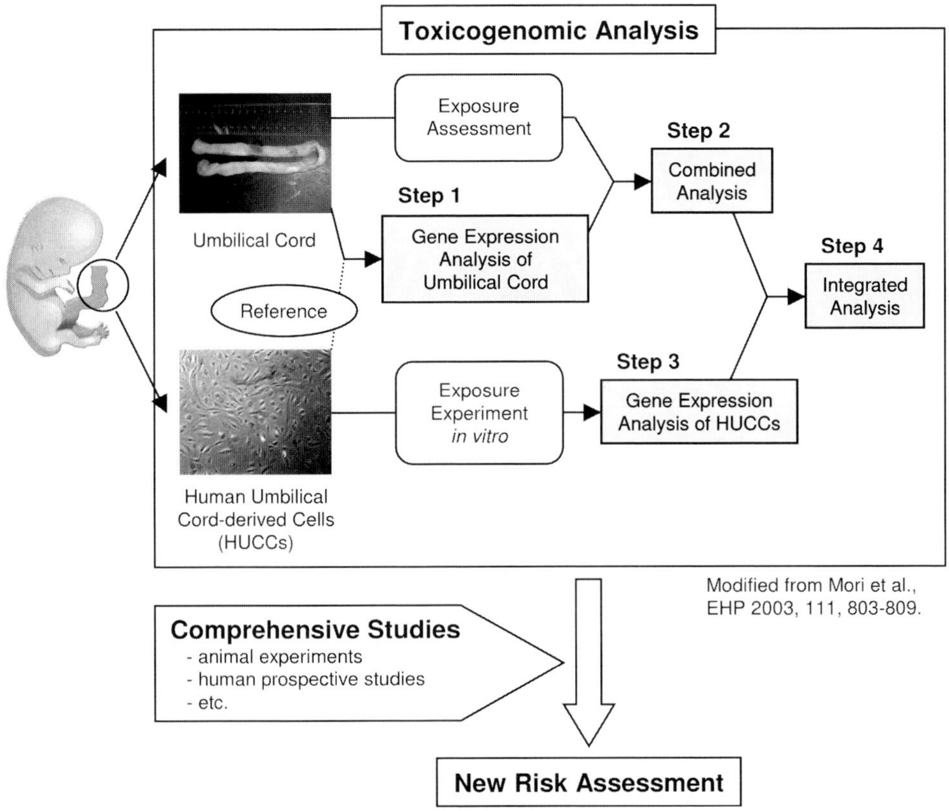

Fig. 20.1 Framework for establishing a new risk-assessment method for assessing human foetal exposure to multiple chemicals by toxicogenomic analysis of umbilical cords (modified from Mori et al. [28]).

To extend the toxicogenomic analysis method to develop a new risk-assessment strategy, comprehensive studies are required to clarify the correlation between data from toxicogenomic analysis of umbilical cords, data from animal experiments in which the adverse effects of chemical exposures are observed, and data from prospective studies of humans (Figure 20.1). These studies are indispensable for linking the gene expression profiles of umbilical cords to the possibly delayed long-term adverse effects of chemicals on individuals. Although there are certain technical and socioethical issues to be solved [28], if the approach shown in Figure 20.1 becomes practical, then toxicogenomic analysis can be used for the early diagnosis and possible prevention of adverse effects caused by multiple chemicals in humans.

20.3
Concentrations of Chemicals in Umbilical Cords of Neonates in Japan

Our study, including measurements of chemical concentrations and analyses of gene expression in umbilical cords, was carried out with the approval of the Congress of Medical Bioethics of Chiba University. We also obtained all the mothers' permission to analyze their blood and their babies' umbilical cords. Nine umbilical cords of Japanese neonates and their maternal blood were used for measurements of concentrations of the following chemicals: PCBs (from mono-PCBs to deca-PCB and total PCBs), hexachlorobenzene (HCB), hexachlorocyclohexane (HCH), *cis*-chlordane, *trans*-chlordane, oxychlordane, *trans*-nonachlor, *p,p*′-dichlorodiphenyltrichloroethane (DDT), *o,p*′-DDT, *p,p*′-dichlorodiphenyldichloroethylene (DDE), *o,p*′-DDE, *p,p*′-dichlorodiphenyldichloroethane (DDD), *o,p*′-DDD, aldrin, endrin, dieldrin, endosulfan, heptachlor, heptachlor epoxide, methoxychlor, and octachlor styrene. The measurement was carried out at SRL Inc. (Tokyo, Japan) using gas chromatography/mass spectrometry, as a part of an assessment by the Ministry of the Environment (Government of Japan). Details of the measurement methods and results are available as a PDF file [29].

Among the chemicals examined, mono-PCBs, nona-PCBs, deca-PCB, *o,p*′-DDE, *o,p*′-DDD, aldrin, endrin, methoxychlor, and octachlor styrene were not detected in any of the samples. PCBs and *p,p*′-DDE were detected in all nine umbilical cords at high concentrations (Table 20.1). Among various components of total PCBs, hexa-PCBs were the main component in most of the umbilical cords, followed by hepta-PCBs. HCB and HCH were also found at high levels in all umbilical cords. The total concentration of the chemicals was highest in sample E and second-highest in sample H. Sample D had the lowest total concentration of the chemicals, and sample B had the second-lowest level.

The chemicals detected in the umbilical cords were also detected in the corresponding maternal blood. Significant correlations were observed between umbilical cords and maternal blood for the concentrations of total-PCBs ($r = 0.893$, $p < 0.005$), HCB ($r = 0.959$, $p < 0.005$), HCH ($r = 0.934$, $p < 0.005$), oxychlordane ($r = 0.821$, $p < 0.01$), *trans*-nonachlor ($r = 0.763$, $p < 0.05$), *p,p*′-DDT ($r = 0.909$, $p < 0.005$), *p,p*′-DDE ($r = 0.967$, $p < 0.005$), dieldrin ($r = 0.857$, $p < 0.005$), and heptachlor epoxide ($r = 0.843$, $p < 0.005$) [30]. These results indicate that these chemicals are transferred from the mothers to their babies. It also suggests that these chemicals are persistent and in equilibrium between the mothers and their babies.

It has been reported that individuals who accumulate PCBs at higher levels also accumulate other persistent chemicals at higher levels [28]. Such a correlation was also observed in this study. Table 20.2 shows the results of correlation analysis between concentrations of total PCBs and other chemicals. In the nine umbilical cords, significant correlations were observed between total PCBs and the following chemicals: HCB ($p < 0.005$), HCH ($p < 0.05$), oxychlordane ($p < 0.05$), *trans*-nonachlor ($p < 0.01$), *p,p*′-DDT ($p < 0.005$), *p,p*′-DDE ($p < 0.005$), and dieldrin ($p < 0.05$) (Table 20.2 and Figure 20.2). Although the differences were not significant, individuals who accumulated higher levels of PCBs tended to also have higher concentra-

Tab. 20.1 Concentration of chemicals detected in human umbilical cords (ng g^{-1} fat weight).

Compound	*A*	*B*	*C*	*D*	*E*	*F*	*G*	*H*	*I*
Total PCBs	73.0	28.0	33.0	19.0	160.0	43.0	53.0	130.0	78.0
– Di-PCBs	1.0	ND	1.1	3.4	1.9	1.8	5.4	2.3	2.5
– Tri-PCBs	4.2	1.1	0.94	2.9	3.8	1.8	3.5	5.5	4.7
– Tetra-PCBs	9.5	ND	ND	0.93	19.0	2.8	5.3	16.0	13.0
– Penta-PCBs	14.0	ND	ND	ND	19.0	ND	ND	25.0	19.0
– Hexa-PCBs	28.0	13.0	14.0	3.6	72.0	18.0	22.0	53.0	26.0
– Hepta-PCBs	14.0	11.0	13.0	6.3	33.0	14.0	14.0	20.0	11.0
– Oct-PCBs	2.9	3.0	4.4	2.3	6.5	3.8	3.1	4.1	2.3
HCB	25.0	17.0	15.0	9.0	42.0	23.0	24.0	27.0	20.0
HCH	16.0	18.0	17.0	15.0	78.0	26.0	32.0	21.0	10.0
cis-Chlordane	0.32	0.48	0.80	ND	0.43	0.73	0.75	0.54	0.59
trans-Chlordane	0.59	1.3	1.3	ND	1.0	1.0	1.2	0.67	0.95
Oxychlordane	3.1	1.6	ND	ND	3.6	ND	3.2	2.4	3.1
trans-Nonachlor	8.0	3.4	5.9	ND	11.0	4.2	7.4	7.6	7.7
p,p'-DDT	3.1	1.6	ND	2.0	11.0	3.4	2.3	11.0	3.7
o,p'-DDT	ND	ND	ND	ND	0.78	ND	0.36	0.77	ND
p,p'-DDE	28.0	28.0	67.0	16.0	180.0	47.0	59.0	140.0	56.0
p,p'-DDD	ND	0.53	ND	ND	1.1	3.6	0.48	0.62	ND
Dieldrin	7.0	2.8	4.1	2.6	12.0	3.1	4.4	3.9	4.3
Endosulfan	2.8	3.1	ND	3.0	2.8	4.2	ND	2.0	1.8
Heptachlor	0.56	0.82	1.3	ND	0.74	1.3	1.1	0.28	0.73
Heptachlor epoxide	2.4	1.2	1.3	ND	3.3	1.1	2.6	1.3	1.3
Total [a]	169.9	107.8	146.7	66.6	507.8	161.6	191.8	349.1	188.2

ND, not detectable.

a) The concentration of total PCBs was used for calculating the total concentration of chemicals in each umbilical cord, and ND was considered = 0 for this purpose.

tions of heptachlor epoxide ($p = 0.066$). Two possible reasons have been suggested for this correlation [28]. One is that people with high accumulation of various chemicals might have been highly exposed because of their eating habits or because they live (or used to live) in an area polluted by these chemicals. Another possible reason is that these people may have lower ability to exclude the chemicals because of their specific genetic backgrounds. The chemicals exhibiting correlations with total PCBs are most of those that show correlations between umbilical cords and maternal blood. Thus, a subset of these chemicals should be focused on in subsequent toxicogenomic analysis.

20.4 Gene Expression in Umbilical Cords

Gene expression was examined in the nine umbilical cords using Human 1 cDNA microarray (Agilent). For reference gene expression data, RNA from HUVEC (Cell Applications, Inc.) was used. HUVEC were cultured according to the manufacture's

Tab. 20.2 Correlation analysis between concentrations of total PCBs and that of other chemical compounds in umbilical cords.

Compound	*Correlation coefficient (r)* [a]	*p Value*
HCB	0.891	<0.005
HCH	0.676	0.046
cis-Chlordane	0.013	0.973
trans-Chlordane	0.006	0.987
Oxychlordane	0.690	0.040
trans-Nonachlor	0.819	0.007
p,p'-DDT	0.940	<0.005
o,p'-DDT	0.864	<0.005
p,p'-DDE	0.910	<0.005
p,p'-DDD	0.040	0.919
Dieldrin	0.767	0.016
Endosulfan	0.049	0.901
Heptachlor	−0.210	0.588
Heptachlor epoxide	0.636	0.066

a) When the compound was not detectable, its concentration was set = 0.

instructions, and the cells were used at the fifth passage. Total RNA was extracted from each umbilical cord or HUVEC using Trizol reagent (Gibco-BRL). Poly(A)$^+$ RNA was purified using Oligotex-dT30 (Takara Shuzo Co.). To generate target DNA for each umbilical cord, Cy5-dUTP (Amersham–Pharmacia Biotech Japan) was incorporated during reverse transcription of poly(A)$^+$ RNA of the umbilical cord using SuperScriptII (Gibco-BRL), primed with an oligo(dT) primer, as described previously [25]. For generation of target DNA of HUVEC, Cy3-dUTP (Amersham–Pharmacia) was incorporated. A mixture of the fluorescent-labelled targets (Cy5 and Cy3) was applied to the microarray surface and covered with a cover slip (24×60 mm). The array was transferred to a hybridization chamber and incubated at 65 °C overnight in a humidified condition. The array was washed and then scanned using a fluorescence laser-scanning device (ScanArray Lite; GSI Lumonics). The fluorescence of all the features on the array was measured using QuantArray software version 2.1 (GSI Lumonics). Each measurement of local background fluorescence was subtracted from the measurement of each feature, and the resulting value was considered the real fluorescence intensity of the feature. During microarray analysis many factors affect the quality of the outcome, and quality control of microarray methods and data is crucial to achieving comparable data [30], as has been recognized in community database initiatives such as MIAME [31]. For this reason, at least replication of analysis is required in microarray analysis. In the present study, however, neither dye swap nor replication of analysis could be performed because of the limited amount of each umbilical cord available.

To compare the fluorescence intensity of a feature between the Cy3 and Cy5 channels, normalization of feature data is necessary. Several methods of normalization exist [32–34]. First, normalization can be done using housekeeping genes such as

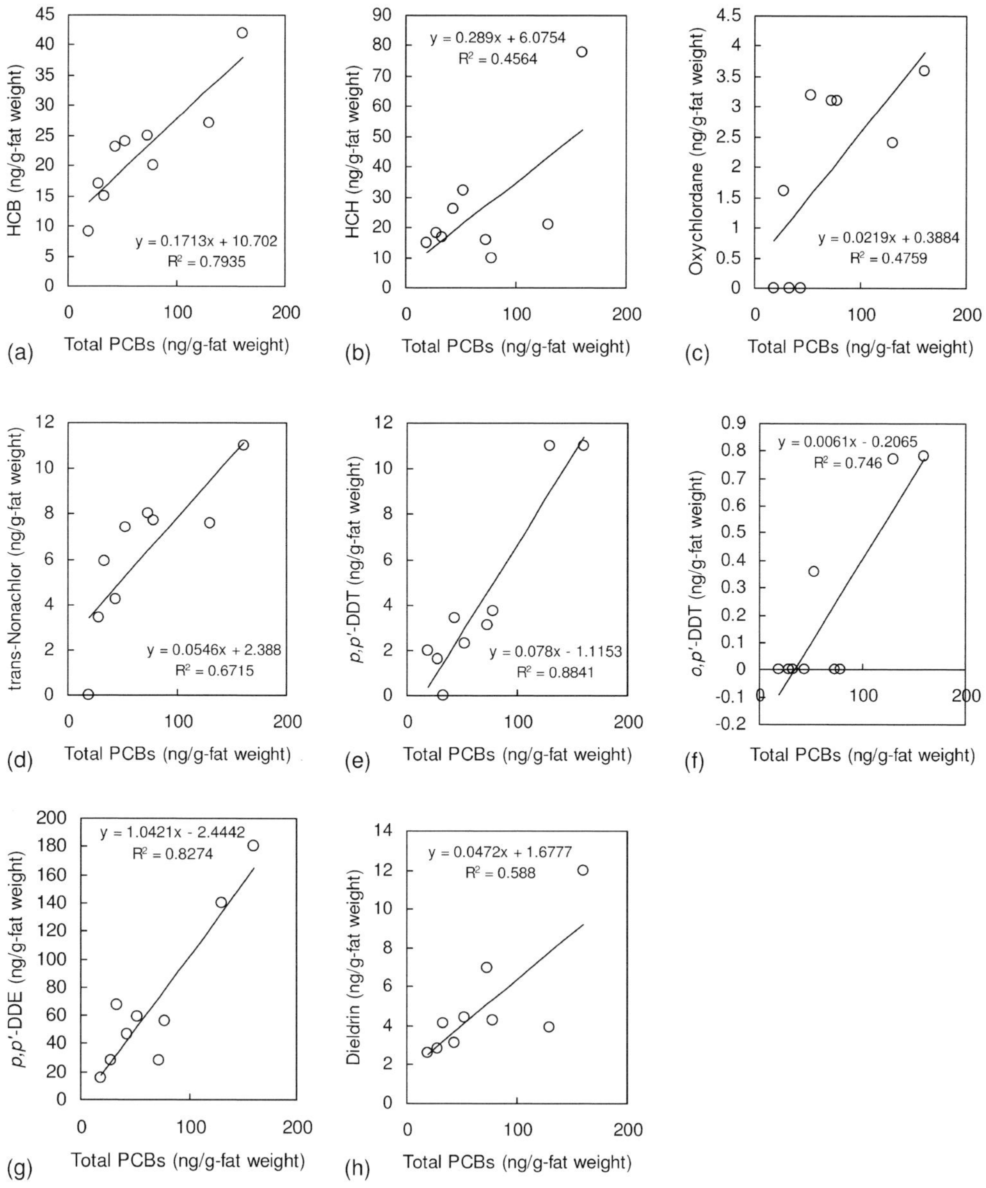

Fig. 20.2 Significant correlations between concentrations of total PCBs and other chemicals in human umbilical cords; (a) HCB, (b) HCH, (c) oxychlordane, (d) *trans*-nonachlor, (e) *p,p'*-DDT, (f) *o,p'*-DDT, (g) *p,p'*-DDE, and (h) dieldrin. Nine umbilical cords were used in each analysis.

β-actin and glyceraldehyde-3-phosphate dehydrogenase (GAPDH). These genes are expressed in most cells, and their expression levels are believed to be almost always constant among various cells. If the fluorescence intensity of these genes differs between the two channels, the values of all features of one channel should be multiplied by a certain coefficient to make the intensity of the housekeeping genes equivalent between the two channels. The second method is global normalization, which is based on the assumption that the total amount of mRNA is the same between the two channels. This method can be applied in many instances but should be avoided when the amount of mRNA is expected to be clearly different between the two channels. The third is to use spike genes (or external controls) such as the luciferase gene. If the microarray carries some spike gene that is not expressed in the samples examined, a certain amount of the spike gene mRNA for both channels can be added prior to the labelling step. This allows us to normalize the fluorescence data using the intensity of the spike gene, which should be the same between both channels. In the present study, we first tried normalization using housekeeping genes, since spike genes were not available. However, when normalization was carried out using β-actin or GAPDH, the bias of signal intensity increased. This must be because expression levels of these genes are actually not the same between umbilical cords and HUVEC. In contrast, the sum of fluorescence intensity of all features in one channel did not differ much from that of the other channel, although the cellular components are different between umbilical cord and HUVEC. Therefore, we used data sets normalized by the global method in later analyses.

Each gene expression level in an umbilical cord was obtained as a ratio with respect to the expression level in HUVEC. However, this ratio does not have meaning unless the fluorescence signal of the gene is higher than the background level in both channels. In the present study, means and standard deviations (SD) of fluorescence measurements of blank spots were calculated in each channel of each array, and only genes that had signals higher than the mean + 2 SD of the blank spots were regarded as genes that were expressed in the umbilical cord or HUVEC. A two-fold difference was used as the cutoff for gene expression; that is, genes that had expression ratios between 0.5 and 2 in all of the umbilical cords were omitted from further analysis, because these genes were expected to exhibit equivalent expression level among all umbilical cords. Thus, we obtained a set of 1765 genes whose expression levels were two-fold (or more) different from those in HUVEC in at least one umbilical cord. In this set, 1081 genes and 652 genes exhibited greater than three-fold and greater than four-fold differences, respectively, in their expression level in umbilical cords relative to that in HUVEC. These genes were used for the subsequent toxicogenomic analysis.

20.5
Toxicogenomic Analysis of Human Umbilical Cords

Two types of general statistical approaches are used for classification of samples based on gene expression. The first is 'supervised' analysis, in which one searches for genes whose expression patterns correlate with an external parameter, such as a pathological feature. The second approach is 'unsupervised' analysis, in which no external feature is used to guide the analysis process. The most common unsupervised analysis method is hierarchical cluster analysis [35, 36]. Unlike in grouping of cancer types or toxicity testing, no phenotype or pathological feature is available for umbilical cords. Therefore we first applied unsupervised analysis using a clustering program, GeneMaths version 1.5 (Applied Maths).

20.5.1 Principal Components Analysis

In the initial phase of analysis, principal components analysis (PCA) is sometimes used to group of genes or samples to see their relative variability [37–40]. Figure 20.3 a shows a three-dimensional view of the PCA visualization, on which the 1765 genes of the nine umbilical cords are plotted. In this visualization, the relative variability of the samples is shown on each axis. The x axis represents the highest contributing factor to the overall variability, which is known as the first component. The y axis shows the second-highest component, and the z axis shows the third-highest component contributing to the variability. The visualization shows that the samples are longitudinally arranged along the x axis. In the left panel, a two-dimensional view of the xy plane of the samples is shown (Figure 20.3 b). The right panel shows how genes contribute to the relative variability of the samples. Window captions above the panels indicate each component and its percentage of contribution. For instance, the first component that is used for the x axis (1 = X in Figure 20.3 b) accounts for 57.4% of the variability contributed by all components. This two-dimensional visualization shows that the samples are arranged in the order of samples E, D, I, G, H, A, F, B, and C along the x axis from right to left. The order and arrangement of samples did not change even when other gene sets (1081 genes of greater than three-fold difference, and 652 genes of greater than four-fold difference) were used.

20.5.2 Hierarchical Cluster Analysis

Next, we carried out hierarchical cluster analysis to group the umbilical cords. In the GeneMaths program, one can chose parameters from several coefficients (Pearson correlation, cosine coefficient, Euclidean distance, and squared Pearson) and clustering algorithms (UPGMA, Ward, single linkage, complete linkage, and neighbour joining), and the clustering results differ somewhat depending on the parameters used. Here, we used the cosine coefficient and the UPGMA algorithm, because the order of resulting clusters under these conditions most resembled the order of the umbilical cords as determined by PCA. Figure 20.4 shows the resulting dendrograms of umbilical cord clusters. The nine umbilical cords were grouped into four main clusters; (1) D and E, or only E; (2) H, G and I, or D, I, G, and H; (3) A and F; and (4) B and C. When the sets of 1765 genes or 1081 genes was used for the analysis, the shapes of the dendrograms were the same for both sets, and the order of umbilical cords from left

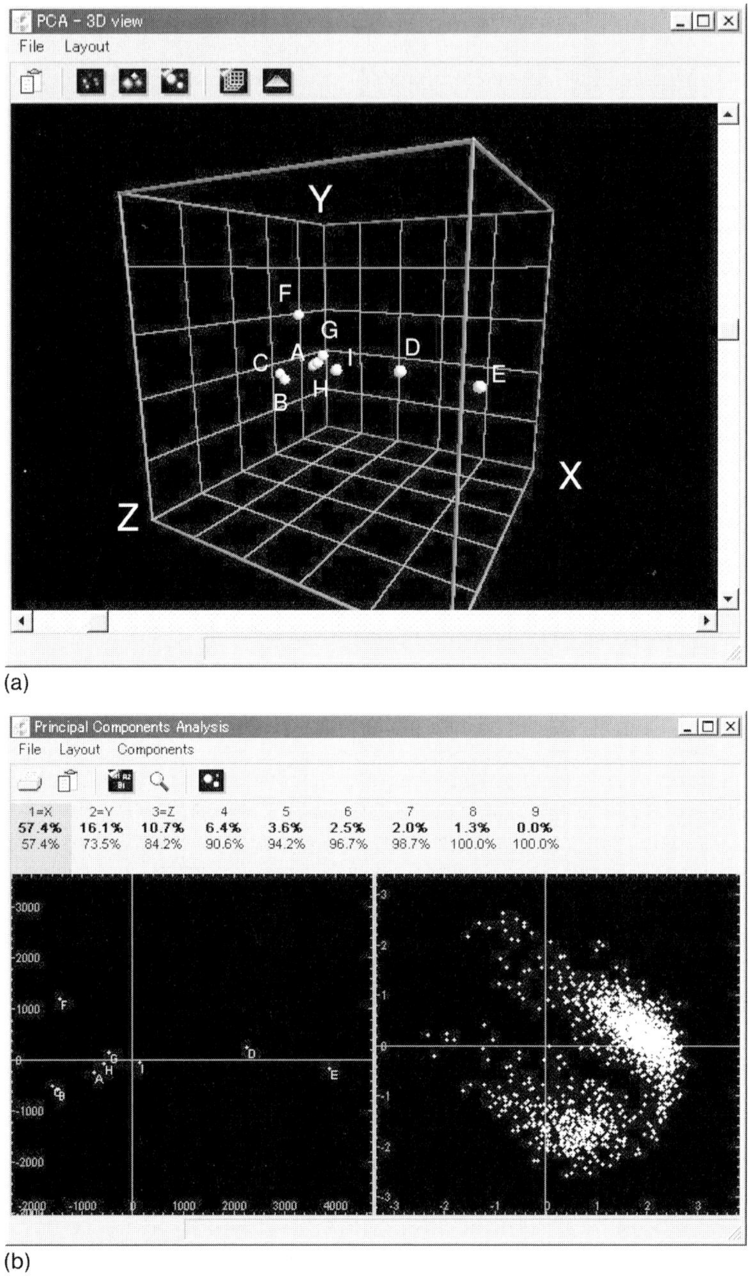

Fig. 20.3 Principal components analysis (PCA) of umbilical cords using 1765 genes. (a) Three-dimensional visualization. (b) Two-dimensional visualization of the *xy* plane, showing the distribution of samples on the left and of genes on the right. By PCA, samples fell in the order E, D, I, G, H, A, F, B, C along the *x* axis from right to left.

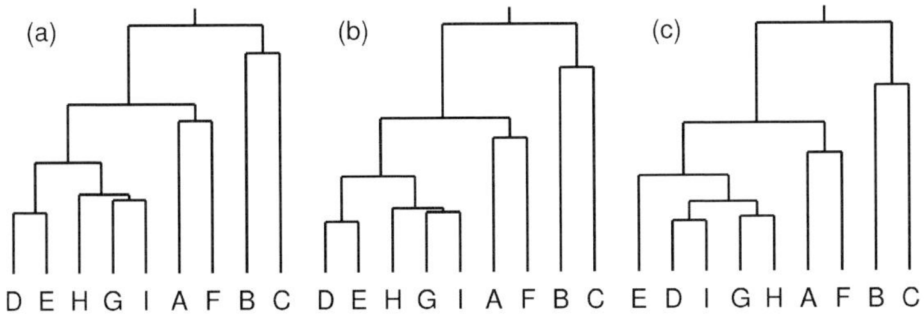

Fig. 20.4 Dendrograms of umbilical cords revealed by hierarchical cluster analysis using (a) 1765, (b) 1081, and (c) 652 genes exhibiting variation across the dataset.

to right was as follows: D, E, H, G, I, A, F, B, and C (Figure 20.4 a, b). When the set of the 652 genes was used, the order of the samples was slightly different from the above, but the same as that obtained by PCA (Figures 20.3 b and 20.4 c).

20.5.3 Relation between Chemical Concentration and Gene Expression in Umbilical Cords

Interestingly, the order of the umbilical cords obtained by cluster analysis using the gene sets showing greater than two-fold or greater than three-fold difference was almost the same as that obtained from the total amounts of chemicals in the umbilical cords, with the exception of sample D (Figure 20.5 a). When the subset of chemicals that exhibited correlation with total PCBs or between umbilical cord and maternal blood was focused on, the order of the sum of concentrations was the same as that for all chemicals (data not shown). In a dendrogram, the left-to-right ordering of objects within a cluster is arbitrary [41]. In the present study, however, PCA clearly showed that samples E and D were farthest from samples B and C. Other samples (H, G, I, A, and F) were between them; the first three were located on the side of D and the latter two were close to B and C. Spearman's rank correlation analysis revealed that there was a significant correlation between the orders of the umbilical cords (without sample D) aligned according to the sum of chemical concentrations and by cluster analysis ($r = 0.976$, $p < 0.005$). These results suggest that gene expression in umbilical cords represent the embryo's exposure levels to those chemicals. Regarding each chemical compound, the alignment of umbilical cords by cluster analysis correlated significantly with that according to the concentration of the following chemicals: total PCBs ($r = 0.905$, $p < 0.005$), HCB ($r = 0.881$, $p < 0.005$), *p,p'*-DDT ($r = 0.821$, $p < 0.01$), oxychlordane ($r = 0.786$, $p < 0.05$), and *trans*-nonachlor ($r = 0.714$, $p < 0.05$). Thus, total PCBs and HCB seem to be the main contributors to the rank correlation, but their correlation coefficients were lower than that for total chemicals. It is thus interesting to note that each gene expression profile may reflect contamination with a mixture of chemicals rather than with each single chemical. This would be an advantage in toxicogenomic analysis for risk assessment of exposure to multiple chemicals.

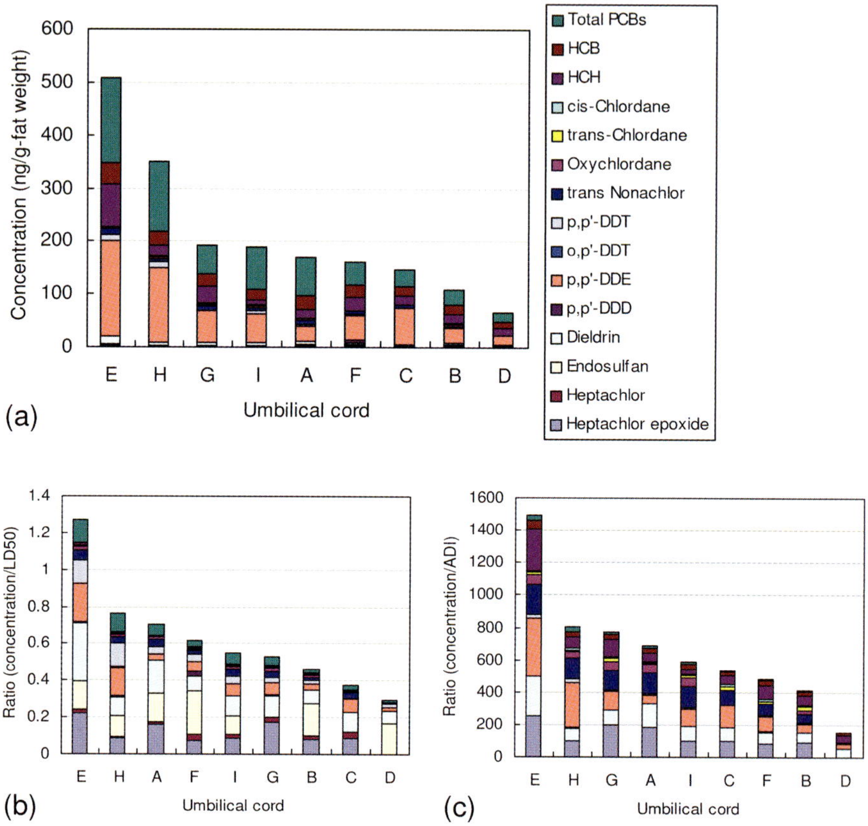

Fig. 20.5 Total concentrations of chemicals before weighting (a) and after weighting the data with the 50% lethal dose (LD_{50}) (b) or the acceptable daily intake (ADI) (c). Samples are arranged in decreasing order of the sum of chemical concentrations/ratios from left to right. Data for LD_{50} (rat, oral) and ADI are from the WebKis-Plus database maintained by the National Institute for Environmental Studies [57]. For *o,p'*-DDT, the minimum lethal dose was used instead of the LD_{50}.

However, the strength of toxicity differs between chemical compounds. Some chemicals may affect gene expression strongly even at low doses and others may not even at high doses. Therefore, we tried to weight the concentration of chemicals with some toxicity parameters, such as the 50% lethal dose (LD_{50}) and the acceptable daily intake (ADI). Figure 20.5 b and c show the results after weighting the chemical concentrations with the LD_{50} (rat, oral) and ADI, respectively. Here, the positions of samples A, C, F, G, and I was slightly different from that in Figure 20.5 a, but that of samples B, D, E, and H was mostly stable in both analyses using all chemicals detected (Figure 20.5 b and c). Rank correlation analysis revealed that there was still significant correlation between the orders of samples after weighting with the LD_{50} ($r = 0.786$, $p < 0.05$) or ADI ($r = 0.905$, $p < 0.005$). Furthermore, the coefficient of the rank correlation for the LD_{50} increased ($r = 0.857$, $p = 0.006$) when the subset of the chemicals was used. This indicates that the correspondence between the order of umbilical cords aligned by concentrations of chemicals and the order obtained by cluster analysis of their gene expression does not change much even after weighting the chemical concentrations with toxicity parameters, especially when the chemicals that exhibit a correlation between umbilical cords and maternal blood were focused on.

Thus, the gene expression profile of each umbilical cord appear to represent its exposure to chemical compounds. Only one exception occurred – sample D. This umbilical cord contained the lowest amount of chemicals, but was grouped in the same cluster as umbilical cord E, which contained the highest chemical amount. There are several possible explanations for this phenomenon. The first is that umbilical cord D may have been highly exposed to other unexamined chemicals or heavy metals such as dioxins, tributyltin, phytoestrogen, lead, or cadmium, which are also detectable in many umbilical cords in Japan [19, 20]. The second possibility is that the baby corresponding to sample D may be more susceptible to the chemicals we examined than the other babies, since susceptibility to chemicals differs between individuals. One may respond strongly to a low level of chemical exposure, and another may not respond much even to a high level of exposure. It seems reasonable to regard higher exposure of foetuses to multiple chemicals as a higher health risk to them [42]. Genetically higher susceptibility is also a risk to health. An important suggestion from the present study is that toxicogenomic analysis can detect a potential high-risk group, because both actually higher exposure levels and genetically higher susceptibility of an individual to multiple chemicals can be regarded as a higher health risk to the individual.

20.5.4
Genes Contributing to Grouping of the Umbilical Cords

What genes are responsible for the grouping of the umbilical cords? This is a common question in supervised analysis. In supervised analysis, an external parameter is necessary. Although one was not available in the present study, we can suppose, for example, that some genes are upregulated in the highly exposed umbilical cords as compared to the low-exposure group. Also, genes in the high-exposure group that were downregulated compared to the low-exposure group may contribute to the grouping of the umbilical cords. Such genes can be revealed by self-organizing map (SOM) analysis [43, 44]. Tables 20.3 and 20.4 show upregulated and downregulated genes, respectively, in samples E and D as compared to B and C.

In Table 20.3, genes for some members of solute-carrier families are listed up as upregulated in umbilical cords E and D. The protein considered member 1 of family 1 (SLC1A1), previously known as HEAAC1, is a neuronal and epithelial glutamate transporter that carries L-glutamate and D-aspartate. It is a sodium-dependent transmembrane protein crucial for terminating the action of the excitatory neurotransmitter glutamate [45, 46]. The gene for member 5 of family 16 (SLC16A5) encodes a member of the monocarboxylate transporter (MCT) family, whose name is MCT6 (previously MCT5) [47]. Although mRNA expression of this transmembrane protein is particularly high in kidney [48], no details are available on the properties of this

Tab. 20.3 Partial list of upregulated genes in umbilical cords E and D as compared to B and C, revealed by SOM analysis.

GenBank[a] *accession no.*	*Gene name*	*Ratios of expression levels relative to HUVEC*								
		E	*D*	*H*	*G*	*I*	*A*	*F*	*B*	*C*
N26306	*Homo sapiens* cDNA FLJ13536 fis, clone PLACE1006521	6.67	5.04	2.2	1.81	2.28	2.19	1.24	1.14	0.94
AK000416	solute-carrier family 16, member 5 (SLC16A5)	6.53	4.84	2.18	2.33	1.59	1.82	1.33	1.1	0.91
M23077	Human pepsinogen gene	6.13	4.51	2.2	2.71	2.19	2.41	1.65	0.98	1.02
AF195765	L2DTL protein	5.88	4.84	1.97	1.5	1.9	2.12	1.43	1.22	0.96
AK001478	novel Ras family protein	5.81	4.22	1.72	2.14	2.51	2.1	1.53	1.11	0.98
AB011096	KIAA0524 protein	5.68	4.06	2.09	1.74	1.98	2.04	1.23	1.06	0.93
D31784	cadherin 6, type 2, K-cadherin	5.54	4.52	2.3	1.7	2.1	1.66	1.23	1.04	0.8
X00419	c-Ha-ras2 oncogene (Harvey ras family)	5.54	4.01	2.37	2.04	2.67	2.38	1.65	1.2	1.01
D86864	acetyl LDL receptor; SREC	5.52	4.78	2.88	1.71	2.14	1.71	1.57	1.11	0.91
AA889740	solute-carrier family 1, member 1 (SLC1A1)	5.42	4.51	2.44	1.47	1.93	1.37	1.76	1	0.99
U55312	G protein-coupled receptor 19	5.38	5.86	1.57	1.98	2.44	1.86	1.36	0.95	1.17
D83174	serine (or cysteine) proteinase inhibitor, clade H (heat shock protein 47), member 2	5.21	4.28	2	2.26	1.98	1.97	2.1	0.94	0.94
AW951503	*trans*-Golgi network protein	5.13	3.54	1.57	1.45	1.81	1.73	1.21	1.01	1.02
AF034632	G protein-coupled receptor 38	4.99	4.15	2.01	2.19	1.89	1.97	1.81	1.35	0.94
AB028970	nuclear receptor corepressor 1	4.81	2.97	1.97	1.68	2.07	2.32	1.4	0.98	1
AI379426	small acidic protein	4.81	2.74	1.86	1.59	2.07	2.26	1.21	1.01	1.12
X14766	GABA A receptor, alpha 1	4.69	4.04	1.7	1.42	1.91	1.72	1.17	1.02	1.1
AA419498	Kallmann syndrome 1 sequence	4.65	2.95	1.66	1.8	1.57	2.19	1.44	0.86	1
AI669338	hypothetical protein similar to mouse HN1	4.53	4.04	1.64	1.84	1.92	2.16	1.47	1.09	1.03
AF165522	ras-related GTP-binding protein 4b	4.52	3.6	1.52	1.74	2.53	1.77	1.25	1.01	1.12
AX017310	Sequence 66 from Patent WO9947669	4.48	3.85	1.93	1.41	1.61	1.65	1.3	1.03	1.02
M28372	zinc finger protein 9	4.47	3.5	2.12	1.46	2.43	2.32	0.95	1.06	1.06
AF077052	translation factor sui1 homolog	4.44	2.95	1.55	1.5	1.78	1.81	1.06	0.98	0.98
D63395	Notch (*Drosophila*) homolog 4	4.4	3.37	1.34	1.14	1.68	1.6	1.03	0.97	0.87
D25304	Rac/Cdc42 guanine exchange factor 6	4.33	4.07	1.63	1.71	1.69	1.94	1.29	1.24	0.83
Z59762	Human CpG island DNA genomic Mse1 fragment, clone 171h5	4.28	2.91	1.57	1.42	1.69	1.69	1.17	0.84	1.06
AK001031	T-box 2	4.21	3.53	1.6	1.94	2.16	2.65	1.43	0.95	1.19
M69238	aryl hydrocarbon receptor nuclear translocator	4.11	3.85	1.78	1.79	1.85	2.04	1.39	0.94	0.97
L02785	solute-carrier family 26, member 3 (SLC26A3)	4.11	3.44	2.16	1.62	2.09	1.72	1.37	1	1.12
AI636514	butyrophilin, subfamily 2, member A2	4.1	3.8	2.2	1.4	1.72	2.06	1.16	0.95	1.16
NM_004577	phosphoserine phosphatase	4.08	3.28	1.91	1.43	2.12	1.8	1.16	0.98	1.1
AI475509	KIAA0782 protein	3.98	3.47	1.77	1.63	1.57	1.67	1.39	0.91	0.85
U14193	general transcription factor IIA, 2 (12-kDa subunit)	3.97	2.81	1.32	1.51	1.46	1.66	0.92	0.7	0.89
AAC32740	F22162_1	3.88	3	1.7	1.61	1.84	1.75	1.35	0.93	1.09

Tab. 20.3 (continued)

GenBank[a) *accession no.*	*Gene name*	*Ratios of expression levels relative to HUVEC* E	D	H	G	I	A	F	B	C
CAB51740	zinc finger 41	3.87	2.67	1.79	1.19	1.59	1.52	1.14	0.91	0.94
BAA97324	contains similarity to acyl-CoA binding protein~gene_id:MYN8.8	3.71	2.63	1.72	1.3	1.47	1.68	0.96	0.87	0.97
AL137661	hypothetical protein DKFZp434P0116	3.69	3.15	1.58	1.44	1.85	1.85	1.22	1.12	0.99
M35878	insulin-like growth factor binding protein 3	3.58	3.06	0.97	1.68	1.83	1.32	1.15	0.82	1.04
U27768	regulator of G-protein signalling 4	3.48	2.87	1.72	1.5	1.65	1.62	1.18	0.84	0.94
D90277	carcinoembryonic antigen-related cell adhesion molecule 3	3.44	3.65	1.55	1.47	1.79	1.62	1.42	1.22	0.99
M11937	immunoglobulin kappa constant	3.37	2.42	1.61	1.54	1.82	1.81	1.13	0.83	0.88
AB047611	macaque brain cDNA, clone: QnpA-11680	3.22	2.97	1.83	1.64	1.97	1.82	1.27	1.06	0.98
AI954732	chromosome 8 open reading frame 2	3.2	2.71	1.23	1.21	1.57	1.83	1.1	1.03	0.85
AJ000479	endothelial differentiation, G-protein-coupled receptor 6	3.19	3.11	1.72	1.07	1.46	1.29	1.58	0.87	1.01
AF191019	hypothetical protein, estradiol-induced	3.05	2.7	1.43	1.31	1.69	1.85	1.15	1.12	1.05
Z49194	POU domain, class 2, associating factor 1	3.03	2.75	1.6	1.36	2.02	1.79	1.14	1.02	0.92
U40490	nicotinamide nucleotide transhydrogenase	3.03	2.46	1.64	1.24	1.7	1.78	1.06	1.2	0.92

a) GenBank database (http://ncbi.nlm.nih.gov/).

Tab. 20.4 Downregulated genes in umbilical cords E and/or D as compared to B and C, revealed by SOM analysis.

GenBank[a) *accession no.*	*Gene name*	*Fold ratios of expression as compared to HUVEC* E	D	H	G	I	A	F	B	C
D50926	KIAA0136 protein	0.22	0.9	0.95	1.23	0.95	1.18	1.01	1.26	0.88
BE206815	G protein, beta polypeptide 2-like 1	0.24	0.29	1.02	0.34	0.88	0.99	1.18	0.85	0.88
AF203815	Human alpha gene sequence	0.29	0.37	0.93	0.71	0.97	1.1	0.88	0.96	0.89
L20688	Rho GDP dissociation inhibitor (GDI) beta	0.36	0.37	0.81	0.74	0.89	0.94	0.53	0.9	0.9
X83703	cardiac ankyrin repeat protein	0.37	0.35	0.72	0.75	0.84	0.99	0.94	0.71	0.87
AF000974	thyroid hormone receptor interactor 6	0.45	0.61	0.82	0.95	0.91	1.07	0.95	0.96	0.74
AK025459	tumour rejection antigen (gp96) 1	0.48	0.49	0.8	0.77	0.99	0.87	0.65	0.86	0.95
AA345289	myosin, light polypeptide, regulatory, non-sarcomeric (20 kDa)	0.57	0.32	0.81	0.53	0.65	0.79	0.93	0.94	0.69
X14787	thrombospondin 1	0.75	0.39	0.7	0.62	0.84	0.81	0.57	0.89	0.55
AF061832	heterogeneous nuclear ribonucleoprotein M	0.97	0.37	0.91	1.08	1.02	0.88	0.67	1.02	0.93
X13293	v-myb avian myeloblastosis viral oncogene homolog-like 2	0.98	0.47	0.93	1.15	0.99	0.85	0.83	1.03	1.08
BE410628	gap junction protein, beta 1, 32 kDa	1.13	0.19	0.97	1.04	0.91	0.92	1.14	1.01	0.99

a) GenBank database (http://ncbi.nlm.nih.gov/).

protein [47]. In solute carrier family 26, member 3 (SLC26A3; previously known as DRA or CLD) is an anion exchanger that is normally abundantly present in the plasma membrane of mature epithelial cells of colon and ileum [49–51]. Although the members are not exactly the same, it is of interest that genes for members of the same solute-carrier family (Slc1a7, Slc16a1, and Slc26a2) are upregulated in the mouse testis after exposure to a putative endocrine disrupter, bisphenol A (unpublished data). The *Slc1a7* gene encodes a sodium-dependent neutral amino acid transporter [52, 53], *Slc16a1* encodes MCT1, whose predominant substrates are lactate, pyruvate, and ketone bodies [47], and *Slc26a2* encodes a sulphate transporter that may also transport multiple anions [51]. It is very likely that these genes for the solute-carrier families are major responders to chemical exposures in various organs, and thus they may be good candidates for biomarkers of exposure.

Genes involved in Ras/MAPK-related signalling pathways, such as those encoding Ki-ras2, guanine nucleotide exchange factor, Ras GAP-1, and MEK5, are upregulated in human hepatoma HepG2 cells after exposure to 10 nM 2,3,7,8-tetrachlorodibenzo-*p*-dioxin [54]. Activation of the *c-Ha-ras* gene by benzo[*a*]pyrene has been also demonstrated in vascular smooth muscle [55, 56]. In the present study, upregulation of a novel Ras family protein, c-Ha-ras2, ras-related GTP-binding protein 4b, and Rac/Cdc42 guanine exchange factor 6 was observed in umbilical cords E and D (Table 20.3). In contrast, the gene for Rho GDP dissociation inhibitor β was downregulated in these umbilical cords (Table 20.4). However, it is not clear whether umbilical cords E and D accumulated higher amounts of dioxins (polychlorinated dibenzo-*p*-dioxins + polychlorinated dibenzofurans + coplanar PCBs) than other cords. In Japan, dioxins are still detectable in many of umbilical cords [19, 20, 28], although there seems to be a tendency to decrease.

20.6 Conclusions

Toxicogenomic analysis of human umbilical cords revealed that the hierarchical order of the umbilical cords clustered according to their gene expression profiles corresponded to their order according to their total concentrations of chemicals, with one exception. In the exceptional umbilical cord, the total concentration of chemicals was lowest, but its gene expression profile was most similar to that of the umbilical cord exhibiting the highest level of total chemical concentrations. These results suggest that gene expression in umbilical cords may reflect their exposure to some persistent chemicals. In addition, the expression profile may reflect contamination with a mixture of chemicals rather than that with each single compound. Furthermore, an important suggestion from this study is that toxicogenomic analysis can detect potential high-risk groups, because genetically higher susceptibility as well as higher exposure of an individual to multiple chemicals can be regarded as a higher health risk to the individual.

To extend the toxicogenomic analysis method to develop a new risk-assessment strategy, comprehensive studies are required to clarify the correlation between data from toxicogenomic analysis of umbilical cords, data from animal experiments in which the adverse effects of exposure to chemicals are observed, and data from prospective studies of humans. These studies are indispensable for linking gene expression profiles of umbilical cords to possible delayed long-term adverse effects of chemicals on individuals. Although certain technical and socioethical issues must be addressed, if this approach becomes practical, toxicogenomic analysis can be used for early diagnosis and possible prevention of adverse effects caused by multiple chemicals in humans.

Acknowledgments

We thank Dr. Hisao Osada (Chiba University) for sampling umbilical cords and Dr. Tetsuya Adachi (Osaka Prefecture University), Ms. Kyoka Takashima (Chiba University), and Mr. Daisuke Nishimura (Chiba University) for their help with the experiments. This work was supported by grants from the Ministry of the Environment (Government of Japan), Ministry of Education, Culture, Sports, Science, and Technology (Government of Japan), New Energy and Industrial Technology Development Organization, and Nanohana Venture Award 2002 (Chiba University).

References

1. Needam, L.L. and Sexton, K.: Assessing children's exposure to hazardous environmental chemicals: an overview of selected research challenges and complexities. *J. Exposure Anal. Environ. Epidermiol.* 2000, **10**, 611–629.
2. Sharpe, R.M. and Skakkebaek, N.E.: Are estrogens involved in falling sperm counts and disorders of the male reproductive tract? *Lancet* 1993, **341**, 1392–1395.
3. Colborn, T., Dumanoski, D. and Mayers, J.P.: *Our Stolen Future.* Plume/Penguin, New York, 1996.
4. Toppari, J., Larsen, J.C., Christiansen, P., Givercman, A., Grandjean, P., Guilette, L.J. Jr., Jegou, B., Jensen, T.K., Jouannet, P., Keiding, N., Leffers, H., McLachlan, J.A., Meyer, O., Muller, J., Rajpert-De Meyts, E., Scheike, T., Sharpe, R., Sumpter, J. and Skakkebaek, N.E.: Male reproductive health and environmental xeno-systems. *Environ. Health Perspect.* 1996, **104**, 741–776.
5. Safe, S.H: Endocrine disruptors and human health: is there a problem? an update. *Environ. Health Perspect.* 2000, **108**, 487–493.
6. Andersson, A.M., Grigor, K.M., Meyts, E.R.D., Leffers, H. and Skakkebaek, N.E. (eds.): *Hormones* and Endocrine Disrupters in Food and Water: Possible Impact on Human Health. Munksgaard, Copenhagen, 2001.
7. Perera, F.P., Illman, S.M., Kinney, P.L., Whyatt, R.M., Kelvin, E.A., Shepard, P., Evans, D., Fullilove, M., Ford, J., Miller, R.L., Meyer, I.H., Rauh, V.A.: The challenge of preventing environmentally related disease in young children: community-based research in New York City. *Environ. Health Perspect.* 2002, **110**, 197–204.
8. Charnley, G. and Putzrath, R.M.: Children's health, susceptibility, and regulatory approaches to reducing risks from chemical carcinogens. *Environ. Health Perspect.* 2001, **109**, 187–192.
9. Needleman, H.L: Lead levels and children's psychologic performance [Letter]. *N. Eng. J. Med.* 1979, **301**, 163.

10. Calabrese, E.J.: *Age and Susceptibility to Toxic Substances.* Wiley, New York, 1986.
11. WHO: *Principles for Evaluating Health Risks from Chemicals during Infancy and Early Childhood: The Need for a Special Approach. Environmental Health Criteria* 59. World Health Organization, Geneva, 1986.
12. Whyatt, R.M. and Perera, F.P.: Application of biologic markers to studies of environmental risks in children and the developing fetus. *Environ. Health Perspect.* 1995, **103** (suppl. 6), 105–110.
13. Jacobson, J.L. and Jacobson, S.W.: Intellectual impairment in children exposed to polychlorinated biphenyls in utero. *N. Eng. J. Med.* 1996, **335**, 783–789.
14. Perera, F.P.: Molecular epidemiology: insights into cancer susceptibility, risk assessment and prevention. *J. Natl. Cancer Inst.* 1996, **88**, 496–509.
15. Moore, K.L. and Persaud, T.V.N.: *The Developing Human*, 6th ed. Saunders, Philadelphia, 1998.
16. Newbold, R.R., Bullock, B.C. and McLachlan, J.A.: Müllerian remnants of male mice exposed prenatally to diethylstilbestrol. *Teratog. Carcinog. Mutagen* 1984, **7**, 337–389.
17. Newbold, R.R.: Effects of developmental exposure to diethylstilbestrol (DES) in rodents: clues for other environmental estrogens. *APMIS* 2001, **109**, S261–S271.
18. Williams, K., McKinnell, C., Saunders, P.T.K., Walker, M., Fisher, J.S., Turner, K.J., Atanassova, N. and Sharpe, R.M.: Neonatal exposure to potent and environmental oestrogens and abnormalities of the male reproductive system in the rat: evidence for importance of the androgen–oestrogen balance and assessment of the relevance to man. *Hum. Reprod. Update* 2001, **7**, 236–247.
19. Mori, C.: Possible effects of endocrine disruptors on male reproductive function. *Acta Anat. Nippon* 2001, **76**, 361–368.
20. Todaka, E. and Mori, C.: Necessity to establish new risk assessment and risk communication for human fetal exposure to multiple endocrine disruptors in Japan. *Congenit. Anom. Kyoto* 2002, **42**, 87–93.
21. National Research Council (NRC): *Risk Assessment in the Federal Government: Managing the Process.* National Academy Press, Washington, DC, 1983.
22. Nuwaysir, E.F., Bittner, M., Trent, J., Barrett, J.C. and Afshari, C.A.: Microarrays and toxicology: the advent of toxicogenomics. *Mol. Carcinogen.* 1999, **24**, 153–159.
23. Iannaccone, P.M.: Toxicogenoics: the call of the wild chip. *Environ. Health Perspect.* 2001, **109**, A8–A11.
24. Shibayama, T., Fukata, H., Sakurai, K., Adachi, T., Komiyama, M., Iguchi, T. and Mori, C.: Neonatal exposure to genistein reduces expression of estrogen receptor alpha and androgen receptor in testes of adult mice. *Endocrine J.* 2001, **48**, 655–663.
25. Adachi, T., Komiyama, M., Ono, Y., Koh, K.-B., Sakurai, K., Shibayama, T., Kato, M., Yoshikawa, T., Seki, N., Iguchi, T. and Mori, C.: Toxicogenomic effects of neonatal exposure to diethylstilbestrol on mouse testicular gene expression in the long term: a study using cDNA microarray analysis. *Mol. Reprod. Dev.* 2002, **63**, 17–23.
26. Adachi, T., Matsuno, Y., Sugimura, A., Takano, K., Koh, K.-B., Sakurai, K., Shibayama, T., Iguchi, T., Mori, C. and Komiyama, M.: ADAM7 (a disintegrin and metalloprotease 7) mRNA is suppressed in mouse epididymis by neonatal exposure to diethylstilbestrol. *Mol. Reprod. Dev.* 2003, **64**, 414–421.
27. Komiyama, M., Adachi, T. and Mori, C.: Analysis of toxicogenomic response to endocrine disruptors in the mouse testis. In: Inoue, T. and Pennie, W.D. (eds.): *Toxicogenomics.* Springer-Verlag Tokyo, Tokyo, 2003, 156–162.
28. Mori, C., Komiyama, M., Adachi, T., Sakurai, K., Nishimura, D., Takashima, K. and Todaka, E.: Application of toxicogenomic analysis to risk assessment of delayed long-term effects of multiple chemicals, including endocrine disruptors in human fetuses. *Environ. Health Perspect.* 2003, **111**, 803–809.
29. Ministry of the Environment (Government of Japan): http://www.env.go.jp/chemi/end/kento04-1.pdf [in Japanese] 2003.

30. Hill, A. and Whitley, M.: Quality control of expression profiling data. In: Burczynski, M.E. (ed.): *An Introduction to Toxicogenomics*. CRC Press, Boca Raton, Florida, 2003, 29–43.

31. Brazma, A., Hingamp, P., Quackenbush, J., Sherlock, G., Spellman, P., Stoeckert, C., Aach, J., Ansorge, W., Ball, C.A., Causton, H.C., Gaasterland, T., Glenisson, P., Holstege, F.C.P., Kim, I.F., Markowitz, V., Matese, J.C., Parkinson, H., Robinson, A., Sarkans, U., Schulze-Kremer, S., Stewart, J., Taylor, R., Vilo, J. and Vingron, M.: Minimum information about a microarray experiment (MIAME): toward standards for microarray data. *Nature Genet.* 2001, **29**, 365–371.

32. Bilban, M., Buehler, L.K., Head, S., Desoye, G. and Quaranta, V.: Normalizing DNA microarray data. *Curr. Issues Mol. Biol.* 2002, **4**, 57–64.

33. Quackenbush, J.: Microarray data normalization and transformation. *Nature Genet. Suppl.* 2002, **32**, 496–501.

34. Microarray Gene Expression Data Society: The MGED Data Transformation and Normalization Working Group. http://www.dnachip.org/mged/normalization.html

35. Eisen, M.B., Spellman, P.T., Brown, P.O. and Botstein, D.: Cluster analysis and display of genome-wide expression patterns. *Proc. Natl. Acad. Sci. USA* 1998, **95**, 14863–14868.

36. Spellman, P.T., Sherlock, G., Zhang, M.Q., Iyer, V.R., Anders, K., Eisen, M.B., Brown, P.O., Botstein, D. and Futcher, B.: Comprehensive identification of cell cycle-regulated genes of the yeast *Saccharomyces cerevisiae* by microarray hybridization. *Mol. Biol. Cell* 1998, **9**, 3273–3297.

37. Hilsenbeck, S.G., Friedrichs, W.E., Schiff, R., O'Connell, P., Hansen, R.K., Osborne, C.K. and Fuqua, S.A.W.: Statistical analysis of array expression data as applied to the problem of tamoxifen resistance. *J. Nat. Cancer Inst.* 1999, **91**, 453–459.

38. Raychaudhuri, S., Stuart, J.M. and Altman, R.B.: Principal components analysis to summarize microarray experiments: application to sporulation time series. *Pac. Symp. Biocomput.* 2000, 455–466.

39. Crescenzi, M. and Giuliani, A.: The main biological determinants of tumor line taxonomy elucidated by a principal component analysis of microarray data. *FEBS Lett.* 2001, **507**, 114–118.

40. Peterson, L.F.: Partitioning large-sample microarray-based gene expression profiles using principal components analysis. *Comput. Methods Programs Biomed.* 2003, **70**, 107–119.

41. Immermann, F. and Huang, Y.: An introduction to cluster analysis. In: Burczynski, M.E. (ed.): *An Introduction to Toxicogenomics*. CRC Press, Boca Raton, Florida, 2003, 45–78.

42. Patandin, S., Lanting, C.I., Mulder, P.G., Boersma, E.R., Sauer, P.J., Weisglas-Kuperus, N.: Effects of environmental exposure to polychlorinated biphenyls and dioxins on cognitive abilities in Dutch children at 42 months of age. *J. Pediatr.* 1999, **134**, 33–41.

43. Tamayo, P., Slonim, D., Mesirov, J., Zhu, Q., Kitareewan, S., Dmitrovsky, E., Lander, E. and Golub, T.: Interpreting patterns of gene expression with self-organizing maps: methods and application to hematopoietic differentiation. *Proc. Natl. Acad. Sci. USA* 1999, **96**, 2907–2912.

44. Kohonen, T.: *Self-Organizing Maps*. Springer, Berlin, 2001.

45. Kanai, Y. and Hediger, M.A.: Primary structure and functional characterization of a high-affinity glutamate transporter. *Nature* 1992, **360**, 467–471.

46. Kanai, Y., Stelzner, M.S., Nussberger, S., Khawaja, S., Hebert, S.C., Smith, C.P. and Hediger, M.A.: The neuronal and epithelial human high affinity glutamate transporter. *J. Biol. Chem.* 1994, **269**, 20599–20606.

47. Halestrap, A.P. and Meredith, D.: The *SLC16* gene family: from monocarboxylate transporters (MCTs) to aromatic amino acid transporters and beyond. *Pflugers Arch. Eur. J. Physiol.* 2003, Online First Publications, http://link.springer.de/link/service/journals/00424/contents/03/01067/paper/s00424-003-1067-2ch000.html

48. Price, N.T., Jackson, V.N. and Halestrap, A.P.: Cloning and sequencing of four new mammalian monocarboxylate transporter (MCT) homologues confirms the existence of a transporter family with an ancient past. *Biochem. J.* 1998, **329**, 321–328.

49. Haila, S., Saarialho-Kere, U., Karjalainen-Lindsberg, M.-L., Lohi, H., Airola, K., Holmberg, C., Hästbacka, J., Kere, J. and Höglund, P.: The congenital chloride diarrhea gene (CLD) is expressed in seminal vesicle, sweat gland, inflammatory colon epithelium, and in some dysplastic cells. *J. Cell Histochem. Biol.* 2000, **113**, 279–286.

50. Jacob, P., Rossmann, H., Lamprecht, G., Kretz, A., Neff, C., Lin-Wu, E., Gregor, M., Groneberg, D.A., Kere, J. and Seidler, U.: Down-regulated in adenoma mediates apical Cl^-/HCO_3^- exchange in rabbit, rat, and human duodenum. *Gastroenterology* 2002, **122**, 709–724.

51. Mount, D.B. and Romero, M.F.: The SCL26 gene family of multifunctional anion exchangers. *Pflugers Arch. Eur. J. Physiol.* 2003, Online First Publications, http://link.springer.de/link/service/journals/00424/contents/03/01090/paper/s00424–003-1090–3ch000.html

52. Liao, K. and Lane, M.D.: Expression of a novel insulin-activated amino acid transporter gene during differentiation of 3T3-L1 preadipocytes into adipocytes. *Biochem. Biophys. Res. Comm.* 1995, **208**, 1008–1015.

53. Utsunomiya-Tate, N., Endou, H. and Kanai, Y.: Cloning and functional characterization of a system ASC-like Na^+-dependent neutral amino acid transporter. *J. Biol. Chem.* 1996, **271**, 14883–14890.

54. Puga, A., Maier, A. and Medvedovic, M.: The transcriptional signature of dioxin in human hepatoma HepG2 cells. *Biochem. Pharmacol.* 2000, **60**, 1129–1142.

55. Sadhu, D.N., Merchant, M., Safe, S.H. and Ramos, K.S.: Modulation of protooncogene expression in rat aortic smooth muscle cells by benzo[*a*]pyrene. *Arch. Biochem. Biophys.* 1993, **300**, 124–131.

56. Bral, C.M. and Ramos, K.S.: Identification of benzo[*a*]pyrene-inducible *cis*-acting elements within c-Ha-ras transcriptional regulatory sequences. *Mol. Pharmacol.* 1997, **52**, 974–982.

57. National Institute for Environmental Studies: WebKis-Plus (Database of chemical compounds). http://w-chemdb.nies.go.jp/

21
Genetic Variability: Implications for Toxicogenomic Research

Gilbert Schönfelder, Dieter Schwarz, Thomas Gerloff, Martin Paul, and Ivar Roots

21.1
Introduction

The toxic potential and molecular mechanisms underlying the action of many environmental pollutants, chemicals, and therapeutic drugs are not well understood. The term 'toxicogenomics' combines profiling of gene expression with knowledge of protein composition (proteomics) and the metabolic constituents ('metabonomics') of the whole organism or a single cell (Rosenblum, 2003). The functional status of the living organism or single cell can be characterized at the molecular level (Rosenblum, 2003). The profiles of gene, protein, and metabolite is increasingly valuable for toxicogenomic research to understand what leads from exposure to hazard.

With the completion of the human genome sequencing project we can evaluate the importance of genetic polymorphisms that alter protein function to the benefit or detriment of individuals upon exposure to many environmental xenobiotics. Toxicologists can catalogue the gene variants that increase or decrease susceptibility to toxicant-induced disease (Simmons and Portier, 2002) and may find more sensitive and characteristic markers of toxicity than conventional toxicological endpoints of reproductive, developmental, carcinogenic, or clinical toxicology testing.

Toxicogenomics may provide a specific molecular 'fingerprint' or 'signature' for multiple pathways, mechanisms, and effects of exposure or toxicological response to toxicants (Roberts et al., 2003).

The molecular fingerprint can be related to expression profiles obtained at multiple dose levels and after single acute exposures compared with long-term chronic exposure. It can demonstrate time courses of gene-expression changes after toxic exposure. These changes can be transient or long-term. Nevertheless, we have to keep in mind that most human exposures are not so simple, because in general, people are exposed to many compounds simultaneously and at low doses (Marchant, 2002). Toxicogenomics has to address more realistic exposure scenarios.

As in pharmacogenomics, toxicogenomics considers gene SNP linkage–disequilibrium (haplotype) mapping and genome-wide SNP linkage–disequilibrium mapping to explain response and toxicity upon xenobiotic exposure, complex disease-sus-

Handbook of Toxicogenomics: Strategies and Applications. Edited by Jürgen Borlak

ISBN: 3-527-30342-1

ceptibility risks, and interactions of the disease with a substance leading to an outcome. Individual variations in drug response or toxicity may not depend only on an SNP in a single gene, but may depend on combinations of polymorphisms in several genes. Our detailed genetic knowledge provides many potential entry points for intervention, including substrate limitation, replacement of a deficient product, using alternative pathways to remove toxic metabolites, and using metabolic inhibitors or inducers. It is a revolution in chemical and drug safety, because it helps to better understand the complexity of gene–environment interactions and has the potential to help prevent adverse drug reactions (Brennan, 2002). On one side, using this new technology we start to understand what leads from exposure to disease. On the other side, where direct quantitative evidence of exposure is lacking (e.g., in forensic cases), toxicogenomics could assist in demonstrating exposure or could disprove arguments that there was no significant exposure (Marchant, 2002). Toxicogenomic assays (i.e., microarrays and real-time PCR) might demonstrate the presence or absence of gene expression (molecular fingerprints) that are characteristic of the toxic substance to which injured victims were allegedly exposed. Nevertheless, in the near future we have to manage the massive amounts of information associated with toxicogenomic approaches. An unprecedented volume of data has to be screened for specific information and linked with data from public databases to produce germane information on gene annotation, protein function, and pathways readily available for data interpretation. Therefore, we have to start to standardize protocols, experiments, vocabularies, and terminology across toxicogenomic technologies (Wakefield, 2003). Bioinformaticians are asked to manage and analyze biological data using advanced computing programs so that any scientist interested in toxicogenomics can benefit from the new databases (Schmidt, 2003; Tong et al., 2003).

21.2
Toxicity Due to Genetic Variability of Xenobiotic-metabolizing Enzymes

The goal of therapeutics is to achieve a beneficial effect with minimal adverse effects. Prior to drug administration it is difficult to predict unexpected severe drug toxicity (adverse effects), because of the genetic heterogeneity of patients. Inter-individual variability in drug toxicity has multiple sources, the most important being genetic polymorphisms in drug-metabolizing enzymes, transporters, and drug targets (Kramer and Kolaja, 2002; Meisel et al., 2003). Polymorphisms are DNA variations occurring in at least 1% of a population. Polymorphisms take the form of SNPs (single nucleotide polymorphisms) or VNTRs (variable numbers of tandem repeats) (Strachan and Read, 2003).

On the one side are the major phase-I reaction enzymes (oxidation, reduction, or hydrolysis). The cytochrome P450 enzymes (CYP450s) and epoxide hydrolase are the most important of these. Many genotype–phenotype studies have shown inter-individual variation in expression levels and activity of CYP450s. On the other side are the phase-II reaction enzymes, which conjugate phase-I products, other reactive intermediates, or the parent compound to form more polar derivatives for renal and biliary elimination. These include UDP-glucuronosyl transferases, N-acetyl transferases, glutathione S-transferases, and sulfotransferases, (Cascorbi et al., 1999; Kerb et al., 1999; Brockmoller et al., 2000; Kerb et al., 2002; Glatt and Meinl, 2004).

21.2.1
Genetic Variability in Carcinogen Activation by CYP450 Enzymes

Many chemical carcinogens are unreactive and require metabolic activation. CYP450s are usually employed for detoxification, but CYP450s can also exert carcinogenic or mutagenic effects. CYP450s share at least 40% sequence homology and are grouped into families (3).

Ubiquitous environmental carcinogens, such as polycyclic aromatic hydrocarbons (e.g., benzo[*a*]pyrene (BaP)), arylamines, heterocyclic amines, and nitroarenes, are oxidized by CYP enzymes to epoxide intermediates in the initial step of activation. After hydrolysis by epoxide hydrolase to dihydrodiol metabolites (diols: e.g., 7,8-dihydrodiol-BaP) they are finally epoxidized again by CYP enzymes to form the ultimate carcinogenic diolepoxides (e.g., DE2, (($\pm$)-BaP-*r*-7,*t*-8-dihydrodiol-*t*-9,10-epoxide) that interact with DNA to initiate carcinogenesis (Conney, 1982).

The most important CYP450s for the activation of procarcinogens are CYP1A1, 1A2, 1B1, 2C9, 2C19, 2E1, and 3A4 (Shimada et al., 1996; Guengerich and Shimada, 1998; Shimada et al., 2001a). CYP1A1 and CYP1B1 are mainly extrahepatically expressed and can be induced by various environmental toxicants (e.g., polychlorinated biphenyls such as 2,3,7,8-tetrachlorodibenzo-*p*-dioxin, TCDD). CYP1A1 is predominantly expressed in the lung, gastrointestinal tract, placenta, brain, and vascular endothelial and smooth muscle cells, whereas CYP1B1 is mainly found in steroidogenic tissues such as breast, uterus, and prostate; both are expressed in breast tumour tissue (Modugno et al., 2003). The latter is the major estradiol hydroxylase and activation of estrogens has been postulated to be a major factor in mammary carcinogenesis. Usually, estrogens are metabolized by CYP1A1 and CYP1B1 to the 2- and 4-hydroxylated products, but both enzymes differ in their regiospecificity: whereas CYP1B1 mainly hydroxylates estrogens in the C4 position, CYP1A1 has its principal site of hydroxylation at C2. Several reports have suggested that the 4-OH catechol estrogens are most important, because they are oxidized to quinones, which represent electrophilic metabolites and are capable of forming DNA adducts (Han and Liehr, 1994). They were also shown to induce endometrial adenocarcinoma (Newbold and Liehr, 2000). However, recent studies support the view that 2-OH–derived metabolites of estrogens also can form DNA adducts with mutagenic properties and therefore may contribute to the development of cancer (Terashima et al., 2001).

An increasing number of epidemiological studies demonstrate association of certain CYP1A1/CYP1B1 genotypes with a higher risk of certain types of cancer in humans (e.g., lung cancer: Drakoulis et al., 1994; Cascorbi et al., 1996; Taioli et al., 1998; Le Marchand et al., 2000; Rojas et al., 2000; oesophagus cancer: Wu et al., 2002; prostate cancer: Suzuki et al., 2003; breast cancer: Firozi et al., 2002; endometrial cancer: Esteller et al., 1997). Particularly, recent pooled and meta-analyses yielded more consistent data and suggest that certain alleles might play a role in carcinogenesis (e.g., Hung et al., 2003; Le Marchand et al., 2003; Taioli et al., 2003; Vineis et al., 2003). Often the variant CYP1A1.2 (Ile462Val), alone or in combination with the *GSTM1-null* genotype, has been identified as important, depending on smoking, gender, and ethnicity. The Ile462Val exchange at 4889 nt (mutation 2) is strictly linked with mutation 1 (Mrozikiewicz et al., 1997). Mutation 1 (CYP1A1.1; T6235C) was the first CYP1A1 mutation detected and correlated with lung cancer. Recent studies with substantial statistical power indicated that certain CYP1B1 genotypes may be at higher risk for endometrial (Sasaki et al., 2003: variants Ala119Ser and Leu432Val) and breast cancer (Rylander-Rudqvist et al., 2003: variant Leu432Val in women who had used hormones for a long time).

It is an attractive hypothesis that individuals with high CYP gene inducibility and/or enzymatic activity and/or low inhibition capability and/or DNA repair capacity may be more susceptible to carcinogens and to developing related types of cancer. Particularly, it has been shown that alterations in catalytic activities are most important. Inter-individual variation in the enzymes involved in carcinogen metabolism can now be extensively studied using recombinant DNA and protein technology. There is optimism that such approaches will be productive in the prediction of cancer risk and toxicity of chemicals. Hence, for instance, the NIEHS has begun an Environmental Genome Project with the long-term goal of associating risks with polymorphisms of the genes involved in carcinogen metabolism (Guengerich, 1998).

Here, we describe recent progress in the *in vitro* characterization of roles of individual polymorphic variants of CYP1A1 and CYP1B1 in metabolism related to carcinogenesis and its inhibition. These studies may be helpful for developing a basis for creating functional analysis systems for comprehensive genomic studies, in which allelic variants of these enzymes can be expressed and examined for parameters relevant to metabolism of carcinogens. We do not consider variations in enzyme induction (expression), detoxification of potentially carcinogenic metabolites by phase-II enzymes, and DNA-repair enzymes, which are also important issues for (individual) cancer-prevention strategies and prediction of toxicity (e.g., Miller et al., 2001).

21.2.1.1 *CYP1A1* and *CYP1B1* Genotype-dependent Carcinogen Activation

CYP1A1

First reports on functional differences considered the two *CYP1A1* variants (wild-type: CYP1A1.1; Ile462Val variant: CYP1A1.2) known at that time and were based on measurements of aryl hydrocarbon hydroxylase activity (AHH) and 7-ethoxyresorufin deethylation activity (EROD). Kawajiri et al. (1993) demonstrated evidence for higher BaP hydroxylation activity in CYP1A1.2 than in the wild-type enzyme. Kiyohara et al. (1998) and Crofts et al. (1994) found increased AHH and EROD activity, respectively, in (human) lymphocytes from individuals homozygous for the *CYP1A1*2* allele. In contrast, Persson et al. (1997) observed no differences in K_m and V_{max} for both CYP1A1-dependent EROD and AHH activity, based on a kinetic study after expression of the two variants in yeast (Table 21.1). Because no differences in substrate affinity or V_{max} were obtained, their preliminary conclusion was that the substrate binding site probably is not affected by the amino acid substitution and that the kinetic properties

Tab. 21.1 Rates and kinetic parameters of CYP1A1-catalyzed formation of resorufin (EROD), 3-OH-BaP, 7,8-diol-BaP, and BaP diolepoxide 2 and of CYP1B1-mediated BaP procarcinogen activation[a)] by naturally occurring CYP variants.

Allele (gene)	*Allelic variant (protein)*	*EROD*			*3-OH-BaP*			*7,8-diol-BaP*			*BaP-DE2 DE2/DE1*	*Refs.*
		K_m	V_{max}	k_{cat}	K_m	V_{max}	k_{cat}	K_m	V_{max}	k_{cat}	V^b	
*CYP1A1 *1*	wild-type	0.12	34.1	284	1.44	44.6	31.0		n. d.		n. d.	Persson et al. (1997)
**2*	Ile462Val	0.12	30.8	257	1.44	39.5	27.4		n. d.		n. d.	
*CYP1A1 *1*	wild-type	2.4	3.1	1.3	appr. equal				0.6[c)]		n. d.	Zhang et al. (1996)
**2*	Ile462Val	2.8	4.4	1.6	„				0.2		n. d.	
*CYP1A1 *1*	wild-type	0.31	16.0	51.6	6.9	2.1	0.304	8.8	1.1	0.125	8.2[b)] 2.95	Schwarz et al. (2001)
**2*	Ile462Val	0.32	19.6	61.3	1.7	0.6	0.353	3.6	0.3	0.083	6.1 3.37	
**4*	Thr461Asn	0.30	22.2	74.0	6.5	1.1	0.169	9.4	0.6	0.064	4.6 3.48	
*CYP1A1 *1*	wild-type				7.3	150	20	1.9	2090	1100		Shimada et al. (2001)[a)]
*CYP1B1 *1*	wild-type				5.1	160	31	1.4	1290	920		
*CYP1B1 *2*	Arg48Gly/ Ala119Ser				7.4	440	60	1.9	1390	730		
*CYP1B1 *3*	Leu432Val				3.8	450	119	2.6	2270	870		
*CYP1B1 *6*	Arg48Gly/ Ala119Ser/ Leu432Val				5.5	220	39	2.2	1940	880		

K_m values are given in μM, V_{max} values and rates V in pmol min^{-1} $pmol^{-1}$ CYP, and catalytic efficiencies k_{cat} in μM^{-1} min^{-1}. n.d. = not determined.

a) Data (K_m in μM and V_{max} in *umu* units min^{-1} $nmol^{-1}$ of CYP) represent kinetic parameters of activation of BaP and 7,8-diol-BaP in *Salmonella typhimurium* NM2009. Substrate concentrations were: 0.6, 1.2, 1.8, and 2.4 μM for BaP and 1, 3.1, 6.2, 12.5, and 25 μM for 7,8-diol-BaP.

b) Rates at 24.5 μM 7,8-diol-BaP.

c) Rates at 40 μM BaP.

of the enzyme are only insignificantly influenced. After that, Zhang et al. (1996) confirmed these data while finding equal rates of BaP hydroxylation and only a slightly increased EROD rate for the CYP1A1.2 variant in a reconstituted system consisting of purified enzymes expressed in *Escherichia coli*. They also found that the wild-type variant CYP1A1.1 variant had the potential to produce up to about three times more bioactivated procarcinogens such as 7,8- and 9,10-dihydrodiol-BaP from BaP (Table 21.1). Because the rates were determined from a single experiment, the authors discussed this difference as not significant but as comparable rates. Nevertheless, these metabolites arise from epoxide hydroxylase-catalyzed hydrolysis of the corresponding CYP1A1-catalyzed BaP-epoxides and represent the ultimate procarcinogenic compounds. Hence, the data of Zhang et al. (1996) constituted the first preliminary evidence for cancer-related functional differences in CYP1A1 variants.

In view of the conflicting results, Schwarz et al. (2001) considered it important to analyze the kinetic properties of the CYP1A1 variants in both BaP and 7,8-dihydrodiol-BaP metabolism. The study was designed to characterize more unambiguously the potential of the respective CYP1A1 variants to produce higher levels of both the ultimate procarcinogenic diol-BaPs and the ultimate carcinogenic BaP-diolepoxides (Table 21.1). Three CYP1A1 variants (http://www.imm.ki.se/CYPalleles/cyp1a1.htm) – including a novel one (CYP1A1.4; Thr461Asn; Cascorbi et al., 1996) – were coexpressed with the redox partner human P450 reductase in insect cells. The assays for EROD activity revealed almost equal K_m values, whereas V_{max} values for both rare variants, CYP1A1.2 and CYP1A1.4, were slightly higher, confirming data obtained by Zhang et al. for CYP1A1.2.

Most active in (total) BaP metabolism was wild-type CYP1A1.1 with 3.3 pmol min^{-1} $pmol^{-1}$ CYP (100%), followed by variants CYP1A1.4 (1.55; ~50%) and CYP1A1.2 (2.3; ~70%) (Schwarz et al., 2001). Here, differential substrate specificity becomes evident, since EROD activity tended to be highest in CYP1A1.4 and lowest in CYP1A1.1. There are interesting differences between the variants in the formation of the procarcinogenic diols. Total diol formation by CYP1A1.1 and CYP1A1.4 was approximately equal, whereas that by CYP1A1.2 was only half (in accordance with data obtained for CYP1A1.2 by Zhang et al.). Interestingly, in comparing the relative diol-to-phenol formation efficiency, it became evident that CYP1A1.4 is the variant exhibiting the highest relative diol formation potency, followed by CYP1A1.1, whereas CYP1A1.2 has the lowest potency (only about half that of CYP1A1.4). With regard to differences in ultimate carcinogen diolepoxide 2 (DE2) formation, it is important to note that wild-type CYP1A1 exhibited the highest production rate. However, comparing the relative formation of DE2-to-DE1, both rare variants show a significantly increased capability for producing the ultimate carcinogenic product DE2.

Taking into account that 2-OH-derived metabolites of estrogens also can form DNA adducts with mutagenic properties (Terashima et al., 2001), we started to examine whether the CYP1A1 polymorphisms lead to differences in oestrogen hydroxylation. Assays were performed using a reconstituted system containing the each purified CYP1A1 variant, purified human P450 reductase, and lipid (Schwarz et al., 2003 a). Confirming the former findings for wild-type CYP1A1, the formation of 2-OH-estradiol significantly exceeded that of 4-OH-estradiol. But with 2-OH/4-OH ratios of 30, 40, and 15, for CYP1A1.1, CYP1A1.2, and CYP1A1.4, respectively, preliminary data demonstrate a remarkable influence of polymorphisms on the regioselectivity of hydroxylation and a significant and markedly increased activity (approximately 5-fold) of the CYP1A1.2 variant for all three hydroxylation sites, C2, C4, and C15, for both estradiol and estrone hydroxylation (D. Schwarz, unpublished results).

In a former study Schwarz et al. (2000) also reported that progesterone and testosterone hydroxylation activities were affected by polymorphisms of the CYP1A1 gene in a regio- and stereoselective manner. CYP1A1.4 had a 3-times higher K_m and V_{max}

for 6β- and 16α-hydroxylation of progesterone than CYP1A1.1 and CYP1A1.2. Testosterone 6β-hydroxylation activity was highest for variants CYP1A1.1 and CYP1A1.4; however, the catalytic efficiencies were essentially similar for all three variants examined. In another study, a kinetic analysis by Chernogolov et al. (2003) showed that wild-type CYP1A1.1 and CYP1A1.2 were equally efficient for formation of all-*trans*-retinoic acid from all-*trans*-retinal, whereas CYP1A1.4 was about half as efficient.

CYP1B1

Compared with CYP1A1, the identification of polymorphisms in the coding region of *CYP1B1* is rather young (http://www.imm.ki.se/CYPalleles/cyp1b1.htm). Several of the mutations resulted in an inactive enzyme and were associated with glaucoma in homozygotes. Four others, however, encoded functional enzymes, and the consequences of these polymorphisms, and certain combinations of them, have been functionally characterized (Table 21.2).

Shimada et al. (1999) assessed four CYP1B1 variants, namely wild-type, Leu432Val (CYP1B1.3), Ala119Ser, and the double mutation Ala119Ser/Leu432Val, to find out whether CYP1B1 polymorphisms affect catalytic activities toward a variety of substrates, including diverse procarcinogens and estrogens (Table 21.2). Kinetic analyses of estradiol hydroxylation showed that V_{max} values for 4-hydroxylation (and 2-hydroxylation) ranged between 0.9 and 1.5 pmol min^{-1} $pmol^{-1}$ CYP (0.3 and 0.6) in these CYP1B1 variants, with K_m values ranging from 1 to 9 μM. Interestingly, the ratio of formation of 4-OH- to 2-OH-estradiol product was higher for the variants containing a Val in position 432 instead of Leu. The same trend was found in the ratio of estrone hydroxylation products. Polymorphisms in the *CYP1B1* gene also affected kinetic parameters of testosterone and progesterone hydroxylation. No effect of these alterations was observed on procarcinogen activation activities of the variants, which were found to be essentially similar, except that the Ala119Ser variant was slightly more active (1.2–1.5-fold).

Li et al. (2000) found that all variants with the Leu432Val substitution showed higher catalytic efficiencies for both 4- and 2-hydroxylation of estradiol. This was mainly due to lower K_m values than for the variants with Leu in position 432 (wild-type and the Asn453Ser variant). Again, no effect of these alterations was observed on properties of other CYP1B1-catalyzed reactions such as EROD, bufuralol hydroxylation, and most important, epoxidation of 7,8-diol-BaP (Table 21.2).

McLellan et al. (2000) expressed wild-type CYP1B1.1 and the double variant CYP1B1.2 (Arg48Gly/Ala119Ser), which is found at a frequency of about 27% in a Caucasian population, in yeast and mammalian COS-1 cells and found no significant kinetic differences in estradiol hydroxylation (Table 21.2). Because the authors also observed similarly stable expression, their conclusion was that these substitutions do not alter function and stability of the protein. Notably, a small but significant kinetic difference was found in the apparent K_m for EROD (data not shown in the table).

Hanna et al. (2000) expressed wild-type and five polymorphic CYP1B1 variants and assayed them in a reconstituted system containing the purified CYP1B1 variant, purified (rat) P450 reductase, and dilaurylphosphatidylcholine, to determine possible differences in oestrogen hydroxylase activity (Table 21.2). Except for the Leu432Val variant, for which K_m was at least twice as high, all CYP1B1 variants exhibited rela-

Tab. 21.2 Kinetic parameters of CYP1B1-catalyzed 2-OH- and 4-OH-estradiol formation and CYP1B1-mediated procarcinogen activation [a)]

Allele	*Allelic Variant*	*BaP-DE2* [b)]			*2-OH-Estradiol*			*4-OH-Estradiol*			*Refs.*
(gene)	*(protein)* [c)]	K_m	V_{max}	k_{cat}	K_m	V_{max}	k_{cat}	K_m	V_{max}	k_{cat}	
CYP1B1 *1 [c)]	wild-type	5.0	3.1	0.62	11.2	0.31	0.028	12.5	1.6	0.128	Li et al. (2000)
*3	Leu432Val	6.2	3.9	0.63	3.6	0.37	0.108	3.8	1.7	0.447	
*4	Asn453Ser	4.8	2.8	0.58	11.5	0.32	0.028	10.7	1.5	0.140	
*6	Arg48Gly/Ala119Ser/ Leu432Val	5.1	3.0	0.59	3.4	0.30	0.088	3.1	1.6	0.516	
	Arg48Gly/Leu432Val		n.d.		4.2	0.40	0.095	3.7	1.6	0.432	
	Ala119Ser/Leu432Val		n.d.		3.5	0.36	0.103	3.3	1.5	0.455	
	Leu432Val/Asn453Ser		n.d.		3.9	0.39	0.100	3.7	1.8	0.487	
CYP1B1 *1	wild-type		n.d.		10.6	0.22	0.020	3.5	0.94	0.27	McLellan et al. (2000)
*2	Arg48Gly/Ala119Ser		n.d.		10.2	0.17	0.017	3.3	0.80	0.24	
CYP1B1 *1 [c)]	wild-type		580 [d)]		6.9	0.42	0.06	5.1	0.91	0.18	Shimada et al. (1999)
*3	Leu432Val		590 [d)]		5.7	0.46	0.08	5.3	1.45	0.27	
	Ala119Ser/Leu432Val		660 [d)]		0.9	0.33	0.37	2.5	1.10	0.44	
	Ala119Ser		720 [d)]		8.4	0.61	0.07	5.2	1.15	0.22	
CYP1B1 *1 [c)]	wild-type		n.d.		21	2.2	0.110	11	3.7	0.33	Hanna et al. (2000) [e)]
*3	Leu432Val		n.d.		34	1.9	0.055	40	4.4	0.11	
*5	Arg48Gly/Leu432Val		n.d.		29	3.2	0.110	19	6.0	0.32	
	Arg48Gly/Ala119Ser/ Asn453Ser		n.d.		29	2.5	0.086	15	4.4	0.29	
	Ala119Ser/Leu432Val		n.d.		18	2.3	0.130	10	3.8	0.37	
	Leu432Val/Asn453Ser		n.d.		39	2.8	0.071	17	4.5	0.27	
CYP1B1 *1	wild-type		2.1 [f)]		16	0.49	0.031	14	2.2	0.16	Shimada et al. (2001)
*2	Arg48Gly/Ala119Ser		2.6 [f)]		9.7	0.31	0.032	9.1	1.1	0.12	
*3	Leu432Val		1.3 [f)]		18	0.47	0.027	15	3.0	0.20	
*5	Arg48Gly/Leu432Val		2.0 [f)]		7.3	0.23	0.032	5.8	1.2	0.21	
*6	Arg48Gly/Ala119Ser/ Leu432Val		1.5 [f)]		8.1	0.29	0.036	6.7	1.7	0.25	
	Arg48Gly		2.9 [f)]		12	0.30	0.025	9.1	1.1	0.12	
	Ala119Ser		2.0 [f)]		17	0.58	0.034	15	2.7	0.18	
	Ala119Ser/Leu432Val		1.1 [f)]		12	0.35	0.030	13	2.6	0.21	

a) K_m values are given in μM, V_{max} values in pmol min^{-1} $pmol^{-1}$ CYP, and catalytic efficiencies k_{cat} in μM^{-1} min^{-1}. n.d. = not determined.

b) The specific metabolite (±)(*r*-7,*t*-8,*t*-9,*c*-10)-7,8,9,10-tetrahydrotetraol-BaP, which is representative for DE2 formation has been determined.

c) In this table we used the nomenclature introduced by the Human Cytochrome P450 (CYP) Allele Committee (http://www.imm.ki.se/CYPalleles/cyp1b1.htm), which is based on the following sequence for wild-type CYP1B1: Arg48, Ala119, Leu432, and Asn453 (*CYP1B1*1*). Note that in the original papers of Li et al. (2000) a nomenclature was used that was based on the amino acid sequence for wild-type CYP1B1 published originally by Sutter et al. (1994).

d) Data represent procarcinogen activation activities of (–)7,8-diol-BaP to DNA-damaging products measured in a *Salmonella typhimurium* NM2009 *umu* response system; activities are given in *umu* units min^{-1} $nmol^{-1}$ CYP.

e) 16α-OH activity was also determined in this study, but the data were not included in this table.

f) Data represent rates (given in pmol min^{-1} $pmol^{-1}$ CYP) of 7,8-diol-BaP formation in presence of rat liver epoxide hydrolase determined at 20 μM BaP.

tively small differences in the kinetic parameters and thus in catalytic efficiencies for estradiol hydroxylation.

In a systematic and detailed study, Shimada et al. (2001 a) compared activities for metabolic activation of a number of PAHs and PAH diols as well as other procarcinogens by CYP1A1, four CYP1B1 variants, and other CYP enzymes (Table 21.1). The four CYP1B1 variants had similar catalytic specificities, except that CYP1B1.3 (Leu432Val variant) had a two to four times the efficiency in catalyzing BaP as the other three variants. We should mention that other variants showed slightly higher activities for activation of certain other procarcinogens also studied in this paper, but not further discussed in this review.

Recently, Shimada et al. (2001 b) summarized the patterns of estradiol and BaP oxidation by expressing eight CYP1B1 variants together with P450 reductase in *E. coli*. A tendency for higher 4-hydroxylation by the Arg48 variants compared to the Gly48 variants was reported, but no significant variations in 2-hydroxylation in all of the variants was found. Interestingly, ratios of formation of 4-OH/2-OH were higher in all variants containing Val432 than in the corresponding Leu432 forms. In contrast, Leu432 variants of CYP1B1 showed higher rates of BaP oxidation to the procarcinogenic product 7,8-diol-BaP.

21.2.1.2 Genotype-dependent Inhibition of Carcinogen Activation

Chemoprevention by dietary intervention will be an important cancer-prevention strategy (Greenwald, 2002; Sabichi et al., 2003; Conney, 2004). Natural polyphenols such as flavonoids are among the promising candidate compounds as they show antioxidative and anticarcinogenic effects in a variety of animal and cell culture experiments (Yang et al., 2001). One mechanism of action in mediating the protective effect may be inhibition of procarcinogen activation (Schwarz et al., 2003 a, b). Recently, a case-control study demonstrated an inverse correlation between lung cancer risk and a diet rich in the flavonoids quercetin (onions, apples) and naringin (white grapefruit) (Le Marchand et al., 2000). The effect of onions was strongest on squamous cell carcinoma and was modified by the *CYP1A1* genotype. These findings suggest that foods rich in certain flavonoids may protect against specific forms of lung cancer and that inhibition of CYP1A1-dependent procarcinogen bioactivation may be the underlying mechanism (Le Marchand et al., 2000).

To test this hypothesis, Schwarz et al. (2004) studied the inhibitory effects of quercetin and naringin on the terminal step in the bioactivation of BaP, the epoxidation of 7,8-dihydrodiol-BaP to the ultimate carcinogenic product, BaP-diolepoxide 2, using different allelic variants of human *CYP1A1* (Table 21.3). Quercetin potently inhibited diolepoxide-2 formation of all CYP1A1 types, with IC_{50} values between 1.6 μM and 7.0 μM (Table 21.2). The differences between the wild-type enzyme and the two variants were statistically significant ($P<0.01$). Kinetic analysis demonstrated that quercetin is a mixed-type inhibitor of CYP1A1.1, CYP1A1.2, and CYP1A1.4 with K_i values of 2.0, 6.4, and 9.3 μM, respectively. In contrast to quercetin, naringin inhibited BaP-diolepoxide-2 formation only slightly.

To our knowledge, this is the first study reporting that inhibition of procarcinogen activation can be a genotype-dependent process. The 7,8-diol-BaP epoxidation activity

Tab. 21.3 IC_{50} values and kinetic parameters of inhibition by quercetin of BaP diolepoxide 2 formation by human CYP1A1 allelic variants.[a)]

	IC_{50} (μM)	K_i (μM)	Type of inhibition[b)]
CYP1A1.1	1.6 ± 0.3	2.0 ± 0.4	mixed type
CYP1A1.2	4.4 ± 0.5	6.4 ± 0.6	mixed type
CYP1A1.4	7.0 ± 1.0	9.3 ± 2.4	mixed type

a) DE2 formation by epoxidation of 7,8-dihydrodiol-BaP was measured in a reconstituted system consisting of purified CYP1A1 variant, purified human P450 reductase, and dilaurylphosphatidylcholine.
b) For all variants the fits for mixed type inhibition were better than those for noncompetitive, although only slightly. Therefore, based on the present data an unambiguous decision cannot be made as to whether inhibition is of mixed type or noncompetitive. Nevertheless, the K_i values determined for both models were not significantly different.

of wild-type CYP1A1 is signifycantly more strongly inhibited by quercetin. Consequently, carriers of the alleles *CYP1A1*2* and *CYP1A1*4* may be at a higher risk of developing lung cancer. Future studies should consider possible genetic variance in both procarcinogen activation and its inhibition caused by polymorphic enzymes.

21.2.1.3 Trends

Summarizing the results, for both CYP1A1 and CYP1B1 several haplotypes occurring in humans have different catalytic properties, as shown by *in vitro* assays using recombinant enzymes. Because a complicating issue with functional relevant polymorphisms is that they can have variable results with different substrates and reactions, it is necessary to study specific cancer-related reactions; otherwise it may be time- and money-wasting. Moreover, in general, these studies should include several reactions – instead of only one – because many of the enzymes, e.g., CYP1A1, catalyze both activation and detoxification pathways – and the balance between these pathways could be decisive. Differences have been found for estradiol, estrone, and BaP procarcinogen metabolism which – although not usually dramatic – may contribute to individual variations in cancer risk. Interestingly, for risk estimation it was found that different allelic variants of CYP1A1 showed differences in the inhibition of carcinogen activation by quercetin, a widely distributed flavonoid in human diets. In our opinion, this might be an important issue to be considered for evaluation of dietary effects on individual disease risk. Further studies will be required to prove the importance of such a genotype-dependent inhibition.

In conclusion, the results obtained in the area of extrahepatic CYP polymorphism and risk of cancer are promising. Further studies are an urgent matter to find correlations between a risk-associated CYP allele and cancer development and finally to propose personalized prevention strategies.

21.2.2
Toxicity by Variants of Thiopurine Methyltransferase (TPMT)

Human thiopurine S-methyltransferase (TPMT; EC 2.1.1.67) is a cytosolic enzyme that catalyses the S-methylation of thiopurine drugs such as 6-thioguanine, 6-mercaptopurine (6-MP), and its pro-drug azathioprine (AZA), which are widely used in treating malignancies (leukaemia), rheumatic diseases, dermatologic conditions, inflammatory bowel disease, and solid organ transplant rejection (Weinshilboum and Sladek, 1980; Woodson and Weinshilboum, 1983; Weinshilboum, 1992; Weinshilboum et al., 1999; Hamdan-Khalil et al., 2003; Nagasubramanian et al., 2003). These pro-drugs undergo metabolic activation, and the therapeutic effect correlates best with concentration of the active 6-thioguanine (6-TGN) metabolites, which are responsible for their therapeutic efficacy and cytotoxicity. Therapeutic response can be maximized when patients achieve therapeutic 6-TGN levels.

A major factor responsible for inter-individual differences in toxicity and therapeutic efficacy of thiopurine drugs in humans are differences in the methylation activity of TPMT. Genetic polymorphisms are associated with decreased activity, which is also associated with increased toxicity. Numerous clinical studies have found intermediate and deficient methylators to be at risk for moderate-to-profound haematopoietic toxicity when treated with standard doses of these medications (Lennard et al., 1987, 1989; Evans et al., 1991; Krynetski et al., 1996; Evans et al., 2001; Nagasubramanian et al., 2003).

TPMT activity is inherited as an autosomal codominant trait. TPMT activity has a trimodal phenotype distribution. ~90% of the African American and Caucasian population have a high methylation activity (high methylator phenotype; HM), 10% have an intermediate activity (intermediate methylator; IM), and 0.3% are devoid of TPMT activity (deficient methylator; DM) owing to homozygousity for alleles with no functional activity (Weinshilboum and Sladek, 1980). Genetic polymorphism of *TPMT* has been observed in many populations, including Caucasians, Asians, Africans and African Americans. The human *TPMT* gene maps to chromosome 6p22.3 and consists of 10 exons, eight of which encode protein (Szumlanski et al., 1996). The polymorphic alleles are characterized by nonsynonymous SNPs in the open reading frame (ORF) that are associated with low enzyme activity owing to enhanced degradation of the mutant protein (Tai et al., 1997). More than 10 *TPMT* alleles have been identified. Three alleles, *TPMT*2* (G238C), *TPMT*3A* (G460A and A719G), and *TPMT*3C* (A719G), represent the most prevalent mutant alleles and account for 80%–95% of the instances of deficient and intermediate enzyme activity in Caucasians and African Americans. Patients heterozygous for these alleles all have intermediate activity, and patients homozygous for these alleles are TPMT-deficient (Yates et al., 1997; Hon et al., 1999). Additionally, compound heterozygotes (*TPMT*2/3A*, *TPMT*2/TPMT*3C* and *TPMT*3A/3C*) are also TPMT-deficient (Yates et al., 1997). *TPMT*3A* is the most prevalent mutant allele in Caucasians, and *TPMT*3C* is the more common mutant allele in Asian, African, and African American populations. In addition, four rare TPMT allelic variants have been identified. Their mutations were located in exon 7 (*G430C*) (Colombel et al., 2000), exon 10 (*T681G*) (Spire-

Vayron de la Moureyre et al., 1998), exon 3 (*A83T*), and exon 6 (*C374T*). The two variants harbouring the Gly144Arg (*TPMT*10*) and His227Gln (*TPMT*7*) substitutions were reported previously in a patient receiving azathioprine (Colombel et al., 2000) and in an individual with intermediate methylating capacity (Spire-Vayron de la Moureyre et al., 1998), respectively. The two other variants are novel and carry the amino acid substitutions, Ser125Leu (*TPMT*12*) and Glu28Val (*TPMT*13*) (Hamdan-Khalil et al., 2003). The His227Gln (*TPMT*7*) variant retained only 10% of the intrinsic clearance value (V_{max}/K_m ratio) of the wild-type enzyme. The Ser125Leu (*TPMT*12*) and Gly144Arg (*TPMT*10*) variants were associated with a significant decrease in intrinsic clearance values, retaining about 30% of the wild-type enzyme, whereas the Glu28Val variant had a more modest decrease (57% of the wild-type enzyme) (Hamdan-Khalil et al., 2003).

Furthermore, a polymorphic locus consisting of a 17- or 18-base-pair repeat element (VNTR) has been identified within the promoter region of the *TPMT* gene. The VNTR lengths varied from three to nine repeats. In Caucasians, mostly polymorphic loci with four or five repeat elements (*VNTR*4* and *VNTR*5*) were found. There was an inverse relationship between the sum of repeat units on the two alleles and the level of TPMT activity, although the effects were quantitatively small. Furthermore, *VNTR*5* and *TPMT*3A* were in linkage disequilibrium. Nevertheless, the potential clinical significance of the VNTR polymorphism remains unclear (Yan et al., 2000).

In summary, the *TPMT* genotype has significant influence on drug disposition and risk of excessive toxicity. Genetically low or deficient TPMT activity is associated with thiopurine drug toxicity (Evans et al., 1991; Schutz et al., 1993; Lennard et al., 1997). Clinical reports from studies in children with acute lymphoblastic leukaemia have confirmed that essentially all homozygous TPMT-deficient patients develop haematopoietic toxicity if treated with conventional doses of thiopurines, whereas most, but not all, patients with a heterozygous TPMT phenotype have intermediate tolerance to thiopurine therapy. Patients with no documented TPMT mutations tolerated 6-mercaptopurine during 84% of scheduled therapy compared with 65% in heterozygous and only 7% in homozygous patients (Relling et al., 1999; Evans et al., 2001; Nagasubramanian et al., 2003).

In summary, to avoid hematotoxicity in TPMT-deficient or heterozygous patients, genetic testing of the TPMT polymorphisms prior to therapy should become routine (Schwab et al., 2002). Especially for the outcome of therapy for childhood lymphoblastic leukaemia, genetically determined TPMT activity may be a substantial regulator of the cytotoxic effect of 6-mercaptopurine (Lennard et al., 1990).

21.2.3
Dihydropyrimidine Dehydrogenase

Dihydropyrimidine dehydrogenase (DPD) is the first and rate-limiting enzyme in the catabolism of the pyrimidine bases uracil and thymidine (Wasternack, 1980; Nagasubramanian et al., 2003) and plays a significant role in the pharmacokinetics of 5-fluorouracil (5-FU). The antimetabolite 5-fluorouracil is used to treat a wide variety of cancers. DPD catabolizes ~80%–90% of an administered dose of 5-FU to the inactive 5,6-dihydro-5-fluorouracil (Heggie et al., 1987; Nagasubramanian et al., 2003) and therefore determines the amount of fluorouracil that is ultimately available to be metabolized to the cytotoxic nucleotide 5-FdUMP (anabolic pathway). Administration of conventional doses of 5-FU can individually result in profound bone marrow and gastrointestinal toxicity. Dihydropyrimidine dehydrogenase is an enzyme that exhibits up to 20-fold variation in activity among individuals (Lu et al., 1993; Etienne et al., 1994; Watters and McLeod, 2003). Therefore, patients who are deficient in DPD (around 0.1% to 3% of the Caucasian population) experience profound systemic toxicity in response to 5-FU (Johnson et al., 1999), because of excessive amounts of 5-FdUMP. Patients with 5-FU-related toxicity of grades 3–4 (haematopoietic, gastrointestinal, or neurological), as graded by the World Health Organization, have decreased peripheral DPD activity, varying from 36% to 59%, as defined by DPD levels <70% of the mean value observed in a normal population (Milano et al., 1999; van Kuilenburg et al., 2001; Nagasubramanian et al., 2003). The molecular basis of the differences in enzyme activity are genetic.

To date, more than 19 mutant alleles have been reported to be associated with reduced DPD activity (McLeod et al., 1998; Innocenti and Ratain, 2002; Watters and McLeod, 2003). The *DPYD* gene has been mapped to chromosome 1p22 and consists of 23 exons (Wei et al., 1998). In the general population, 3%–5% of individuals are heterozygous carriers of mutations that inactivate DPD, and 0.1% of individuals are homozygous for mutations that inactivate DPD (Lu, Zhang, and Diasio, 1993; Gonzalez and Fernandez-Salguero, 1995; Ridge et al., 1998a,b). The most frequent mutation in patients with partial or complete DPD deficiency accounts for about 50% of known nonfunctional alleles and is caused by a G → A transition within the 5′-splicing site of intron 14 (exon 14-skipping mutation, *DPYD*2A*), resulting in loss of exon 14 and production of a nonfunctional protein truncated by 55 amino acids with virtually no enzyme activity (Johnson et al., 1999; van Kuilenburg et al., 2001). The frequency of the *DPYD*2A* allele in the Caucasian populations is 0.9% (Raida et al., 2001; van Kuilenburg et al., 2001). Family studies in paediatric patients with DPD-deficiency phenotypes and in cancer patients experiencing moderate to severe toxicity after 5-FU administration show poor genotype–phenotype concordance. Nearly 25% of cancer patients who had grade 3–4 toxicity following 5-FU treatment were heterozygous for the *DPYD*2A* allele (Raida et al., 2001). However, *DPYD*2A* is not the only mechanism for severe 5-FU toxicity. Indeed, many patients with severe 5-FU toxicity have no detected mutations in the coding region of the *DPYD* gene (Collie-Duguid et al., 2000). Whereas 57% of cancer patients with 5-FU toxicity had a molecular basis for reduced DPD activity in one study (van Kuilenburg et al., 2000), only 17% of patients in another study had a molecular basis for their deficient DPD phenotype (Collie-Duguid et al., 2000).

Despite the controversial results, the apparently high prevalence of the *DPYD* mutation associated with lack of DPD activity in the normal population warrants genetic screening for the presence of these mutations in cancer patients before administration of 5-FU. Toxico- and pharmacogenomics has the challenge of identifying early those patients likely to experience severe 5-FU toxicity.

21.2.4
UDP-glucuronosyl Transferase Enzymes

Glucuronidation can also occur as a toxification step, especially acylglucuronidation, as found in the metabolism of valproic acid, diclofenac, and others. UDP-glucuronosyltransferase (UGT) is a microsomal enzyme that is responsible for glucuronidation reactions (Nagasubramanian et al., 2003) and is thus a key enzyme in humans and other mammalian species for detoxification of a diverse range of endogenous compounds, including bilirubin and steroid hormones, and of toxicants (i. e., chemicals, drugs, carcinogens, and environmental pollutants) (Miners et al., 2002).

Several studies found inter-individual differences in the content of UGTs in the liver and other organs, such as in the kidney, intestine, and steroid target tissues, most likely caused by differential *UGT* gene expression (Miners et al., 2002). UGT proteins exist as a superfamily of enzymes (UGT 1A, 2A, and 2B subfamilies) (Mackenzie et al., 1997). UGT 1A isoforms are encoded by a single gene locus on chromosome 2q37 (Owens and Ritter, 1995; Mackenzie et al., 1997; Miners et al., 2002). *UGT1A* comprises at least 12 promoters and first exons, which are spliced separately to common exons 2–5. The *UGT1A* locus encodes nine functional enzymes: UGT 1A1, 1A3, 1A4, 1A5, 1A6, 1A7, 1A8, 1A9, and 1A10 (Miners et al., 2002). The substrate specificities of the various isoforms include bilirubin, amines, and planar and bulky phenols. UGT2 mRNAs are transcribed from individual genes, because UGT2 enzymes are encoded by separate genes clustered on chromosome 4. UGT2 enzymes exhibit differences in amino acid sequence throughout the entire polypeptide chain. Family-2 human enzymes include UGT 2A1, 2B4, 2B7, 2B10, 2B11, 2B15, and 2B17. The numerous members of the family-2 enzymes catalyze glucuronidation of diverse chemicals, including steroids, bile acids, and opioids.

Genetic polymorphisms of UGT isoforms are potentially of toxicological and physiological signifycance. Several genetic polymorphisms have been described, namely UGT 1A1, 1A6, 1A7, 2B4, 2B7, and 2B15. UGT1A1 is primarily responsible for glucuronidation of bilirubin *in vivo*. Polymorphisms in UGT1A1 often result in altered expression and activity of this enzyme, leading to decreased capacity to glucuronidate bilirubin (Burchell, 2003). The frequencies of individual UGT1A1 polymorphisms show extensive variability across ethnic groups. Three forms of inheritable unconjugated hyperbilirubinaemia exist, leading to constitutional unconjugated jaundice, Crigler–Najjar type I and II, or Gilbert syndrome (Mackenzie et al., 1997; Burchell and Hume, 1999). The prevalence of Gilbert syndrome is 3%–10% in Caucasians; and based on genotyping, the prevalence of Crigler–Najjar type I and II is 7%–19%.

There is evidence to suggest that individuals with Gilbert syndrome may be at greater risk of toxicity from xenobiotics metabolised by UGT1A1. Gilbert syndrome usually arises from a polymorphism in the *UGT1A1* promoter, which contains a variable number of tandem repeats (VNTR). These TA repeat elements, $(TA)_{5-8}TAA$, influence UGT1A1 expression by altering transcriptional activity (Bosma et al., 1995; Beutler et al., 1998; Burchell and Hume, 1999). In contrast, a six-repeat allele $(TA)_6TAA$ is the most common wild-type *UGT1A1*1*, leading to normal UGT1A1 expression and normal toxicity risk. *UGT1A1* expression decreases with increasing number of TA repeats (Beutler et al., 1998; Iyer et al., 1999). Homozygousity for the TA-insertion alleles $(TA)_{7/8}TAA$ is required for Gilbert syndrome (Bosma et al., 1995; Monaghan et al., 1996; Akaba et al., 1998; Ando et al., 1998; Maruo et al., 1999), although not necessarily for manifestation of hyperbilirubinaemia, probably because of nongenetic factors including bilirubin production, hepatic uptake, diet, and therapeutic drug use. In individuals of African origin, an uncommon $(TA)_5TAA$ variant has been reported, which appears to function normally. Although the frequency of the TA-insertion alleles is low (~3%) in Japanese and Chinese people, missense mutations (particularly Gly71Arg) in the *UGT1A1* coding region lead to Gilbert syndrome in these populations.

Irinotecan is an anticancer drug with strong activity through an inhibition of topoisomerase I. Irinotecan itself is a pro-drug, which requires activation to its active metabolite, SN-38. SN-38 is glucuronidated by UGT1A1 to form an inactive metabolite (SN-38 glucuronide), which is excreted in the small intestine. With increased levels of SN-38, dose-limiting toxicity of irinotecan is observed (Gupta et al., 1994). There is evidence from several studies that glucuronidation of the active metabolite of the anticancer drug irinotecan was decreased in livers homozygous for the $(TA)_7$-TAA allele (the *UGT1A1*28* allele), and patients with mutant *UGT1A1* alleles are over-represented amongst those experiencing severe toxicity (Iyer et al., 1999; Ando et al., 2000). Therefore, it seems that polymorphism in UGT1A1 can influence the outcome of irinotecan therapy. Indeed, the presence of seven repeats, in contrast to the wild-type allele *UGT1A1*1*, results in the variant allele *UGT1A1*28*. The *UGT1A1*28* allele is associated with reduced *UGT1A1* expression, leading to reduced SN-38 glucuronidation (Fisher et al., 2000, 2001; Iyer et al., 1998, 1999, 2002). This leads to an increase in the active metabolite SN-38 and a higher risk of developing toxicity and an increased chance of developing diarrhoea and leucopoenia.

Determination of the *UGT1A1* genotypes may be clinically useful for predicting severe toxicity not only to irinotecan.

21.3
Involvement of Xenobiotic Transporter Systems in Toxicogenomics

Xenobiotic transporters are major factors in the distribution of toxicants and carcinogens; therefore, their polymorphic expression can also be postulated to be an important modulator in the defence against toxic compounds and carcinogens.

Active transport processes of substrates through biological membranes have now become a key concept in the disposition of diverse compounds. Transport proteins are located ubiquitously throughout the body, but many carriers are found preferentially in several absorptive and excretory tissues, including the intestinal epithelia, the liver, and tubular epithelial cells of the kidneys (Lee, 2000; Ayrton and Morgan, 2001). By analogy to phase-I and phase-II reactions of xenobiotic and drug metabolism, transporter-mediated active gastrointestinal, biliary, and renal excretion of compounds is now considered a phase-III reaction. Moreover, transporters are essential components of blood–tissue barrier sites, including the blood–brain, blood–placenta-, and blood–

testis barriers (Cordon-Cardo et al., 1990; Rao et al., 1999). In these sensitive organs, transporters serve as a defence mechanism to protect the tissue against toxic substrates.

According to their principal direction of substrate passage into or out of the cell, transmembrane transporters can be subdivided into uptake and efflux systems. However, under physiological conditions some carriers can mediate substrate passage in either direction. Important members of uptake carrier systems include organic anion transporters (OATPs, SLCO), organic cation transporters (OCTs, SLC22A), dipeptide transporters (PEPTs, SLC15A), nucleoside transporters (CNTs, SLC28A), and monocarboxylate carriers (MCTs, SLC28A). The ATP binding cassette (ABC) family of transmembrane transporters are mainly efflux carrier systems that are supposed to play a major role in detoxification processes. This large and phylogenetically ancient protein family can be found ubiquitously in bacteria, archaea, and eukaryotes (Higgins, 2001). Efflux carriers of the ABC family have been recognized as major factors in the disposition of xenobiotics and drugs. Currently, members of the ABCB and ABCC subfamilies of ABC transporters are the focus of toxicological investigations.

21.3.1 MDR1 (ABCB1)

The most extensively investigated efflux transporter is the product of the *MDR1* gene (*ABCB1*), P-glycoprotein (Pgp). Pgp is one of the major mediators of the multidrug-resistance phenotype of cancer cells against a variety of antitumor drugs (Juranka et al., 1989). By overexpressing this efflux carrier, cells protect themselves from the accumulation of cytotoxic drugs in the cytosol. Pgp is localized in diverse excretory and absorptive tissues, such as the canalicular (apical) membrane of hepatocytes, the brush border membrane of proximal tubular cells of the kidney, and the apical membrane of the intestinal lining (Tanigawara, 2000). This localization implies that the physiological function of Pgp is to diminish the absorption of toxicants and to mediate their biliary and renal excretion. Pgp is also localized in capillary endothelial cells of blood–tissue barrier sites, most importantly at the blood–brain barrier (de Lang et al, 1998). There Pgp helps to prevent the passage of toxicants into sensitive tissues. The substrate specificity of Pgp is extraordinarily broad and includes structurally diverse compounds (Table 21.4). Interestingly, Pgp shares a variety of substrates with the phase-I metabolizing enzyme CYP3A4. This and the strong colocalization of Pgp and CYP3A4 indicate their combined action in a coordinated defence mechanism against xenobiotics (Wacher et al., 1995).

Genetic polymorphisms of *MDR1* either alter the transport function or the level of Pgp expression. The transport function determines the efficiency and substrate specificity of a carrier protein, which is most accurately expressed by the substrate concentration at half maximal transport velocity, designated K_m. The amount of transport protein expressed is a key parameter of transport capacity. Induction of Pgp by, e.g., rifampin, significantly alters blood plasma levels of the cardiac glycoside digoxin after oral application (Greiner et al., 1999). Thus, variations in intestinal Pgp expression levels apparently influence the individual exposure to xenobiotics.

Tab. 21.4 Substrates of P-glycoprotein.

Category	*Drug*	*Category*	*Drug*
Antineoplastic agents	Actinomycin D	β blocker	Bunitrolol
	Daunorubicin		Celiprolol
	Doxorubicin		Talinolol
	Doxetaxel	CNS drugs	Fluphenazine
	Irinotecan		Perphenazin
	Mitomycin C		Perphenazine
	Mitoxantrone		Phenoxazine
	Paclitaxel		Phenytoin
	Tamoxifen	H_1 antihistamines	Fexofenadine
	Tenoposide		Terfenadine
	Topotecan	H_2 antihistamines	Cimetidine
	Vinblastine		Ranitidine
	Vincristine	HIV protease inhibitors	Amprenavir
Antibiotics	Cefazolin		Indinavir
	Cefoperazon		Nelfinavir
	Erythromycin		Ritonavir
	Levofloxacin		Saquinavir
	Sparfloxacin	Immunosuppressants	Cyclosporine A
Antiemetics	Domperidon		Tacrolimus
	Ondansetron	Lipid-lowering drugs	Atorvastatine
Cardiac drugs	Amiodaron		Lovastatine
	Digitoxin	Morphins	Morphine
	Digoxin		Loperamide
	Propafenone	Steroids	Aldosterone
	Quinidine		Dexamethasone
Ca blockers	Diltiazem		Hydrocortisone
	Mibefradil	Others	Colchicine
	Nicardipine		Debrisoquine
	Verapamil		Losartan
			Sestamibi

Up to now, more than 20 single nucleotide polymorphisms (SNPs) of *MDR1* have been identified (Hoffmeyer et al., 2000; Cascorbi et al., 2001; Kim et al., 2001; Marzolini et al., 2004). Most of them are either intronic or noncoding. One silent SNP in exon 26 3435C>T was linked to a nonsynonymous SNP in exon 21 2677G>T and to a synonymous SNP in exon 12 1236C>T (Johne et al., 2002). Interestingly, nonsynonymous *MDR1* polymorphisms appear to be rare in the white population, except for the SNP in exon 21 2677G>T. This SNP shows the peculiarity of a triple variant with 2677A in 1.9% of alleles, coding for Thr893 (Cascorbi et al., 2001).

Homozygous persons carrying the T-allele in *MDR1* exon 26 3435 had significantly lower intestinal Pgp expression levels than heterozygous individuals or homozygous carriers of the wild-type allele (Hoffmeyer et al., 2000; Figure 21.1A). Consequently, in comparison to the CC-wild type, steady-state plasma levels of the model compound digoxin were higher in persons homozygous for the T-allele (Figure 21.1B). In $CD56^+$

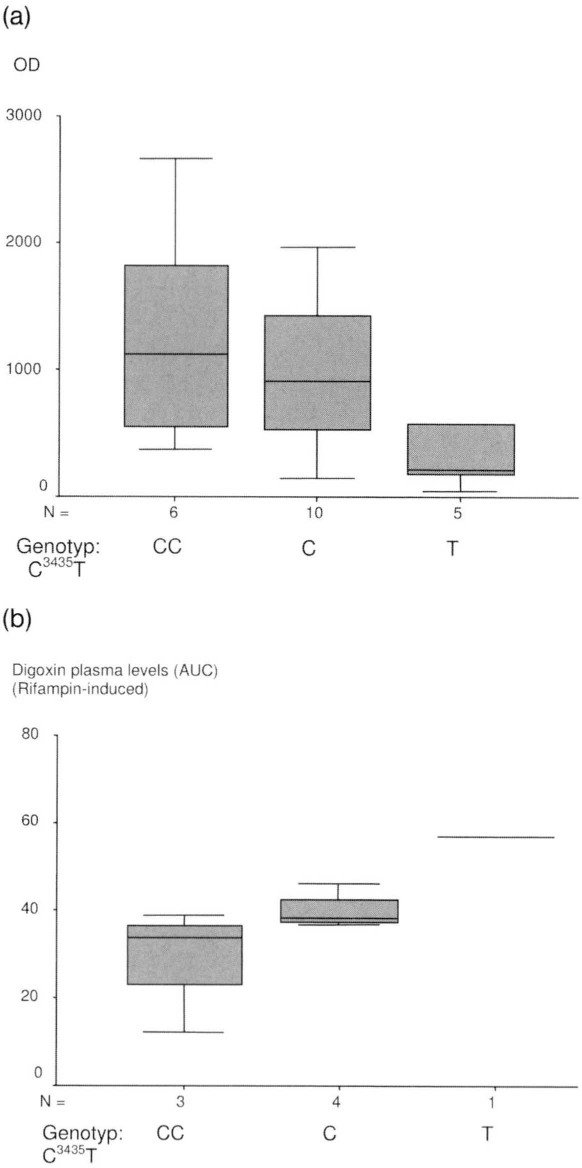

Fig. 21.1 Intestinal MDR1 expression levels and transport function according to the genotype in exon 26 3435C>T [51]. (A) Genotype-dependent Pgp content in the villous epithelia of the duodenum and (B) *in vivo* Pgp activity determined by plasma levels of digoxin; area under the curve (AUC, $\mu g\ h^{-1}\ L^{-1}$) after induction with rifampin. Digoxin plasma levels are inversely correlated with Pgp expression levels in the same individuals (Hoffmeyer et al., 2000). This finding has been confirmed in two more comprehensive studies (Hoffmeyer et al., 2000; Johne et al., 2002)

natural killer cells, Pgp function, as determined by rhodamine-123 efflux, was also correlated with the exon 26 3435C>T genotype in the rank order CC > CT > TT according to efflux activity (Hitzl et al., 2001). These results were in good agreement with *MDR1* genotype-related MDR1 mRNA and Pgp expression levels on peripheral blood mononuclear cells of HIV patients (Fellay et al., 2002). Pgp content and mRNA steady-state levels were highest in individuals of the CC genotype in exon 26 3435 compared to the CT or TT group. However, published results are quite controversial, as discussed in Johne et al. (2002) and Marzolini et al. (2004). This may point to the impact of haplotypes that may not yet be sufficiently elucidated.

In a recent case-control study, the contribution of the *MDR1* exon 26 3435C>T polymorphism to susceptibility of renal cell carcinomas was investigated (Siegesmund et al., 2002). From the lower Pgp expression levels and diminished transport activity in *MDR1* exon 26 3435 T-allele carriers, it was inferred that this allele may be associated with diminished local detoxification capabilities of carcinogens and thus with increased risk of developing renal cell tumours. Indeed, the results of this study provided good evidence for a *MDR1* exon 26 3435 genotype-dependent influence in the development of renal epithelial tumours. Persons carrying at least one T allele appeared to be predisposed to acquiring papillary and chromophobe renal cell carcinomas or oncocytic adenomas.

21.3.2
Multidrug Resistance-related Proteins (MRPs, ABCC)

Family members of the MRP and ABCC ABC transporters are very likely to participate in the removal of xenobiotics and toxicants, not only in vertebrates, but also in other species, including yeast, nematodes, and plants. Substrate compounds of MRPs include mycotoxins, heavy metals, agrochemicals, and lipid metabolites (Table 21.5). Therefore, these transporters are assumed to belong to a widely distributed defence system against xenobiotics.

Tab. 21.5 Xenobiotics transported by MRP1 (according to Leslie et al., 2001).

Substrate
Aflatoxin B1-epoxide-GS
Chlorambucil-GS
2,4-Dinitrophenyl-GS
Doxorubicin-GS
Estrone 3-sulphate
Etoposid-glucuronide
4-Hydroxynonenol-GS
Melphalan-GS
Methotresate
Metolachlor-GS

MRP2 is predominantly expressed in canalicular (apical) membranes of hepatocytes but can also be found in apical membranes of enterocytes (van Aubel et al., 2000) and epithelial cells of proximal tubules of the kidney (Schaub et al., 1997). However, an excretory function in the latter two could not be demonstrated. MRP2 mediates the biliary excretion of conjugated compounds but also some non-conjugated substrates, including pravastatin and methotrexate. Impaired MRP2 transport function can be seen in patients suffering from Dubin–Johnson syndrome (DJS), a rare autosomal-recessive disorder resulting in diminished biliary excretion of conjugated anions from phase-II metabolic reactions, mild conjugated hyperbilirubinaemia, and melanine-like dispositions in the liver (Paulsusma and Elferink, 1997). DJS patients are at considerable risk of adverse reactions and toxicity in drug treatments and xenobiotic exposure.

Currently, five SNPs in coding regions (exons) and one SNP in the promoter of *MRP2* are known from a screening of the *MRP2* gene in a sample of Japanese persons (Ito et al., 2001). Most frequent SNPs were C24T (18.8%) of the promoter region and the two exonic SNPs G1249A (12.5%, exon 10) and C3972T (21.9%, exon 28). Further investigations of cell lines derived from samples of liver resections of 72 Japanese patients resulted in four SNPs located in the promoter region and 23 exonic SNPs (Itoda et al., 2002). However, the functional consequences of *MRP2* SNPs are not yet clear.

MRP1 (ABCC1) could be identified as an additional carrier mediating a multidrug resistance phenotype in a small-cell lung carcinoma cell line that does not overexpress MDR1 (ABCB1) (Cole et al., 1992). The substrate spectrum of this carrier is similar to that of MDR1, except that MRP1 transports only conjugated compounds (Konig et al., 1999). Additionally, MRP1 is ubiquitously expressed in normal tissues throughout the body, although in the liver only low expression levels were detected (Cherrington et al., 2002). MRP1 is also an efflux pump for glutathione, glucuronate, and sulphate conjugates of many xenobiotics. Thus, this transporter is very likely to determine exposure to toxicants. Deletion of regions of the *MRP1* gene coding for the first membrane-spanning domain (MSD1) (Gao et al., 1998) or blockade of parts of the first nucleotide-binding fold (NBD1) by monoclonal antibodies (Hipfner et al., 1999) resulted in a decay of MRP1 transport function. SNPs located in these functionally important regions are of potential interest in toxicogenetic studies.

Our knowledge of functionally relevant MRP1 genetic polymorphisms is currently limited. Several SNPs in Caucasian and a Japanese people could be identified in the *MRP1* gene (Conrad et al., 2001; Ito et al., 2001). Most of them were noncoding or located in intronic regions adjacent to exon–intron boundaries. A total of six nonsynonymous *MRP1* SNPs were detected, but their allelic frequencies were low, so that all carriers of the missense mutations were heterozygous for the wild-type allele. Mutations located in sensitive regions for MRP1 transport function included G128C, C218T (MSD1), and G671V, G2168A (NBD1). Noncoding and intronic SNPs were detected at frequencies between 0.01 and 0.375 (31) (Ito et al., 2001).

The functional consequences of the *MRP1* SNPs G671V, within NBD1, and of Arg433Ser, located in a putative cytoplasmic loop, was determined in *in vitro* transport assays (Conrad et al., 2002). Although the first had no impact on MRP1 transport activity, the Arg433Ser polymorphism diminished transport of leukotriene C4 and estrone sulphate by half, due to a decrease in V_{max} for both compounds (the K_m remained unchanged). In addition, doxorubicin resistance of cells overexpressing the mutant Arg433Ser MRP1 was twice as high as in the wild-type.

References

Akaba K, Kimura T, Sasaki A, Tanabe S, Ikegami T, Hashimoto M, Umeda H, Yoshida H, Umetsu K, Chiba H, Yuasa I, and Hayasaka K (1998) Neonatal hyperbilirubinemia and mutation of the bilirubin uridine diphosphate-glucuronosyltransferase gene: a common missense mutation among Japanese, Koreans and Chinese. *Biochem. Mol. Biol. Int.* **46**:21–26.

Ando Y, Chida M, Nakayama K, Saka H, and Kamataki T (1998) The *UGT1A1*28* allele is relatively rare in a Japanese population. *Pharmacogenetics* **8**:357–360.

Ando Y, Saka H, Ando M, Sawa T, Muro K, Ueoka H, Yokoyama A, Saitoh S, Shimokata K, and Hasegawa Y (2000) Polymorphisms of UDP-glucuronosyltransferase gene and irinotecan toxicity: a pharmacogenetic analysis. *Cancer Res.* **60**:6921–6926.

Ayrton A and Morgan P. (2001) Role of transport proteins in drug absorption, distribution and excretion. *Xenobiotica* **31**:469–497.

Beutler E, Gelbart T, and Demina A (1998) Racial variability in the UDP-glucuronosyltransferase 1 (UGT1A1) promoter: a balanced polymorphism for regulation of bilirubin metabolism? *Proc. Natl. Acad. Sci. USA* **95**:8170–8174.

Bosma PJ, Chowdhury JR, Bakker C, Gantla S, de Boer A, Oostra BA, Lindhout D, Tytgat GN, Jansen PL, Oude Elferink RP. (1995) The genetic basis of the reduced expression of bilirubin UDP-glucuronosyltransferase 1 in Gilbert's syndrome. *N. Engl. J. Med.* **333**:1171–1175.

Brauch H et al. (1999) Trichloroethylene exposure and specific somatic mutations in patients with renal cell carcinoma. *J. Natl. Cancer Inst.* **91**:854–861.

Brennan P (2002) Gene–environment interaction and aetiology of cancer: what does it mean and how can we measure it? *Carcinogenesis* **23**:381–387.

Brockmoller J, Cascorbi I, Henning S, Meisel C, and Roots I (2000) Molecular genetics of cancer susceptibility. *Pharmacology* **61**:212–227.

Burchell B (2003) Genetic variation of human UDP-glucuronosyltransferase: implications in disease and drug glucuronidation. *Am. J. Pharmacogenomics* **3**:37–52.

Burchell B and Hume R (1999) Molecular genetic basis of Gilbert's syndrome. *J. Gastroenterol. Hepatol.* **14**:960–966.

Cascorbi I, Brockmoller J, and Roots I (1996) A C4887A polymorphism in exon 7 of human *CYP1A1*: population frequency, mutation linkages, and impact on lung cancer susceptibility. *Cancer Res.* **56**:4965–4969.

Cascorbi I, Brockmoller J, Mrozikiewicz PM, Muller A, and Roots I (1999) Arylamine N-acetyltransferase activity in man. *Drug Metab Rev.* **31**:489–502.

Cascorbi I, Gerloff T, Johne A, Meisel C, Hoffmeyer S, Schwab M, Schaeffeler E, Eichelbaum M, Brinkmann U, and Roots I (2001) Frequency of single nucleotide polymorphisms in the P-glycoprotein drug transporter MDR1 gene in white subjects. *Clin. Pharmacol. Ther.* **69**:169–174.

Chernogolov A, Behlke J, Schunck W H, Roots I, Schwarz D. (2003) Human CYP1A1 allelic variants: baculovirus expression and purification, hydrodynamic, spectral and catalytical properties and their potency in the formation of all-*trans*-retinoic acid. *Prot. Expr. Purif.* **28**, 259–269.

Cherrington NJ et al. (2002) Organ distribution of multidrug resistance proteins 1, 2, and 3 (Mrp1, 2, and 3) mRNA and hepatic induction of Mrp3 by constitutive androstane receptor activators in rats. *J. Pharmacol. Exp. Ther.* **300**:97–104.

Cole SPC et al. (1992) Overexpression of a transporter gene in a multidrug-resistant human lung cancer cell line. *Science* **258**:1650–1654.

Collie-Duguid ES, Etienne MC, Milano G, and McLeod HL (2000) Known variant DPYD alleles do not explain DPD deficiency in cancer patients. *Pharmacogenetics* **10**:217–223.

Colombel JF, Ferrari N, Debuysere H, Marteau P, Gendre JP, Bonaz B, Soule JC, Modigliani R, Touze Y, Catala P, Libersa C, and Broly F (2000) Genotypic analysis of thiopurine S-methyltransferase in patients with Crohn's disease and severe myelosuppression during azathioprine therapy. *Gastroenterology* **118**:1025–1030.

Conney AH. (1982) Induction of microsomal enzymes by foreign chemicals and carcinogenesis by polycyclic aromatic hydrocarbons. *Cancer Res.* **42**, 4875–4917.

Conney AH (2004) Tailoring cancer chemoprevention regimens to the individual. *J. Cell Biochem.* **91**:277–286.

Conrad S et al. (2001) Identification of human multidrug resistance protein 1 (MRP1) mutations and characterization of a G671V substitution. *J. Hum. Genet.* **46**:656–663.

Conrad S et al. (2002) A naturally occurring mutation in MRP1 results in a selective decrease in organic anion transport and in increased doxorubicin resistance. *Pharmacogenetics* **12**:321–330.

Cordon-Cardo C et al. (1990) Expression of the multidrug resistance gene product (P-glycoprotein) in human normal and tumor tissues. J. *Histochem. Cytochem.* **38**:1277–1287.

Crofts F, Taioli E, Trachman J, Cosma G N, Currie DM, Toniolo P and Garte, SJ. (1994) Functional significance of different human CYP1A1 genotypes. *Carcinogenesis* **15**, 2961–2963.

de Lange EC et al. (1998) BBB transport and P-glycoprotein functionality using MDR1A (–/–) and wild-type mice. Total brain versus microdialysis concentration profiles of rhodamine-123. *Pharm. Res.* **15**:1657–1665.

Drakoulis N, Cascorbi I, Brockmoller J, Gross CR, and Roots I (1994) Polymorphisms in the human CYP1A1 gene as susceptibility factors for lung cancer: exon-7 mutation (4889 A to G), and a T to C mutation in the 3′-flanking region. *Clin. Investig.* **72**:240–248.

Esteller M, Garciua A, Martinez-Palonas JM, Xercavins J, and Reventos J. (1997) Germ line polymorphism in cytochrome P450 1A1 (C4887 CYP1A1) and methylenetetrahydrofolate reductase (MTHFR) genes and endometrial cancer. *Carcinogenesis* **18**, 2307–2311.

Etienne MC, Lagrange JL, Dassonville O, Fleming R, Thyss A, Renee N, Schneider M, Demard F, and Milano G (1994) Population study of dihydropyrimidine dehydrogenase in cancer patients. *J. Clin. Oncol.* **12**:2248–2253.

Evans WE, Horner M, Chu YQ, Kalwinsky D, and Roberts WM (1991) Altered mercaptopurine metabolism, toxic effects, and dosage requirement in a thiopurine methyltransferase-deficient child with acute lymphocytic leukemia. *J. Pediatr.* **119**:985–989.

Evans WE, Hon YY, Bomgaars L, Coutre S, Holdsworth M , Janco R, Kalwinsky D, Keller F, Khatib Z, Margolin J, Murray J, Quinn J, Ravindranath Y, Ritchey K, Roberts W, Rogers ZR, Schiff D, Steuber C, Tucci F, Kornegay N, Krynetski EY, and Relling MV (2001) Preponderance of thiopurine S-methyltransferase deficiency and heterozygosity among patients intolerant to mercaptopurine or azathioprine. *J. Clin. Oncol.* **19**: 2293–2301.

Fellay J et al. (2002) Response to antiretroviral treatment in HIV-1–infected individuals with allelic variants of the multidrug resistance transporter 1: a pharmacogenetics study. *Lancet* **359**:30–36.

Firozi PF et al. (2002) Aromatic DNA adducts and polymorphisms of *CYP1A1, NAT2,* and *GSTM1* in breast cancer. *Carcinogenesis* **23**, 301–306.

Fisher MB, Vandenbranden M, Findlay K, Burchell B, Thummel KE, Hall SD, and Wrighton SA (2000) Tissue distribution and interindividual variation in human UDP-glucuronosyltransferase activity: relationship between UGT1A1 promoter genotype and variability in a liver bank. *Pharmacogenetics* **10**: 727–739.

Fisher MB, Paine MF, Strelevitz TJ, and Wrighton SA (2001) The role of hepatic and extrahepatic UDP-glucuronosyltransferases in human drug metabolism. *Drug Metab. Rev.* **33**:273–297.

Gao M et al. (1998) Multidrug resistance protein. *J. Biol. Chem.* **273**:10733–10740.

Glatt H and Meinl W (2004) Pharmacogenetics of soluble sulfotransferases (SULTs). *Naunyn Schmiedebergs Arch. Pharmacol.* **369**:55–68.

Gonzalez FJ and Fernandez-Salguero P (1995) Diagnostic analysis, clinical importance and molecular basis of dihydropyrimidine dehydrogenase deficiency. *Trends Pharmacol. Sci.* **16**:325–327.

GREENWALD P (2002) Cancer chemoprevention. *Br. Med. J.* **321**, 714–718.

GREINER B et al. (1999) The role of intestinal P-glycoprotein in the interaction of digoxin and rifampin. *J. Clin. Invest.* **104**:147–153.

GUENGERICH FP (1998) The environmental genome project: functional analysis of polymorphisms. *Environ. Health Perspect.* **106**, 365–368.

GUENGERICH FP. (2000) Metabolism of chemical carcinogens. *Carcinogenesis* **21**, 345–351.

GUENGERICH FP, and SHIMADA T. (1998) Activation of procarcinogens by human cytochrome P450 enzymes. *Mutation Res.* **400**, 201–213.

GUPTA E, LESTINGI TM, MICK R, RAMIREZ J, VOKES EE, and RATAIN MJ (1994) Metabolic fate of irinotecan in humans: correlation of glucuronidation with diarrhea. *Cancer Res.* **54**:3723–3725.

HAMDAN-KHALIL R, ALLORGE D, LO-GUIDICE JM, CAUFFIEZ C, CHEVALIER D, SPIRE C, HOUDRET N, LIBERSA C, LHERMITTE M, COLOMBEL JF, GALA JL, and BROLY F (2003) In vitro characterization of four novel non-functional variants of the thiopurine S-methyltransferase. *Biochem. Biophys. Res. Commun.* **309**:1005–1010.

HAN X, and LIEHR JG. (1994) DNA single-strand breaks in kidneys of Syrian hamsters treated with steroidal estrogens: hormone-induced free radical damage preceding renal malignancy. *Carcinogenesis* **15**, 997–1000.

HANNA IH, DAWLING S, ROODI N, GUENGERICH FP, and PARL FF. (2000) Cytochrome P450 1B1 (CYP1B1) pharmacogenetics: association of polymorphisms with functional differences in estrogen hydroxylation activity. *Cancer Res.* **60**, 3440–3444.

HEGGIE GD, SOMMADOSSI JP, CROSS DS, HUSTER WJ, and DIASIO RB (1987) Clinical pharmacokinetics of 5-fluorouracil and its metabolites in plasma, urine, and bile. *Cancer Res.* **47**:2203–2206.

HIGGINS CF (2001) ABC transporters: physiology, structure and mechanism: an overview. *Res. Microbiol.* **152**:205–210.

HIPFNER DR et al. (1999) Monoclonal antibodies that inhibit the transport function of the 190-kDa multidrug resistance protein, MRP. *J. Biol. Chem.* **274**:15420–15426.

HITZL M et al. (2001) The C3435T mutation in the human MDR1 gene is associated with altered efflux of the P-glycoprotein substrate rhodamine 123 from CD56+ natural killer cells. *Pharmacogenetics* **11**:1–6.

HOFFMEYER S, BURK O, VON RICHTER O, ARNOLD HP, BROCKMOLLER J, JOHNE A, CASCORBI I, GERLOFF T, ROOTS I, EICHELBAUM M, and BRINKMANN U (2000) Functional polymorphisms of the human multidrug-resistance gene: multiple sequence variations and correlation of one allele with P-glycoprotein expression and activity *in vivo*. *Proc. Natl. Acad. Sci. USA* **97**:3473–3478.

HON YY, FESSING MY, PUI CH, RELLING MV, KRYNETSKI EY, and EVANS WE (1999) Polymorphism of the thiopurine S-methyltransferase gene in African-Americans. *Hum. Mol. Genet.* **8**:371–376.

HUNG RJ et al. (2003) CYP1A1 and GSTM1 genetic polymorphisms and lung cancer risk in Caucasian non-smokers: a pooled analysis. *Carcinogenesis* **24**, 875–882.

INGELMAN-SUNDBERG M (2001) Genetic variability in susceptibility and response to toxicants. *Toxicol. Lett.* **120**, 259–268.

INNOCENTI F and RATAIN MJ (2002) Update on pharmacogenetics in cancer chemotherapy. *Eur. J. Cancer* **38**:639–644.

ITO S et al. (2001) Polymorphism of the ABC transporter genes, MDR1, MRP1 and MRP2/cMOAT, in healthy Japanese subjects. *Pharmacogenetics* **11**:175–184.

ITODA M et al. (2002) Polymorphisms in the ABCC2 (cMOAT/MRP2) gene found in 72 established cell lines derived from Japanese individuals: an association between single nucleotide polymorphisms in the 5′-untranslated region and exon 28. *Drug Metab. Dispos.* **30**:363–364.

IYER L, KING CD, WHITINGTON PF, GREEN MD, ROY SK, TEPHLY TR, COFFMAN BL, and RATAIN MJ (1998) Genetic predisposition to the metabolism of irinotecan (CPT-11): role of uridine diphosphate glucuronosyltransferase isoform 1A1 in the glucuronidation of its active metabolite (SN-38) in human liver microsomes. *J. Clin. Invest.* **101**:847–854.

IYER L, HALL D, DAS S, MORTELL MA, RAMIREZ J, KIM S, DI RIENZO A, and RATAIN MJ (1999) Phenotype–genotype correlation of *in vitro* SN-38 (active metabolite of irinotecan) and bilirubin glucuronidation in human liver tissue with UGT1A1 promoter polymorphism. *Clin. Pharmacol. Ther.* **65**:576–582.

IYER L, DAS S, JANISCH L, WEN M, RAMIREZ J, KARRISON T, FLEMING GF, VOKES EE,

Schilsky RL, and Ratain MJ (2002) *UGT1A1*28* polymorphism as a determinant of irinotecan disposition and toxicity. *Pharmacogenomics. J.* **2**:43–47.

Johne A, Kopke K, Gerloff T, Mai I, Rietbrock S, Meisel C, Hoffmeyer S, Kerb R, Fromm MF, Brinkmann U, Eichelbaum M, Brockmoller J, Cascorbi I, and Roots I (2002) Modulation of steady-state kinetics of digoxin by haplotypes of the P-glycoprotein MDR1 gene. *Clin. Pharmacol. Ther.* **72**: 584–594.

Johnson MR, Hageboutros A, Wang K, High L, Smith JB, and Diasio RB (1999) Life-threatening toxicity in a dihydropyrimidine dehydrogenase-deficient patient after treatment with topical 5-fluorouracil. *Clin. Cancer Res.* **5**:2006–2011.

Juranka PF et al. (1989) P-glycoprotein: multidrug-resistance and a superfamily of membrane-associated transport proteins. *FASEB J.* **3**:2583–2592.

Kawajiri K, Nakachi K, Imai K, Watanabe J, and Hayashi S. (1993) The CYP1A1 gene and cancer susceptibility. *Crit. Rev. Oncol. Hematol.* **14**, 77–87.

Kerb R, Brockmoller J, Sachse C, and Roots I (1999) Detection of the *GSTM1*0* allele by long polymerase chain reaction. *Pharmacogenetics* **9**:89–94.

Kerb R, Brockmoller J, Schlagenhaufer R, Sprenger R, Roots I, and Brinkmann U (2002) Influence of *GSTT1* and *GSTM1* genotypes on sunburn sensitivity. *Am. J. Pharmacogenomics* **2**:147–154.

Kim RB et al. (2001) Identification of functionally variant *MDR1* alleles among European Americans and African Americans. *Clin. Pharmacol. Ther.* **70**:189–199.

Kiyohara C, Nakanishi Y, Inutsuka S, Takayama K, Hara N, Motohiro A, Tanaka K, Kono S, and Hirohata T. (1998) The relationship between CYP1A1 aryl hydrocarbon hydroxylase activity and lung cancer in a Japanese population. *Pharmacogenetics* **8**, 315–323.

Konig J et al. (1999) Conjugate export pumps of the multidrug resistance protein (MRP) family : localization, substrate specificity, and MRP2-mediated drug resistance. *Biochim. Biophys. Acta* **1461**:377–394.

Kramer JA and Kolaja KL (2002) Toxicogenomics: an opportunity to optimise drug development and safety evaluation. *Expert. Opin. Drug Saf.* **1**:275–286.

Krynetski EY, Tai HL, Yates CR, Fessing MY, Loennechen T, Schuetz JD, Relling MV, and Evans WE (1996) Genetic polymorphism of thiopurine S-methyltransferase: clinical importance and molecular mechanisms. *Pharmacogenetics* **6**:279–290.

Lee VHL. (2000) Membrane transporters. *Eur. J. Pharm. Sci.*, **11**, Suppl. 2, S41–S50.

Le Marchand L, Murphy SP, Hankin JH, Wilkens LR, Kolonel N. (2000) Intake of flavonoids and lung cancer. *J. Natl. Cancer Inst.* **92**, 154–160.

Le Marchand L et al. (2003) Pooled analysis of the *CYP1A1* exon 7 polymorphism and lung cancer (United States). *Cancer Causes Control* **14**, 339–346.

Lennard L, Van Loon JA, Lilleyman JS, and Weinshilboum RM (1987) Thiopurine pharmacogenetics in leukemia: correlation of erythrocyte thiopurine methyltransferase activity and 6-thioguanine nucleotide concentrations. *Clin. Pharmacol. Ther.* **41**:18–25.

Lennard L, Van Loon JA, and Weinshilboum RM (1989) Pharmacogenetics of acute azathioprine toxicity: relationship to thiopurine methyltransferase genetic polymorphism. *Clin. Pharmacol. Ther.* **46**:149–154.

Lennard L, Lilleyman JS, Van Loon J, and Weinshilboum RM (1990) Genetic variation in response to 6-mercaptopurine for childhood acute lymphoblastic leukaemia. *Lancet* **336**:225–229.

Lennard L, Welch JC, and Lilleyman JS (1997) Thiopurine drugs in the treatment of childhood leukaemia: the influence of inherited thiopurine methyltransferase activity on drug metabolism and cytotoxicity. *Br. J. Clin. Pharmacol.* **44**:455–461.

Leslie EM, Deeley RG, and Cole SP (2001) Toxicological relevance of the multidrug resistance protein 1, MRP1 (ABCC1) and related transporters. *Toxicology* **167**, 3–23.

Li DN, Seidel A, Pritchard MP, Wolf CR, and Friedberg T. (2000) Polymorphisms in P450 CYP1B1 affect the conversion of estradiol to the potentially carcinogenic metabolite 4-hydroxyestradiol. *Pharmacogenetics* **10**, 343–353.

Lu Z, Zhang R, and Diasio RB (1993) Dihydropyrimidine dehydrogenase activity in human peripheral blood mononuclear cells and liver: population characteristics, newly identified deficient patients, and clinical implication in 5-fluorouracil chemotherapy. *Cancer Res.* **53**:5433–5438.

Mackenzie PI, Owens IS, Burchell B, Bock KW, Bairoch A, Belanger A, Fournel-Gigleux S , Green M, Hum DW, Iyanagi T, Lancet D, Louisot P, Magdalou J, Chowdhury JR, Ritter JK, Schachter H, Tephly TR, Tipton KF, and Nebert DW (1997) The UDP glycosyltransferase gene superfamily: recommended nomenclature update based on evolutionary divergence. *Pharmacogenetics* 7: 255–269.

Marchant GE (2002) Toxicogenomics and toxic torts. *Trends Biotechnol.* **20**:329–332.

Maruo Y, Nishizawa K, Sato H, Doida Y, and Shimada M (1999) Association of neonatal hyperbilirubinemia with bilirubin UDP-glucuronosyltransferase polymorphism. *Pediatrics* **103**:1224–1227.

Marzolini C, Paus E, Buclin T, and Kim RB (2004) Polymorphisms in human MDR1 (P-glycoprotein): recent advances and clinical relevance. *Clin. Pharmacol. Ther.* **75**:13–33.

McLellan RA, Oscarson M, Hidestrand M, Leidvik B, Jonsson E, Otter C, and Ingelman-Sundberg M. (2000) Characterization and functional analysis of two common human cytochrome P450 1B1 variants. *Arch. Biochem. Biophys.* **378**, 175–181.

McLeod HL, Collie-Duguid ES, Vreken P, Johnson MR, Wei X, Sapone A, Diasio RB, Fernandez-Salguero P, van Kuilenberg AB, van Gennip AH, and Gonzalez FJ (1998) Nomenclature for human DPYD alleles. *Pharmacogenetics* **8**:455–459.

Meisel C, Gerloff T, Kirchheiner J, Mrozikiewicz PM, Niewinski P, Brockmoller J, and Roots I (2003) Implications of pharmacogenetics for individualizing drug treatment and for study design. *J. Mol. Med.* **81**:154–167.

Milano G, Etienne MC, Pierrefite V, Barberi-Heyob M, Deporte-Fety R, and Renee N (1999) Dihydropyrimidine dehydrogenase deficiency and fluorouracil-related toxicity. *Br. J. Cancer* **79**:627–630.

Miller III, MC, Mohrenweiser HW, and Bell DA (2001) Genetic variability in susceptibility and response to toxicants. *Toxicol. Lett.* **120**, 269–280.

Miners JO, McKinnon RA, and Mackenzie PI (2002) Genetic polymorphisms of UDP-glucuronosyltransferases and their functional significance. *Toxicology* **181–182**:453–456.

Modugno F, Knoll C, Kanbour-Shakir A, and Romkes M. (2003) A potential role for the estrogen-metabolizing cytochrome P450 enzymes in human breast carcinogenesis. *Breast Cancer Res. Treat.* **82**, 191–197.

Monaghan G, Ryan M, Seddon R, Hume R, and Burchell B (1996) Genetic variation in bilirubin UPD-glucuronosyltransferase gene promoter and Gilbert's syndrome. *Lancet* **347**:578–581.

Mrozikiewicz PM, Cascorbi I, Brockmöller J, and Roots I (1997) CYP1A1 mutations 4887A, 4889G, 5639C and 6235C in the Polish population and their allelic linkage, determined by peptide nucleic acid-mediated PCR clamping. *Pharmacogenetics* **7**:303–307.

Nagasubramanian R, Innocenti F, and Ratain MJ (2003) Pharmacogenetics in cancer treatment. *Annu. Rev. Med.* **54**:437–452.

Newbold RR, and Liehr JG. (2000) Induction of uterine adenocarcinoma in CD-1 mice by catechol estrogens. *Cancer Res.* **60**, 235–237.

Owens IS and Ritter JK (1995) Gene structure at the human *UGT1* locus creates diversity in isozyme structure, substrate specificity, and regulation. *Prog. Nucleic Acid Res. Mol. Biol.* **51**:305–338.

Paulusma CC and Oude Elferink RP (1997) The canalicular multispecific organic anion transporter and conjugated hyperbilirubinemia in rat and man. *J. Mol. Med.* **75**:420–428.

Persson I, Johansson I, and Ingelman-Sundberg M. (1997) In vitro kinetics of two human CYP1A1 variant enzymes suggested to be associated with interindividual differences in cancer susceptibility. *Biochem. Biophys. Res. Commun.* 231, 227–230.

Raida M, Schwabe W, Hausler P, van Kuilenburg AB, van Gennip AH, Behnke D, and Hoffken K (2001) Prevalence of a common point mutation in the dihydropyrimidine dehydrogenase (DPD) gene within the 5′-splice donor site of intron 14 in patients with severe 5-fluorouracil (5-FU)-related toxicity compared with controls. *Clin. Cancer Res.* **7**:2832–2839.

Rao VV, et al. (1999) Choroid plexus epithelial expression of MDR1 P glycoprotein and multidrug resistance-associated protein contribute to the blood–cerebrospinal-fluid drug-permeability barrier. *Proc. Natl. Acad. Sci. USA* **96**:3900–3905.

Relling MV, Hancock ML, Rivera GK, Sandlund JT, Ribeiro RC, Krynetski EY, Pui CH, and Evans WE (1999) Mercaptopurine therapy intolerance and heterozygosity at the thiopurine S-methyltransferase gene locus. *J. Natl. Cancer Inst.* **91**:2001–2008.

Ridge SA, Sludden J, Brown O, Robertson L, Wei X, Sapone A, Fernandez-Salguero PM, Gonzalez FJ, Vreken P, van Kuilenburg AB, van Gennip AH, and McLeod HL (1998 a) Dihydropyrimidine dehydrogenase pharmacogenetics in Caucasian subjects. *Br. J. Clin. Pharmacol.* **46**:151–156.

Ridge SA, Sludden J, Wei X, Sapone A, Brown O, Hardy S, Canney P, Fernandez-Salguero P, Gonzalez FJ, Cassidy J, and McLeod HL (1998 b) Dihydropyrimidine dehydrogenase pharmacogenetics in patients with colorectal cancer. *Br. J. Cancer* **77**: 497–500.

Roberts R, Cain K, Coyle B, Freathy C, Leonard JF, and Gautier JC (2003) Early drug safety evaluation: biomarkers, signatures, and fingerprints. *Drug Metab Rev.* **35**:269–275.

Rojas M, Cascorbi I, Alexandrov K, Kriek E, Auburtin G, Mayer L, Kopp-Schneider A, Roots I and Bartsch H. (2000) Modulation of benzo[*a*]pyrene diolepoxide-DNA adduct levels in human white blood cells by *CYP1A1, GSTM1* and *GSTT1* polymorphism. *Carcinogenesis* **21**, 35–41.

Rosenblum IY (2003) Toxicogenomic applications to drug risk assessment. *Environ. Health Perspect.* **111**:A804–A805.

Rylander-Rudqvist T. et al. (2003) Cytochrome P450 1B1 gene polymorphisms and postmenopausal breast cancer risk. *Carcinogenesis* **24**, 1533–1539.

Sabichi AL, Demierre MF, Hawk ET, Lerman CE, and Lipman SM. (2003) Frontiers in cancer prevention research. *Cancer Res.* **63**, 5649–5655.

Sasaki M, Tanaky Y, Kaneuchi M, Sakuragi N, and Dahiya R. (2003) CYP1B1 gene polymorphisms have higher risk for endometrial cancer, and positive correlations with estrogen receptor α and estrogen receptor β expressions. *Cancer Res.* **63**, 3913–3918.

Schaub TP et al. (1997) Expression of the conjugate export pump encoded by the *mrp2* gene in the apical membrane of kidney proximal tubules. *J. Am. Soc. Nephrol.* **8**:1213–1221.

Schmidt CW (2003) Toxicogenomics: an emerging discipline. EHP. *Toxicogenomics* **111**: A20–A25.

Schutz E, Gummert J, Mohr F, and Oellerich M (1993) Azathioprine-induced myelosuppression in thiopurine methyltransferase deficient heart transplant recipient. *Lancet* **341**:436.

Schwab M, Schaffeler E, Marx C, Fischer C, Lang T, Behrens C, Gregor M, Eichelbaum M, Zanger UM, and Kaskas BA (2002) Azathioprine therapy and adverse drug reactions in patients with inflammatory bowel disease: impact of thiopurine S-methyltransferase polymorphism. *Pharmacogenetics* **12**:429–436.

Schwarz D, and Roots I. (2003 a) In vitro assessment of inhibition by natural polyphenols of metabolic activation of procarcinogens by human CYP1A1. *Biochem. Biophys. Res. Commun.* **303**, 902–907.

Schwarz D, Kisselev P, Schunck WH, Chernogolov A, Boidol W, Cascorbi I, and Roots I. (2000) Allelic variants of human cytochrome P450 1A1 (CYP1A1): effect of T461N and I462V substitutions on steroid hydroxylase specificity. *Pharmacogenetics* **10**, 519–530.

Schwarz D, Kisselev P, Cascorbi I, Schunck WH, and Roots I (2001) Differential metabolism of benzo[*a*]pyrene and benzo[*a*]-pyrene-7,8-dihydrodiol by human CYP1A1 variants. *Carcinogenesis* **22**:453–459.

Schwarz D, Kisselev P, and Roots I. (2004) *CYP1A1* genotype-selective inhibition of benzo[*a*]pyrene activation by quercetin. *Eur. J. Cancer* **40**, in press.

Schwarz D, Kisselev P, and Roots I. (2003 b) St. John's wort extracts and some of their constituents potently inhibit ultimate carcinogen formation from benzo[a]pyrene-7,8-dihydrodiol by human CYP1A1. *Cancer Res.* **63**, 8062–8068.

Shimada T, Hayes CL, Yamazaki H, Amin S, Hecht SS, Guengerich FP, and Sutter TR. (1996) Activation of chemically diverse procarcinogens by human cytochrome P450 1B1. *Cancer Res.* **56**, 2979–2984.

Shimada T, Watanabe J, Kawajiri K, Sutter TR, Guengerich FP, Gillam EMJ, and Inoue K. (1999) Catalytic properties of polymorphic human cytochrome P450 1B1 variants. *Carcinogenesis* **20**, 1607–1614.

Shimada T, Oda Y, Gillam EMJ, Guengerich FP, and Inoue K. (2001 a) Metabolic activation of polycyclic aromatic hydrocarbons and other procarcinogens by cytochrome P450 1A1 and P450 1B1 allelic variants and other human cytochromes P450 in *Salmonella typhimurium* NM2009. *Drug Metab. Dispos.* **29**, 1176–1182.

Shimada T, Watanabe J, Inoue K, Guengerich FP, and Gillam EMJ. (2001 b) Specificity of 17β-oestradiol and benzo[*a*]pyrene oxidation by polymorphic human cytochrome P4501B1 variants substituted at residues 48, 119, and 432. *Xenobiotica* **31**, 163–176.

Siegsmund M et al. (2002) Association of the P-glycoprotein transporter MDR1 (C4545T) polymorphism with the susceptibility to renal epithelial tumors. *J. Am. Soc. Nephrol.* **13**:1847–1854.

Simmons PT and Portier CJ (2002) Toxicogenomics: the new frontier in risk analysis. *Carcinogenesis* **23**:903–905.

Spire-Vayron de la Moureyre, Debuysere H, Mastain B, Vinner E, Marez D, Lo Guidice JM, Chevalier D, Brique S, Motte K, Colombel JF, Turck D, Noel C, Flipo RM, Pol A, Lhermitte M, Lafitte JJ, Libersa C, and Broly F (1998) Genotypic and phenotypic analysis of the polymorphic thiopurine S-methyltransferase gene (TPMT) in a European population. *Br. J. Pharmacol.* **125**:879–887.

Strachan T and Read A (2004) *Human Molecular Genetics 3*. Garland Science, Chap. 11, pp. 315–349.

Sutter TR, Tang YM, Hayes CL, Wo YP, Jabs EW, Li X, Yin H, Cody CW, and Greenlee WF. (1994) Complete cDNA sequence of a human dioxin-inducible mRNA identifies a new gene subfamily of cytochrome p450 that maps to chromosome 2. *J. Biol. Chem.* **269**, 13092–13099.

Suzuki K. et al. (2003) Association of the genetic polymorphism in cytochrome P450 (CYP) 1A1 with risk of familial prostate cancer in a Japanese population: a case-control study. *Cancer Lett.* **195**, 177–183.

Szumlanski C, Otterness D, Her C, Lee D, Brandriff B, Kelsell D, Spurr N, Lennard L, Wieben E, and Weinshilboum R (1996) Thiopurine methyltransferase pharmacogenetics: human gene cloning and characterization of a common polymorphism. *DNA Cell Biol.* **15**:17–30.

Tai HL, Krynetski EY, Schuetz EG, Yanishevski Y, and Evans WE (1997) Enhanced proteolysis of thiopurine S-methyltransferase (TPMT) encoded by mutant alleles in humans (*TPMT*3A, TPMT*2*): mechanisms for the genetic polymorphism of TPMT activity. *Proc. Natl. Acad. Sci. USA* **94**: 6444–6449.

Taioli E, Ford J, Trachman J, Li Y, Demopoulos R, and Garte S. (1998) Lung cancer risk and *CYP1A1* genotype in African Americans. *Carcinogenesis* **19**, 813–817.

Taioli E. et al. (2003) Polymorphisms in *CYP1A1, GSTM1, GSTT1* and lung cancer below the age of 45 years. *Int. J. Epidemiol.* **32**, 60–63.

Tanigawara Y (2000) Role of P-glycoprotein in drug disposition. *Ther. Drug Monit.* **22**: 137–140.

Terashima I, Suzuki M, and Shibutani S. (2001) Mutagenic properties of estrogen quinone-derived DNA adducts in simian kidney cells. *Biochemistry* **40**, 166–172.

Tong W, Cao X, Harris S, Sun H, Fang H, Fuscoe J, Harris A, Hong H, Xie Q, Perkins R, Shi L, and Casciano D (2003) ArrayTrack: supporting toxicogenomic research at the U.S. Food and Drug Administration National Center for Toxicological Research. *Environ. Health Perspect.* **111**: 1819–1826.

van Aubel RA et al. (2000) Expression and immunolocalization of multidrug resistance protein 2 in rabbit small intestine. *Eur. J. Pharmacol.* **400**:195–198.

van Kuilenburg AB, Haasjes J, Richel DJ, Zoetekouw L, Van Lenthe H, De Abreu RA, Maring JG, Vreken P, and van Gennip AH (2000) Clinical implications of dihydropyrimidine dehydrogenase (DPD) deficiency in patients with severe 5-fluorouracil-associated toxicity: identification of new mutations in the *DPD* gene. *Clin. Cancer Res.* **6**:4705–4712.

van Kuilenburg AB, Muller EW, Haasjes J, Meinsma R, Zoetekouw L, Waterham HR, Baas F, Richel DJ, and van Gennip AH (2001) Lethal outcome of a patient with a complete dihydropyrimidine dehydrogenase (DPD) deficiency after administration of 5-fluorouracil: frequency of the common IVS14+1G>A mutation causing DPD deficiency. *Clin. Cancer Res.* **7**:1149–1153.

Vineis P. et al. (2003) CYP1A1 T3801 C polymorphism and lung cancer: a pooled analysis of 2451 cases and 3358 controls. *Int. J. Cancer* **104**, 650–657.

Wacher VJ et al. (1995) Overlapping substrate specificities and tissue distribution of cytochrome P450 3A and P-glycoprotein: implications for drug delivery and activity in cancer chemotherapy. *Mol. Carcinog.* **13**:129–134.

Walker VE and Meng Q. (2000) 1,3-butadiene: cancer, mutations, and adducts. III. In vivo mutation of the endogenous *hprt* genes of mice and rats by 1,3-butadiene and its metabolites. *Res. Rep. Health. Eff. Inst.* **92**:89–138.

Wakefield J (2003) Toxicogenomics: roadblocks and new directions. *Environ. Health Perspect.* **111**:A334.

Wasternack C (1980) Degradation of pyrimidines and pyrimidine analogs: pathways and mutual influences. *Pharmacol. Ther.* **8**: 629–651.

Watters JW and McLeod HL (2003) Cancer pharmacogenomics: current and future applications. *Biochim. Biophys. Acta* **1603**:99–111.

Wei X, Elizondo G, Sapone A, McLeod HL, Raunio H, Fernandez-Salguero P, and Gonzalez FJ (1998) Characterization of the human dihydropyrimidine dehydrogenase gene. *Genomics* **51**:391–400.

Weinshilboum RM (1992) Methylation pharmacogenetics: thiopurine methyltransferase as a model system. *Xenobiotica* **22**:1055–1071.

Weinshilboum RM and Sladek SL (1980) Mercaptopurine pharmacogenetics: monogenic inheritance of erythrocyte thiopurine methyltransferase activity. *Am. J. Hum. Genet.* **32**:651–662.

Weinshilboum RM, Otterness DM, and Szumlanski CL (1999) Methylation pharmacogenetics: catechol O-methyltransferase, thiopurine methyltransferase, and histamine N-methyltransferase. *Annu. Rev. Pharmacol. Toxicol.* **39**:19–52.

Woodson LC and Weinshilboum RM (1983) Human kidney thiopurine methyltransferase. Purification and biochemical properties. *Biochem. Pharmacol.* **32**:819–826.

Wu MT, Lee JM, Wu DC, Ho CK, Wang YT, Lee YC, Hsu HK, and Kao EL. (2002) Genetic polymorphisms of cytochrome P4501A1 and oesophageal squamous-cell carcinoma in Taiwan. *Br. J. Cancer* **87**, 529–532.

Yan L, Zhang S, Eiff B, Szumlanski CL, Powers M, O'Brien JF, and Weinshilboum RM (2000) Thiopurine methyltransferase polymorphic tandem repeat: genotype–phenotype correlation analysis. *Clin. Pharmacol. Ther.* **68**:210–219.

Yang CS, Landau MJ, Huang MT, and Newmark HL. (2001) Inhibition of carcinogenesis by dietary polyphenolic compounds. *Annu. Rev. Nutr.* **21**, 381–406.

Yates CR, Krynetski EY, Loennechen T, Fessing MY, Tai HL, Pui CH, Relling MV, and Evans WE (1997) Molecular diagnosis of thiopurine S-methyltransferase deficiency: genetic basis for azathioprine and mercaptopurine intolerance. *Ann. Intern. Med.* **126**: 608–614.

Zhang ZY, Fasco MJ, Huang L, Guengerich FP, and Kaminsky LS. (1996) Characterization of purified human recombinant cytochrome P4501A1-Ile^{462} and -Val^{462}: Assessment of a role for the rare allele in carcinogenesis. *Cancer Res.* **56**, 3926–3933.

22
Profiling of Peripheral Blood Gene Expression to Search for Biomarkers

Arno Kalkuhl and Mario Beilmann

22.1
Introduction

One of the greatest single limitations of modern toxicological practice is the uncertainty of extrapolating from laboratory models to humans. Thus, there is a need for 'bridging biomarkers' of damage that can be used to compare toxic responses among species [1]. Toxicogenomics is one of the most promising approaches to identifying such markers. Peripheral blood is of specific interest, as blood is easily available from both animals and humans. A sufficient number of nucleated cells supplying mRNA offers the possibility to use peripheral blood for gene expression studies, and blood cells were successfully used to classify B-cell chronic leukemias [2, 3], to investigate renal diseases in which circulating blood cells play a role [4], and to get new insight into immunity and immunopathology [5–7].

After compound administration, blood cells are exposed to significant concentrations of this agent because drugs or chemicals are distributed via the bloodstream and 'direct' blood functions such as immunomodulation can be studied by gene expression analysis. More intriguing is the search for bridging biomarkers in the blood that are predictive for toxic events in other target organs, which cannot regularly be studied by gene expression analysis in humans, e.g., the liver. The first step in identifying cross-species biomarkers is to identify cross-organ biomarkers in model animals. One class of cross-organ biomarkers consists of genes that are simultaneously altered in both the blood and the target organ. In this class, nucleated cells of peripheral blood and the cells of the 'true' target organ must have – at least in part – an identical transcriptional response. Since basic mechanisms of toxicity, for instance oxidative stress, are described in a variety of organs, it is likely that different cell types show some overlapping gene expression responses to toxic stimuli. An additional class of biomarkers can be identified by studying pathways instead of single genes; however, the number of genes and their signalling pathways that have been linked to toxicological mechanisms is rather small at present. Finally, peripheral blood is systemically delivered to almost all organs throughout the body, allowing communication between blood cells and diverse target or effector cells of the entire

Handbook of Toxicogenomics: Strategies and Applications. Edited by Jürgen Borlak

ISBN: 3-527-30342-1

organism. Therefore, gene expression in blood cells may respond to changes in other organs.

Compared to gene expression studies using solid organs like the liver, there are some specific issues in analyzing peripheral blood. First, peripheral blood is not a closed system, but one of several pools in which the cells of interest (nucleated blood cells) are located. Second, this circulating pool can be altered by processes like recruitment of cells from the bone marrow storage pool. The cellular composition of peripheral blood can be changed by a variety of stimuli, and the blood picture (hemogram) is frequently affected after administration of high doses of drugs or chemicals. Therefore, one has to carefully analyze whether a measured effect in gene expression is caused by 'real' gene expression changes of responding cells or by changes in the cell composition.

22.2
Objective

The aim of this study was to analyze gene expression patterns of peripheral blood cells after administration of three different compounds (cyclosporin A, gentamicin, and WY-14643) to rats and to compare these patterns with those in the liver and/or the kidney of the same animals. The comparisons should identify genes that respond similarly in blood cells and in the liver or kidney after compound administration.

The three compounds were chosen because of their well described side effects. The renal toxicity of gentamicin is characterized by an early impairment in proximal tubular function. The hypolipidemic agent WY-14643 causes rat liver changes typically associated with peroxisome proliferation such as an increase of the liver weight, elevation in hepatic palmitoyl CoA oxidation, and CYP4a induction [8]. The main complication of treatment with the immunosuppressive drug cyclosporin A is nephrotoxicity. In addition, hepatic complications are reported [9]. The pharmacological effect of cyclosporin A made it likely to cause significant gene expression changes in peripheral blood cells, and it was therefore considered a positive control within this study.

The high doses were chosen so as to cause toxic effects in the respective target organ; whereas the selected low dose reflected pharmacological dosage. The early time-point (one day after a single administration) was chosen to compare the acute response of the compounds, the late time-point (7 days or 14 days) was chosen to analyze samples at a time point at which histopathological changes in the respective target organ could be shown. As very limited data on drug induced gene expression patterns in peripheral blood have been published so far, we decided to use a broad approach (with three compounds, two time points, and two doses per compound) rather than an in-depth analysis for a 'final' identification of biomarkers in the blood (using only three replicates, analysis of gene expression by one method).

22.3 Methods

22.3.1 Animal Study

Male Han Wistar rats (CrlGlxBrlHan) (13–15 weeks) (Charles River) were housed in polycarbonate cages with food and water ad libitum. Cyclosporin A (Biomol Research Laboratories) was suspended in olive oil and administered by oral gavage at a low-dose (LD) of 5 mg kg^{-1} d^{-1} and a high-dose (HD) of 50 mg kg^{-1} d^{-1}, respectively. Gentamicin sulphate (Sigma) was given i.m. in a 0.9% saline solution at doses of 2 mg kg^{-1} d^{-1} (LD) or 80 mg kg^{-1} d^{-1} (HD). For WY-14643 (Alexis Biochemicals), a suspension in 0.5% natrosol 250 HX was prepared and given by oral gavage at a dose of 1 mg kg^{-1} d^{-1} (LD) and 50 mg kg^{-1} d^{-1} (HD). Three rats per group were treated with one of the test compounds or with the respective vehicle. Necropsy was performed 24 h after a single administration (all compounds) or 24 h after a 7-day treatment (gentamicin sulphate and WY-14643) or a 14-day treatment (cyclosporin A). A brief summary of the study design is presented in Table 22.1. Animals were anesthetized with sodium pentobarbital via intraperitoneal injection. Blood samples for RNA isolation and haematology were taken from the aorta abdominalis. Standard haematology was performed for white blood cell count, differential leukocyte count (lymphocytes, neutrophils, basophils, eosinophils, and monocytes), red blood cells,

Tab. 22.1 Study design.

Compound	*Route of administration*	*Dosage [mg kg^{-1} d^{-1}]*	*Group*	*Administration time [days]*	*Organ(s) used for DGE*
Cyclosporin A	p.o.	0	control	1	blood/kidney/liver
Cyclosporin A	p.o.	5	low-dose (LD)	1	blood/kidney/liver
Cyclosporin A	p.o.	50	high-dose (HD)	1	blood/kidney/liver
Cyclosporin A	p.o.	0	control	14	blood/kidney
Cyclosporin A	p.o.	5	low-dose (LD)	14	blood/kidney
Cyclosporin A	p.o.	50	high-dose (HD)	14	blood/kidney
Gentamicin	i.m.	0	control	1	blood/kidney
Gentamicin	i.m.	2	low-dose (LD)	1	blood/kidney
Gentamicin	i.m.	80	high-dose (HD)	1	blood/kidney
Gentamicin	i.m.	0	control	7	blood/kidney
Gentamicin	i.m.	2	low-dose (LD)	7	blood/kidney
Gentamicin	i.m.	80	high-dose (HD)	7	blood/kidney
WY-14643	p.o.	0	control	1	blood/liver
WY-14643	p.o.	1	low-dose (LD)	1	blood/liver
WY-14643	p.o.	50	high-dose (HD)	1	blood/liver
WY-14643	p.o.	0	control	7	blood/liver
WY-14643	p.o.	1	low-dose (LD)	7	blood/liver
WY-14643	p.o.	50	high-dose (HD)	7	blood/liver

p.o.: per os (by gavage); i.m.: intra muscular; DGE: differential gene expression.

reticulocytes, haemoglobin, haematocrit, MCH, MCHC, and MCV using an ADVIA (Bayer Diagnostics). After blood collection, the liver and kidneys were immediately removed and weighed. For RNA isolation the right part of the median lobe (lobus dexter medialis) of the liver was snap-frozen in liquid nitrogen. The left part of the median lobe (lobus sinister medialis) was fixed in 10% neutral buffered formalin for histopathological examination. Kidney samples for RNA isolation were collected by hemidissection of the kidneys. One half of each kidney was snap-frozen in liquid nitrogen, the remaining half was fixed in formalin as described above.

22.3.2 RNA Isolation

22.3.2.1 From Whole Blood

For gene expression analysis, blood was sampled in PAXgene blood RNA tubes (PreAnalytiX) and analyzed according to the manufacturer's instructions. Briefly, blood samples (2.5 mL) were collected in PAXgene blood RNA tubes and stored for 1 day at room temperature. RNA isolation began with centrifugation to pellet nucleic acids in the PAXgene blood RNA tube. The pellet was washed, and proteinase K was added to digest proteins. Alcohol was added to adjust binding conditions, and the sample was applied to a PAXgene RNA spin column. During a brief centrifugation, RNA was selectively bound to the PAXgene silica gel membrane as contaminants passed through. After washing steps, RNA was eluted in an optimized buffer. Total RNA was stored at −80 °C.

22.3.2.2 From Peripheral Blood Mononuclear Cells (PBMCs)

To separate PBMCs from whole blood-containing BD Vacutainer™ CPT™ tubes, a centrifugation for 25 min at 1800 × g and RT was performed, and erythrocytes and neutrophils were pelleted below a gel barrier. Directly above the gel barrier PBMCs were visible as a white suspension. After discarding two-thirds of the upper phase, the BD Vacutainer CPT tubes were inverted repeatedly to resuspend PBMCs, which were then transferred into a fresh 15-mL tube. PBMCs were pelleted subsequently by centrifugation for 10 min at 300 × g at 4 °C. After discarding the supernatant, PBMCs were lysed by addition of RLT lysis buffer (Qiagen) containing 1% beta-mercaptoethanol. RNA was extracted with a Qiagen RNeasy kit according to the manufacturer's protocol for RNA isolation from animal cells. In detail, for complete lysis and homogenization, PBMC lysate was applied to a QIAshredder spin column (Qiagen) and was centrifuged at maximum speed. One volume of 70% ethanol was added to the homogenized sample, and the whole suspension was applied to an Rn.easy mini spin-column placed in a 2 mL collection tube. Thereafter, a centrifugation was performed for 15 s at ≥8000 × g. Flowthrough was discarded. To remove DNA contamination, the spin-column membrane was incubated with DNase I prepared with RDD buffer for 15 min at room temperature. The spin-column was washed with RW1 buffer and thereafter transferred to a new collection tube. RPE buffer was passed twice through the spin column by centrifugation for 2 min at ≥10 000 × g. The spin-column was then transferred to a new collection tube, and

RNA was eluted from the spin-column by pipetting water onto the spin-column membrane with subsequent centrifugation for 1 min at $\geq 8000 \times g$. RNA was then analyzed for quality assessment using the Bioanalyzer and RNA chips (Agilent).

22.3.2.3 From Liver and Kidney

After withdrawal of rat liver (right medial lobe) and kidney, samples (one half, prepared by sagittal transection) were wrapped in aluminium foil, frozen in liquid nitrogen, and stored at −80 °C. For homogenization, liver samples were reduced to small pieces by grinding in a mortar filled with liquid nitrogen. Liver pieces as well as kidney samples (each approx. 250 mg) were thawed in RLT lysis buffer (Qiagen) containing beta-mercaptoethanol and homogenized immediately using an Ultrathurrax for 45 s. After homogenization, total RNA was isolated from each sample with an RNeasy Midi Kit (Qiagen), according to the manufacturer's protocol, which is similar to that for the RNeasy Mini Kit described in detail above. To avoid major contamination with genomic DNA, a DNase incubation step was included.

22.3.3 Differential Gene Expression Analysis and Statistics

For differential gene expression analysis GeneChip® (Affymetrix) arrays were used. The principle of this system is to hybridize mRNA transcripts onto a microarray chip (GeneChip) that contains thousands of coding DNA sequences from rats. Thereafter, the hybridized mRNA transcripts were labelled by fluorescence staining, allowing the relative detection of transcripts present in the sample.

In detail: total RNA was converted into double-stranded cDNA by using the Superscript Choice System (Invitrogen). Briefly, 5 µg of total RNA was reverse-transcribed with Superscript II reverse transcriptase and a T7-(dT)24 primer. Second-strand synthesis was then performed with *Escherichia coli* DNA ligase, *E. coli* DNA polymerase and RNase H, and finally with T4 DNA polymerase. To obtain double-stranded DNA, phenol–chloroform–isoamylalcohol extraction was performed by using phase-lock gels (Brinkmann) and ethanol precipitation.

In vitro transcription and biotin labelling was performed with the Bioarray High Yield RNA Transcript Labeling Kit (Enzo). cRNA was then purified with an RNeasy Mini Kit (Qiagen) and then fragmented.

Fragmented labelled cRNA (15 µg) together with control cRNA spikes (BioB, BioC, BioD, cre) were loaded onto Affymetrix rat GeneChip array RGU35A, which contains coding DNA sequences of nearly 8800 transcripts, for overnight hybridization. After hybridization, the arrays were washed and stained with streptavidin–phycoerythrin. The GeneChip arrays were analyzed at a resolution of 3 µm with a Hewlett-Packard GeneArray Scanner.

For calculation of the GeneChip hybridization signals, the Affymetrix Microarray Suite software (MAS 5.0) was employed using default settings. Briefly, standard background correction was carried out, and each GeneChip array was scaled to a target intensity of 100 in order to compare the different arrays. For an absolute expression analysis, MAS 5.0 uses an algorithm that results in a 'detection call', which indicates whether a particular transcript is present (detected) or absent (undetected). Another algorithm calculates a 'signal' value for each probe set, which indicates the relative abundance of the respective transcript.

Since each experiment was done in triplicate, the median signal value of each set of triplicates was used for differential analysis of untreated samples versus treated samples. This analysis resulted in a 'fold change' value for each transcript after treatment.

In addition to the values derived from MAS 5.0 analysis, we performed calculations with the Statistical Analyses System SAS (version 6.12). To compare the difference between untreated and treated samples a nonparametric Mann–Whitney U test (two-sided) was employed. With a confidence interval of 95% (p value of 0.05) the Mann–Whitney U test extracted only those probe sets from the treatment group for which the single values from a triplicate were either all higher or all lower than the respective values of the control group.

To extract significantly differentially expressed genes, we defined the following cut-off criteria. The extracted genes must have a p value of 0.05 according to the Mann–Whitney U test, and they must have at least two 'present' calls out of six 'detection' calls (each three for treated and untreated samples). In addition, each probe set (gene) was considered to have a fold change value of at least 1.2.

This set of cut-off criteria resulted in a set of differentially expressed genes that were the basis for our functional classification. Due to the limited number of animals per treatment group (three), there is a probability that false negatives occur (especially when one animal did not respond). Therefore, particular genes of interest (e.g., according to their known relation to adverse events) were evaluated by analyzing the respective raw values rather than by doing an automated analysis based on the defined cut-off criteria.

22.4 Results and Discussion

22.4.1 Comparison of Analyzing Two Different Blood Cell Populations

Peripheral blood contains nucleated cells (predominantly neutrophils, lymphocytes, and monocytes), as well as non-nucleated cells (platelets and reticulocytes), which contain residual transcripts. As each of the cell types has a variety of functions, the cell/RNA isolation method substantially affects the outcome of the study. For the main part of the study we decided to use the PAXgene Blood RNA system, by which the RNA profile is immediately stabilized at the point of collection. This minimizes changes in gene expression due to storage, transportation, and manipulation of the sample. In addition, the inclusion of all blood cell types may be an advantage for the search of biomarkers. The disadvantage of this approach is that low-abundance mRNA (especially if the cell type is rare within peripheral blood, e.g., monocytes) may fall below the detection limit of the GeneChips.

For a limited number of control samples, we used Vacutainer cell preparation tubes (CPT) as a second method; these allow isolation of the peripheral blood mononuclear cells (PBMCs) by density gradient centrifugation. The enrichment of these important immunologically relevant and nucleated cells should increase the gene detection sensitivity for them, making it possible to monitor transcripts that are expressed at low levels especially in these cell types.

So far it is not clear whether the expression of certain genes may be altered during processing of the blood samples due to *in vitro* transcription.

Table 22.2 shows the differences of the cell types that were analyzed by the two applied methods. Vacutainer centrifugation resulted in elimination of red blood cells, decrease in the amount of neutrophils (the dominant cell type), and therefore enrichment of PBMCs. Interestingly, in this rat experiment the monocytes were also largely eliminated.

According to product information (joint letter between PreAnalytiX and Affymetrix, 2003; http://www.affymetrix.com/), human blood shows 10%–15% fewer 'present calls' and a ~1.5-fold decrease in signal intensity for whole blood RNA prepared by the PAXgene method compared with PBMC RNA obtained with the Vacutainer CPT system. To assess the difference of expression sensitivity within rat blood, we compared gene expression results performed with RNA from the two different methods. We found an increase of 'present calls' in rat blood from 13.5% for the PaxGene method to 35.6% for the Vacutainer CPT method. This high difference may be due to the different composition of rat blood compared to human blood. When comparing three independent GeneChip arrays for PBMCs and three for whole blood, we detected 1258 genes as 'present' in all three PBMCs arrays and 'absent' in all three whole blood arrays, indicating a significant gain in sensitivity. However, we cannot exclude the possibility that a number of genes were unregulated by the isolation process. We found only 16 genes that were 'present' in all whole blood samples and at the same time 'absent' in the PBMC analysis. The occurrence of genes present only in whole blood may be explained by genes predominantly expressed in neutrophils, which were depleted in the PBMC fraction. It is known that non-nucleated reticulocytes carry large numbers of RNA molecules (tRNA, rRNA, mRNA). Although this cell type represents only 0.5% to 2% of the

Tab. 22.2 Hemogram of rat peripheral blood.

Cell type	*Rat blood cells* [a)] *% of WBC*	*Rat PBMC* [b)] *% of WBC*
Neutrophils	10.9	3.2
Lymphocytes	85.9	95.5
Monocytes	1.3	0.1
Eosinophils	1.3	1.1
Basophils	0.3	0

PBMC: peripheral blood cells; WBC: white blood cells
a) Derived from whole peripheral blood.
b) Derived from Vacutainer CPT centrifugation.

red blood cells, their RNA may contribute up to 70% of total RNA from whole blood, because of the very high number of red blood cells in blood (Technical Note, 2003, Affymetrix).

In summary, the choice of blood cell population and RNA isolation method has a major impact on gene expression results. Therefore, all results have to be discussed in the context of the underlying cell and RNA separation techniques.

22.4.2 Hemogram/Histopathology in the Animal Study

Hemograms of blood derived from samples taken at each time point and each dose reveal that the compounds did not induce significant changes in the proportions of blood cell populations. Therefore, detected gene expression changes are not due to changes in the blood picture. We cannot however exclude the possibility that the composition of lymphocyte subtypes may have changed.

Pathology induced in the kidney or the liver after administration of the test compounds reflected the findings published in the literature and showed that the high doses of the test compounds used can be considered toxic. In the kidneys of animals given 50 mg kg^{-1} cyclosporin for 14 days, the cells of the juxtaglomerular apparatus were hyperplastic. The epithelium of renal tubules showed degenerative and regenerative changes. Gentamicin administration at 80 mg kg^{-1} for seven days caused adverse effects in the kidney. Tubular epithelial cells, laden with massive amounts of eosinophilic granular material, underwent necrosis. Hyaline casts were present in markedly affected tubules and the epithelium showed regenerative changes. There was no, or only minimal, interstitial inflammatory reaction. A seven-day administration of 50 mg kg^{-1} WY-14643 caused a moderate hepatocellular hypertrophy with an increased number of mitotic figures.

22.4.3 Analysis of the Number of Significantly Deregulated Genes

22.4.3.1 Blood

First we analyzed the number of genes that showed a significant compound-induced expression change in both peripheral blood and the respective target organs.

In the peripheral blood samples collected 24 h after a single administration, the number of deregulated genes was comparable for all compounds and was in the range of 1.2% to 2.2% of the 8800 analyzed probe sets. This number of detected genes must be interpreted in light of the fact that the gene expression analysis of whole rat blood (PaxGene protocol) results in only 13.5% 'present calls'. As the 'present call' is one of the selection criteria we used (see Methods) the number of 'truly' changed genes might be underestimated in our analysis due to limited sensitivity of the procedure for RNA isolation and subsequent GeneChip analysis. Interestingly, neither an increase in the number of deregulated genes nor an increase in the magnitude of the deregulation was observed in the high-dose groups relative to the low-dose groups at this time point (Table 22.3).

Tab. 22.3 Numbers of deregulated genes in blood cells after treatment with cyclosporin A, gentamicin, or WY-14643.

	1 d LD			*1 d HD*			*7d/14d* LD*			*7d/14d* HD*		
	FC≥1.2	*FC≥2*	*FC≥5*	*FC≥1.2*	*FC≥2*	*FC≥5*	*FC≥1.2*	*FC≥2*	*FC≥5*	*FC≥1.2*	*FC≥2*	*FC≥5*
						Cyclosporin A*						
Up	64		0	56	0	0	52	0	0	153	58	13
Down	52	4	0	36	5	0	44	1	0	133	12	0
Total	116	4	0	92	5	0	96	1	0	286	70	13
						Gentamicin						
Up	85	16	0	50	3	0	43	1	0	96	1	0
Down	101	7	0	66	8	0	42	0	0	60	0	0
Total	186	23	0	116	11	0	85	1	1	156	1	0
						WY-14643						
Up	76	7	0	88	7	2	42	0	0	56	3	0
Down	98	7	0	110	10	0	32	2	1	36	2	0
Total	174	14	0	198	17	2	74	2	1	92	5	0

LD = low-dose; HD = high-dose; d = day; FC = fold change.

After 7 or 14 days of administration of WY-14643 or gentamicin, the number and extent of deregulated genes was in the same range as described for day one. In contrast, a 14-day administration of 50 mg kg^{-1} cyclosporin A (high-dose) caused a strong increase in the number of affected genes. In addition, the number of genes whose expression was changed more than 2-fold or 5-fold relative to controls was significantly increased. It is likely that this gene expression response is due to the pharmacological effect of cyclosporin A on blood cells and their precursors. However, as a 14-day administration of 50 mg kg^{-1} cyclosporin A causes nephrotoxicity, some of the changes may also reflect toxic effects in the target organ.

When comparing the genes that were deregulated in both the low- and the high-dose groups by a particular compound after 24 h, we found an overlap of about 20% for all compounds tested (Table 22.4). In addition, the majority of these genes were deregulated in the identical direction. This high percentage of overlapping genes be-

Tab. 22.4 Percentage of deregulated genes in blood overlapping in different doses and time points when treated with cyclosporin A, gentamicin or WY-14643.

	*Cyclosporin A**		*Gentamicin*		*WY-14643*	
Overlap (dose)	% of LD	% of HD	% of LD	% of HD	% of LD	% of HD
1 d LD + HD	19.82	25	15.59	25	22.98	20.2
7d/14d* LD + HD	14.58	4.89	14.11	7.69	13.51	10.86
Overlap (time)	% of 1d	% of 14d	% of 1d	% of 7d	% of 1d	% of 7d
LD 1 d + 7d/14d*	10.34	12.5	3.76	8.23	1.72	4.05
HD 1 d + 7d/14d*	6.52	2.09	7.75	5.76	7.57	16.3

d = day; LD = low-dose; HD = high-dose

Tab. 22.5 Numbers of deregulated genes in the kidney after treatment with cyclosporin A or gentamicin.

	1 d LD			*1 d HD*			*7d/14d* LD*			*7d/14d* HD*		
	FC≥1.2	*FC≥2*	*FC≥5*	*FC≥1.2*	*FC≥2*	*FC≥5*	*FC≥1.2*	*FC≥2*	*FC≥5*	*FC≥1.2*	*FC≥2*	*FC≥5*
						Cyclosporin A*						
Up	114	1	0	117	13	1	122	0	0	210	21	3
Down	78	1	0	107	4	0	156	0	0	234	21	4
Total	192	2	0	224	17	1	278	0	0	444	42	7
						Gentamicin						
Up	233	5	0	182	6	0	52	4	0	590	113	17
Down	114	2	0	94	0	0	40	3	0	344	29	0
Total	347	7	0	276	6	0	92	7	0	934	142	17

LD = low-dose; HD = high-dose; d = day; FC = fold change.

tween the low- and the high-dose groups indicates that the observed gene expression response of peripheral blood cells is compound-specific. We did not identify any single gene that was significantly affected by all three drugs after 24 h.

The numbers of genes deregulated in the identical direction at both dosages of each of the compounds were remarkably decreased after 7 or 14 days of administration (Table 22.4). This decrease may be due to diversification of the gene expression response over time. As the high-dose treatments caused adverse effects in the respective target organ (kidney and/or liver), the decreased overlap between the low- and high-dose groups after 7 or 14 days compared to the overlap after one day may also reflect the pathophysiological situation.

22.4.3.2 Kidney

The highest number of deregulated genes in the kidney was observed in the high-dose groups after 7 days of gentamicin and 14 days of cyclosporin A administration, the time points at which histopathological changes in the liver were observed (Table 22.5). Cyclosporin A induced an increase of deregulated genes after a single dose of 50 mg kg^{-1}. In contrast, a single dose of 80 mg kg^{-1} gentamicin did not cause an increase in changing genes compared to the low-dose (2 mg kg^{-1}). Overall, the kidney as the toxicological target organ responded to toxic doses of cyclosporin A or gentamicin with significant changes in gene expression.

22.4.3.3 Liver

Analysis of the liver samples revealed a strong gene expression response after administration of WY-14643. The number of affected genes rose from the low-dose group (1 mg kg^{-1}) to the high-dose group (50 mg kg^{-1}) from about 6% to 13% (Table 22.6). In contrast to the observations in the kidney after cyclosporin A and gentamicin administration, the strongest response to WY-14643 was seen after one day, a time point at which histopathological changes were not observed.

An evident and dose-dependent gene expression response in the liver was observed after cyclosporin A administration, consistent with the cyclosporin A-dependent hepatic side effects reported in the literature.

Tab. 22.6 Numbers of deregulated genes in the liver after treatment with cyclosporin A or WY-14643.

	1 d LD			*1 d HD*			*7 d LD*			*7 d HD*		
	FC≥1.2	*FC≥2*	*FC≥5*	*FC≥1.2*	*FC≥2*	*FC≥5*	*FC≥1.2*	*FC≥2*	*FC≥5*	*FC≥1.2*	*FC≥2*	*FC≥5*
					Cyclosporin A							
Up	83	2	1	209	10	0						
Down	89	5	0	150	7	3		n. d.			n. d.	
Total	172	7	1	359	17	3						
					WY-14643							
Up	181	23	7	438	112	25	199	46	11	189	92	17
Down	361	43	2	712	157	7	221	12	1	640	118	10
Total	542	66	9	1150	269	32	420	58	12	829	210	27

LD = low-dose; HD = high-dose; d = day; FC = fold change; n. d. = not done.

22.4.4
Analysis of Deregulated Genes in Blood after Cyclosporin A Administration

The immunosuppressive drug cyclosporin A was used as a positive control for gene expression changes in blood. The mechanism of action of cyclosporin A was recently reviewed [10].

In Table 22.7, all genes that were differentially regulated after administration of 50 mg kg^{-1} cyclosporin A for 14 days, according to the defined criteria, are classified into functional classes. Many genes regulated in blood can be functionally linked to immunomodulation, as is likely after administration of an immunosuppressant drug. Many of them can be assigned to T-cell response (for example, cytokine components or immunoglobulins). Several genes are related to activities of the innate immune system (for example, Kupffer cell receptor), indicating that the cyclosporin A response is not only T-cell specific.

Expression of the hepatocyte growth factor (HGF), and the ligand of the receptor tyrosine kinase MET was down-regulated by cyclosporin A (Table 22.7). The signalling pathway controlled by these two genes is involved in many inflammatory processes [11–13]. Rat studies have shown that HGF, which is low in the liver under physiological conditions, is highly induced by liver damage [14, 15]. HGF is secreted into serum, binds after activation to the receptor MET, and enhances liver regeneration. HGF activity is often regulated on the protein level by release from cell repositories and the extracellular matrix, or by proteolytic cleavage of HGF precursor [16, 17], but can also be regulated by transcription [18, 19]. In addition, the transcription is also inducible, especially through inflammatory stimulation. Although specialized liver cells (Ito cells) seem to be the main producer under these conditions, the secretion of HGF from intracellular vesicles of neutrophils, as well as the presence of HGF transcripts within this cell type, was shown recently [20]. Expression of *c-met*, the gene for the HGF receptor MET, in mononuclear blood cells is low or even absent under physiological conditions, but is highly inducible through stimulation by mediators of inflammation [21, 22]. The observed down-regulation of both HGF

Tab. 22.7 Deregulated genes[a)] in blood after treatment with cyclosporin A (14 days, high-dose).

Sequence ID (Affymetrix)	*Description*	*Fold change*
Immune response/inflammation		
U17919	allograft inflammatory factor 1	1.8
U72350	B cell lymphoma 2 like	–1.53
rc_AA818072	bcl-2 associated death agonist	1.38
M61875	CD44 antigen	1.84
rc_AA818025	CD59 antigen	1.71
rc_AA818025	CD59 antigen	2.21
U90610	chemokine receptor (LCR1)	–1.29
AJ009698	embigin	1.53
rc_AA891690	ESTs, highly similar to tumour necrosis factor (ligand) superfamily, member 13 [*Mus musculus*]	5.03
rc_AA893235	ESTs, highly similar to G0S2_MOUSE putative lymphocyte G0/G1 switch protein 2 (G0S2-like protein) [*M. musculus*]	13.04
rc_AA799861	ESTs, highly similar to IRF7_MOUSE Interferon regulatory factor 7 (IRF-7) [*M. musculus*]	–1.68
rc_AA799861	ESTs, highly similar to IRF7_MOUSE Interferon regulatory factor 7 (IRF-7) [*M. musculus*]	–1.55
M21622	Fc fragment of Ige, high affinity I, receptor for, alpha polypeptide	–2.05
M32062	Fc receptor, IgG, low affinity III	5.03
M32062	Fc receptor, IgG, low affinity III	5.94
X54400	hepatocyte growth factor	–2.02
AJ223184	immunoglobulin superfamily, member 6	1.97
AJ223184	immunoglobulin superfamily, member 6	3.1
X65036	integrin alpha 7	–1.57
AF003598	Integrin beta 7	1.33
X52140	integrin, alpha 1	–1.46
rc_AI177366	Integrin, beta 1	1.96
rc_AI014163	interferon-related developmental regulator 1	2.77
M98820	interleukin 1 beta	1.59
M55532	Kupffer cell receptor	–1.81
rc_AI232078	latent transforming growth factor beta binding protein 1	–1.56
U53184	LPS-induced TNF-alpha factor	1.35
U65007	met proto-oncogene	–1.61
rc_AA924542	p38 mitogen activated protein kinase	–1.41
M18853	rat T-cell receptor active alpha-chain C-region mRNA, partial cds, clone TRA29	–1.37
AF029240	*Rattus norvegicus* partial mRNA for BM1k MHC class Ib antigen, strain SHR	–1.23
Stress/oxidative stress		
D78308	calreticulin	–1.47
M21060	superoxide dismutase 1, soluble	1.44
rc_AA891286	thioredoxin reductase 1	1.94
J03752	microsomal glutathione S-transferase 1	2.61
Unclassified		
V01217	actin, beta	1.25
M63282	activating transcription factor 3	–1.42

Tab. 22.7 (continued)

Sequence ID (Affymetrix)	Description	Fold change
Unclassified (continued)		
D12771	adenine nucleotide translocator 2, fibroblast isoform (ATP–ADP carrier protein)	3.61
M64780	agrin	–1.61
M12919mRNA#2	aldolase A	1.5
M12919mRNA#2	aldolase A	1.6
X73911	amiloride binding protein 1	–1.59
X52196cds	arachidonate 5-lipoxygenase activating protein	1.92
rc_AI104781	arachidonate 5-lipoxygenase-activating protein	3.24
D13120	ATP synthase subunit δ	1.44
rc_AA799778	ATP synthase, H^+ transporting, mitochondrial F_0 complex, subunit β, isoform 1	1.5
X54510	ATP synthase, H^+ transporting, mitochondrial F_0 complex, subunit F6	1.58
rc_AA800212	ATPase, Ca^{2+} transporting, cardiac muscle, slow twitch 2	–1.45
U43175	ATPase, vacuolar, 14 kDa	1.23
rc_AA891035	beclin 1 (coiled-coil, myosin-like BCL2-interacting protein)	2.14
M81681	biliverdin reductase A	2.66
AJ132230	bradykinin receptor B1	–1.64
rc_AA799418	calcitonin gene-related peptide-receptor component protein	1.37
rc_AI010725	calnexin	1.6
L13039	calpactin I heavy chain	2.75
L07578	casein kinase 1, delta	–1.3
M38135	cathepsin H	1.85
X60769mRNA	CCAAT/enhancer binding protein (C/EBP), beta	6.04
M65149	CCAAT/enhancer binding, protein (C/EBP) delta	3.6
U23056	C-CAM4 protein	1.26
rc_AA925473	cell division cycle 42 homolog (S. cerevisiae)	1.53
U42976	cholinergic receptor, nicotinic, beta polypeptide 4	–1.55
AJ224680	cyclic nucleotide-gated channel beta subunit 1	–1.36
U18729	cytochrome b558 alpha subunit	4.15
AF076183	cytosolic sorting protein PACS-1	–1.57
AF045564	development-related protein	–2.49
X59267	drebrin 1	–1.77
U42627	dual specificity phosphatase 6	2.29
rc_AI104012	dual specificity Yak1-related kinase	–1.47
X98377	emerin	1.45
rc_AI639247	EST, moderately similar to T17296 hypothetical protein DKFZp434I092.1 – human (fragment) [*Homo sapiens*]	–1.2
rc_AA799654	ESTs, highly similar to f-box and WD-40 domain protein 5; F-box protein Fbw5 [*M. musculus*]	–1.26
rc_AA874999	ESTs, highly similar to protein translocation complex beta; protein transport protein SEC61 beta subunit [*H. sapiens*]	1.62
rc_AA891790	ESTs, highly similar to RIKEN cDNA 2310005G07 [*M. musculus*]	–1.49
rc_AA933158	ESTs, highly similar to superkiller viralicidic activity 2-like (*Saccharomyces cerevisiae*) [*M. musculus*]	–1.36
rc_AA956114	ESTs, highly similar to ubiquitin conjugating enzyme [*R. norvegicus*]	1.82

Tab. 22.7 (continued)

Sequence ID (Affymetrix)	Description	Fold change
Unclassified (continued)		
rc_AA891717	ESTs, highly similar to upstream transcription factor 1 [*R. norvegicus*]	−1.2
rc_AA893173	ESTs, highly similar to vacuolar protein sorting 29 (S. *pombe*); vacuolar protein sorting 29 (yeast); vacuolar sorting protein 29 [*M. musculus*]	4.01
rc_AA893741	ESTs, highly similar to zinc finger protein 289; RIKEN cDNA 2310032E02 gene [*M. musculus*]	−1.43
rc_AA891920	ESTs, highly similar to A chain A, structural basis for the recognition of a nucleoporin Fg repeat by the Ntf2-like domain of Tap-P15 Mrna nuclear export factor [*H. sapiens*]	−2.07
rc_AA874874	ESTs, Highly similar to ADHX_RAT alcohol dehydrogenase class III (alcohol dehydrogenase 2) (glutathione-dependent formaldehyde dehydrogenase) (fdh) (faldh) (alcohol dehydrogenase-B2) [*R. norvegicus*]	−1.32
rc_AA892179	ESTs, highly similar to CIKS_HUMAN adapter protein CIKS (Connection to IKK and SAPK/JNK) [*H. sapiens*]	−1.36
rc_AA875523	ESTs, highly similar to MLES_RAT myosin light chain alkali, smooth-muscle isoform (MLC3SM) [*R. norvegicus*]	−1.99
rc_AA866276	ESTs, highly similar to MYDM_MOUSE myeloid-associated differentiation marker (myeloid up-regulated protein) [*M. musculus*]	2.37
rc_AI639387	ESTs, highly similar to RT06_MOUSE mitochondrial 28S ribosomal protein S6 (MRP-S6) [*M. musculus*]	1.42
rc_AI639518	ESTs, highly similar to S55370 RNA polymerase II chain hRPB17 [*H. sapiens*]	−1.51
rc_AI178828	eukaryotic translation initiation factor 4E binding protein 1	−2.1
U05014	eukaryotic translation initiation factor 4E binding protein 1	1.74
D90109	fatty acid coenzyme A ligase, long chain 2	1.92
AB012933	fatty acid coenzyme A ligase, long chain 5	1.96
X05834	fibronectin 1	3.07
X16145	fucosidase, alpha-L-1, tissue	1.54
rc_AI009191	Fyn proto-oncogene	1.69
L14684	G elongation factor	−1.3
rc_AI232477	G protein gamma-5 subunit	2.5
D13518	GATA-binding protein 1 (globin transcription factor 1)	−1.43
X74402	GDP-dissociation inhibitor 1	1.59
L28801	general transcription factor III C 1	−1.64
X07467	glucose-6-phosphate dehydrogenase	1.31
U08259	glutamate receptor, ionotropic, NMDA2C	−1.89
M91652complete_seq	glutamine synthetase (glutamate-ammonia ligase)	1.67
M91652complete_seq	glutamine synthetase (glutamate-ammonia ligase)	1.77
U96130	glycogenin	1.91
L02896	glypican 1	−1.47
rc_AI175208	golgi SNAP receptor complex member 2	−1.24
D49847	growth factor receptor bound protein 2	−1.6
U53475	GTPase Rab8b	2.02

Tab. 22.7 (continued)

Sequence ID (Affymetrix)	*Description*	*Fold change*
Unclassified (continued)		
M12672	GTP-binding protein (G-alpha-i2)	1.2
M17526	guanine nucleotide binding protein, alpha o	–1.46
U88324	guanine nucleotide-binding protein beta 1	1.43
U88324	guanine nucleotide-binding protein beta 1	1.46
rc_AA875512	hemoglobin Y, beta-like embryonic chain	–1.52
rc_AA965147	heterogeneous nuclear ribonucleoprotein A1	2.25
rc_AI070026	homeo box A2	–2.3
AB017140	homer, neuronal immediate early gene, 1	–1.59
rc_AI137583	Inhibitor of DNA binding 2, dominant negative helix-loop-helix protein	2.42
M54926	lactate dehydrogenase A	1.33
U19614	lamina-associated polypeptide 1C	1.52
J02962	lectin, galactose binding, soluble 3	2.93
L03294	lipoprotein lipase	–1.38
Z11995cds	low density lipoprotein receptor-related protein associated protein 1	2.02
rc_AA892775	lysozyme	1.41
rc_AI010480	malate dehydrogenase mitochondrial	1.49
M93401	methylmalonate semialdehyde dehydrogenase gene	–1.67
U75920	microtubule-associated protein, RP/EB family, member 1	–1.8
AB017655	muscarinic receptor m2	–1.79
U31367	myelin and lymphocyte protein	4.49
M62992	nuclear pore glycoprotein 62	–1.51
M25804	nuclear receptor subfamily 1, group D, member 1	–1.3
U10995	nuclear receptor subfamily 2, group F, member 1	–1.43
AF003926	nuclear receptor subfamily 2, group F, member 6	–1.52
rc_AA866472	nucleosome assembly protein 1-like 1	–1.33
M58369	pancreatic lipase	–1.56
AF065438	peptidylprolyl isomerase C-associated protein	–3.72
U25651	phosphofructokinase, muscle	–1.64
X59601	plectin	1.21
X76724	potassium voltage gated channel, shaker related subfamily, beta member 2	–1.38
U57362	procollagen, type XII, alpha 1	–1.78
rc_AI235492	proline rich 2	–1.56
rc_AA875233	prosaposin (sulphated glycoprotein, sphingolipid hydrolase activator)	2.26
M19936	prosaposin (sulphated glycoprotein, sphingolipid hydrolase activator)	3.05
AB017188	proteasome (prosome, macropain) 26S subunit, non-ATPase, 4	–1.24
X02918	protein disulfide isomerase (Prolyl 4-hydroxylase, beta polypeptide)	1.44
U06230	protein S	–1.62
D45412	protein tyrosine phosphatase, receptor type, O	2.2
U28938	protein tyrosine phosphatase, receptor type, O	2.94
U73458	protein tyrosine phosphatase, receptor-type, N polypeptide 2	–1.42
X63675	proviral integration site 1	–1.33
M75153	RAB11a, member RAS oncogene family	1.56

Tab. 22.7 (continued)

Sequence ID (Affymetrix)	*Description*	*Fold change*
Unclassified (continued)		
AA799389	Rab3B protein	−1.42
rc_AA893443	RAP1B, member of RAS oncogene family	1.87
X85183	Ras-related GTP-binding protein ragA	−1.24
rc_AA892146	*R. norvegicus* Tclone4 mRNA	2.42
rc_AA900505	rhoB gene	2.38
rc_AI639490	ribosomal protein S10	−1.69
AF100470	ribosome associated membrane protein 4	1.9
M10094	RT1 class Ib gene	−1.87
X06916	S100 calcium-binding protein A4	3.85
rc_AA957003	S100 calcium-binding protein A8 (calgranulin A)	4.23
U33472	serine/threonine kinase 10	1.29
M83143	sialyltransferase 1 (beta-galactoside alpha-2,6-sialytransferase)	−1.39
rc_AI232096	solute carrier family 15, member 2	−1.56
D13962	solute carrier family 2 A3 (neuron glucose transporter)	−1.33
rc_AA859666	solute carrier family 25 (mitochondrial carrier; dicarboxylate transporter), member 10	−1.37
D82883	solute carrier family 26 (sulphate transporter), member 2	−1.44
M96601	solute carrier family 6, member 6	2.14
AF052596	synaptosomal-associated protein, 23 kDa	1.29
L20822	syntaxin 5a	−1.41
X56228	thiosulfate sulphur transferase (rhodanese)	−1.59
U09256	transketolase	2.01
rc_AA860030	tubulin, beta 5	−1.59
AB015432	tumour-associated protein 1	−1.37
rc_AI180424	tyrosine 3-monooxygenase/tryptophan 5-monooxygenase activation protein, zeta polypeptide	1.47
rc_AI103698	UDP-glucose dehydrogenase	−1.86
AB013732	UDP-glucose dehydrogenase	−1.43
X52311	unr protein	1.8
rc_AI237654	up-regulated by 1,25-dihydroxy vitamin D-3	1.55
rc_AI059963	vacuolar protein sorting homolog r-vps33b	−1.45
X62952	vimentin	2.68

a) Sequences with unknown function or ESTs with moderate or weak similarity to known genes are not included.

and MET is in line with the immunosuppressive effect of cyclosporin A. The physiological relevance of the down-regulation in healthy animals without signs of inflammation or infection and hence with low expression levels of HGF and MET in blood has to be clarified.

Several genes, such as those encoding microsomal glutathione S-transferase 1 and superoxide dismutase 1 (Table 22.7), which are associated with antioxidant defence mechanisms, were up-regulated in blood cells after cyclosporin A administration. Glutathione S-transferases are induced by a variety of extracellular stimuli, such as hormones, chemical carcinogens, and cellular stress-inducing agents. Several observations imply reactive oxygen as a transduction signal [23]. Superoxide dismutase is an important protective enzyme against the superoxide anion. Interestingly, there is some evidence that reactive oxygen species take part in the cyclosporin A-induced pathogenesis of the kidney [10]. Oxidative stress is a common toxic mechanism, and marker genes for this effect are good candidates for bridging biomarkers. Recently, simultaneous differential gene expression of genes indicative of oxidative stress was described in the blood and the heart of rats after administration of adriamycin [24].

22.4.5
Analysis of Genes Deregulated in Blood and Target Organ

To search for biomarkers of toxicity in blood we looked for genes that are simultaneously deregulated in both peripheral blood cells and the respective target organ of WY-14643 (liver), cyclosporin A (kidney and liver), and gentamicin (kidney). Table 22.8 shows the percentage of deregulated genes in whole blood that were also deregulated in the liver or kidney at the identical time points and dose. Between 0.9% (cyclosporin A, one day, low-dose) and 28% (WY-14643, one day, high-dose) of the genes found to be deregulated in whole blood were also significantly regulated in the liver or kidney. The higher overlap in the high-dose groups occurred mainly because more genes were found to be deregulated in the defined target organ.

Tab. 22.8 Percentage of deregulated genes in blood also deregulated in other organs.

		Kidney		*Liver*	
		Cyclosporin A %[a)]	*Gentamicin* %[a)]	*Cyclosporin A* %[a)]	*WY-14643* %[a)]
1 day	LD	0.9	5.9	2.6	13.8
	HD	4.3	8.6	8.7	28.3
7/14 days	LD	7.3	1.2		10.6
	HD	9.8	12.2		16.3

a) Percentage of genes detected in blood and overlapping with kidney or liver detection.
LD = low-dose; HD = high-dose.

22.4.5.1 WY-14643

Table 22.9 shows the genes that were significantly deregulated in identical directions in both blood and liver after one day of administration of 50 mg kg^{-1} WY-14643.

TSC-22

One of these genes is the gene for transforming growth factor-β–stimulated clone 22 (*TSC-22*). We have frequently observed down-regulation of *TSC-22* after administration of toxins in several organs (unpublished results), suggesting that changes in *TSC-22* expression may be an unspecific marker of toxicity in several organs. *TSC-22* encodes a leucine zipper-containing protein that represses transcription [25]. *TSC-22*

Tab. 22.9 Genes deregulated in an identical direction in blood and liver after treatment with WY-14643 (one day, high-dose).

Sequence ID	*Description*	*Fold change (blood)*	*Fold change (liver)*
AB003515	GABA(A) receptor-associated protein like 2	−1.33	−1.2
D78308	calreticulin	−1.44	−2.12
J02962	lectin, galactose binding, soluble 3	−2.04	−1.36
K03250	ribosomal protein S11	1.21	1.47
L15618	casein kinase II, alpha 1 polypeptide	−1.39	−1.48
L25785	transforming growth factor beta stimulated clone 22	−1.57	−2.47
M11670	catalase	−1.51	−1.36
M17419	ribosomal protein L5	1.35	1.35
M25804	nuclear receptor subfamily 1, group D, member 1	1.29	1.6
M91597	nucleoside diphosphate kinase	1.36	1.36
rc_AA891068	peptidylglycine alpha-amidating monooxygenase	−1.76	−1.34
rc_AA892831	ESTs, Highly similar to JC6524 26S proteasome regulatory complex chain p44.5 [*H. sapiens*]	1.46	1.47
rc_AI014135	ESTs	1.65	1.91
rc_AI172162	proteasome (prosome, macropain) subunit, beta type 4	1.38	1.53
rc_AI178207	ribosomal protein S21	1.42	1.44
rc_AI639394	–	1.79	1.48
S48325	–	1.49	1.32
U00926	ATP synthase, H^+ transporting, mitochondrial F_1 complex, δ subunit	1.42	1.64
U23769	PDZ and LIM domain 1	−1.37	−1.27
U76714	solute carrier family 39 (iron-regulated transporter), member 1	−1.43	−1.97
V01217	actin, beta	−1.23	−1.26
X53363cds	calreticulin	−1.68	−2.29
X53773	adaptor protein complex AP-2, alpha 2 subunit	−1.22	−1.39
X57529cds	–	1.32	1.24
X62146cds	–	1.35	1.21
X95850mRNA	–	1.71	−1.36
Z78279	collagen, type 1, alpha 1	1.35	−1.59

was originally isolated as a TGF-β-induced gene; however, the *TSC-22* promoter was not activated by the enhanced TGF-β signalling. Therefore it was suggested that up-regulation of TSC-22 mRNA by TGF-β 1 is achieved by mRNA stabilization, not by transcriptional activation [26]. Nakashiro et al. [27] found that *TSC-22* is induced by anticancer drugs in a human salivary gland cancer cell line. In addition, *TSC-22* negatively regulates the growth of these cells, and down-regulation of *TSC-22* in these cells plays a major role in salivary gland tumourigenesis. Overexpression of *TSC-22* markedly enhances 5-fluorouracil–induced apoptosis [28]. Interestingly, the therapeutic activity of PPARgamma agonists against prostate cancer was also associated with increased expression of *TSC-22* [29]. Taking these results together, *TSC-22* seems to play a role in the control of proliferation and apoptosis. Its observed down-regulation in blood and liver cells (1.6- and 2.5-fold respectively, Table 22.9) may be a sign of WY-14643-induced proliferative and transcription-controlled effects.

Calreticulin

Calreticulin is found in every cell of higher organisms, with the exception of erythrocytes. Calreticulin was first identified as a Ca^{2+}-binding protein of the muscle sarcoplasmic reticulum [30]. Over the past several years a large number of cellular functions have been proposed for calreticulin, which include cell adhesion and gene expression, as well as endoplasmatic reticulum-related functions like chaperone activity and Ca^{2+} storage [31]. This variety of functions makes it difficult to interpret the effect of the observed down-regulation of its gene one day after WY-14643 treatment. We observed that the calreticulin gene is also down-regulated after 14 days of cyclosporin A treatment. The frequent regulation of this gene after administration of compounds in toxic doses (unpublished data) is in accordance with other studies [32], and suggests that calreticulin is an unspecific stress marker.

22.4.5.2 Gentamicin

One of the genes that is significantly regulated in the identical direction in both blood and kidney after seven days administration of gentamicin at 80 mg kg^{-1} was that for glutathione peroxidase 1 (data for other identified genes not shown). This gene was significantly down-regulated (1.3-fold) in both kidney and peripheral blood cells. A persistent decrease in glutathione peroxidase activity in rat liver after gentamicin treatment was shown by Soejima et al. [33]. In addition, reduced activity of glutathione peroxidase was also reported in the kidney and the heart of guinea pigs [34, 35]. As gentamicin seems to induce oxidative stress in different organs and different species, glutathione peroxidase 1 can be considered to be a candidate gene for gentamicin-related toxicity.

22.4.5.3 Cyclosporin A

Calbindin

A biomarker of toxicity is ideally directly connected with the specific toxic mechanism of the evaluated compound. One candidate is calbindin-D28kDa, a protein whose expression was found to be down-regulated after cyclosporin A administration to rats, in a proteome-wide approach [36]. This decrease was shown to be a consequence of a decreased mRNA level [37]. One indication that this decrease in calbindin-D28kDa is caused by cyclosporin A-induced nephrotoxicity came from studies with dogs and monkeys. These species are generally devoid of cyclosporin A-mediated nephrotoxicity, and their levels of renal calbindin-D28kDa were not affected when they were treated with cyclosporin A [38]. In contrast, a marked decrease in calbindin-D28kDa levels was found in most kidney biopsy sections from cyclosporin A-treated human kidney-transplant recipients with renal vascular or tubular toxicity. This strongly suggests that calbindin-D28kDa is a marker for human cyclosporin A-nephrotoxicity.

Therefore, we looked at mRNA levels for calbindin-D28kDa in the kidney and blood of cyclosporin A-treated rats (Table 22.10). Affymetrix rat chip RGU-34A in-

Tab. 22.10 Differential gene expression analysis of calbindin 1 probe sets in kidney and blood after cyclosporin A treatment.

Probe set	***Name***	***Fold change***	***Detection call***					
			C 1	***C 2***	***C 3***	***T 1***	***T 2***	***T 3***
Kidney		**1 d LD vs. C**						
M31178_at	calbindin 1	1.03	P	P	P	P	P	P
M31178_g_at	calbindin 1	**–2.55**	**P**	**P**	**P**	**P**	**P**	**P**
rc_AI102839_at	calbindin 1	–1.14	P	P	P	P	P	P
rc_AI102839_g_at	calbindin 1	–1.09	P	P	P	P	P	P
Kidney		**1 d HD vs. C**						
M31178_at	calbindin 1	1.33	P	P	P	P	P	P
M31178_g_at	calbindin 1	**–10.57**	**P**	**P**	**P**	**P**	**P**	**P**
rc_AI102839_at	calbindin 1	–1.06	P	P	P	P	P	P
rc_AI102839_g_at	calbindin 1	–1.04	P	P	P	P	P	P
Blood		**1 d LD vs. C**						
M31178_at	calbindin 1	1.05	P	A	A	A	A	A
M31178_g_at	calbindin 1	–3.6 #	A	A	A	A	A	A
rc_AI102839_at	calbindin 1	1.18	A	A	A	A	A	A
rc_AI102839_g_at	calbindin 1	1.06	P	P	P	P	P	P
Blood		**1 d HD vs. C**						
M31178_at	calbindin 1	1.01	M	A	A	A	A	A
M31178_g_at	calbindin 1	–1.27	A	A	A	A	A	A
rc_AI102839_at	calbindin 1	–2.75	A	A	A	A	A	A
rc_AI102839_g_at	calbindin 1	**–1.82**	**P**	**P**	**P**	**P**	**P**	**P**

d = day; LD = low-dose; HD = high-dose; C = control sample; T = treated sample; A = absent; M = marginal; P = present; # = not significant due to very low signal values.

cludes four different probe sets of the calbindin-D28kDa gene. All of them differ largely in the 3′-UTR, indicating different mRNA molecules. We found that one of the probe sets (M31178_g_at) was down-regulated in the kidney, indicating a marked decrease of one specific mRNA. This regulation was visible after one day of high-dose cyclosporin A administration (2.8-fold) and was enhanced after a 14-day application (10.6-fold). This time-dependent regulation is in line with the findings of Steiner et al. [36] on the protein level.

We also observed down-regulation of calbindin after cyclosporin A administration in blood cells. However, this was seen in a probe set (rc_AI102839_g_at) that showed no deregulation in the kidney samples. In contrast, the probe set showing down-regulation in the kidney was not affected in blood. According to Affymetrix customer information and our own analysis, all probe sets are specific for calbindin-D28kDa protein but hybridize with different 3′-UTR regions. This suggests that different transcripts of calbindin RNA, for example through alternative splicing, exist and that regulation of the transcripts is organ-specific. The existence of distinct genes is also possible, but not yet known.

Cyclophilin

It has been shown that cyclosporin A binds to cyclophilin A [39]. As the binding target of the cyclophilin–cyclosporin A complex, the phosphatase calcineurin was identified. The inactivation of the phosphatase activity of calcineurin resulting from binding of the cyclophilin–cyclosporin A complex led to inhibition of the calcineurin-dependent activation of transcription factors, which ultimately regulate transcription of the IL-2 gene [40, 41]. We therefore analyzed whether cyclophilin A, as an important pharmacological target protein, is regulated on the mRNA level in the kidney and peripheral blood.

Four probe sets on the RGU34A chip are designed to detect cyclophilin A. The RNA of cyclophilin A is highly abundant in the blood and kidney. In the blood samples, three of the four probe sets detecting cyclophilin A showed a significant increase (between 1.7- and 2-fold) after 14 days of cyclosporin A administration at 50 mg kg^{-1} in two of the three animals (Table 22.11). This observed induction could be explained as a compensatory response to the decreased concentration of free cyclophilin A due to its binding to cyclosporin A. In the kidney all probe sets showed an increase in cyclophilin A mRNA (three of them considered statistically significant) in both the

Tab. 22.11 Differential gene expression analysis of cyclophilin A probe sets in blood and kidney after cyclosporin A treatment.

Probe set	*Name*	*Fold change*	*Detection Call*					
			C 1	*C 2*	*C 3*	*T 1*	*T 2*	*T 3*
Kidney		1 d LD vs. C						
M19533mRNA_i_at	cyclophilin A	**1.44**	P	P	P	P	P	P
rc_AA818152_f_at	cyclophilin A	**1.24**	P	P	P	P	P	P
rc_AA818858_s_at	cyclophilin A	1.14	P	P	P	P	P	P
rc_AI228674_s_at	cyclophilin A	**1.27**	P	P	P	P	P	P
Kidney		1 d HD vs. C						
M19533mRNA_i_at	cyclophilin A	**1.35**	P	P	P	P	P	P
rc_AA818152_f_at	cyclophilin A	**1.21**	P	P	P	P	P	P
rc_AA818858_s_at	cyclophilin A	1.13	P	P	P	P	P	P
rc_AI228674_s_at	cyclophilin A	**1.28**	P	P	P	P	P	P
Blood		1 d LD vs. C						
M19533mRNA_i_at	cyclophilin A	–1.16	P	P	P	P	P	P
rc_AA818152_f_at	cyclophilin A	1.21	P	P	P	P	P	P
rc_AA818858_s_at	cyclophilin A	–1.13	P	P	P	P	P	P
rc_AI228674_s_at	cyclophilin A	–1.17	P	P	P	P	P	P
Blood		1 d HD vs. C						
M19533mRNA_i_at	cyclophilin A	**1.96**	P	P	P	P	P	P
rc_AA818152_f_at	cyclophilin A	1.14	P	P	P	P	P	P
rc_AA818858_s_at	cyclophilin A	**1.7**	P	P	P	P	P	P
rc_AI228674_s_at	cyclophilin A	**1.47**	P	P	P	P	P	P

d = day; LD = low-dose; HD = high-dose; C = control sample; T = treated sample; A = absent; M = marginal; P = present.

low- (5 mg kg^{-1}) and the high-dose (50 mg kg^{-1}) groups after the 14-day administration period. This finding is in agreement with a previous report that cyclosporin A treatment increases the level of cytosolic cyclophilin A as measured by confocal microscopy and quantitative immunofluorescence [42]. It was also reported that cyclosporin A modifies the subcellular distribution of cyclophilin A [43].

To date, it is not clear whether the nephrotoxic effects of cyclosporin A are mediated through binding to renal immunophilin and inhibition of calcineurin phosphatase, as suggested by Su et al. [44]. However, the concomitant increase of cyclophilin A in blood cells and the kidney after cyclosporin A treatment demonstrates the possibility of assessing effects in the toxicological target organ by analyzing blood cells.

22.5 Summary

In this study we analyzed gene expression patterns in peripheral blood samples after administration of three different compounds (cyclosporin A, gentamicin, and WY-14643) to rats and compared these patterns with that in liver and/or kidney samples. Our results suggest that peripheral blood can be used for biomarker identification in a toxicogenomic approach. Several candidate genes for potential biomarkers were identified. Further studies with a greater number of replicates will be needed to establish the boundaries of the observed correlation. More detailed time course studies will also be necessary for better understanding of the observed effects. There is also a need to develop RNA isolation methods that overcome the current limitations, for example, in sensitivity. Increased knowledge of the function and regulation of genes will be the base for a challenging safety assessment – not to understand molecular processes in the analyzed cell but rather to study effects in a different organ. However, the urgent need to identify bridging biomarkers will encourage rapid development in this field.

References

[1] M.J. Aardema and J.T. MacGregor: Toxicology and genetic toxicology in the new era of 'toxicogenomics': impact of '-omics' technologies, Mutat Res 499 (2002) 13–25.

[2] A.A. Alizadeh, M.B. Eisen, R.E. Davis, C. Ma, I.S. Lossos, A. Rosenwald, J.C. Boldrick, H. Sabet, T. Tran, X. Yu, J.I. Powell, L. Yang, G.E. Marti, T. Moore, J. Hudson, Jr., L. Lu, D.B. Lewis, R. Tibshirani, G. Sherlock, W.C. Chan, T.C. Greiner, D.D. Weisenburger, J.O. Armitage, R. Warnke, R. Levy, W. Wilson, M.R. Grever, J.C. Byrd, D. Botstein, P.O. Brown and L.M. Staudt: Distinct types of diffuse large B-cell lymphoma identified by gene expression profiling, Nature 403 (2000) 503–511.

[3] C. Stratowa, G. Loffler, P. Lichter, S. Stilgenbauer, P. Haberl, N. Schweifer, H. Dohner and K.K. Wilgenbus: CDNA microarray gene expression analysis of B-cell chronic lymphocytic leukemia proposes potential new prognostic markers involved in lym-

phocyte trafficking, Int J Cancer 91 (2001) 474–480.
[4] D. Alcorta, G. Preston, W. Munger, P. Sullivan, J.J. Yang, I. Waga, J.C. Jennette and R. Falk: Microarray studies of gene expression in circulating leukocytes in kidney diseases, Exp Nephrol 10 (2002) 139–149.
[5] R.J. Glynne and S.R. Watson: The immune system and gene expression microarrays: new answers to old questions, J Pathol 195 (2001) 20–30.
[6] L.W. Ellisen, R.E. Palmer, R.G. Maki, V.B. Truong, P. Tamayo, J.D. Oliner and D.A. Haber: Cascades of transcriptional induction during human lymphocyte activation, Eur J Cell Biol 80 (2001) 321–328.
[7] H. Hamalainen, H. Zhou, W. Chou, H. Hashizume, R. Heller and R. Lahesmaa: Distinct gene expression profiles of human type 1 and type 2 T helper cells, Genome Biol 2 (2001) RESEARCH0022.
[8] D.E. Amacher, R. Beck, S.J. Schomaker and C.V. Kenny: Hepatic microsomal enzyme induction, beta-oxidation, and cell proliferation following administration of clofibrate, gemfibrozil, or bezafibrate in the CD rat, Toxicol Appl Pharmacol 142 (1997) 143–150.
[9] M.D. Pickrell, R. Sawers and J. Michael: Pregnancy after renal transplantation: severe intrauterine growth retardation during treatment with cyclosporin A, Br Med J (Clin Res Ed) 296 (1988) 825.
[10] T. Parra Cid, J.R. Conejo Garcia, F. Carballo Alvarez and G. de Arriba: Antioxidant nutrients protect against cyclosporine A nephrotoxicity, Toxicology 189 (2003) 99–111.
[11] Y. Yoshinaga, Y. Matsuno, S. Fujita, T. Nakamura, M. Kikuchi, Y. Shimosato and S. Hirohashi: Immunohistochemical detection of hepatocyte growth factor/scatter factor in human cancerous and inflammatory lesions of various organs, Jpn J Cancer Res 84 (1993) 1150–1158.
[12] J. Maeda, N. Ueki, T. Hada and K. Higashino: Elevated serum hepatocyte growth factor/scatter factor levels in inflammatory lung disease, Am J Respir Crit Care Med 152 (1995) 1587–1591.
[13] Y. Shimada, M. Yoshiyama, S. Jissho, K. Kamimori, Y. Nakamura, H. Iida, K. Takeuchi and J. Yoshikawa: Hepatocyte growth factor production may be related to the inflammatory response in patients with acute myocardial infarction, Circ J 66 (2002) 253–256.
[14] P.M. Lindroos, R. Zarnegar and G.K. Michalopoulos: Hepatocyte growth factor (hepatopoietin A) rapidly increases in plasma before DNA synthesis and liver regeneration stimulated by partial hepatectomy and carbon tetrachloride administration, Hepatology 13 (1991) 743–750.
[15] C. Selden, R. Johnstone, H. Darby, S. Gupta and H.J. Hodgson: Human serum does contain a high molecular weight hepatocyte growth factor: studies pre- and post-hepatic resection, Biochem Biophys Res Commun 139 (1986) 361–366.
[16] E. Gak, W.G. Taylor, A.M. Chan and J.S. Rubin: Processing of hepatocyte growth factor to the heterodimeric form is required for biological activity, FEBS Lett 311 (1992) 17–21.
[17] A. Masumoto and N. Yamamoto: Sequestration of a hepatocyte growth factor in extracellular matrix in normal adult rat liver, Biochem Biophys Res Commun 174 (1991) 90–95.
[18] R. Zarnegar: Regulation of HGF and HGFR gene expression, Exs 74 (1995) 33–49.
[19] K. Matsumoto, H. Okazaki and T. Nakamura: Novel function of prostaglandins as inducers of gene expression of HGF and putative mediators of tissue regeneration, J Biochem 117 (1995) 458–464.
[20] A. Grenier, S. Chollet-Martin, B. Crestani, C. Delarche, J. El Benna, A. Boutten, V. Andrieu, G. Durand, M.A. Gougerot-Pocidalo, M. Aubier and M. Dehoux; Presence of a mobilizable intracellular pool of hepatocyte growth factor in human polymorphonuclear neutrophils, Blood 99 (2002) 2997–3004.
[21] Q. Chen, M.C. DeFrances and R. Zarnegar: Induction of met protooncogene (hepatocyte growth factor receptor) expression during human

monocyte-macrophage differentiation, Cell Growth Differ 7 (1996) 821–832.
[22] M. Beilmann, M. Odenthal, W. Jung, G.F. Vande Woude, H.P. Dienes and P. Schirmacher: Neoexpression of the c-met/hepatocyte growth factor-scatter factor receptor gene in activated monocytes, Blood 90 (1997) 4450–4458.
[23] V. Daniel: Glutathione S-transferases: gene structure and regulation of expression, Crit Rev Biochem Mol Biol 28 (1993) 173–207.
[24] H.R. Brown, H. Ni, G. Benavides, L. Yoon, K. Hyder, J. Giridhar, G. Gardner, R.D. Tyler and K.T. Morgan: Correlation of simultaneous differential gene expression in the blood and heart with known mechanisms of adriamycin-induced cardiomyopathy in the rat, Toxicol Pathol 30 (2002) 452–469.
[25] H.A. Kester, C. Blanchetot, J. den Hertog, P.T. van der Saag and B. van der Burg: Transforming growth factor-beta–stimulated clone-22 is a member of a family of leucine zipper proteins that can homo- and heterodimerize and has transcriptional repressor activity, J Biol Chem 274 (1999) 27439–27447.
[26] D. Uchida, F. Omotehara, K. Nakashiro, Y. Tateishi, S. Hino, N.M. Begum, T. Fujimori and H. Kawamata: Posttranscriptional regulation of TSC-22 (TGF-beta-stimulated clone-22) gene by TGF-beta 1, Biochem Biophys Res Commun 305 (2003) 846–854.
[27] K. Nakashiro, H. Kawamata, S. Hino, D. Uchida, Y. Miwa, H. Hamano, F. Omotehara, H. Yoshida and M. Sato: Down-regulation of TSC-22 (transforming growth factor beta-stimulated clone 22) markedly enhances the growth of a human salivary gland cancer cell line *in vitro* and *in vivo*, Cancer Res 58 (1998) 549–555.
[28] D. Uchida, H. Kawamata, F. Omotehara, Y. Miwa, S. Hino, N.M. Begum, H. Yoshida and M. Sato: Over-expression of TSC-22 (TGF-beta stimulated clone-22) markedly enhances 5-fluorouracil-induced apoptosis in a human salivary gland cancer cell line, Lab Invest 80 (2000) 955–963.
[29] Y. Xu, S. Iyengar, R.L. Roberts, S.B. Shappell and D.M. Peehl: Primary culture model of peroxisome proliferator-activated receptor gamma activity in prostate cancer cells, J Cell Physiol 196 (2003) 131–143.
[30] T.J. Ostwald and D.H. MacLennan: Isolation of a high affinity calcium-binding protein from sarcoplasmic reticulum, J Biol Chem 249 (1974) 974–979.
[31] K.H. Krause and M. Michalak: Calreticulin, Cell 88 (1997) 439–443.
[32] R.J. Kaufman: Stress signaling from the lumen of the endoplasmic reticulum: coordination of gene transcriptional and translational controls, Genes Dev 13 (1999) 1211–1233.
[33] A. Soejima, S. Ishizuka, M. Suzuki, N. Miyake, K. Fukuoka and T. Nagasawa: Biochemical renal manifestations induced by consecutive administration of gentamicin in rats, Nephron 80 (1998) 331–339.
[34] M. Kavutcu, O. Canbolat, S. Ozturk, E. Olcay, S. Ulutepe, C. Ekinci, I.H. Gokhun and I. Durak: Reduced enzymatic antioxidant defense mechanism in kidney tissues from gentamicin-treated guinea pigs: effects of vitamins E and C, Nephron 72 (1996) 269–274.
[35] H.S. Ozturk, M. Kavutcu, M. Kacmaz, O. Canbolat and I. Durak: The effects of gentamicin on the activities of glutathione peroxidase and superoxide dismutase enzymes and malondialdehyde levels in heart tissues of guinea pigs, Curr Med Res Opin 14 (1997) 47–52.
[36] S. Steiner, L. Aicher, J. Raymackers, L. Meheus, R. Esquer-Blasco, N.L. Anderson and A. Cordier: Cyclosporine A decreases the protein level of the calcium-binding protein calbindin-D28kDa in rat kidney, Biochem Pharmacol 51 (1996) 253–258.
[37] O. Grenet, M.C. Varela, F. Staedtler and S. Steiner: The cyclosporine A-induced decrease in rat renal calbindin-D28kDa protein as a consequence of a decrease in its mRNA, Biochem Pharmacol 55 (1998) 1131–1133.
[38] L. Aicher, D. Wahl, A. Arce, O. Grenet and S. Steiner: New insights into cyclosporine A nephrotoxicity by pro-

teome analysis, Electrophoresis 19 (1998) 1998–2003.

[39] R.E. Handschumacher, M.W. Harding, J. Rice, R.J. Drugge and D.W. Speicher: Cyclophilin: a specific cytosolic binding protein for cyclosporin A, Science 226 (1984) 544–547.

[40] D.A. Fruman, C.B. Klee, B.E. Bierer and S.J. Burakoff: Calcineurin phosphatase activity in T lymphocytes is inhibited by FK 506 and cyclosporin A, Proc Natl Acad Sci USA 89 (1992) 3686–3690.

[41] S.J. O'Keefe, J. Tamura, R.L. Kincaid, M.J. Tocci and E.A. O'Neill: FK-506- and CsA-sensitive activation of the interleukin-2 promoter by calcineurin, Nature 357 (1992) 692–694.

[42] M.L. McDonald, T. Ardito, W.H. Marks, M. Kashgarian and M.I. Lorber: The effect of cyclosporine administration on the cellular distribution and content of cyclophilin, Transplantation 53 (1992) 460–466.

[43] M. Demeule, A. Laplante, A. Sepehr-Arae, G.M. Murphy, R.M. Wenger and R. Beliveau: Association of cyclophilin A with renal brush border membranes: redistribution by cyclosporine A, Kidney Int 57 (2000) 1590–1598.

[44] Q. Su, L. Weber, M. Le Hir, G. Zenke and B. Ryffel: Nephrotoxicity of cyclosporin A and FK506: inhibition of calcineurin phosphatase, Ren Physiol Biochem 18 (1995) 128–139.

23
How Things Could Be Done Better Using Toxicogenomics: A Retrospective Analysis

Laura Suter and Rodolfo Gasser

23.1
Introduction

Failure of compounds due to safety issues in late preclinical development or in the clinic represent an important economic burden for the pharmaceutical industry. The commonly used strategy of pharmaceutical research organizations of concentrating efforts in increasing efficacy might be a one reason for this development, since increasing potency does not reduce toxicity and might even enhance it. Thus, to minimize the risk of uncovering safety issues late in development, efficacy and safety should ideally be determined simultaneously and at very early stages [1, 1 a]. To achieve this ideal situation, a change in the traditional drug discovery process must take place. Toxicogenomics is one of the means that could enable scientists to integrate toxicology into the earlier discovery phases by including sensitive parameters that would recognize liabilities at lower doses (pharmacological rather than toxicological doses) or after short exposure times (acute rather than chronic exposures). Hence, possible liability flags will be raised at the time of lead selection or shortly thereafter. Genomics approaches are already having a great impact in pharmacology and toxicology, since they allow the prediction and differentiation of species-specific responses and also identify populations of responders and nonresponders [2]. Advances in the use of genomics technologies in relation to therapy have been widely reported in the field of cancer research. Optimistic estimates foresee that the replacement of current methods by toxicogenomics may shorten the safety assessment for a NDA from years to days and therefore reduce the costs by a factor of four to six [3]. A more realistic picture with the data currently available suggest that toxicogenomics will reduce failure rates by helping select the right compounds for development and by accelerating toxicology testing. One of the main requirements for this goal is the use of the data to accurately predict toxic potential and to discover and apply suitable biomarkers amenable to screening using the generated data [4].

Substantial quantities of data have been generated with known hepatotoxicants. In addition, global gene expression analysis has also been considered for evaluation of

Handbook of Toxicogenomics: Strategies and Applications. Edited by Jürgen Borlak

ISBN: 3-527-30342-1

nephrotoxicity [5], genotoxicity [6], testicular toxicity [7] (and see other chapters in this book).

Generally, global gene expression results have been analyzed by following two major approaches: A 'holistic' approach, including as many genes as possible to obtain a profile or fingerprint, and a mechanistic approach, focused on subsets of genes believed to bear mechanistic relevance. Both approaches can be seen as complementary and have advantages and disadvantages. Analyses concentrating in gene expression profiles identify fingerprints that allow compounds to be classified according to mechanisms of action (toxicity or pharmacology) using a variety of statistical tools. The advantage of this approach lies in the unbiased selection of the genes driving the classification and in the ability to use gene expression information with unknown biological relevance (i. e., ESTs). The main disadvantage is the need for a robust database of gene expression data that serves as the model to which newly interrogated compounds are compared. Databases can be generated by each user or can be acquired from commercial providers, but either way, they are very costly. Mechanistic analyses usually concentrate on genes of mechanistic interest and investigate the cellular and molecular mechanisms related to the compound. This analysis procedure provides very useful information that allows for the generation of hypotheses regarding the primary molecular target of a compound. It has the disadvantage of allowing the scientist to introduce knowledge-driven bias into the data. Hence, it is vital that the generated mechanistic hypothesis be corroborated by appropriately designed follow-up experiments. In addition, mechanistic analyses rely on the availability of accurate functional information on the affected genes and may thus disregard important gene expression changes, due to a lack of knowledge regarding their biological function. Fingerprint and mechanistic analyses have proven very useful and have shown that gene expression analysis provides sufficient information to classify compounds according to their mechanism of toxicity and also to identify cellular processes related to the toxic event [8–14].

23.2
Case Example: Two 5-HT_6 Receptor Antagonists Displaying Similar Pharmacological Activity and Different Toxicity Profiles

23.2.1
Pharmacological Characteristics of the Compounds

Serotonin (5-hydroxytryptamine, 5-HT) is involved in the pathogenesis of a number of disorders in the central nervous system [15]. The serotonin receptor family is a member of the larger family of G-protein coupled receptors [16]. The genes for several serotonin receptors (5-HT receptors) have been cloned and characterized, including the 5-HT_6 receptor [17]. Northern blot analysis has shown that the 5-HT_6 receptor is expressed mainly in brain, with very weak to no expression in the periphery [17, 18]. This receptor appears to be involved in certain anxiety disorders, and functional studies have demonstrated that blocking the receptor enhances acetylcholine neurotransmission in the rat brain [19, 20]. Furthermore, experiments performed with antisense oligonucleotides and with specific 5-HT_6 receptor antagonists showed that blocking this receptor type produced an increase in the retention of learning in rats [21]. From behavioural studies, the 5-HT_6 receptor is a potential target for treatment of memory deficit, as in patients with Alzheimer's disease. Moreover, its exclusive localization in the central nervous system implies that molecules that specifically target this receptor should cause no or few side effects in the periphery. A possible clinical candidate was 4-amino-*N*-(6-bromo-1 *H*-indol-4-yl)–benzenesulfonamide (Ro-Cmp A). This compound binds to the 5-HT_6 receptor and elicits its pharmacological activity as a specific antagonist. No effects due to exaggerated pharmacology were anticipated, as often occurs with commonly used therapies such as acetylcholinesterase inhibitors or muscarinic agonists.

23.2.2
Toxicological Findings in Rats and Dogs

Ro-Cmp A caused hepatic lipid accumulation although the receptor is not expressed in liver. Hepatotoxicity was observed in rodents (rats, 1-, 2- and 4-week toxicity studies) and in nonrodents (dogs, 2-week exposure) and led eventually to the discontinuation of the experimental drug.

Rats treated daily for a week with increasing doses of Ro-Cmp A displayed hepatic steatosis at doses of 100 mg kg^{-1} d^{-1} or higher, accompanied by an increase in relative liver weight. Histological examination of the tissue of the affected animals showed hepatocellular vacuolation, characterized by multiple small discrete periacinar vacuoles that sometimes coalesced to form larger ones and which stained positive for lipids (microsteatosis) (Figure 23.1). In addition, these animals displayed lower circulating levels of triglycerides and cholesterol, indicating disturbances in lipid/steroid homeostasis. Pharmacokinetic studies over a one-week period demonstrated a low potential for accumulation of the compound; therefore, accumulation was not the cause of the observed toxicological findings. An additional observation was that the findings were consistently more severe in female animals than in males. This could not be explained by differences in exposure to the compound, since pharmacokinetic analyses indicated no consistent gender differences that could account for the bias in the toxicological findings.

The compound was discontinued relatively late in the development process after a considerable amount of time, effort, and funds had already been spent on preclinical testing. Hence, earlier detection of the hepatic liability of Ro-Cmp A would have made it possible to redirect resources to the development of other chemical entities with higher chances of success. Also, understanding the cellular and molecular mechanisms leading to toxicity would have been immensely useful in the selection of follow-up clinical candidates without this hepatic liability. From a mechanistic point of view, the lack of expression of 5-HT_6 receptor in the liver provided a strong argument against toxicity due to a pharmacologically mediated process. Furthermore, other 5-HT_6 antagonists, such as 4-(2-brom-6-pyrrolidine-1-ylpyridine-4-sulfonyl)-phenylamine (Ro-Cmp B), did not cause hepatic steatosis. Ro-Cmp B is closely related to Ro-

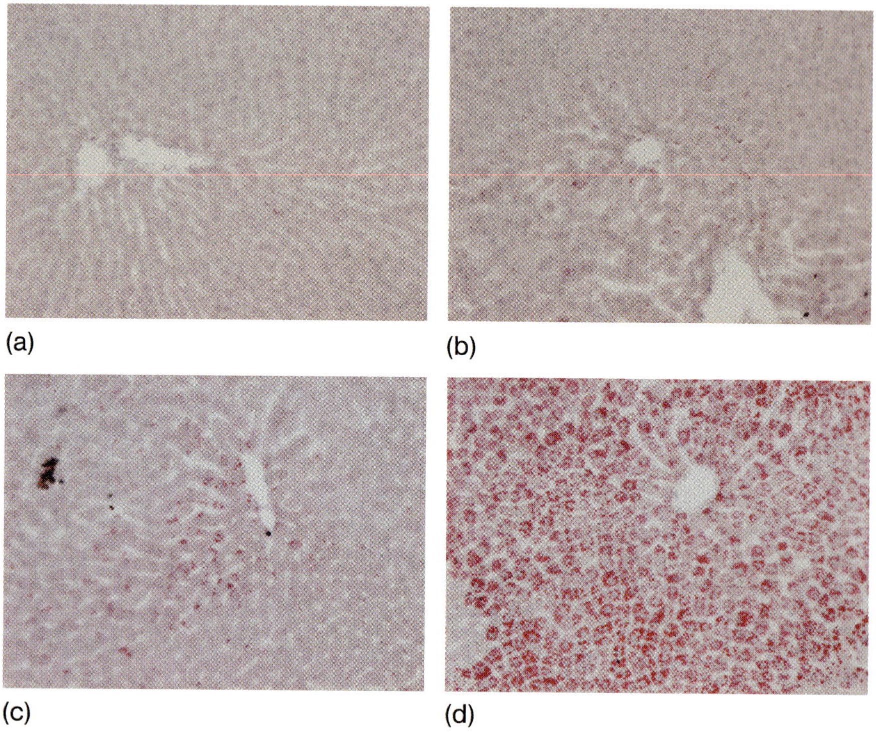

Fig. 23.1 Photomicrographs of histological findings in liver after seven days of treatment with several doses of Ro-Cmp A. Representative liver sections stained with haematoxylin–eosin and with Fat-Red-O for visualization of lipids (red). (a) Control; (b) low dose (30 mg kg^{-1} d^{-1}; (c) medium dose (100 mg kg^{-1} d^{-1}); (d) high dose (400 mg kg^{-1} d^{-1})

Cmp A in its pharmacological profile. Thus, the mechanism by which Ro-Cmp A causes hepatic steatosis is different from those that lead to its pharmacological efficacy.

23.3 The use of Toxicogenomics (Retrospectively) to Evaluate Hepatic Liability

The open issues of hepatic liability and of its underlying mechanisms could not be addressed with sufficient depth by using conventional toxicology assays. Thus, a toxicogenomics approach was initiated to better understand the molecular mechanisms leading to or related to the observed findings. The main goals of the study were to

- obtain additional data supporting toxicogenomics analysis as a useful tool to detect hepatotoxicants,
- differentiate two pharmacologically closely related compounds with dissimilar toxicological characteristics,

– evaluate the potential use of toxicogenomics if employed as a predictive tool early in the development process,
– gain insight into the possible molecular mechanisms underlying the described hepatic findings.

For the toxicogenomic studies, male Wistar rats were dosed for seven days with several doses of Ro-Cmp A. Based on previous toxicological studies under similar conditions, hepatic steatosis appeared to be dose-dependent. It was therefore of interest to determine if gene expression changes also reflected this dose dependence and if subchronic administration of Ro-Cmp A combined with gene expression analysis would be adequate to detect this liability. In parallel, groups of male rats were also dosed acutely (single dose, necropsy at 6 or 24 h) with a high dose of Ro-Cmp A or Ro-Cmp B, to investigate whether or not these two compounds could be distinguished based on their gene expression profiles after acute exposure (Table 23.1).

The chosen study design allowed the comparison of a compound eliciting hepatotoxicity (steatosis) with a compound lacking this effect and also permitted the evalua-

Tab. 23.1 Treatment groups and summary of results from conventional endpoints. Each treatment group was composed of five male Wistar rats.

Group	*Dosing scheme*	*Histopathology*		*Lipid content*		*Serum enzymes*
		General	*Fatty change*	*Liver tissue*	*Serum*	
Ro-Cmp A control, 7 d	repeated, daily 7 d	no finding	+	control	control	control
Ro-Cmp A 30 $mg\ kg^{-1}$, 7 d	repeated, daily 7 d	no finding	+	NC	NC	NC
Ro-Cmp A 100 $mg\ kg^{-1}$, 7 d	repeated, daily 7 d	no finding	++	NC	NC	NC
Ro-Cmp A 400 $mg\ kg^{-1}$, 7 d	repeated, daily 7 d	vacuolation	+++	↑	↓ TG[a)] ↓ chol.[a)]	NC
Ro-Cmp A control, 6 h	single dose	no finding	+	control	control	control
Ro-Cmp A 400 $mg\ kg^{-1}$, 6 h	single dose	no finding	+	NC	NC	NC
Ro-Cmp B 400 $mg\ kg^{-1}$, 6 h	single dose	no finding	+	NC	NC	NC
Ro-Cmp A control, 24 h	single dose	no finding	+	control	control	NC
Ro-Cmp A 400 $mg\ kg^{-1}$, 24 h	single dose	↑mitosis vacuolation	++	↑	↑ TG ↓chol.	NC
Ro-Cmp B 400 $mg\ kg^{-1}$, 24 h	single dose	no finding	+	NC	NC	NC

a) Decrease was not statistically significant as assessed with *t* test.

TG = triglycerides, chol. = cholesterol, control = values from control-treated animals used as baseline reference, NC = no change.

tion of subchronic (with clear histopathology) and acute (without histopathology) exposures. Analysis of the obtained data allowed us to assess the use of toxicogenomics for the detection of toxic liabilities quickly and accurately. In addition, the identification and evaluation of genes differentially regulated by the compounds made it possible to draw mechanistic conclusions related to the toxic manifestation, in spite of confounding similar pharmacological profiles.

In addition to conventionally evaluated toxicological endpoints, gene and protein expression analyses were also performed, as described elsewhere [22]. Briefly, total RNA was obtained by standard laboratory protocols, using a commercially available kit. Total RNA was either used as template for the synthesis of double-stranded cDNA, followed by *in vitro* transcription, or for the synthesis of single-stranded cDNA for subsequent RT–PCR analysis using specific primers and the SYBR Green PCR Master Mix (Applied Biosystems). Labelled *in vitro* transcripts were hybridized onto Affymetrix Microarrays (RG-U34A) and the obtained image files analyzed with the Microarray Suite software, version 5.0 (Affymetrix). RT–PCR was performed and measured using the ABI-PRISM 7700 sequence detection system (Applied Biosystems). In addition to gene expression analysis, protein levels were also evaluated. Total liver protein was denatured and separated by SDS–PAGE. Nitrocellulose membranes were incubated with specific first and second antibodies, and the intensities of the protein bands were assessed by densitometry.

23.4 Classification of Compounds with the Use of a Reference Gene Expression Database

Liver gene expression profiles from all animals treated with Ro-Cmp A were compared to the Roche Toxicogenomics database using a variety of data analysis tools. In the Roche Toxicogenomics database, compounds are divided into several subcategories according to associated histopathological manifestations, amongst them 'steatosis'. Classification analysis showed that Ro-Cmp A could be identified as steatotic, based on the gene expression profile elicited by subchronic exposure (seven consecutive days). This held true when we used a variety of public (hierarchical clustering, principal components analysis: PCA) and in-house developed (correlation analysis, support vector machines: SVM) statistical analysis procedures, demonstrating the robustness of the dataset. It was clearly shown that analysis of gene expression profiles is capable of accurately reflecting histopathology and clinical chemistry, commonly used endpoints in toxicological studies (Table 23.2). Moreover, liver expression patterns from animals dosed acutely with Ro-Cmp A and killed 6 or 24 h after administration were also correctly classified as steatotic, in spite of the fact that no clear histopathology or clinical chemistry manifestations were observed 6 h after a single dose. At the earliest evaluated time point (6 h) the classification relied on a selection of marker genes rather than on the gene expression profile, as described later in this chapter.

Tab. 23.2 Classification of the treated animals using gene expression profiles. Each treatment group was composed of five male animals; depending on the analysis method, either individual animals or group means were used for classification.

Group	*Toxicity*	*Conventional endpoints*	*PCA* [a]	*Similarity index*	*SVM*	*Cluster* [a]
Ro-Cmp A control, 7 d	control	+	no toxic	ND	control	no toxic
Ro-Cmp A 30 mg kg^{-1}, 7 d	steatotic	+	toxic	CYP inducer, steatotic	ND	toxic
Ro-Cmp A 100 mg kg^{-1}, 7 d	steatotic	++	toxic	CYP inducer, steatotic	ND	toxic
Ro-Cmp A 400 mg kg^{-1}, 7 d	steatotic	+++	toxic	CYP inducer, steatotic	steatotic	toxic
Ro-Cmp A Control, 6 h	control	+	no toxic	ND	control	no toxic
Ro-Cmp A 400 mg kg^{-1}, 6 h	steatotic	+	toxic	CYP inducer, steatotic	control	toxic
Ro-Cmp B 400 mg kg^{-1}, 6 h	no toxic	+	no toxic	no match in database	ND	no toxic
Ro-Cmp A control, 24 h	control	+	no toxic	ND	control	no toxic
Ro-Cmp A 400 mg kg^{-1}, 24 h	steatotic	++	toxic	CYP inducer, steatotic	steatotic	toxic
Ro-Cmp B 400 mg kg^{-1}, 24 h	no toxic	+	no toxic	no match in database	ND	no toxic

a) PCA and clustering analysis are relative analyses that assess if the treated groups aggregate with the controls or not, relying on a subset of modulated probe sets. ND = not determined.

PCA = principal components analysis (SIMCA-P, Umetrics); similarity index: in-house developed algorithm for the generation of similarity indexes; SVM = supervised algorithm based on support vector machines; clustering = hierarchical clustering using a correlation algorithm and average linkage method.

23.4.1 Differentiation of Two Pharmacologically Closely Related Compounds

Inclusion of the nonhepatotoxic compound Ro-Cmp B in the analysis allowed comparison of the gene expression profiles of two compounds displaying similar pharmacology and different toxicology. Gene expression profiles of animals treated with Ro-Cmp B grouped with the time matched controls, while gene expression profiles from animals treated acutely with Ro-Cmp A grouped with those subchronically exposed to Ro-Cmp A and associated with steatosis (Figure 23.2).

Hence, both compounds were differentiated by the induced gene expression changes also at time points as early as 6 h, when no other indications of toxicity were evident. These findings strongly support the assumption that gene expression analysis can provide insights into toxicity potential much faster than conventional end-

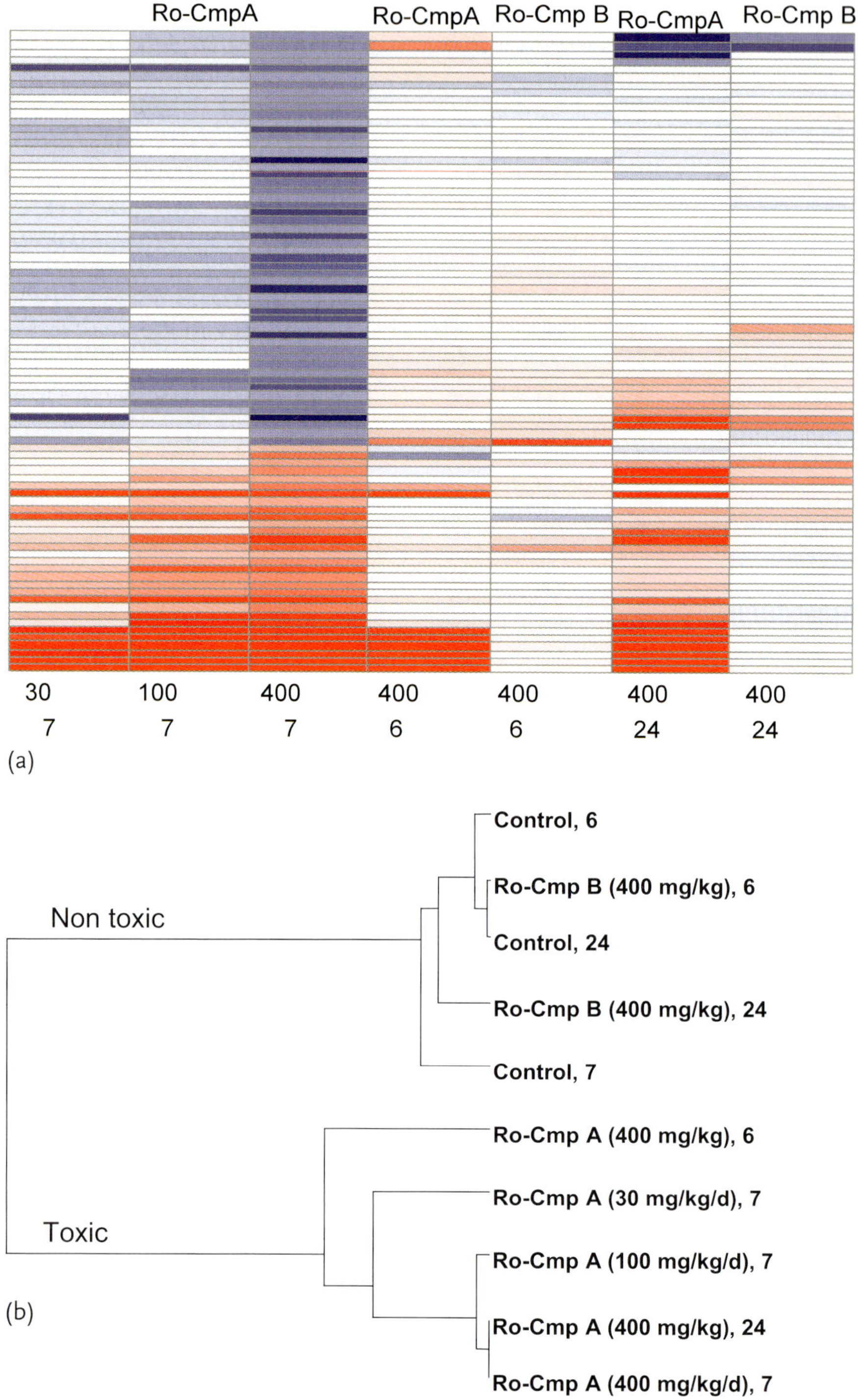
Ro-CmpA
Ro-CmpA
Ro-Cmp B
Ro-CmpA
Ro-Cmp B
30
7
100
7
400
7
400
6
400
6
400
24
400
24
(a)
Non toxic
Toxic
Control, 6
Ro-Cmp B (400 mg/kg), 6
Control, 24
Ro-Cmp B (400 mg/kg), 24
Control, 7
Ro-Cmp A (400 mg/kg), 6
Ro-Cmp A (30 mg/kg/d), 7
Ro-Cmp A (100 mg/kg/d), 7
Ro-Cmp A (400 mg/kg), 24
Ro-Cmp A (400 mg/kg/d), 7
(b)

points. Here, acute exposure of rats to the compound was sufficient to detect its toxic potential. The results also demonstrate that two very closely related compounds can be differentiated by using toxicogenomics. Moreover, unwanted side effects can be detected earlier with gene expression analysis than with conventional toxicology measurements, which usually involve longer exposure periods and require large amounts of compound and resources. Thus, toxicogenomics can improve the process of detecting toxic liabilities of compounds under evaluation.

23.4.2
Use of Gene Expression for Mechanistic Hypothesis Generation

Among the genes induced specifically by Ro-Cmp A were several specific to cytochromes P450 (CYP2B1/2 and CYP3A1), while genes for ornithine aminotransferase (AA893325), alcohol sulfotransferase (D14987), hepatocyte nuclear factor 3 gamma (*HNF-3gamma*, AB017044), and serine dehydratase (J03863) were repressed (see Table 23.3). In addition, several genes related to lipid and cholesterol homeostasis, such as those encoding hydroxymethylglutaryl-CoA synthase (HMGCoA synthase, X52625) and the CYP7 family, were deregulated by treatment with this compound. An additional group of genes showed moderate to weak modulation of their expression levels, but this regulation was consistent among biological replicates and is therefore believed to bear biological relevance. In particular, genes encoding senescence marker protein (D31662), hepatocyte nuclear factor 1-alpha (HNF-1alpha, J03170), and the epidermal and the hepatic forms of fatty acid binding protein (S69874 and V01235) were significantly repressed, while those for malic enzyme (AI171506) and epoxide hydrolase (M26125) were induced.

The analysis of complex gene expression changes has allowed us to identify a subset of genes that may be associated with the toxic event under investigation. In particular, expression of CYP2B2 was consistently associated with liver toxicity events elicited by Ro-Cmp A, since a dose-dependent induction of CYP2B2 mRNA after seven days of treatment was noted. Induction of this gene was observed already 6 and 24 h after a single-dose administration of this compound, while the nonhepatotoxic Ro-Cmp B did not elicit any effect detectable with microarrays. Therefore, a novel link between the induction of CYP2B2 in the rat and microvesicular steatosis can be postulated. It remains to be established whether induction of this gene is a cause or effect of the underlying mechanisms or merely an adaptive response. Induction of the cytochrome P450 CYP2B family genes, described for phenobarbital-type CYP indu-

◀ **Fig. 23.2** Cluster analysis using gene expression data. (a) Cluster analysis (by probe sets) based on modulated genes. Blue boxes represent down-regulated genes and red boxes represent up-regulated genes. Intensity of the colour relates to the relative change. Note the dose dependence observed at seven days of treatment (lanes 1 through 3) and the minimal changes caused by the nontoxic compound Ro-Cmp B after acute exposure (lanes 5 and 7). (b) Cluster analysis (by treatment groups) based on modulated genes. Control animals and animals treated with Ro-Cmp B group together, and samples from animals treated with any dose of Ro-Cmp A group in a separate branch, demonstrating that the two compounds can clearly be distinguished.

Tab. 23.3 Expression of selected genes obtained after in-vivo exposures and assessed by using microarrays.

Affymetrix probe set ID	*Genebank acc. no.*	*Gene symbol*	*Short name*	*Max. signal*	*Ro-Cmp A 30 mg/kg/d 7 days*		*Ro-Cmp A 100 mg/kg/d 7 days*		*Ro-Cmp A 400 mg/kg/d 7 days*		*Ro-Cmp A 400 mg/kg 6 hours*		*Ro-Cmp B 400 mg/kg 6 hours*		*Ro-Cmp A 400 mg/kg 24 hours*		*Ro-Cmp B 400 mg/kg 24 hours*	
					FChg	*p-value*	*FChg*	*p-value*	*FChg*	*p-value*	*FChg*	*p-value*	*FChg*	*p-value*	*FChg*	*p-value*	*FChg*	*p-value*
Pharmacological target																		
S62043_s_at	S62043	*NA*	5-HT6 receptor	67	0.6	0.061	0.6	0.124	0.7	0.131	1.4	0.330	1.6	0.267	1.1	0.793	1.5	0.314
Calcium signaling, aging																		
D31662exon#4_s_at	D31662	*NA*	SMP-30	2116	1.1	0.561	0.8	0.087	0.7	0.032	0.8	0.391	1.0	0.784	0.7	0.028	1.2	0.234
Energy																		
rc_AI171506_g_at	AI171506	Me1	Malic enzyme	996	2.0	0.025	2.1	0.021	2.9	0.045	1.6	0.063	2.3	0.070	2.2	0.077	1.2	0.300
rc_AA893325_at	AA893325	Oat	Ornithine aminotrans-ferase	315	1.0	0.911	0.8	0.548	0.4	0.011	1.2	0.550	1.0	0.728	0.9	0.819	1.1	0.788
J03863_at	J03863	Sdh	Serine dehydratase	1671	0.9	0.693	0.6	0.067	0.5	0.032	1.6	0.296	1.1	0.828	0.3	0.034	0.4	0.068
J03865mRNA_f_at	J03865	*NA*	Serine dehydratase	437	0.7	0.204	0.5	0.059	0.4	0.040	1.4	0.047	1.0	0.984	0.8	0.298	0.7	0.302
X13119cds_s_at	X13119	*NA*	Serine dehydratase	307	0.8	0.395	0.6	0.113	0.4	0.036	2.6	0.217	0.8	0.708	0.4	0.046	0.4	0.040
Lipid metabolism and transport																		
M26125_at	M26125	Ephx1	Epoxide hydrolase	10075	1.4	0.020	1.5	0.008	1.9	0.003	1.2	0.134	1.1	0.095	1.9	0.021	1.0	0.809
rc_AI104882_s_at	AI104882	Ephx2	Epoxide hydrolase	258	1.4	0.077	1.3	0.208	1.3	0.049	0.9	0.829	1.1	0.692	1.0	0.925	0.9	0.839
X60328_g_at	X60328	Ephx2	Epoxide hydrolase	199	1.7	0.052	1.4	0.266	1.4	0.034	0.8	0.454	0.7	0.046	0.8	0.027	1.0	0.930
S69874_s_at	S69874	*NA*	FABP (epidermal)	792	0.9	0.730	0.5	0.045	0.4	0.018	1.3	0.177	1.2	0.484	0.9	0.590	1.1	0.693
V01235_at	V01235	Fabp1	FABP (liver)	8695	0.8	0.038	0.7	0.010	0.7	0.016	0.8	0.209	0.8	0.126	0.9	0.438	1.1	0.410
S62097_s_at	S62097	*NA*	Geranyl-geranyl transferase	122	0.8	0.009	0.7	0.009	0.6	0.001	1.1	0.650	1.3	0.185	1.4	0.192	1.1	0.635

rc_AI171090_g_at	AI171090	Hmgcl	HMG-CoA lyase	459	0.9	0.430	0.7	0.003	0.7	0.002	0.9	0.323	0.9	0.562	1.3	0.452	1.4	0.076
M33648_at	M33648	*NA*	HMG-CoA synthase	9080	0.9	0.111	0.8	0.018	0.8	0.014	0.9	0.136	0.8	0.087	0.9	0.411	1.1	0.390
X52625_at	X52625	Hmgcs1	HMG-CoA synthase	1469	1.6	0.008	1.4	0.320	2.0	0.023	0.7	0.138	0.9	0.764	0.7	0.055	1.2	0.215
Metabolism																		
D14987_f_at	D14987	Sth2	Alcohol Sulfono-transferase	3292	0.5	0.045	0.5	0.046	0.4	0.038	1.0	0.895	1.5	0.068	1.0	0.844	1.0	0.792
D14988_f_at	D14988	Sth2	Alcohol Sulfono-transferase	6654	0.5	0.072	0.6	0.078	0.5	0.049	1.1	0.618	1.4	0.108	1.3	0.282	1.2	0.370
rc_AA818122_f_at	AA818122	Sth2	Alcohol Sulfono-transferase	3948	0.5	0.067	0.5	0.065	0.3	0.031	1.4	0.271	1.6	0.046	1.5	0.106	0.8	0.469
L24896_s_at	L24896	Gpx4	Glutathione peroxidase	1100	0.6	0.004	0.8	0.147	0.7	0.000	0.9	0.752	1.0	0.850	1.0	0.840	0.9	0.750
U73174_at	U73174	Gsr	Glutathione reductase	118	1.0	0.915	1.2	0.586	1.6	0.136	0.9	0.759	1.1	0.652	2.5	0.054	1.4	0.159
U73174_g_at	U73174	Gsr	Glutathione reductase	248	1.5	0.175	1.4	0.116	2.1	0.007	1.1	0.837	1.3	0.238	1.8	0.160	0.8	0.240
K00136mRNA_at	K00136	Gsta2	Glutathione S-transferase ya	7805	1.5	0.014	2.1	0.004	2.5	0.010	1.4	0.061	1.5	0.097	1.5	0.130	0.8	0.285
M13506_at	M13506	*NA*	UDPGT	5809	3.1	0.001	4.3	0.003	5.6	0.002	1.5	0.181	1.3	0.204	3.0	0.003	0.9	0.757
Metabolism/Cytochromes P450																		
K03241cds_s_at	K03241	*NA*	CYP1A2	3384	1.2	0.494	1.9	0.000	2.0	0.029	1.2	0.413	1.3	0.304	1.8	0.119	0.8	0.261
M11251cds_f_at	M11251	*NA*	CYP1B	17769	3.6	0.002	9.6	0.028	13.3	0.000	10.7	0.002	1.1	0.775	9.8	0.001	0.8	0.531
D17349cds_f_at	D17349	*NA*	CYP2B15	4160	3.1	0.003	5.0	0.028	6.7	0.002	4.7	0.001	1.2	0.245	5.2	0.001	1.0	0.987
J00728cds_f_at	J00728	*NA*	CYP2B2	27994	3.4	0.000	4.9	0.002	5.4	0.000	5.8	0.002	1.1	0.782	4.7	0.002	1.2	0.287
K00996mRNA_s_at	K00996	*NA*	CYP2B2	18428	6.5	0.001	15.8	0.028	20.8	0.002	11.3	0.006	1.2	0.193	17.5	0.001	1.3	0.268
K01721mRNA_s_at	K01721	Cyp2b15	CYP2B2	27043	4.0	0.000	4.3	0.014	3.2	0.025	9.6	0.000	1.5	0.044	3.5	0.031	1.4	0.233
M13234cds_f_at	M13234	*NA*	CYP2B2	26127	4.2	0.002	7.3	0.007	9.2	0.000	8.2	0.002	1.4	0.166	8.3	0.000	1.2	0.558
J02657_s_at	J02657	Cyp2c	CYP2C11	29188	1.1	0.310	1.2	0.105	1.1	0.370	1.0	0.989	1.1	0.305	0.7	0.108	0.7	0.111
M18363cds_s_at	M18363	*NA*	CYP2C11	11716	1.5	0.001	1.4	0.036	1.3	0.055	1.0	0.961	1.1	0.595	0.7	0.129	0.7	0.097
X79081mRNA_f_at	X79081	*NA*	CYP2C11	6716	1.4	0.221	1.4	0.132	1.3	0.312	1.2	0.179	1.2	0.341	0.8	0.211	0.8	0.127

Tab. 23.3 (continued)

Affymetrix probe set ID	*Genebank acc. no.*	*Gene symbol*	*Short name*	*Max. signal*	*Ro-Cmp A 30 mg/kg/d 7 days*		*Ro-Cmp A 100 mg/kg/d 7 days*		*Ro-Cmp A 400 mg/kg/d 7 days*		*Ro-Cmp A 400 mg/kg 6 hours*		*Ro-Cmp B 400 mg/kg 6 hours*		*Ro-Cmp A 400 mg/kg 24 hours*		*Ro-Cmp B 400 mg/kg 24 hours*	
					FChg	*p-value*	*FChg*	*p-value*	*FChg*	*p-value*	*FChg*	*p-value*	*FChg*	*p-value*	*FChg*	*p-value*	*FChg*	*p-value*
M14776_f_at	M14776	*NA*	CYP2C6	11687	2.1	0.008	2.4	0.009	2.5	0.007	1.2	0.560	1.0	0.889	1.7	0.005	0.9	0.643
rc_AA945571_s_at	AA945571	Cyp2c37	CYP2C6	20736	2.2	0.000	2.4	0.000	2.7	0.000	1.1	0.159	0.8	0.018	1.6	0.006	0.9	0.510
D13912_s_at	D13912	Cyp3a3	CYP3A1	11790	1.5	0.017	3.6	0.048	5.7	0.009	1.5	0.035	1.2	0.077	3.6	0.026	0.8	0.320
L24207_i_at	L24207	Cyp3a3	CYP3A1	716	1.4	0.056	1.5	0.085	2.6	0.048	1.1	0.181	1.2	0.026	3.1	0.078	1.2	0.237
L24207_r_at	L24207	Cyp3a3	CYP3A1	601	1.7	0.162	2.9	0.010	4.2	0.029	1.3	0.216	1.6	0.035	4.3	0.035	1.2	0.394
X64401cds_s_at	X64401	Cyp3a3	CYP3A1	27871	1.8	0.002	3.0	0.024	3.1	0.005	1.2	0.210	1.0	0.982	1.6	0.029	0.8	0.384
U36992_at	U36992	Cyp7b1	CYP7B1	189	0.8	0.227	0.7	0.097	0.5	0.004	1.3	0.284	1.0	0.833	1.6	0.221	1.3	0.338
L00320cds_f_at	L00320	*NA*	CYP2B, exon 9	16700	5.1	0.005	12.6	0.027	17.2	0.002	13.5	0.002	1.4	0.235	11.0	0.001	1.1	0.749
Nuclear receptors																		
AF082124_s_at	AF082124	Ahr	AhR	98	2.1	0.112	1.6	0.367	2.3	0.071	2.2	0.139	0.7	0.614	1.1	0.894	0.3	0.038
AF082125_s_at	AF082125	Ahr	AhR	244	3.0	0.174	0.8	0.299	5.1	0.106	2.3	0.211	0.3	0.089	2.5	0.353	0.3	0.215
U61184_at	U61184	Arnt1	AhR nuclear translocator (ARNT)	163	0.9	0.666	0.8	0.051	0.7	0.024	1.2	0.019	1.6	0.000	0.9	0.616	1.0	0.737
J03170_at	J03170	Tcf1	HNF1-α	268	0.8	0.077	0.7	0.050	0.7	0.038	1.3	0.024	1.3	0.079	1.3	0.028	1.4	0.109
AB017044exon_at	AB017044	*NA*	HNF3-γ	210	0.8	0.022	0.8	0.468	0.5	0.000	0.9	0.745	1.0	0.986	0.8	0.282	0.9	0.622

a) GenBank accession number, gene symbol, and short name were extracted and adapted from Affymetrix descriptions (www.affymetrix.com).
NA = not available. Max. signal: the average intensity of the treatment group with the highest signal. This parameter indicates whether a gene was highly or poorly expressed. Probe sets with intensity lower than 100 were considered to be nondetectable. FChg = Induction/repression expressed as fold change with respect to the time-matched control; *p* value = significance level obtained from a *t* test.

cers, occurs prior to the appearance of major histological findings, at a low dose of 30 mg kg^{-1} after 7 days of treatment, as well as at the earliest tested time point (400 mg kg^{-1}, 6 h).

As mentioned above, Ro-Cmp A shows gender-specific toxic manifestations, females being more susceptible than males. The gene expression results collected in the toxicogenomics study and the observed reduction in circulating cholesterol suggest that cholesterol and steroids such as estrogens contribute to the mechanism of toxicity. In support of this, Kawamoto and coworkers provided evidence that estrogens are activators of the constitutive androstane receptor (CAR), a nuclear receptor that induces transcription of the CYP2B family after exposure to xenobiotics such as phenobarbital [22]. Also, Kocarek and coworkers described induction of rat CYP2B in association with inhibition of cholesterol synthesis [24]. Further supporting evidence was recently published, indicating that an endogenous molecule related to cholesterol homeostasis interacts with the PB-response enhancer sequences of some phenobarbital-induced cytochromes P450 [25]. These reports, taken together with the observed induction of CYPs and serum cholesterol reduction, suggest a possible causal relation between impairment of the sterol metabolic pathway (possibly by inhibition of cholesterol synthesis), induction of CYP2B, and fat accumulation in the hepatocytes.

23.4.3
Corroboration of the Mechanistic Hypothesis I: Validation of the Technology

The validity of the detected gene expression changes for the selected marker genes needs to be assessed further. Gene expression data from microarrays are generally statistically unsound, presenting biostatistics with a challenge that has not yet been resolved adequately. Biological experiments that do not involve the use of microarray-based platforms usually deal with a relatively large number of biological replicates and a relatively small number of parameters. Microarray data represent the opposite situation. On the one hand – due to the relatively high costs involved – most microarray experiments minimize the number of biological replicates, sometimes even resorting to pooling samples to minimize the number of microarrays needed. On the other hand, a typical microarray experiment generates thousands of data points. Conventional statistics (such as variance analysis and pair-wise comparisons with parametric tests) assumes that a number of prerequisites were met, such as normal distribution of the data and independence of the observations. Nevertheless, it is known that groups of genes can be coregulated by a stimulus and that redundancy in the microarray designs leads to several probes detecting the same mRNA. In addition, expression of certain genes may be turned on or off, rather than following a normal distribution pattern within a population. Additional confounding factors are time and dose responses. Thus, the datasets are very complex and highly multivariate. Several approaches are currently used to analyze this kind of data, and many publications on statistical microarray data analysis are available, but to date, there is no one-size-fits-all solution [26–32]. The statistical pitfalls can lead to a number of false-positive results that are erroneously believed to be statistically significant. It is also noteworthy that microarray platforms can also provide misleading results

Tab. 23.4 *In vivo* PCR results measured using specific primers and SYBR Green as a reporter fluorophore.

Description	***GenBank acc. no.***	***7 d***			***6 h***		***24 h***		***Affymetrix Results (Ro-Cmp A)***			
		Ro-Cmp A (30 mg kg^{-1})	Ro-Cmp A (100 mg kg^{-1})	Ro-Cmp A (400 mg kg^{-1})	Ro-Cmp A (400 mg kg^{-1})	Ro-Cmp B (400 mg kg^{-1})	Ro-Cmp A (400 mg kg^{-1})	Ro-Cmp B (400 mg kg^{-1})	Affy ID	Max. Signal	Max. FChg	*p* value (*t* test)
Alzheimer's disease amyloid a4 protein (homolog)	X07648	ND	ND	2.0	1.0	1.0	1.7	1.4	X07648cds_at	329	2.0	0.009
Aryl hydrocarbon receptor (AhR)	AF082124	ND	ND	2.0	2.7	1.7	1.1	1.2	AF082125_s_at	244	4.1	**0.106**
btg2 protein (ngf-inducible anti-proliferative protein pc3) [a]	M60921	ND	ND	1.1	0.5	0.4	2.6	0.6	M60921_g_at	175	0.9	**0.076**
Carboxyl-esterase	AB010635;	2.9	6.3	12.3	1.1	1.3	5.0	2.8	AB010635_s_at	2177	5.1	0.017
Cytochrome P450 CYP2B2	J00728	20.2	27.5	3.6	31.4	3.1	72.0	4.4	M13234cds_f_at	26126	8.2	0.000
Cytochrome P450 CYP3A1	D13912	ND	ND	3.5	1.1	0.9	2.3	0.8	D13912_s_at	11790	4.7	0.009
Cytochrome P450 CYP2B, exon 9	L00320	20.5	87.9	210.5	90.6	0.7	95.1	0.9	L00320cds_f_at	16699	16.2	0.002
Glutathione reductase	U73174	ND	ND	1.4	1.2	1.1	1.9	1.0	U73174_g_at	248	2.1	0.007
UDP-glucuronosyl transferase 2b1	RNUD2A10 M35086; J05482	3.4	3.0	5.9	4.1	0.1	5.0	1.8	M13506_at	5809	4.6	0.002

a) For *btg2*, maximal induction (measured by microarrays and RT–PCR) occurred 24 h after acute administration. For all other genes, maximal induction was generally achieved in the animals treated with 400 mg kg^{-1} Ro-Cmp A for 7 days. The induction observed for *btg2* and *AhR* using microarrays was considered statistically not significant (*p* values in **bold**).

per se. Despite the advances in sequencing efforts for several species – including human and rat – sequence mistakes, unspecific cross-hybridization, and annotation errors increase the possibility for misinterpretation of the data. It is thus prudent to relate and corroborate gene expression data obtained from microarrays to those obtained by other analytical procedures, in order to identify reliable marker genes for a given cellular event. One of the most commonly used methods of confirming gene expression changes is quantitative RT–PCR, using fluorescent reporters of product amplification. In the present example, gene expression modulation of nine genes of interest, among them two exons of CYP2B, was evaluated by using QRT–PCR with SYBR Green as the reporting fluorophore. The results obtained (Table 23.4) agreed with the microarray results and confirmed the observed gene expression changes.

Confirmation of transcriptional changes with methods such as RT–PCR does not necessarily prove (or validate) the biological relevance of the findings, but allows one to eliminate the possibility of technical error. This does not guarantee that the observed changes in messenger RNA are reflected in concomitant altered protein synthesis and/or activity. To clarify whether the induction of messenger RNA from CYP2B led to an increase in protein levels, microsomal levels of this cytochrome P450 were quantified by Western blot analysis (Figure 23.3). An increase in enzyme content was established after subchronic exposure (seven consecutive days) and 24 h after a single administration of Ro-Cmp A. No change in the levels of immunoreactive CYP2B was observed in animals killed 6 h after a single administration of Ro-Cmp A or in any of the rats treated with Ro-Cmp B. Thus, protein levels generally paralleled the levels of mRNA, with the exception of the earliest tested time point. Here, we assumed that the time lag between increased mRNA production and protein synthesis is responsible for the observation.

The results obtained from this toxicogenomics approach show that there is a subset of genes whose expression levels are reliably altered after exposure to Ro-Cmp A but not Ro-Cmp B. Moreover, we confirmed that the transcriptional induction of CYP2B leads to an increase in immunoreactive protein. These results allow for the generation of mechanistic hypotheses of biological relevance that relate cytochrome P450 induction and impairment of steroidogenesis to the hepatic steatosis caused by Ro-Cmp A.

23.4.4 Corroboration of the Mechanistic Hypothesis II: *in vitro* Studies

The increased expression of genes, such as CYP2B, regulated via activation of nuclear receptors and the decrease in circulating cholesterol observed in rats, as well as the data published by Kocarek and coworkers, suggested a possible interaction of Ro-Cmp A with the cholesterol biosynthesis pathway and steroid metabolism in general [24, 33]. Supplementary experiments were initiated to explore the relationships further (Boess et al., in preparation). Rat primary hepatocytes obtained from male animals and cultured in monolayer configuration were exposed to the two compounds investigated in the whole animals for a period of up to 24 h, at two doses (20 and 100 μM). Cytotoxicity, cellular lipid accumulation, and gene expression

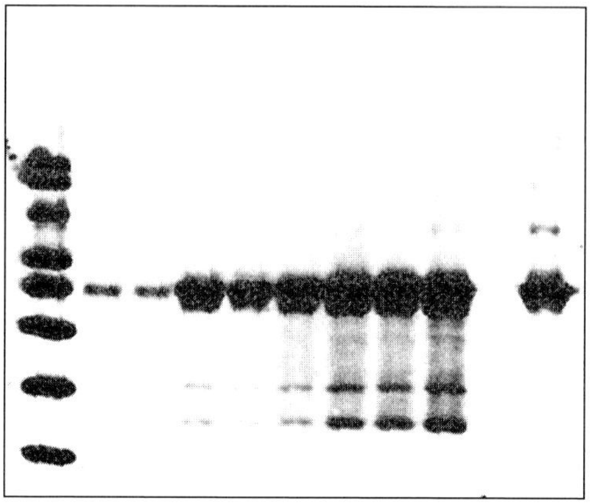

(a)

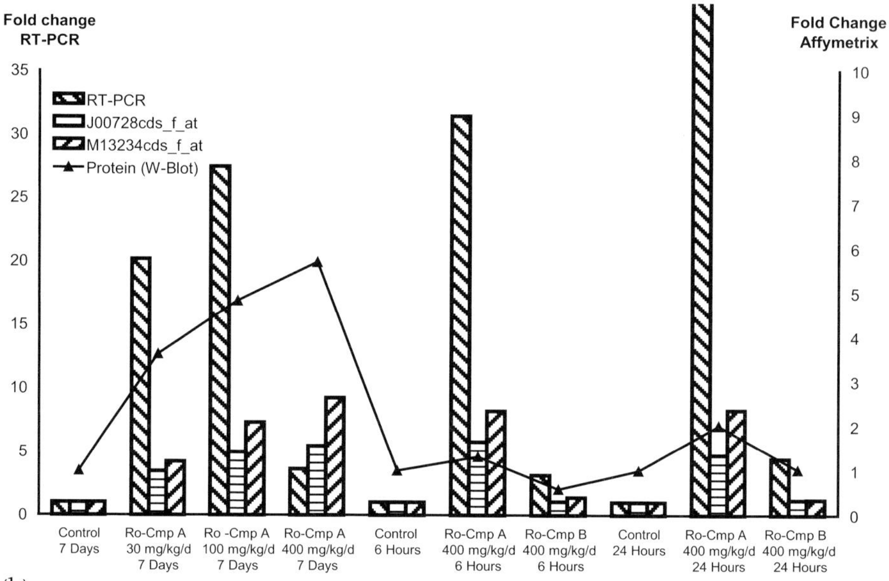

(b)

Fig. 23.3 Western blot results for CYP2B family. (a) Western blot after seven days of exposure to the compound, displaying results from two representative animals of each treatment group. (b) Graphical representation of gene expression levels for CYP2B assessed by RT–PCR and microarray (bars) and protein levels measured from Western blots by densitometry.

changes were assessed. Increased LDH release into the medium was observed at the highest tested concentration of Ro-Cmp A (100 µM), indicating compound-induced cytotoxicity. No cytotoxicity was observed at lower concentrations of Ro-Cmp A (20 µM) nor at any tested concentration of Ro-Cmp B. In addition, Ro-Cmp A was able to induce lipid accumulation, as assessed by Nile red staining of cultured hepatocytes, in a dose-dependent manner. Conversely, Ro-Cmp B failed to induce lipid accumulation *in vitro*. Additional experiments indicated that the observed lipid accumulation was most probably due to inhibition of lipid beta oxidation, which is a common mechanism associated with steatosis and steatohepatitis [34–36]. The effects of both compounds on beta oxidation were assessed, and the obtained results showed that Ro-Cmp A at concentrations of 100 µM or higher inhibited lipid oxidation, as reflected by decreased amounts of TCA-precipitable products from ^{14}C-labelled palmitic acid in cultured rat hepatocytes [34]. An equal concentration (100 µM) of Ro-Cmp B did not cause inhibition of beta oxidation. In addition, the cellular ATP content was decreased by of Ro-Cmp A, indicating an effect on mitochondria, but no effect on the levels of cellular ATP was produced by Ro-Cmp B.

Furthermore, Ro-Cmp A inhibited cholesterol biosynthesis in primary rat hepatocyte cultures as well as in the human hepatoma cell line HepG2. These results confirmed an effect of the compound in steroidogenesis and indicate that inhibition of cholesterol biosynthesis is not related to the metabolic activation of the compound, as it occurs in both primary hepatocytes that are metabolically competent and in HepG2 cells, which display strongly diminished drug-metabolizing ability.

Gene expression results obtained from hepatocytes exposed to the compounds generally supported the findings observed in the whole animals (Boess et al., in preparation). In spite of this qualitative agreement, and contrary to the *in vivo* results, modulation of the genes *in vitro* did not show dose dependence under the experimental design used (Table 23.5). Induction of the selected genes was highest at the

Tab. 23.5 Gene expression *in vitro*. Expression of selected marker genes as assessed by using microarrays (Affymetrix GeneChips) or RT–PCR. Values are expressed as fold changes with respect to the control. Note that Ro-Cmp A elicited maximal gene induction at a concentration of 20 µM, but the cytotoxic concentration of 100 µM had a weaker effect. Conversely, the low concentration of Ro-Cmp B did not induce these genes, but the high concentration (100 µM) caused a weak effect.

Gene name	*20 µM Ro-Cmp A*		*100 µM Ro-Cmp A*		*20 µM Ro-Cmp B*		*100 µM Ro-Cmp B*	
	Affymetrix FChg	*PCR FChg*	*Affymetrix FChg*	*PCR FChg*	*Affymetrix FChg*	*PCR FChg*	*Affymetrix FChg*	*PCR FChg*
Cytochrome P450 CYP2B2	23.69	259.87	3.25	2.37	1.43	3.06	4.50	14.30
Cytochrome P450 CYP2B, exon 9	29.17	241.07	5.19	10.09	1.34	2.63	2.61	5.82
Cytochrome P450 CYP3A1	3.86	8.46	1.62	2.33	1.42	1.73	2.59	2.51
UDP-glucuronosyl transferase 2b1	3.25	101.59	1.12	4.90	1.13	2.41	2.37	2.01

low dose of Ro-Cmp A (20 μM) and less at the high dose (100 μM), probably due to emerging cytotoxicity. Unspecific cytotoxicity is an additional confounding factor that needs to be carefully evaluated when interpreting gene expression results from cell culture systems. It is also noteworthy that the high dose of the nonsteatotic compound Ro-Cmp B caused a mild, yet significant, induction of CYP2B, CYP3A1, and UDP2B. Nevertheless, this induction was several times less pronounced than that caused by the low dose of Ro-Cmp A. The cytotoxic effect of the high dose (100 μM) of Ro-Cmp A on the hepatocytes was not only evident according to increased LDH release into the culture medium, but was also reflected by the transcriptional induction of genes related to cellular damage. Among the genes induced at a high dose of Ro-Cmp A were IGFBP-1, the heme oxygenase gene, and Gadd45, in addition to a weaker induction of genes such as CYP2B and CYP3A1 (among others) that appeared to be specific markers of the steatosis associated with the exposure to this compound. The down-regulation of genes for enzymes involved in the steroideogenic pathway, such as the CYP7 family and HMG-CoA synthase, relates to the deregulation of cholesterol homeostasis, a hallmark of the hepatotoxicity caused by Ro-Cmp A.

The experiments performed in primary rat hepatocyte cultures confirmed the steatotic potential of Ro-Cmp A, since accumulation of intracellular lipids was elicited by exposing the cell cultures to this compound and not to Ro-Cmp B. The effect on lipid homeostasis appeared at concentrations lower than those leading to overt cytotoxicity, as determined by measuring LDH release. At higher concentrations, the accumulation of cellular lipids caused by Ro-Cmp A is accompanied by cytotoxicity, as assessed by LDH leakage and gene expression analysis. With respect to the inhibition of cholesterol synthesis, the results of the *in vitro* tests also corroborated the hypothesis generated from the *in vivo* observations, indicating an effect of Ro-Cmp A on cholesterol biosynthesis. Conversely, Ro-Cmp B did not cause any fat accumulation, inhibition of cholesterol biosynthesis, or cytotoxicity under identical experimental conditions. Regarding gene expression analysis, the expression changes elicited by Ro-Cmp A in CYP2B, CYP3A1, and UDP2B *in vitro* were in good agreement with the effects on the same genes in the livers of the treated animals. Thus, transcriptional effects on a subset of appropriately selected marker genes provide information regarding potential liability *in vivo*.

23.5 Conclusions and Outlook

The main goals of this retrospective toxicogenomics evaluation, as enumerated above, were met:

- Regarding the detection of hepatotoxicants by using transcript profiles, data supporting the usefulness of gene expression analysis for the classification and detection of hepatoxins were provided. The obtained results supplied ample proof of the suitability of gene expression analysis to classify the compound under investigation (Ro-Cmp A) as steatotic when compared to the reference Roche Toxicogenomics database. The main prerequisite for meeting this goal is the availability of a high-quality reference database.

- The data also demonstrate that the two compounds with similar pharmacological profiles and distinct toxicological characteristics can be distinguished based on the gene expression profiles elicited in a given target organ. By including a known hepatotoxic and a nonhepatotoxic compound in the evaluation process, results were generated *in vivo* and *in vitro* that stressed this point. This is a pivotal finding, since test compounds that are intended to become medicines have inherent pharmacological activities that induce a response that is not indicative of the toxic potential of the drug. This pharmacological response is a confounding factor that, if not carefully taken into consideration, might mask the toxic response, generating false-negative results. Alternatively, the pharmacological effect might be erroneously considered to be related to toxicity, generating false-positive results. Both outcomes would be detrimental to the drug development process.
- The presented case study provides arguments supporting the use of toxicogenomics in early phases of drug development. It was shown that acute *in vivo* exposures, as well as *in vitro* approaches, were able to reveal the liability associated with Ro-Cmp A. Short-term *in vivo* studies, as well as a reliable *in vitro* screening tool, could easily be employed during the early phases of clinical candidate selection. The specificity of this response is shown by the concomitant evaluation of the nontoxic pharmacological analogue. As previously mentioned, *in vitro* results need to be evaluated carefully, since confounding factors such as cytotoxicity due to unrealistically high exposures can confound the interpretation of the data.
- The careful evaluation of modulated genes with known biological functions and the subsequent design of *in vitro* studies that corroborated the findings strongly support the usefulness of toxicogenomics for generating mechanistic hypotheses that need biological validation. Within this context, it is vital to clearly understand that technical data confirmation through additional gene expression analysis tools, as well as considering biological relevance through functional assays, is necessary. In this case example, induction of CYP2B and impairment of the cholesterol biosynthesis pathway were confirmed. Further studies may clarify whether these compound-related processes are involved in initiation of the toxic phenomenon or are adaptive responses useful as surrogate diagnostic markers for the hepatosteatosis elicited by this class of compounds.

The knowledge extracted from the presented retrospective analysis suggests that the selected subset of genes would have been a sufficient indicator for the possible liability of the compound. Had we possessed this information prior to the selection and discontinuation of these two 5-HT_6 receptor antagonists, we could have performed exposure tests with primary rat hepatocytes followed by gene expression analysis by PCR at a very early phase, in parallel with determination of the pharmacological efficacy parameters. The pattern of gene modulation would have raised a red flag regarding the steatotic potential of Ro-Cmp A, and suitable confirmatory experiments could have been promptly designed. On the one hand, *in vitro* evaluation of the ability of the compound to produce fat accumulation, inhibition of beta oxidation, and inhibition of cholesterol synthesis could have been promptly performed. On the other hand, short-term, acute exposures of animals would have provided additional information regarding the transferability of the *in vitro* findings to the *in vivo* situation; ruling out an *in vitro*–specific finding. A test program as described could have been performed within days or weeks, sparing the time and resources dedicated to the relatively long toxicology analyses.

In summary, our experience provides an additional piece of support for the use of gene expression analysis as a powerful tool for assessing biological effects, such as toxic or pharmacologic responses *in vivo* as well as *in vitro*. In this example, gene expression analysis *in vivo* provided interesting results regarding the mechanisms underlying toxicological findings in the rat. Transcript profiles alone provided sufficient information to identify the liability of the compound when compared to an existing toxicogenomics database. From a mechanistic point of view, it becomes clear that gene expression analysis does not provide easy answers to complex matters. Nevertheless, in this example, we were able to identify a group of genes modulated mainly via nuclear receptor activation. This group of genes provides insights into the underlying mechanisms and is amenable to being measured via higher-throughput assays such as RT–PCR. Hence, once genes of interest are identified, testing of toxicological potential can be greatly shortened and simplified by evaluating the effects after short exposure times and by developing appropriate assays *in vitro* as well as *in vivo*.

Acknowledgements

We thank all the scientific and technical staff who were at some point involved in evaluation of the compounds and who provided much of the information regarding routine toxicology and pharmacokinetics results. In particular, we thank Dr. F. Boess and coworkers for careful design and performance of the *in vitro* studies and Dr. M. C. de Vera for evaluation of the histopathology slides. Additional thanks go to the Toxicogenomics and the Bioinformatics groups at F. Hoffmann-La Roche, for without their help none of these results could have been obtained or analyzed. We also thank N. Flint and M. Haiker for critical reading of the manuscript.

References

1. Ulrich R, Friend SH. Toxicogenomics and drug discovery: will new technologies help us produce better drugs? *Nat Rev Drug Discov* 2002; **1**: 84–88.
1a. Suter L, Babiss LE, Wheeldon EB. Toxicogenomics in Predictive Toxicology in Drug Development. *Chemistry & Biology* 2004; 11(2): 161–171.
2. Watters JW, McLeod HL. Cancer pharmacogenomics: current and future applications. *Biochim Biophys Acta* 2003; **1603**: 99–111.
3. Boggs WM. *Toxicogenomics: Genome-Based Assessment of Drug Toxicity.* Decision Resources Inc., Walthanm, MA; 2003.
4. Goodsaid FM. Genomic biomarkers of toxicity. *Curr Opin Drug Discov Dev* 2003; **6**: 41–49.
5. Huang Q, Dunn RT, 2nd, Jayadev S, DiSorbo O, Pack FD, Farr SB, et al. Assessment of cisplatin-induced nephrotoxicity by microarray technology. *Toxicol Sci* 2001; **63**: 196–207.
6. Aardema MJ, MacGregor JT. Toxicology and genetic toxicology in the new era of 'toxicogenomics': impact of '-omics' technologies. *Mutat Res* 2002; **499**: 13–25.
7. Cheng RY, Alvord WG, Powell D, Kasprzak KS, Anderson LM. Microarray analysis of altered gene expression in the TM4 Sertoli-like cell line exposed to chromium(III) chloride. *Reprod Toxicol* 2002; **16**: 223–236.
8. Amin RP, Hamadeh HK, Bushel PR, Bennett L, Afshari CA, Paules RS. Genomic interrogation of mechanism(s) underlying cellular responses to toxicants. *Toxicology* 2002; **181–182**: 555–563.
9. Bartosiewicz MJ, Jenkins D, Penn S, Emery J, Buckpitt A. Unique gene expression patterns in liver and kidney associated with exposure to chemical toxicants. *J Pharmacol Exp Ther* 2001; **297**: 895–905.
10. Bulera SJ, Eddy SM, Ferguson E, Jatkoe TA, Reindel JF, Bleavins MR, et al. RNA expression in the early characterization of hepatotoxicants in Wistar rats by high-density DNA microarrays. *Hepatology* 2001; **33**: 1239–1258.
11. Hamadeh HK, Bushel PR, Jayadev S, DiSorbo O, Bennett L, Li L, et al. Prediction of compound signature using high density gene expression profiling. *Toxicol Sci* 2002; **67**: 232–240.
12. Morgan KT. Gene expression analysis reveals chemical-specific profiles. *Toxicol Sci* 2002; **67**: 155–156.
13. Hamadeh HK, Bushel PR, Jayadev S, Martin K, DiSorbo O, Sieber S, et al. Gene expression analysis reveals chemical-specific profiles. *Toxicol Sci* 2002; **67**: 219–231.
14. Waring JF, Ciurlionis R, Jolly RA, Heindel M, Ulrich RG. Microarray analysis of hepatotoxins *in vitro* reveals a correlation between gene expression profiles and mechanisms of toxicity. *Toxicol Lett* 2001; **120**: 359–368.
15. Mossner R, Schmitt A, Syagailo Y, Gerlach M, Riederer P, Lesch KP. The serotonin transporter in Alzheimer's and Parkinson's disease. *J Neural Transm Suppl* 2000; **60**: 345–350.
16. Saudou F, Hen R. 5-Hydroxytryptamine receptor subtypes in vertebrates and invertebrates. *Neurochem Int* 1994; **25**: 503–532.
17. Ruat M, Traiffort E, Arrang JM, Tardivel-Lacombe J, Diaz J, Leurs R, et al. A novel rat serotonin (5-HT6) receptor: molecular cloning, localization and stimulation of cAMP accumulation. *Biochem Biophys Res Commun* 1993; **193**: 268–276.
18. Yoshioka M, Matsumoto M, Togashi H, Mori K, Saito H. Central distribution and function of 5-HT6 receptor subtype in the rat brain. *Life Sci* 1998; **62**: 1473–1477.
19. Sleight AJ, Monsma FJ, Jr., Borroni E, Austin RH, Bourson A. Effects of altered 5-ht6 expression in the rat: functional studies using antisense oligonucleotides. *Behav Brain Res* 1996; **73**: 245–248.
20. Bourson A, Borroni E, Austin RH, Monsma FJ, Jr., Sleight AJ. Determination of the role of the 5-ht6 receptor in the rat brain: a study using antisense

oligonucleotides. *J Pharmacol Exp Ther* 1995; **274**: 173–180.

21. Woolley ML, Bentley JC, Sleight AJ, Marsden CA, Fone KC. A role for 5-ht6 receptors in retention of spatial learning in the Morris water maze. *Neuropharmacology* 2001; **41**: 210–219.
22. Kawamoto T, Kakizaki S, Yoshinari K, Negishi M. Estrogen activation of the nuclear orphan receptor CAR (constitutive active receptor) in induction of the mouse Cyp2b10 gene. *Mol Endocrinol* 2000; **14**: 1897–1905.
23. Suter L, Haiker M, De Vera MC, Albertini S. Effect of two 5-HT(6) receptor antagonists on the rat liver: a molecular approach. *Pharmacogenomics J* 2003; **3**(6): 320–334.
24. Kocarek TA, Kraniak JM, Reddy AB. Regulation of rat hepatic cytochrome P450 expression by sterol biosynthesis inhibition: inhibitors of squalene synthase are potent inducers of CYP2B expression in primary cultured rat hepatocytes and rat liver. *Mol Pharmacol* 1998; **54**: 474–484.
25. Ourlin JC, Handschin C, Kaufmann M, Meyer UA. A Link between cholesterol levels and phenobarbital induction of cytochromes P450. *Biochem Biophys Res Commun* 2002; **291**: 378–384.
26. Raychaudhuri S, Stuart JM, Altman RB. Principal components analysis to summarize microarray experiments: application to sporulation time series. *Pac Symp Biocomput* 2000: 455–466.
27. Butte A. The use and analysis of microarray data. *Nat Rev Drug Discov* 2002; **1**: 951–960.
28. Ambroise C, McLachlan GJ. Selection bias in gene extraction on the basis of microarray gene-expression data. *Proc Natl Acad Sci USA* 2002; **99**: 6562–6566.
29. Liu A, Zhang Y, Gehan E, Clarke R. Block principal component analysis with application to gene microarray data classification. *Stat Med* 2002; **21**: 3465–3474.
30. Eisen MB, Spellman PT, Brown PO, Botstein D. Cluster analysis and display of genome-wide expression patterns. *Proc Natl Acad Sci USA* 1998; **95**: 14863–14868.
31. Schoelkopf B. *Advances in Kernel Methods: Support Vector Learning.* MIT Press, Cambridge, MA; 1999.
32. Salter AH, Nilsson KC. Informatics and multivariate analysis of toxicogenomics data. *Curr Opin Drug Discov Dev* 2003; **6**: 117–122.
33. Kocarek TA, Reddy AB. Negative regulation by dexamethasone of fluvastatin-inducible CYP2B expression in primary cultures of rat hepatocytes: role of CYP3A. *Biochem Pharmacol* 1998; **55**: 1435–1443.
34. Fromenty B, Pessayre D. Inhibition of mitochondrial beta-oxidation as a mechanism of hepatotoxicity. *Pharmacol Ther* 1995; **67**: 101–154.
35. Freneaux E, Labbe G, Letteron P, The Le D, Degott C, Geneve J, et al. Inhibition of the mitochondrial oxidation of fatty acids by tetracycline in mice and in man: possible role in microvesicular steatosis induced by this antibiotic. *Hepatology* 1988; **8**: 1056–1062.
36. Fromenty B, Berson A, Pessayre D. Microvesicular steatosis and steatohepatitis: role of mitochondrial dysfunction and lipid peroxidation. *J Hepatol* 1997; **26**(Suppl 1): 13–22.

24
Toxicogenomics Applied to Hematotoxicology

Yoko Hirabayashi and Tohru Inoue

24.1
Introduction: Forward and Reverse Genomics

Microarray [1, 2] and/or gene chip [3] technologies have enabled the survey of a large number of gene expressions. Specifically, along with the progress in the human and the mouse whole-genome sequencing projects [4, 5], nearly complete gene expression profiling for not only cellular physiological phenotypes, but also for pathological and clinical phenotypes, can also be done with the newly developed genomics methodology. In contrast, prediction and identification of a variety of physiological and pathologic phenotypes solely by gene expression profiling, that is, predictive genomics, is also presumed to be possible by this strategy, once a comprehensive database has been established. The former is called forward genomics, and the latter reverse genomics (Figure 24.1) [6]. The application of microarray and gene chip technologies in toxicology is called toxicogenomics [7]. Toxicogenomics can contribute to elucidating the toxicological mechanism (inductive toxicogenomics) and to predicting various possible toxic phenotypes solely on the basis of similarity in gene expression profiling without annotation of chemical characteristics (deductive toxicogenomics). The former is intended to define an unknown gene profiling marker, and consequently, proteomics markers, whereas the latter is intended to predict various possible toxicological phenotypes even without annotative information. The predictability of the latter strategy should be enhanced by using a database resulting from collaboration between the above-mentioned inductive and deductive approaches. These are analogous to the clinical use of genomics for human tissue samples and using informatics on clinical data to predict the diagnosis of diseases, responses to treatment, and consequent individual prognoses. Such medical and medicinal genomics information (including knowledge of single nucleotide polymorphisms; SNPs) may eventually make custom-made personal treatment protocols possible, and the newly established methodology should also make SNP-oriented human ecotoxicological risk evaluation possible.

In the toxicological application of toxicogenomics using experimental animals, toxicogenomics appears to have two definitive advantages: first, a reduction in the number of test animals and a shortening of the test period, and second, the use of

Handbook of Toxicogenomics: Strategies and Applications. Edited by Jürgen Borlak

ISBN: 3-527-30342-1

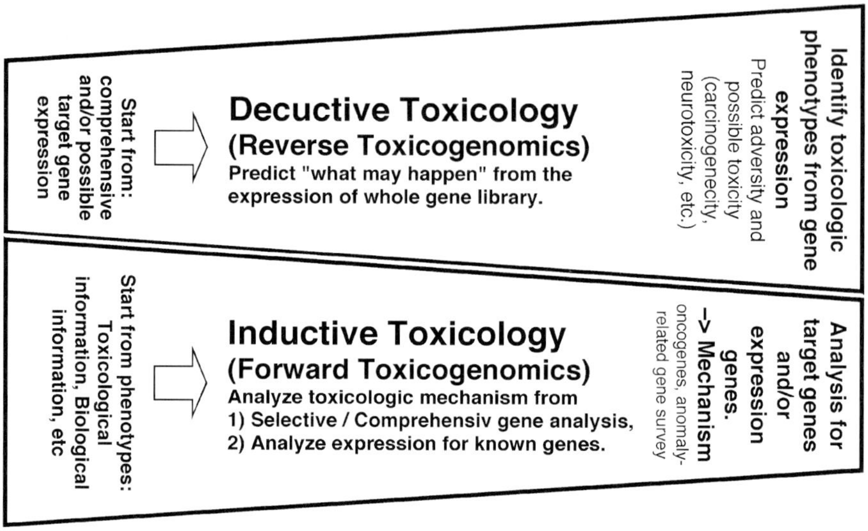

Fig. 24.1 Structures of inductive toxicology vs. deductive toxicology. The former begins its analyses from various toxicological phenotypes, including gross and/or pathological findings, and laboratory information, and proceeds toward the mechanism, whereas the latter focuses on predicting toxicological phenotypes solely on the basis of similarities in gene expression profiles without annotation of chemical characteristics. Nominally, the information on various phenotypes can be more diverse and far larger than the information on original gene expression profiling.

simpler technologies applying established expression profiles as new biomarkers, rather than sophisticated technologies requiring skills and experience. Since various phenotypes, including animal behaviour, are ultimately linked to the expression of genes and appear in consequence of the expression of a limited number of genes, much information can be condensed into a gene expression profile. At this moment, generalized reverse toxicogenomics is still a theory, except for the use of chips for customized purposes. However, the general applicability of species differences, including the extrapolation of responses from experimental animals to humans, the extrapolation of changes *in vitro* to responses *in vivo*, the possibility of analyzing multiple of toxicities from multiple toxicants, as well as the ability to extrapolate from high-dose markers to possible low-dose responses, and the discovery of early gene markers for long-term endpoints, are all promising future challenges [7].

In hematotoxicological applications, because the cellular targets of hematopoietic repertoires vary depending on the position of hierarchical structures along with their immaturity (that is, their 'stemness') and differentiation status, an accurate cell-separation technique for obtaining a reliable homogeneous fraction for relevant and repeatable comparison is necessary, such as flow-cytometric cell sorting with or without various markers for cellular identification or differentiation. Although it is generally accepted that such profiling differences are affected by sampling timing in various tissues in living animals, the hematopoietic tissue, as a continuously proliferating tissue, specifically shows a significantly different and labile profile in the microarray between the tissues immediately after damage and other tissues in the recovery phase. Furthermore, controversial time-sequenced responses differ between immature and differentiated cell compartments; thus, the timing of tissue sampling and the relevant comparison of fractionated blood cell compartments are critical for establishing a repeatable outcome [7].

In the following section, first, a brief overview of the physiological characteristics of hematopoietic stem/progenitor cells is given as a cellular biological basis of hematotoxicology. This is followed by a review of gene expression profiling, that is, molecular signatures, for stem cells. Two case studies on hematotoxicological toxicogenomics, involving radiation and benzene hematotoxicities, are then described so as to review two human ultimate leukemogens and their leukemogenic/hematotoxic profiling obtained by using a microarray. In the section on benzene exposure, gene expression profiling is specifically focused on in comparing p53 knockout (KO) and wild-type (WT) mice.

24.2 Hematopoietic Stem/Progenitor Cells in Hematotoxicology

Since the hematopoietic system consists of a mixture of heterogeneous cells with respect to not only functionally different cellular lineages, but also different stages in differentiation, an unfractionated blood sample may give differing gene expression profiles, and microarray data may not always provide an efficient and predictable outcome. As briefly described in the Introduction, specific attention should be paid to the preparation and interpretation of microarray data; thus, this section provides an overview of the hematopoietic system with respect to the nature of hematopoietic stem/progenitor cells and with special reference to microarray data processing and its interpretation.

The concept of a multipotent hematopoietic stem cell dates back to the radiation studies of Jacobson and coworkers in 1949–1950 [8–10], who observed autonomous hematopoietic recovery in lethally irradiated mice whose spleen or bone marrow had been shielded during otherwise lethal radiation exposure. In 1961, Till and McCulloch discovered that when normal bone marrow cells are transplanted into lethally irradiated mice, their spleens develop macroscopically visible colonies originating from regenerated hematopoietic cells and that the number of colonies directly correlates with the number of bone marrow cells injected, based on the hypothesis that each colony is derived from a single stem (termed spleen colony-forming unit, CFU-S) [11]. In 1965, they confirmed the clonogenic nature of CFU-S and then developed the currently used spleen colony assay for hematopoietic clonality [12]. Since Till and McCulloch's discovery, CFU-S was assumed to be the hematopoietic stem cells for more than 40 years; however, after the discovery of cells possessing a long-term repopulating ability in lethally irradiated mice, which were in addition found not to produce spleen colonies [13], CFU-Ss were renamed pluripotent hematopoietic progenitor cells, and the name of the cells in the common stem/progenitor cell compartment discussed here was changed to hematopoietic stem/progenitor cells.

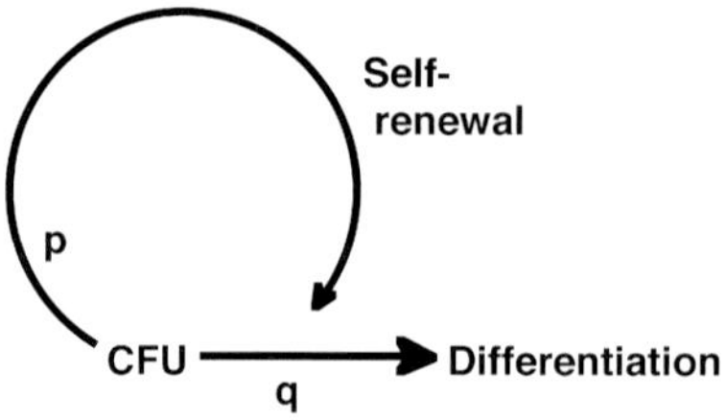

Fig. 24.2 Stem cell capability. Stem cells are capable of both proliferation (p) and differentiation (q), where p and q are independent variables; the ratio between the two is probabilistic. In the steady state, $p + q = 1$ [16].

Hematopoietic stem/progenitor cells, by definition, are targets of toxicological effects [14, 15]. Stem cells are capable of undergoing self-renewal (p) and/or differentiation (q), where p and q are independent variables. In the steady state, $p + q = 1$ (Figure 24.2) [16]. The progeny of hematopoietic stem/progenitor cells can be represented as a hierarchy of self-replicating, differentiating, and/or maturing daughter cells whose frequency depends on the relative probability of self-renewal during colony growth [16–19]. Relatively primitive hematopoietic stem cells, termed long-term repopulating stem cells (LTRCs), possess a relatively high capacity for multilineage differentiation and tend to generate mixed lymphomyeloid colonies in culture [18]. The mechanism of molecular switching of lineage-specific differentiation is not yet fully understood, but over-expression of TAL-1, a transcription factor involved in myeloid differentiation, inhibits lymphoid differentiation in ectopic over-expressing mice [20]. The mechanism of molecular switching was extensively studied by Lemischka's group [21] (see next section). The uncommitted hematopoietic progenitor cell, termed the *in vitro* colony-forming unit (CFU-C), can generate various lineage-specific colonies in semisolid culture, depending on the specific hematopoietic growth factors used to supplement the culture medium [16, 22].

Primitive stem cells and differentiating progenitor cells differ in kinetic characteristics. A method of evaluating stem cell kinetics *in vivo*, called the BUUV method, is available, and its use is introduced in Section 24.5.1. Once primitive stem cells (which tend to be predominantly in G_0) enter the cell cycle, they tend to proliferate at a more rapid rate than early progenitor cells [23]. Thus, elucidation of stemness is of special interest (see next section). One particular characteristic of the stem/progenitor function is explained by the significance of the activity of telomerase, a reverse transcriptase, as it is associated with the replicating potential of stem/progenitor cells. That is, primitive stem cells have a lower telomerase activity than do early progenitor cells, whereas early progenitor cells have high telomerase activity; however, as they mature or after repeated bone marrow transplantation, progenitor cells lose their telomerase activity [24, 25].

The shape of a hematopoietic colony growing in semisolid culture reflects its differentiation characteristics which, in turn, depend on the receptors expressed by its stem/progenitor cells and on the growth factor(s) used to supplement the culture medium (Figure 24.3). Colonies derived from immature stem cells are characterized by compactness, a high self-renewal capability, and a relatively low differentiation activity. Early uncommitted CFU-C generate an aggregation of several subcolonies called a mixed colony, indicating coexistence of a high self-renewal capacity and active differentiation ability. Although these colony-forming units in culture are

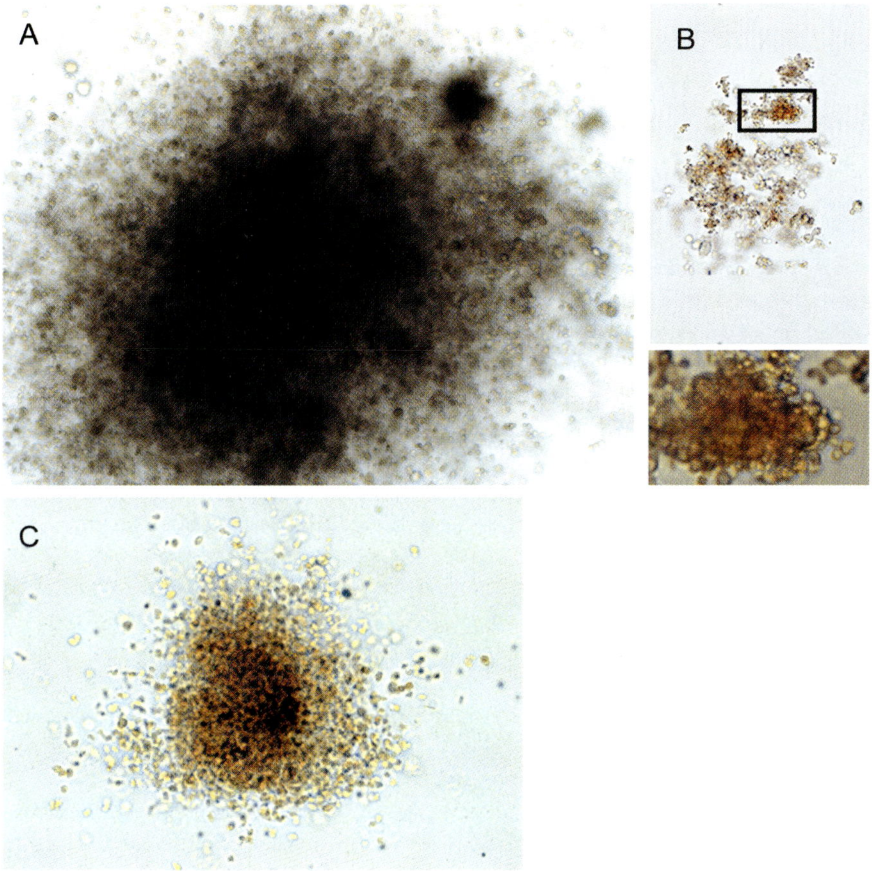

Fig. 24.3 Various hematopoietic colonies. Cultures of colonies were started from bone marrow cells, 2×10^4 cells mL^{-1}, grown in semisolid media with 0.8% methylcellulose in alpha MEM supplemented with 30% FCS (HyClone Lab.), 1% BSA, 10^{-4} M 2-mercaptoethanol, 1 μg mL^{-1} interleukin 3, and 2 U mL^{-1} erythropoietin. (A) Colony-forming unit with granulo–macrophage–megakaryocyte elements (original magnification, ×15); (B) burst colony-forming unit composed of erythroid elements (the inset at the bottom is a higher-magnification view of the boxed daughter aggregate at the top) (original magnification, ×15, top; and ×225 bottom); (C) colony-forming unit granulo–macrophage in the right (original magnification, ×15).

thought to be more differentiated progenitors than CFU-S, there are more primitive stem/progenitor cells, which are thought not to produce spleen colonies but which support the survival of lethally irradiated mice (LTRCs) [18, 26]). The hierarchy of the hematopoietic stem/progenitor cells mentioned above appears to express their own gene-expression profiling (see next section).

Correlating patterns of hematopoietic colony growth with changes in rates of hematopoietic stem/progenitor cell self-renewal and differentiation may be a useful tool for toxicological evaluation. That is, a large colony is derived from a progenitor cell whose progeny has a high rate of both proliferation and differentiation, whereas an aggregate of numerous smaller colonies indicates derivation from a stem/progenitor cell with a high rate of self-renewal but a low rate of differentiation. Early stem/progenitor cells tend to generate compact colonies, whereas the more mature (committed) progenitor cells tend to produce dispersed colonies. The differentiation status may also reflect specific gene expression profiling (see next section). The shape and size of a hematopoietic colony can be an index of a stem/progenitor cell's kinetic status [23].

Current progress in the study of stem-cell plasticity is significant. The capability of stem cells to differentiate into various tissues is virtually unlimited. Not only have embryonic stem cells been shown to be able to differentiate into hematopoietic stem cells [27] or neuronal stem cells [28] and adipocytes [29], but hematopoietic stem cells have also been shown to be able to differentiate into hepatic oval cells [30] and hemangioendothelial cells [31]. Moreover, bone marrow stromal cells appear to be capable of differentiating into neuronal stem cells [32], hematopoietic stem cells [33], and cardiac muscle cells [34]. Such transorganic tissue stem cell systems may express common gene profiling on one hand, but each tissue stem cell system, including embryonic stem cells, expresses its own specific gene profiling [35] (see next section).

24.3 Molecular Signature of Stemness of Hematopoietic Stem/Progenies

Hematopoietic tissue consists of various blood cells and stromal cells, which form the hierarchy of the blood family. The proliferation and differentiation of blood cells are regulated by the interaction between blood cells, between blood cells and stromal cells, and between stromal cells indirectly through various cytokine secretions. Various blood lineages originate from each progenitor, which are different from common hematopoietic stem cells. Importantly, each progenitor cell expresses different molecular signatures (gene profiles), which enable them to maintain their particular characteristics. In this section, some trials to determine such particular gene-expression profiling of physiological stem/progenitor cells are introduced.

To elucidate the molecular signatures of hematopoietic stem/progenitor cells, it is important to characterize each expression profile that is specifically linked to each cell compartment, which is fractionated into various groups of bone marrow cells along with their differentiation from stem cells through progenitor cells to terminally differentiated cells. Thus, before microarray analyses, obtaining the expression profile of the specific fraction of the hematopoietic compartment provides essential information useful in future microarray analysis. Lemischka and coworkers analyzed a genome-wide gene expression defining regulatory pathways in stem cells [35] (Figure 24.4A). They fractionated $Sca^{pos}AA4.1^{pos}Kit^{pos}Lin^{neg/lo}$ [21, 36] and obtained cells from the fraction. cDNA libraries were obtained by removing of the $AA4.1^{neg}$ fraction [21]. According to the report of Phillips et al. [21], 42% of the genes studied either exactly matched data in PubMed queries or were homologous to known protein sequences, 39% were found in a list of expression sequence tag (EST) homology, and 14% of the genes studied found no match. Based on the functions predicted

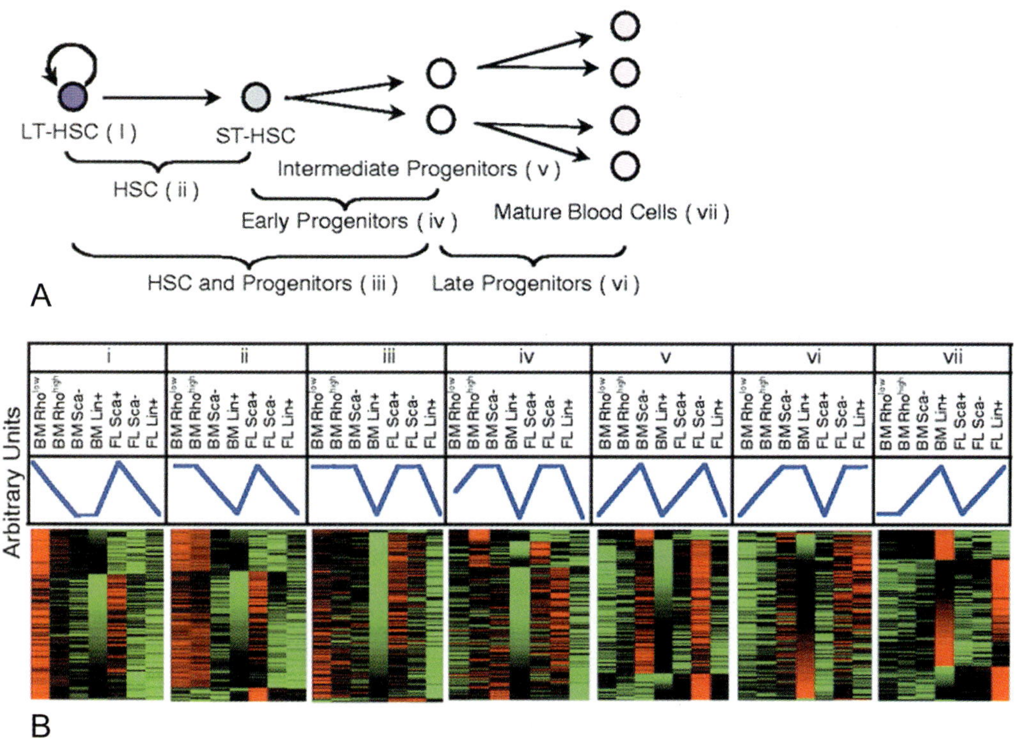

Fig. 24.4 (A) Hematopoietic hierarchy subgrouped into different stem and progenitor populations with their corresponding expression clusters (i to vii.). (B) Individual genes were assigned to expression clusters as described elsewhere, and relative expression levels are displayed in red (highest) to green (lowest) correlation. Predicted cellular roles of identified hematopoietic-specific gene products are shown [35]. (Reprinted with permission from Ivanova et al., *Science* 298: 601–604, 2002. Copyright 2002 AAAS.)

on the basis of the possible amino acid sequences mentioned above, the 39% EST consist of 32% genes for cell signalling, 24% for RNA synthesis, 18% for metabolism, 13% for protein synthesis, 7% for cell division, 4% for cell structure, and 2% for cell defence. The major functional categories of the entire subtracted genes consist of the following: five genes for transcription factors and chromatin-binding proteins (*ALL-1, AML-1/CBF, Dnmt-3b, Evi-1,* and *macroH2A 1.2*), with 10 novel related molecules; five genes for surface molecules (*Flk-2, Smoothened, Hem-1, CD34,* and *CD27*) with 10 novel related molecules; five genes for secreted proteins (angiopoietin, *IL-12 p35, MIP2, IL-16,* and MIP-related protein 2), with 10 novel non-annotated molecules; five genes for signalling molecules (*Dishevelled-1, Manic Fringe, Ski, DOKL, p56Dok-2*), with 10 novel related molecules; 10 genes homologous to *Caenorhabditis elegans* orthologs; and 10 genes homologous to *Drosophila* orthologs [21]. Recently, gene expression profiles for the stem cell fraction were directly observed [35]. On the basis of the expression profiles of the stem cell fraction separated by a cell sorter (Sca^{pos}AA4.1^{pos}Kit^{pos}Lin$^{neg/lo}$), Ivanova and coworkers observed the microarray profiles of each bone marrow fraction separated into seven subgroups, from stem cell through progenitor cell to terminally differentiated cells, using cell-surface markers (Figure 24.4 B) [35]. According to information on the function of gene expression profiling specifically related to primitive hematopoietic stem/progenitor cells, the LT-HSC (long-term hemopoietic stem cells; Sca^{pos}Kit^{pos}Rho^{low}Lin^{neg}) fraction possesses two particular functions, transcription, such as *Hox* gene family, and cell-cell communication. The later consists of signalling ligands, receptors, extracellular matrix, and adhesion molecules, tends to be overexpressed in the HSC-specific gene set, and includes such LT-HSC–specific ligands as *Bmp8a*, *Wnt10A*, EGF family members *Ereg* and *Hegfl*, the angiogenesis-promoting factor *Agpt*, a ligand for the ROBO receptor family *Slit2*, and the ephrin receptor ligand *EfnB2*. The corresponding genes are recognized as involved in stem–stromal cell interactions in general, but *Wnt10A/Frizzled* and *Agpt/Tek* are, on the other hand, known to be expressed solely in stem cells. (Further, expression of these genes are also known to be common in the early development of embryonic stem cells.) In their reports [35], a large amount of supporting online materials and raw data including those for 4289 genes were attached, which were obtained by using Affymetrix systems (the above is excerpted with permission from NB Ivanova et al., *Science* 298: 601–604 (2002); copyright 2002 AAAS). Similar trials were performed by Park et al. [37], Ma et al. [38], and Attia et al. [39]; however, the data obtained cannot be compared among the reports, because the microarray systems and fractionation methods used were different. Also, overlapping genes were rarely observed because the stem cell compartments sorted out were different. Changes in the above-mentioned expression profiles diagnostic of stemness due to hematotoxicity are of special interest to analyze as a possible stem cell-specific response (see Sections 24.5.3, 24.5.5, and the Summary).

Interestingly, when gene expression was compared among embryonic, neuronal, and hematopoietic stem cells, 283 genes were commonly expressed in these three stem cell systems among the 2359 genes in the HSCs (Figure 24.5) [35]. Future mi-

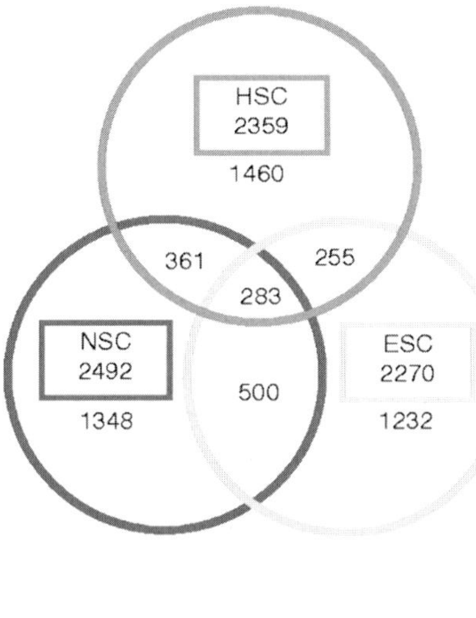

Fig. 24.5 Overlapping gene expressions in diverse murine stem cells. Venn diagram showing shared and distinct gene expressions among neuronal stem cells (NSCs), embryonic stem cells (ESCs), and hematopoietic stem cells (HSCs) [35]. (Reprinted with permission from Ivanova et al., *Science* 298: 601–604, 2002. Copyright 2002 AAAS.)

croarray studies on stem cells from different tissues and embryonic stem cells may elucidate the molecular mechanism underlying the plasticity of stem cell differentiation described in this section.

24.4 Radiation Hematotoxicity and Leukemogenesis

24.4.1 Radiation Effects on Hematopoietic Stem/Progenitor Cells

The idea that radiation can cause leukaemia was first raised in 1911 by von Jagie et al. [40], who described an increased incidence of leukaemia among clinical radiologists working with radiography and radioisotopes. This concept was reinforced by the high incidence of leukaemia among nuclear-bomb victims in Hiroshima and Nagasaki [41]. As indicated elsewhere, multiple hits are required for acute myeloid leukaemia (AML) to develop in this setting [41]. This suggests that younger individuals are potentially at greater risk of leukaemia because they have a greater risk for a secondary hit within their lifetime than do older individuals, although such a trend can be seen only when risks are broken down into age classes. In the setting of chronic myeloid leukaemia (CML), which presumably requires only a single hit or a few hits, younger individuals are also at higher risk than are older members of the general population [41].

The evolution of leukaemia from hematopoietic stem/progenitor cells has been well documented by a number of investigators [42–44]. Consequently, the incidence of radiation-induced leukaemia can be represented by a convex curve in which the incidence of leukaemia decreases at doses of radiation higher than 400 cGy [43], since high-dose radiation exposure does not induce leukaemia but instead causes excessive stem cell killing. If one takes into account stem cell survival after radiation, it is possible that the least number of stem cells is required for induction; thus, increased risk correlates with radiation dose [45]. One can calculate the actual risk by incorporating the total number of bone marrow stem/progenitor cells into the calculated survival curve for hematopoietic stem/progenitor cells (Figure 24.6 A): The integral (shaded area) between the two lines corresponds to a high leukaemia risk. As the radiation dose approaches zero or exceeds 500 cGy, the respective integral areas increase or decrease, and the exponential risk approaches but never reaches zero, even with an infinite number of experimental subjects.

Interestingly, there are two settings in which the incidence of radiation leukaemia increases continuously with increasing radiation dose, namely, during fractionated radiation exposure and with p53 gene deficiency. With fractionated radiation exposure, using 100 divided doses, a different risk curve is obtained [45]. Using hematopoietic spleen colony assays, we found much flatter curves for both stem cell survival and leukaemia risk after single-dose radiation rather than after fractionated-dose radiation, even at high doses (Figure 24.6B). What type of gene expression profiles participates in these particular settings is of special interest (see next subsection).

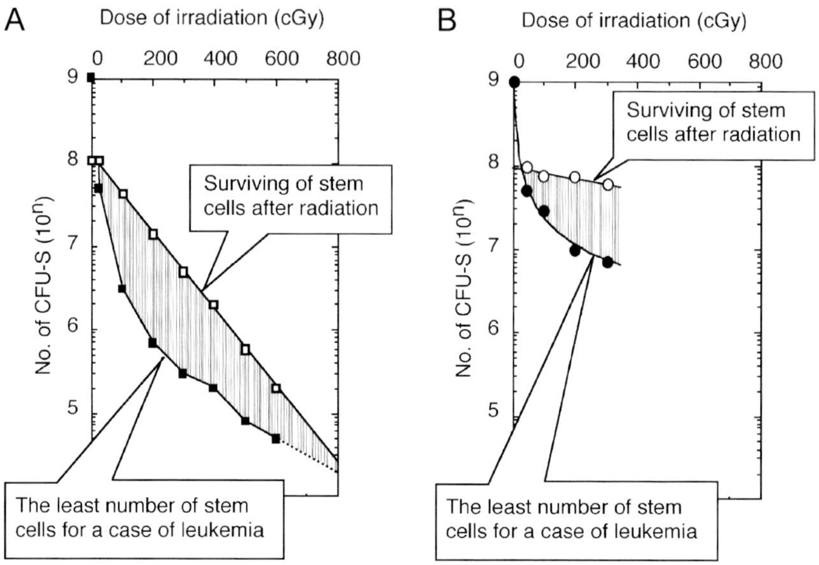

Fig. 24.6 Risk of radiation-induced leukaemia. Incidence of radiation-induced leukaemia and possible risk calculation represented by the shaded area between survival of stem cells (open symbols) and the fewest stem cells needed for a leukaemia case (closed symbols) as a function of radiation dose. (A) Single dose of radiation and (B) 100 split doses, were given [45].

Radiation induces apoptosis in mouse hematopoietic stem/progenitor cell compartments. Using p53-deficient (p53 KO) mice, we determined whether p53 deficiency blocks apoptosis. As expected, the stem/progenitor cell survival curves were flatter in p53 KO than in WT mice, demonstrating that p53 deficiency induces resistance to apoptosis and, consequently, a higher incidence of leukaemia [46]. (Comparative graph on radiation leukaemogenesis using p53 KO mice similar to Figure 24.6 is not shown.) The increased incidence of leukaemogenesis associated with p53 deficiency is consistent with the observation of increased leukaemogenesis at high radiation doses (for example, 500 cGy) in these animals [47].

Primitive stem cells require cytokines, the stem cell factor (SCF), and interleukin-3 (IL-3) to proliferate and generate hematopoietic colonies *in vitro* [48]. Moreover, we should note that primitive hematopoietic stem cells, but not more mature progenitor cells, express the growth-inhibitory signalling molecule, the tumour growth factor (TGF) beta receptor [49, 50]. TGF-beta does not increase the number of colonies generated in culture from WT stem/progenitor cells. Interestingly, such negative regulation of TGF-beta for primitive stem/progenitor cells fails when bone marrow cells are harvested from p53 KO [50]. It is also of interest that mice overexpressing the SV40-large T gene and made p53-deficient can suffer from a myelodysplastic syndrome, in which lack of regulation of growing potential in the primitive stem/progenitor cells is presumably induced by dysfunction of the negative regulator TGF-beta [51].

24.4.2
Radiation Exposure and Gene Expression Microarray

Irradiation of the hematopoietic system induces graded dose-dependent impairment of blood cells based on different radiation sensitivities at different stages of differentiation or with different positions in the cell cycle. Whereas common gene profiles among the doses were observed (40–50%), most of the genes did not overlap at different doses. To determine whether microarrays are useful for identifying these dose-related changes in gene expression, gene expressions at two doses, namely, 100 and 300 cGy, of gamma rays were compared with those in a nonirradiated control (Figure 24.7A). Although a possible common gene profile should be useful tool to search for biomarkers for dose–risk assessments, a unique gene profile at different irradiation doses should be useful for analyzing unique gene repertoires functioning at each radiation dose.

Among the genes expressed in the bone marrow one month after 100 or 300 cGy irradiation were those for *Mus musculus* p53-variant mRNA (U59758), cyclin G1 (L49507), cyclin-dependent kinase inhibitor 1C (*p57*; U22399), *M. musculus* mRNA for cyclin B1 for cell cycle (X64713), *M. musculus* apoptosis-inducing factor AIF mRNA (AF100927), *M. musculus* mRNA for caspase-12 for apoptosis-related genes

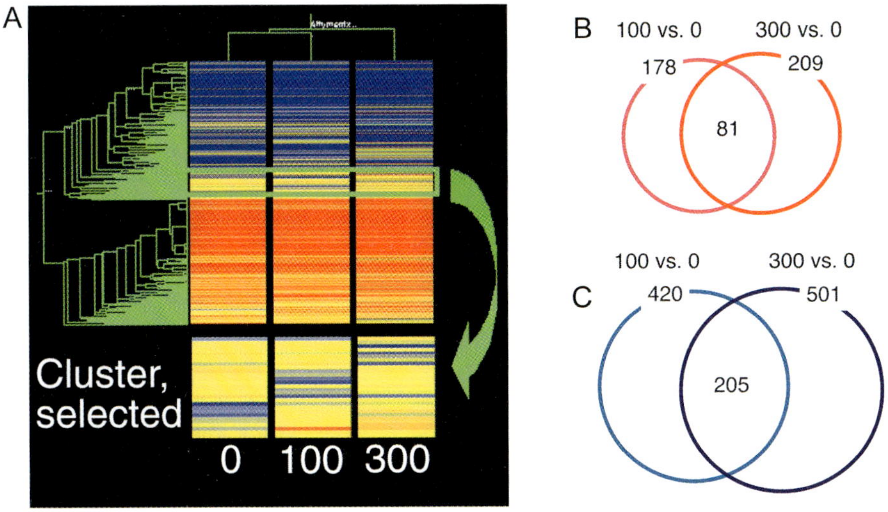

Fig. 24.7 (A) Cluster diagrams of gene trees, comparing the expression profiles among the groups (0, 100, and 300 cGy). GeneSpring software was used to normalize absolute gene expressions for each dose; the lowest expression level is shown in blue, the highest in red, and the intermediate in yellow. Most of expression profile patterns among the groups here seem to be similar in spectra, except in the region indicated by the green box, where the cluster regions selected show different expression profiles for each dose group, as shown on the bottom. (B) and (C) Venn diagrams showing (B) the numbers of genes expressed greater than twice the control levels and (C) the number of genes expressed less than half the control levels. The size of each circle is relative to the number of genes with changed expression, revealing that a larger number of genes was down-modulated (C) by irradiation, and one third of genes were up-regulated (B) by irradiation.

(Y13090), *M. musculus N-myc* gene, 3′ end and MoMuLV-like endogenous provirus, 5′ end (M29211), *Mago-nashi homolog*, a proliferation-associated *Drosophila* ortholog (AF035939) for proliferation-related genes, *M. musculus* thioredoxin mRNA (U85089), a nuclear gene encoding a mitochondrial protein, and *M. musculus* thioredoxin-related protein mRNA (AF052660) for oxidative-stress–related genes. Dose-related gene expression showed that many genes, that is, *M. musculus* endogenous retroviral sequence Mu ERV-*L gag, pol*, and dUTPase genes (Y12713), *M. musculus schlafen3* (Slfn3) mRNA (AF099974), and *Ul-M-BH0-ajy-d-09–0-Ul.s1 M. musculus* cDNA, 3′ end (A1853444), are potential common genes for indicating radiation exposure, and that the mouse germline IgH-chain gene (DJC region segment D-FL16.1; J00475) and *caspase-12* (Y13090) are dose-dependent gene markers. Whether expression of the genes Y12713, AF099974, and A1853444 is altered at much lower radiation doses is of interest for their use as possible gene markers for low-dose radiation (Figure 7 B and C).

The gene expression profiles in spontaneous and radiation-induced tumours differed, which is another interesting finding. Since C3H/He mice produce less than 1% of spontaneous myeloid leukemias, if spontaneous myeloid leukaemia tissue is obtained from such rare cases by the subtraction method, such a method would provide a specific gene profile difference between these types of tumours and would contribute a unique gene marker for identifying leukemias possibly induced by radiation.

24.5 Benzene-induced Hematotoxicity and Leukemogenesis

24.5.1 Benzene Exposure and Cell Cycle in Hematopoietic Stem/Progenitor Cells

The first report on leukaemia induced by benzene inhalation was made by Delore and Borgomano in 1928 [52] who described in a case of leukaemia in a French pharmacist. However, experimental induction of leukaemia by benzene exposure was not successful for more than half a century, until Snyder et al. and our group reported it over two decades ago [53–55]. Nevertheless, the mechanistic background of benzene-induced leukaemia remained an enigma until the peculiar benzene-induced cell kinetics of stem/progenitor cells was recently elucidated in our study, in which we demonstrated a marked, continuous oscillatory decrease in peripheral blood and bone marrow cellularities during and after benzene exposure [14], which epigenetically preceded and led to the development of leukaemia more than a year later.

The BUUV method[1)] enables the determination of stem/progenitor-cell–specific cellular kinetics [56], such as labelling rate, cycling fraction of clonogenic progenitor

1) The BUUV method involves incorporation of bromodeoxyuridine (BrdU) through an osmotic minipump, followed by specific purging of BrdU-containing cells by exposure to ultraviolet light at a specific wavelength, followed by assaying the ratio of hemopoietic colonies between the purged and the control. Hemopoietic stem/progenitor cell-specific parameters for cell kinetics, such as a doubling time, size of the cycling (i.e., DNA-synthesizing) or quiescent cell fractions, and also the size of cycling fraction per unit time-interval can be obtained (Figure 24.8A).

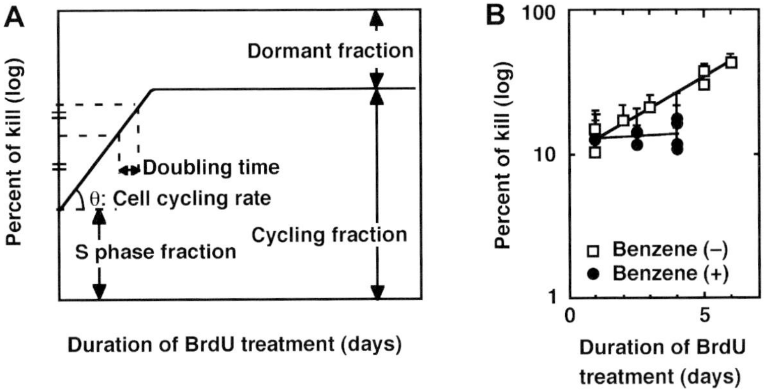

Fig. 24.8 (A) BUUV method of measuring cycling stem cells: model and parameters. Method for evaluating stem cell kinetics. Continuous infusion of bromodeoxyuridine via an osmotic minipump was used to label cycling cells, followed by UV exposure to kill the labelled cells. Then the surviving stem cells formed hematopoietic colonies [56]. (B) Cell cycle of granulo–macrophage colony-forming unit (CFU-GM) during exposure of normal mice to benzene. Note the significant suppression of the cell cycle fraction during benzene exposure with respect to the nonexposed control (closed circles and open squares, respectively).

cells, and other cell cycle parameters (Figure 24.8A). The cycling fraction of stem/progenitor cells was found not to undergo active haematopoiesis but rather to remain low in bromodeoxyuridine (BrdU) incorporation during benzene inhalation (Figure 24.8B). Furthermore, we found evidence that the decrease in the cycling fraction may be mediated in part by a slowing of stem/progenitor cell cycling per se or by p21 up-regulation [14].

Benzene-induced leukaemogenicity seem to differ between mice lacking p53 (p53 KO) and mice carrying WT p53. In p53 KO mice, DNA damage due to weak mutagenicity and/or chromosomal damage is retained, and those types of damage participate in the activation of protooncogenes and similar species, which leads cells to undergo further neoplastic changes. In contrast, in WT mice, a marked oscillatory change in the cell cycle of the stem cell compartment seems to be an important factor for these mice to experience a possible consequent mutagenic event.

Another interesting observation was the controversial experimental data concerning the level of actively cycling hematopoietic cells after benzene exposure. Although many investigators observed suppression of peripheral blood and bone marrow cellularities, some observed a suppression of cell cycling in the bone marrow, as measured by a decrease in tritiated thymidine incorporation [57], whereas others observed a marked increase in the number of cycling stem/progenitor cells in bone marrow and peripheral blood [55, 58, 59]. Careful analysis of these apparently conflicting data revealed increased cell cycling occurring at least two hours after the termination of benzene exposure. Thus, the higher tritiated thymidine incorporation documented by Cronkite et al. [55] 18 hours after the termination of benzene exposure probably reflected a recovery phase.

Based on the above-mentioned findings, we initiated a series of studies in 1997 to elucidate the leukaemogenic effect of benzene in mice. Using the p53 KO mouse, we confirmed that benzene has a moderate genotoxic effect, as measured by a micronucleus test performed four weeks after the initiation of benzene inhalation. Moreover, p53-deficient mice manifested increased susceptibility to benzene-induced leukaemogenicity [60]. Similar findings regarding increased leukaemogenicity after benzene exposure have been documented by French et al. at the National Institute of Environmental Health Sciences [61]. Presumably, benzene-induced leukaemia was not detected in earlier animal studies because its manifestations was masked by either pancytopenia due to severe myelosuppression or by the use of a benzene dose too low to induce pancytopenia and/or leukaemia.

24.5.2 Gene-expression Profile after Benzene Exposure in WT Mice

Based on the background of benzene-induced hematotoxicity and its leukaemogenesis, the cDNA microarray analysis was focused on to determine whether it can elucidate the underlying mechanism. The results of cDNA microarray analysis showed a broad consensus that the p53 tumour-suppressor gene is central to the mechanism of action of benzene, by strictly regulating specific genes involved in the pathways of cell cycle arrest, apoptosis, and DNA repair. Such a close association of p53 gene function and benzene toxicity raises the question regarding the fate of mice whose p53 gene was knocked out after benzene exposure; thus, cDNA microarray analysis data from p53 KO and WT mice were analyzed with Genespring software. In p53 WT mice, the expression profiles of genes encoding many proteins involved in benzene metabolism (CYP2E1 [62] and myeloperoxidase (MPO) [63]), cell cycle or cell proliferation (p53, $p21^{waf1}$, cyclin G1, and Gadd45 [64]), and apoptosis (Bax-alpha [64]) were generally consistent with the cDNA microarray data for C57BL/6 mice described elsewhere (Table 24.1). A difference was noted in the expression patterns of specific genes taken during and after exposure of C57BL/6 mice to 300 ppm benzene for two weeks, as determined using the Incyte GEM cDNA microarray system (Figure 24.9). Figure 24.9A

Tab. 24.1 Genes reported to be up-regulated after benzene inhalation.

Category	*Gene name*	*Reference*
Metabolic enzyme	CYP 2E1	62
	myeloperoxidase (MPO)	63
Cell cycle	p53	64
	p21 (waf 1)	64
	cyclin G	64
	Gadd 45	64
Apoptosis	Bax-alpha	64
Oncogene	c-fos	82

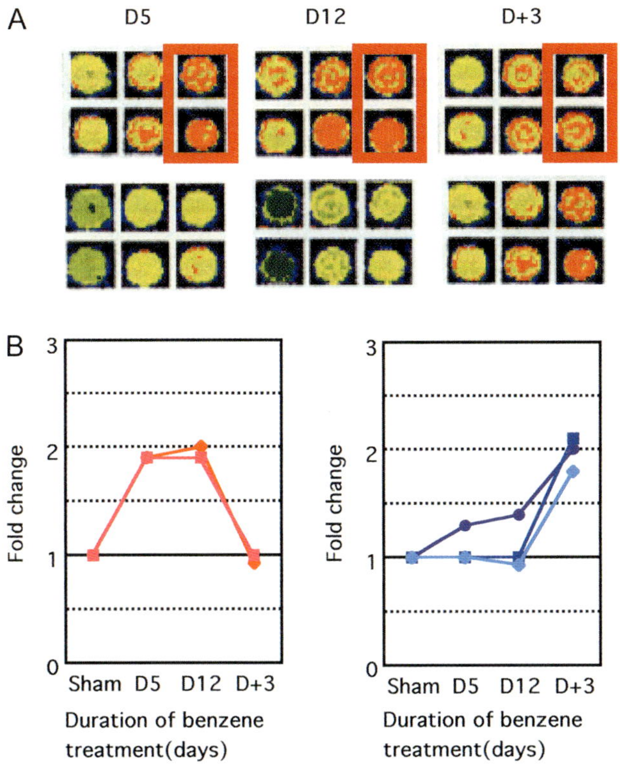

Fig. 24.9 Time course of microarray assays. Mice were exposed to benzene at 300 ppm for 1 week (D5) and 2 weeks (D12). D+3 designates the recovery group. The Incyte GEM system was used. Background-subtracted element signals were used to calculate the Cy3:Cy5 ratio. (A) Colour images of selected genes (two spots on the top right in each group) up-regulated (relative to nonexposed control) during and after benzene inhalation in red, down-regulated expression in green, and unchanged expression in yellow. Note that *MPO* (GenBank accession number X15378) shows up-regulation during benzene exposure followed by immediate down-regulation after exposure. (B) Time sequence of changes in expression of two different gene sets. *Left panel:* Genes up-regulated during benzene exposure followed by immediate down-regulation after benzene exposure: *MPO* genes (GenBank accession numbers X15313 and X15378, the same genes as in (A); squares and diamonds, respectively). *Right panel:* Genes up-regulated, gradually or immediately, after benzene exposure, chiefly represented by genes for DNA repair and proliferation during the recovery phase; *MCLP* (squares), *cdc2* (diamonds), and *lipocalin 2* (circles).

shows that the expression of MPO increased during exposure to benzene (right top square consisting two spots at D5 and D12) and then decreased three days after the termination of benzene exposure (right top square consisting two spots at D+3). Figure 24.9B (left) shows graphic expression of fold changes in the expression of MPOs (X15313 based on the mRNA sequence and X15378 based on the genomic sequence) mentioned above. There are corresponding spots for D5, D12, and D+3, revealing various expression patterns along the time course. A particular expression of the aryl-hydrocarbon receptor (AhR) was stably observed; its expression and the relationship to benzene exposure could not be specified; however, as we previously observed, sensitivity to benzene toxicity is innate in AhR KO mice, implying that AhR transmits this sensitivity to benzene toxicity [15].

Also, a number of genes not previously reported show specific expression profiles after benzene exposure. We discovered the following points associated with the mechanism of action of benzene [65]: (1) benzene induces DNA damage in cells in any phase of the cell cycle; (2) for G1–S cell cycle arrest, not only the p53-mediated pathway but also the pRb gene-mediated pathway is involved; (3) p53-mediated *caspase 11* activation, aside from p53-mediated *Bax* gene induction, might be an important pathway for cellular apoptosis after benzene exposure; (4) *p58*, elongation factor-1 delta and Wee1-kinase may participate in G2–M cell cycle arrest induced by benzene; (5) DNA repair genes such as *Rad51, Rad 54* and *topoisomerase III* are activated after benzene exposure (Clastogenesis-related *topo-II* depression was insignificant.).

24.5.3
Cell-cycle–related Genes in p53 KO and WT Mice

Mice lacking the p53 gene generally had expression patterns similar to those of WT mice for genes involved in benzene metabolism (CYP2E1 [62, 66] and MPO [63]) and haemopoiesis, suggesting that p53 KO mice are also affected by benzene exposure to a similar extent, as also proposed previously based on the high number of micronuclei in benzene-exposed p53-deficient mice [67] (Table 24.2; see lines for up- or down-regulated both simultaneously in p53 KO and WT). To elucidate the difference in expression between p53 KO and WT mice, clustering analysis was performed [65]. The genes expressed include cell cycle- and apoptosis-associated genes. Table 24.3 shows

Tab. 24.2 Gene expression changes during and after benzene inhalation in the presence or absence of p53 gene.

Change in gene expression after benzene inhalation		***Category***
WT	***p53 KO***	
No change	No change	No relationship
	Up-regulated Down-regulated	Levelled by WT p53 during/after the benzene inhalation.
Up-regulated	No change	Genes up-regulated during/after benzene inhalation.
	Up-regulated	Genes up-regulated during/after benzene inhalation without any correlation of the p53 gene.
	Down-regulated	Genes levelled and also up-regulated by WT p53 with some other genes during/after benzene inhalation.
Down-regulated	No change	Genes down-regulated during/after benzene inhalation.
	Up-regulated	Genes levelled and also down-regulated by WT p53 with some other genes during/after benzene inhalation.
	Down-regulated	Genes down-regulated during/after benzene inhalation without any correlation of the p53 gene.

Tab. 24.3 Major changes in gene expression profiles in wild-type (WT) and p53-knockout (KO) mice. Mice exposed to 300 ppm benzene for 6 h d^{-1}, 5 d wk^{-1}, for almost 2 weeks and killed on day 12.[a)]

Gene name or name of protein encoded by the gene	*Fold change* WT	KO	*Accession number*
Aldehyde dehydrogenase 4	1.07	2.44	U14390
Apoptotic protease activating factor 1 (Apaf-1)	1.16	1.75	AF064071
Bax-alpha	1.20	1.21	L22472
Bcl-2 alpha	0.91	1.66	L31532
Calcyclin	1.08	1.89	X66449
Caspase-9	0.83	1.59	AB019600
Caspase-9S	0.84	2.26	AB019601
Caspase-11	2.49	1.22	Y13089
Caspase-12	0.86	0.18	Y13090
c-fos	1.57	0.94	V00727
Cyclin B1	0.85	1.48	X64713
Cyclin D1[b)]	0.44	(–)	M64403
Cyclin D3	0.83	1.20	M86186
cyclin G1	1.67	1.32	L49507
CYP2E1	2.13	1.72	X01026
Cyclin D-interacting myb-like protein (Dmp1)	2.01	2.81	U70017
Elongation factor 1[b)]	3.12	(–)	AF304351
Gadd 45[b)]	1.63	(–)	U00937
Glyceraldehyde-3-phosphate dehydrogenase	1.06	3.34	M32599
G protein-coupled receptor (GPCR/EB11)	0.01	0.97	L31580
JNK2	1.07	1.82	AB005664
KSR1, protein kinase related to Raf protein kinase	1.11	2.57	U43585
Lactate dehydrogenase 1 (LDH1)	1.13	2.34	AW123952
Lactate dehydrogenase 2 (LDH2)	0.97	1.72	X51905
Metallothionein 1	4.89	0.93	V00835
Metaxin2	0.95	1.55	AF053550
mLimk1, *Mus musculus* protein kinase	2.67	1.18	X86569
Mph1/Rae 28, polycomb binding protein	4.97	0.06	U63386
Myeloperoxidase (MPO)	1.68	1.49	X15378
p21[b)]	1.37	(–)	U09507
p53, variant mRNA	1.03	0.13	U59758
p58, protein kinase inhibitor (PKI)	1.55	0.81	U28423
PERK, ER resident kinase	0.81	1.63	AF076681
PI3K catalytic subunit p110 delta	2.36	0.18	U86587
RAB17, member of RAS oncogene family	2.42	1.53	X70804
Rad50	1.23	0.40	U66887
Rad51	0.72	0.08	AV311591
Rad54[b)]	1.50	(–)	AV311591
Siva, pro-apoptotic protein	0.88	1.62	AF033115
Smad6	1.36	1.92	AF010133
Serum inducible kinase (SNK)	1.68	1.02	M96163
Superoxide dismutase, Cu/Zn	1.19	1.63	M35725
Topoisomerase III[b)]	1.90	(–)	AB006074
Tuberous sclerosis 2 (Tsc-2)	2.00	1.25	U37775

Tab. 24.3 (continued)

Gene name or name of protein encoded by the gene	*Fold change*		*Accession number*
	WT	*KO*	
Wee-1 [b)]	1.95	(–)	D30743
Wig-1, p53-inducible zinc finger protein	1.83	0.07	AF012923
WISP1	0.68	1.26	AF100777
WISP2	0.83	8.32	AF100778
Wnt-1/INT-1	1.72	1.23	M11943

a) The studies involved two to four animals and the data were obtained by using Affymetrix gene chips. Mice were killed on day 12 immediately after benzene exposure.
b) No data available for p53 KO mice.

major selected genes whose expression showed p53-dependent benzene-induced decrease or increase (gene for G protein-coupled receptor 1), or in which gene expression was abolished in p53 KO mice. Cyclin genes, such as *cyclin B1* and *cyclin D3*, were generally activated in p53 KO mice by benzene exposure; in contrast, cell-cycle suppressor genes, including the G2–M cycle checkpoint gene, *p58* [68], were up-regulated in WT mice. These findings are compatible with the idea that the hematopoietic cell cycle continues in p53 KO mice even during benzene exposure, whereas it is arrested due to alterations in the expression of cell-cycle checkpoint genes, particularly the p53 gene, in WT mice. Such information may be very important for understanding yet-unknown toxicity mechanisms of chemicals. It is important to note here that such conclusions may be drawn by carefully and simultaneously screening different expression patterns of many genes having interrelated functions, even genes that show only small changes in expression level (about 1.5 to 2 fold). Investigation of the expression of a limited number of genes generally may not provide an insight into the main mechanism of action of chemicals or clues about the particular role of each of the investigated genes involved in the mechanism. Toxicogenomics may have a strong advantage from that point of view, as is also well described in the literature [7].

Ivanova et al. listed 17 genes including three EST genes in the cell cycle regulators among the genes profiled as stemness indicators [35]. Among them, 12 genes were confirmed in the list of genes expressed in the steady-state bone marrow of our present study. The expression levels of these 12 genes were all nearly comparable to that of beta actins; that is, comparable to the percent of the 'stem cell' concentration.

Two cell cycle regulator genes, *Wee 1* (D30743; one of the 17 mentioned above [35]) and *Mph1/Rae28/Edr1* (U63386; a member of polycomb, classified as one of the chromatin regulator genes in the stemness profile [35]), were significantly expressed after benzene exposure and were identified as possible candidates of marker genes for benzene exposure. Whether these possible marker genes for benzene exposure represent a change in an expression profile of stemness or are genes expressed in new, reacting progenitor cells after benzene exposure is not known; however, a possible role of these two genes as marker genes for benzene exposure is of much interest.

24.5.4
Apoptosis-related Genes in p53 KO and WT Mice

The microarray analysis results of p53 KO mice reminded us of the important role of the p53 gene in the mechanism of action of benzene. The genes regulated by the p53 gene, including *p21* [64], *caspase 11* [69], *PIK3K* [70] and *cyclin G1* [71], were distinctly up-regulated in the benzene-exposed WT mice (Table 24.3). It is of great interest that *caspase 11* rather than *caspase 9* was highly expressed after benzene exposure, suggesting that the p53-mediated activation of *caspase 11* is an important signalling pathway for apoptosis of bone marrow cells triggered by benzene exposure. This novel observation associated with the benzene toxicity mechanism, together with down-modulation of *caspase 12*, was similarly addressed in a study of the mechanism of chronic obstructive urinary disturbances, in which p53 KO and p53 WT mice were used [69]. On the other hand, the up-regulation and down-modulation of genes associated with oxidative stress was shown in p53 KO mice, which suggests that benzene may have produced oxidative stress in these mice (Table 24.3) [65]. It is not clear why oxidative-stress–associated genes are activated in p53 KO mice but not in WT mice; this may reflect deregulation of the redox cycle due to the absence of the p53 gene and the consecutive counteractivation of antioxidant enzymes [72]. The genes encoding apoptotic protease activating factor 1 (*Apaf-1*) and metaxin and the *Siva* gene were also up-regulated in the benzene-exposed p53 KO mice [65]. The expression of these genes may suggest that pro-apoptotic conditions are induced by benzene exposure of p53 KO mice. It was, however, found that survival or anti-apoptosis genes such as *bcl-2*, *caspase 9S* (an endogenous dominant-negative form of *caspase-9* [73]), and *Smad6* (an antagonist of the TGF-beta signalling [74]) gene, were also activated in p53-KO mice (Table 24.3) [65]. The up-regulation of the gene for PERK (ER transmembrane protein kinase) in p53 KO mice [65] indicates a triggering of the unfolded protein response (UPR) signalling pathway, resulting in a loss of *cyclin D1* [75] (which was statistically less confident in the present data).

24.5.5
DNA-repair–related Genes in the p53 Gene Network

Despite the possible DNA damage in bone marrow cells from p53 KO mice, the DNA repair system is not likely to be functioning efficiently in these mice, since DNA repair genes that were actively functioning in the WT mice exposed to benzene were not activated but rather suppressed in the p53 KO mice [65]. In association with cell proliferation and apoptosis, high expression levels of the *tuberous sclerosis* gene (*Tsc-2*), a tumour-suppressor gene encoding tuberin, and the gene encoding metallothionein 1 were noted in the WT mice (Table 24.3), raising the possibility that these genes are regulated by p53. The association of metallothionein with p53 transcriptional activity was recently postulated after study of an *in vitro* system in which metallothionein acts as a potent chelator to remove zinc from p53, thereby modulating p53 transcriptional activity [76]. The *Tsc-2* gene was recently reported to regulate the insulin signalling pathway mediated by AKT/PKB for cell growth [77, 78]. It is noteworthy that *Tsc-2* is a target gene of 2,3,5-tris(glutathione-*S*-y) hydroquinone, a metabolite of hydroquinone for renal cell transformation [79]. The high expression level of the *mph1* (rae28) gene in the WT mice (Table 24.3) [65] along with severe depression of bone marrow cells was interesting in association with the sustained activity of hematopoietic stem cells [80]. Furthermore, the *Wnt-1* signalling pathway was also likely to be activated by benzene exposure. Aberrant expression of downstream genes such as *WISP1* and *WISP2* did not occur in the WT mice, but such expression was evident in the p53 KO [65]. Since the Wnt-1 signalling pathway is reported to regulate the proliferation and survival of various types of stem cells, including B-lymphocytes [81], the activation of both the *mph1* and *Wnt-1* genes may be associated with the rapid recovery of suppressed bone marrow cellularity after termination of benzene exposure. Some upstream genes encoding p53, such as those encoding cyclin D-interacting myb-like protein (*Dmp1*) and *KSR1* (protein kinase related to *Raf*) in the p53 KO mice, compared with those of the corresponding experimental group of WT mice, were up-regulated to a similar extent or even strongly enhanced in their expression (Table 24.3) [65]. This is another indication of the role of the p53-mediated pathway in the mechanism of action of benzene associated with cell cycle regulation.

Finally, by analyzing gene expression profiles, one can elucidate the mechanisms underlying benzene hematotoxicity. The next step is to further analyze the fractionated stem cell compartment and compare the results with those reported by Ivanova et al. [35]. For example, *CYP2E1* is known to be constitutively expressed in the WT mice [62], which was confirmed in the present investigation (Table 24.3). Interestingly, *CYP2E1* gene expression is in the list of Ivanova et al. [35]. Since the list was established by subtraction of the expression of cells other than stem cells from the expression in stem cell compartment, the expression of the *CYP2E1* gene targeted by benzene toxicity is assumed to be an exact reflection of benzene-induced stemness toxicity.

24.6 Summary

Molecular biology has enabled the elucidation of biological subjects by two strategies, namely, inductive and deductive approaches. The progress in the mouse whole-genome sequencing project has enabled the elucidation of bilateral interrelationships between toxicological phenotypes related to particular toxicants and expression profiles of pertinent genes induced by exposure to toxicants [7]. Since all the phenotypes observed through various traditional toxicological tests should be eventually linked to gene expression profiles, translation between phenotypes and gene expression profiles provides a promising tool for predictive toxicology, despite some phenotypes being expressed due to various nongenomic signal transductions. In fact, many gene expression trials have been performed to provide adequate molecular biological information on the underlying mechanism of such phenotypes. In this chapter, hematotoxic gene expression profiles after a single dose of 300 cGy irradiation or repeated inhalation of 300 ppm benzene for 6 h a day, 5 days a week, for 2 weeks were introduced as an inductive approach of toxicogenomics. Then, a couple of plausible genes were selected with respect to the 'stemness profile' and discussed as a deductive approach for possible hematotoxicological applications of toxicogenomics. We did not incorporate data on clinical diagnosis, responsiveness to treatment, nor prognosis in this chapter, but considerable predictability has been shown in such trials elsewhere [83, 84].

Two major unresolved questions that we may have to pay specific attention to at this time are how one can define a specific mechanistic interpretation of the expression profiles for each discontinuous independent parameter; and how one can define a possible predictability of gene expression profiles (for carcinogenicity, for example) not only for the chemical group for which data were compiled during establishment of a database, but also for a group for which data were not incorporated into the database, that is, unknown chemicals. These unknown subjects should be given focus in future trials in toxicogenomics.

Finally, we have to note that the application of toxicogenomics to hematotoxicology should eventually focus on changes in the expression profiles of the hematopoietic stem cell/progenitor compartment, although the presented case study did not fully focus on this issue. In the WT mice, up-regulation of the *p53* gene did not appear in two weeks after intermittent benzene exposure, but was weakly detected a month after 300 cGy irradiation. Up-regulation of *cyclin G1*, downstream of *p53*, was observed after both benzene inhalation and 300 cGy irradiation, implying that the up-regulation of *cyclin G1* may be a relevant reflection of prolonged DNA damage.

When benzene was administered, down-regulation of *caspase 12* and up-regulation of *cyclin B1* was seen only when *p53* was knocked out (these gene changes may be hidden by *p53* gene regulation in WT mice) [65]. Participation of the same gene repertoire as in benzene exposure is observed even in the WT mice one month after 300-cGy irradiation, suggesting that the result may reflect a possible *p53* dysfunction in these irradiated mice.

For the future, more precise comparison between common gene expressions in the expression profiles in hematopoietic stem/progenitor cells after radiation exposure and benzene inhalation and the expression of genes on the stemness list compiled by Ivanova et al. [35] may lead to a clearer understanding of a possible marker repertoire of stem/progenitor cells for general hematotoxicological responses.

Acknowledgements

The article is dedicated to the late Dr. Eugene P. Cronkite. Financial support was received from the Japan Health Sciences Foundation (Research on Health Sciences focusing on Drug Innovation, KH31034) and the fund from Nuclear Research of the MEXT, Japan.

References

1 M. Schena, D. Shalon, R. W. Davis, P. O. Brown. *Science* **1995**, *270*, 467–470.

2 M. Schena, D. Shalon, R. Heller, A. Chai, P. O. Brown, R. W. Davis. *Proc Natl Acad Sci USA* **1996**, *93*, 10614–10619.

3 S. P. Fodor, R. P. Rava, X. C. Huang, A. C. Pease, C. P. Holmes, C. L. Adams. *Nature* **1993**, *364*, 555–556.

4 J. C. Venter, M. D. Adams, E. W. Myers, P. W. Li, R. J. Mural, G. G. Sutton, H. O. Smith, M. Yandell, C. A. Evans, R. A. Holt, J. D. Gocayne, P. Amanatides, R. M. Ballew, D. H. Huson, J. R. Wortman, Q. Zhang, C. D. Kodira, X. H. Zheng, L. Chen, M. Skupski, G. Subramanian, P. D. Thomas, J. Zhang, G. L. Gabor Miklos, C. Nelson, S. Broder, A. G. Clark, J. Nadeau, V. A. McKusick, N. Zinder, A. J. Levine, R. J. Roberts, M. Simon, C. Slayman, M. Hunkapiller, R. Bolanos, A. Delcher, I. Dew, D. Fasulo, M. Flanigan, L. Florea, A. Halpern, S. Hannenhalli, S. Kravitz, S. Levy, C. Mobarry, K. Reinert, K. Remington, J. Abu-Threideh, E. Beasley, K. Biddick, V. Bonazzi, R. Brandon, M. Cargill, I. Chandramouliswaran, R. Charlab, K. Chaturvedi, Z. Deng, V. Di Francesco, P. Dunn, K. Eilbeck, C. Evangelista, A. E. Gabrielian, W. Gan, W. Ge, F. Gong, Z. Gu, P. Guan, T. J. Heiman, M. E. Higgins, R. R. Ji, Z. Ke, K. A. Ketchum, Z. Lai, Y. Lei, Z. Li, J. Li, Y. Liang, X. Lin, F. Lu, G. V. Merkulov, N. Milshina, H. M. Moore, A. K. Naik, V. A. Narayan, B. Neelam, D. Nusskern, D. B. Rusch, S. Salzberg, W. Shao, B. Shue, J. Sun, Z. Wang, A. Wang, X. Wang, J. Wang, M. Wei, R. Wides, C. Xiao, C. Yan, A. Yao, J. Ye, M. Zhan, W. Zhang, H. Zhang, Q. Zhao, L. Zheng, F. Zhong, W. Zhong, S. Zhu, S. Zhao, D. Gilbert, S. Baumhueter, G. Spier, C. Carter, A. Cravchik, T. Woodage, F. Ali, H. An, A. Awe, D. Baldwin, H. Baden, M. Barnstead, I. Barrow, K. Beeson, D. Busam, A. Carver, A. Center, M. L. Cheng, L. Curry, S. Danaher, L. Davenport, R. Desilets, S. Dietz, K. Dodson, L. Doup, S. Ferriera, N. Garg, A. Gluecksmann, B. Hart, J. Haynes, C. Haynes, C. Heiner, S. Hladun, D. Hostin, J. Houck, T. Howland, C. Ibegwam, J. Johnson, F. Kalush, L. Kline, S. Koduru, A. Love, F. Mann, D. May, S. McCawley, T. McIntosh, I. McMullen, M. Moy, L. Moy, B. Murphy, K. Nelson, C. Pfannkoch, E. Pratts, V. Puri, H. Qureshi, M. Reardon, R. Rodriguez, Y. H. Rogers, D. Romblad, B. Ruhfel, R. Scott, C. Sitter, M. Smallwood, E. Stewart, R. Strong, E. Suh, R. Thomas, N. N. Tint, S. Tse, C. Vech, G. Wang, J. Wetter, S. Williams, M. Williams, S. Windsor, E. Winn-Deen, K. Wolfe, J. Zaveri, K. Zaveri, J. F. Abril, R. Guigo, M. J. Campbell, K. V. Sjolander, B. Karlak, A. Kejariwal, H. Mi, B. Lazareva, T. Hatton, A. Narechania, K. Diemer, A. Muruganujan, N. Guo, S. Sato, V. Bafna, S. Istrail, R. Lippert, R. Schwartz, B. Walenz, S. Yooseph, D. Allen, A. Basu, J. Baxendale, L. Blick, M. Caminha, J. Carnes-Stine, P. Caulk, Y. H. Chiang, M. Coyne, C. Dahlke, A. Mays, M. Dombroski, M. Donnelly, D. Ely, S. Esparham, C. Fosler, H. Gire, S. Glanowski, K. Glasser, A. Glodek, M. Gorokhov, K. Graham, B. Gropman, M. Harris, J. Heil, S. Henderson, J. Hoover, D. Jennings, C. Jordan, J. Jordan, J. Kasha, L. Kagan, C. Kraft, A. Levitsky, M. Lewis, X. Liu, J. Lopez, D. Ma, W. Majoros, J. McDaniel, S. Murphy, M. Newman, T. Nguyen, N. Nguyen, M. Nodell, S. Pan, J. Peck, M. Peterson, W. Rowe, R. Sanders, J. Scott, M. Simpson, T. Smith, A. Sprague, T. Stockwell, R. Turner, E. Venter, M. Wang, M. Wen, D. Wu, M. Wu, A. Xia, A. Zandieh, X. Zhu. *Science* **2001**, *291*, 1304–1351.

5 R. H. Waterston, K. Lindblad-Toh, E. Birney, J. Rogers, J. F. Abril, P. Agarwal, R. Agarwala, R. Ainscough, M. Alexandersson, P. An,

S. E. Antonarakis, J. Attwood, R. Baertsch, J. Bailey, K. Barlow, S. Beck, E. Berry, B. Birren, T. Bloom, P. Bork, M. Botcherby, N. Bray, M. R. Brent, D. G. Brown, S. D. Brown, C. Bult, J. Burton, J. Butler, R. D. Campbell, P. Carninci, S. Cawley, F. Chiaromonte, A. T. Chinwalla, D. M. Church, M. Clamp, C. Clee, F. S. Collins, L. L. Cook, R. R. Copley, A. Coulson, O. Couronne, J. Cuff, V. Curwen, T. Cutts, M. Daly, R. David, J. Davies, K. D. Delehaunty, J. Deri, E. T. Dermitzakis, C. Dewey, N. J. Dickens, M. Diekhans, S. Dodge, I. Dubchak, D. M. Dunn, S. R. Eddy, L. Elnitski, R. D. Emes, P. Eswara, E. Eyras, A. Felsenfeld, G. A. Fewell, P. Flicek, K. Foley, W. N. Frankel, L. A. Fulton, R. S. Fulton, T. S. Furey, D. Gage, R. A. Gibbs, G. Glusman, S. Gnerre, N. Goldman, L. Goodstadt, D. Grafham, T. A. Graves, E. D. Green, S. Gregory, R. Guigo, M. Guyer, R. C. Hardison, D. Haussler, Y. Hayashizaki, L. W. Hillier, A. Hinrichs, W. Hlavina, T. Holzer, F. Hsu, A. Hua, T. Hubbard, A. Hunt, I. Jackson, D. B. Jaffe, L. S. Johnson, M. Jones, T. A. Jones, A. Joy, M. Kamal, E. K. Karlsson, D. Karolchik, A. Kasprzyk, J. Kawai, E. Keibler, C. Kells, W. J. Kent, A. Kirby, D. L. Kolbe, I. Korf, R. S. Kucherlapati, E. J. Kulbokas, D. Kulp, T. Landers, J. P. Leger, S. Leonard, I. Letunic, R. Levine, J. Li, M. Li, C. Lloyd, S. Lucas, B. Ma, D. R. Maglott, E. R. Mardis, L. Matthews, E. Mauceli, J. H. Mayer, M. McCarthy, W. R. McCombie, S. McLaren, K. McLay, J. D. McPherson, J. Meldrim, B. Meredith, J. P. Mesirov, W. Miller, T. L. Miner, E. Mongin, K. T. Montgomery, M. Morgan, R. Mott, J. C. Mullikin, D. M. Muzny, W. E. Nash, J. O. Nelson, M. N. Nhan, R. Nicol, Z. Ning, C. Nusbaum, M. J. O'Connor, Y. Okazaki, K. Oliver, E. Overton-Larty, L. Pachter, G. Parra, K. H. Pepin, J. Peterson, P. Pevzner, R. Plumb, C. S. Pohl, A. Poliakov, T. C. Ponce, C. P. Ponting, S. Potter, M. Quail, A. Reymond, B. A. Roe, K. M. Roskin, E. M. Rubin, A. G. Rust, R. Santos, V. Sapojnikov, B. Schultz, J. Schultz, M. S. Schwartz, S. Schwartz, C. Scott, S. Seaman, S. Searle, T. Sharpe, A. Sheridan, R. Shownkeen, S. Sims, J. B. Singer, G. Slater, A. Smit, D. R. Smith, B. Spencer, A. Stabenau, N. Stange-Thomann, C. Sugnet, M. Suyama, G. Tesler, J. Thompson, D. Torrents, E. Trevaskis, J. Tromp, C. Ucla, A. Ureta-Vidal, J. P. Vinson, A. C. Von Niederhausern, C. M. Wade, M. Wall, R. J. Weber, R. B. Weiss, M. C. Wendl, A. P. West, K. Wetterstrand, R. Wheeler, S. Whelan, J. Wierzbowski, D. Willey, S. Williams, R. K. Wilson, E. Winter, K. C. Worley, D. Wyman, S. Yang, S. P. Yang, E. M. Zdobnov, M. C. Zody, E. S. Lander. *Nature* **2002**, *420*, 520–562.

6 T. Inoue, W. D. Pennie. (Eds.), *Toxicogenomics*, Springer-Verlag, Tokyo, **2003**.

7 T. Inoue, Introduction, toxicogenomics: a new paradigm of toxicology, in *Toxicogenomics*, T. Inoue, W. D. Pennie (Eds.), Springer-Verlag Tokyo, **2003**.

8 L. O. Jacobson, E. K. Marks, E. O. Gaston, M. J. Robson, R. E. Zirkle. *Proc Soc Exp Biol Med* **1949**, *70*, 740–742.

9 L. O. Jacobson, E. L. Simmons, W. F. Bethard, E. K. Marks, M. J. Robson. *Proc Soc Exp Biol Med* **1950**, *73*, 455–459.

10 L. O. Jacobson, E. L. Simmons, E. K. Marks, M. J. Robson, W. F. Bethard, E. O. Gaston. *J Lab Clin Med* **1950**, *35*, 746–770.

11 J. E. Till, E. A. McCulloch. *Radiat Res* **1961**, *14*, 213–222.

12 A. J. Becker, E. A. McCulloch, L. Siminovitch, J. E. Till. *Blood* **1965**, *26*, 296–308.

13 M. Osawa, K. Nakamura, N. Nishi, N. Takahasi, Y. Tokuomoto, H. Inoue, H. Nakauchi. *J Immunol* **1996**, *156*, 3207–3214.

14 B. I. Yoon, Y. Hirabayashi, Y. Kawasaki, Y. Kodama, T. Kaneko, D. Y. Kim, T. Inoue. *Exp Hematol* **2001**, *29*, 278–285.

15 B. I. Yoon, Y. Hirabayashi, Y. Kawasaki, Y. Kodama, T. Kaneko, J. Kanno, D. Y. Kim, Y. Fujii-Kuriyama, T. Inoue. *Toxicol Sci* **2002**, *70*, 150–156.

16 L. G. Lajtha, R. Schofield. *Adv Gerontol Res* **1971**, *3*, 131–146.

17 T. Nakahata, A. J. Gross, M. Ogawa. *J Cell Physiol* **1982**, *113*, 455–458.

18 T. Suda, J. Suda, M. Ogawa. *J Cell Physiol* **1983**, *117*, 308–318.

19 T. Shibagaki, T. Inoue, N. Kubota, M. Kanisawa. *Exp Hematol* **1986**, *14*, 794–797.

20 N. Goardon, A. Schuh, I. Hajar, X. Ma, H. Jouault, E. Dzierzak, P. H. Romeo, L. Maouche-Chretien. *Blood* **2002**, *100*, 491–500.

21 R. L. Phillips, R. E. Ernst, B. Brunk, N. Ivanova, M. A. Mahan, J. K. Deanehan, K. A. Moore, G. C. Overton, I. R. Lemischka. *Science* **2000**, *288*, 1635–1640.

22 I. Nishijima, T. Nakahata, S. Watanabe, K. Tsuji, I. Tanaka, Y. Hirabayashi, T. Inoue, K. Arai. *Blood* **1997**, *90*, 1031–1038.

23 Y. Hirabayashi, M. Matsuda, S. Aizawa, Y. Kodama, J. Kanno, T. Inoue. *Exp Biol Med (Maywood)* **2002**, *227*, 474–479.

24 C. P. Chiu, W. Dragowska, N. W. Kim, H. Vaziri, J. Yui, T. E. Thomas, C. B. Harley, P. M. Lansdorp. *Stem Cells* **1996**, *14*, 239–248.

25 R. C. Allsopp, S. Cheshier, I. L. Weissman. *J Exp Med* **2001**, *193*, 917–924.

26 S. J. Morrison, I. L. Weissman. *Immunity* **1994**, *1*, 661–673.

27 N. Hole. *Cells Tissues Organs* **1999**, *165*, 181–189.

28 D. I. Gottlieb, J. E. Huettner. *Cells Tissues Organs* **1999**, *165*, 165–172.

29 C. Dani. *Cells Tissues Organs* **1999**, *165*, 173–180.

30 B. E. Petersen, W. C. Bowen, K. D. Patrene, W. M. Mars, A. K. Sullivan, N. Murase, S. S. Boggs, J. S. Greenberger, J. P. Goff. *Science* **1999**, *284*, 1168–1170.

31 I. Hamaguchi, X. L. Huang, N. Takakura, J. Tada, Y. Yamaguchi, H. Kodama, T. Suda. *Blood* **1999**, *93*, 1549–1556.

32 G. C. Kopen, D. J. Prockop, D. G. Phinney. *Proc Natl Acad Sci USA* **1999**, *96*, 10711–10716.

33 A. Umezawa, T. Maruyama, K. Segawa, R. K. Shadduck, A. Waheed, J. Hata. *J Cell Physiol* **1992**, *151*, 197–205.

34 S. Makino, K. Fukuda, S. Miyoshi, F. Konishi, H. Kodama, J. Pan, M. Sano, T. Takahashi, S. Hori, H. Abe, J. Hata, A. Umezawa, S. Ogawa. *J Clin Invest* **1999**, *103*, 697–705.

35 N. B. Ivanova, J. T. Dimos, C. Schaniel, J. A. Hackney, K. A. Moore, I. R. Lemischka. *Science* **2002**, *298*, 601–604.

36 K. A. Moore, H. Ema, I. R. Lemischka. *Blood* **1997**, *89*, 4337–4347.

37 I. K. Park, Y. He, F. Lin, O. D. Laerum, Q. Tian, R. Bumgarner, C. A. Klug, K. Li, C. Kuhr, M. J. Doyle, T. Xie, M. Schummer, Y. Sun, A. Goldsmith, M. F. Clarke, I. L. Weissman, L. Hood, L. Li. *Blood* **2002**, *99*, 488–498.

38 X. Ma, T. Husain, H. Peng, S. Lin, O. Mironenko, N. Maun, S. Johnson, D. Tuck, N. Berliner, D. S. Krause, A. S. Perkins. *Blood* **2002**, *100*, 833–844.

39 M. A. Attia, J. P. Welsh, K. Laing, P. D. Butcher, F. M. Gibson, T. R. Rutherford. *Br J Haematol* **2003**, *122*, 498–505.

40 N. von Jagie, G. Schwarz, L. von Sievenrock. *Berl Klin Wchnschr* **1911**, *48*, 1220–1222.

41 M. Ichimaru, T. Ishimaru. *Radiation Effects Research Foundation* technical report draft document. Hiroshima, Japan, RERF publication. **1977**, February 2, 262–282.

42 E. A. McCulloch. *Blood* **1983**, *62*, 1–13.

43 K. Yoshida, K. Nemoto, M. Nishimura, I. Hayata, T. Inoue, M. Seki. *Int J Cell Cloning* **1986**, *4*, 91–102.

44 Y. Hirabayashi, T. Inoue, K. Yoshida, H. Sasaki, S. Kubo, M. Kanisawa, M. Seki. *Int J Cell Cloning* **1991**, *9*, 24–42.

45 E. P. Cronkite, V. P. Bond, A. L. Carsten, T. Inoue, M. E. Miller, J. E. Bullis. *Radiat Environ Biophys* **1987**, *26*, 103–114.

46 Y. Hirabayashi, M. Matsuda, T. Matumura, H. Mitsui, H. Sasaki, T. Tukada, S. Aizawa, K. Yoshida, T. Inoue. *Leukemia* **1997**, *11 Suppl 3*, 489–492.

47 K. Yoshida, S. Aizawa, K. Watanabe, Y. Hirabayashi, T. Inoue. *Leuk Res* **2002**, *26*, 1085–1092.

48 P. A. Lowry, K. M. Zsebo, D. H. Deacon, C. E. Eichman, P. J. Quesenberry. *Exp Hematol* **1991**, *19*, 994–996.

49 I. K. McNiece, I. Bertoncello, J. R. Keller, F. W. Ruscetti, C. A. Hartley, K. M. Zsebo. *Int J Cell Cloning* **1992**, *10*, 80–86.

50 H. Sasaki, M. Matsuda, Y. Lu, K. Ikuta, S. Matsuyama, Y. Hirabayashi, H. Mitsui, T. Matsumura, M. Muramatsu, T. Tsukada, S. Aizawa, T. Inoue. *Leukemia* **1997**, *11*, 239–244.

51 T. Inoue, Y. Hirabayashi, H. Sasaki, M. Matsuda, Y. Furuta, S. Aizawa. *Int J Pediatric Hematol/Oncol* **1997**, *4*, 221–230.

52 P. Delore, C. Borgomano. *J. de méd de Lyon* **1928**, *9*, 227–223.

53 C. A. Snyder, B. D. Goldstein, A. R. Sellakumar, I. Bromberg, S. Laskin, R. E. Albert. *Toxicol Appl Pharmacol* **1980**, *54*, 323–331.

54 E. P. Cronkite, J. Bullis, T. Inoue, R. T. Drew. *Toxicol Appl Pharmacol* **1984**, *75*, 358–361.

55 E. P. Cronkite, T. Inoue, A. L. Carsten, M. E. Miller, J. E. Bullis, R. T. Drew. *J Toxicol Environ Health* **1982**, *9*, 411–421.

56 Y. Hirabayashi, T. Matsumura, M. Matsuda, K. Kuramoto, K. Motoyoshi, K. Yoshida, H. Sasaki, T. Inoue. *Mech Ageing Dev* **1998**, *101*, 221–231.

57 S. Moeschlin, B. Speck. *Acta Haematol* **1967**, *38*, 104–111.

58 R. D. Irons, H. Heck, B. J. Moore, K. A. Muirhead. *Toxicol Appl Pharmacol* **1979**, *51*, 399–409.

59 G. M. Farris, S. N. Robinson, K. W. Gaido, B. A. Wong, V. A. Wong, W. P. Hahn, R. S. Shah. *Fundam Appl Toxicol* **1997**, *36*, 119–129.

60 Y. Kawasaki, Y. Hirabayashi, B. I. Yoon, Y. Huo, T. Kaneko, Y. Kurokawa, T. Inoue. *Jpn J Cancer Re.* **2001**, *92 Suppl*, 71.

61 J. E. French, G. D. Lacks, C. Trempus, J. K. Dunnick, J. Foley, J. Mahler, R. R. Tice, R. W. Tennant. *Carcinogenesis* **2001**, *22*, 99–106.

62 U. Bernauer, B. Vieth, R. Ellrich, B. Heinrich-Hirsch, G. R. Janig, U. Gundert-Remy. *Arch Toxicol* **1999**, *73*, 189–196.

63 D. G. Schattenberg, W. S. Stillman, J. J. Gruntmeir, K. M. Helm, R. D. Irons, D. Ross. *Mol Pharmacol* **1994**, *46*, 346–351.

64 S. E. Boley, V. A. Wong, J. E. French, L. Recio. *Toxicol Sci* **2002**, *66*, 209–215.

65 B. I. Yoon, G. X. Li, K. Kitada, Y. Kawasaki, K. Igarashi, Y. Kodama, T. Inoue, K. Kobayashi, J. Kanno, D. Y. Kim, Y. Hirabayashi. *Environ Health Perspect* **2003**, *111*, 1411–1420.

66 U. Bernauer, B. Vieth, R. Ellrich, B. Heinrich-Hirsch, G. R. Janig, U. Gundert-Remy. *Arch Toxicol* **2000**, *73*, 618–624.

67 L. N. Healy, L. J. Pluta, R. A. James, D. B. Janszen, D. Torous, J. E. French, L. Recio. *Mutagenesis* **2001**, *16*, 163–168.

68 S. Zhang, M. Cai, S. Xu, S. Chen, X. Chen, C. Chen, J. Gu. *J Biol Chem* **2002**, *277*, 35314–35322.

69 Y. J. Choi, L. Mendoza, S. J. Rha, D. Sheikh-Hamad, E. Baranowska-Daca, V. Nguyen, C. W. Smith, G. Nassar, W. N. Suki, L. D. Truong. *J Am Soc Nephrol* **2001**, *12*, 983–992.

70 B. Singh, P. G. Reddy, A. Goberdhan, C. Walsh, S. Dao, I. Ngai, T. C. Chou, O. C. P, A. J. Levine, P. H. Rao, A. Stoffel. *Genes Dev* **2002**, *16*, 984–993.

71 A. Shimizu, J. Nishida, Y. Ueoka, K. Kato, T. Hachiya, Y. Kuriaki, N. Wake. *Biochem Biophys Res Commun* **1998**, *242*, 529–533.

72 N. S. Chandel, M. G. Vander Heiden, C. B. Thompson, P. T. Schumacker. *Oncogene* **2000**, *19*, 3840–3848.

73 D. W. Seol, T. R. Billiar. *J Biol Chem.* **1999**, *274*, 2072–2076.

74 T. Imamura, M. Takase, A. Nishihara, E. Oeda, J. Hanai, M. Kawabata, K. Miyazono. *Nature* **1997**, *389*, 622–626.

75 J. W. Brewer, J. A. Diehl. *Proc Natl Acad Sci USA* **2000**, *97*, 12625–12630.

76 C. Meplan, M. J. Richard, P. Hainaut. *Oncogene* **2000**, *19*, 5227–5236.

77 X. Gao, D. Pan. *Genes Dev* **2001**, *15*, 1383–1392.

78 C. J. Potter, L. G. Pedraza, T. Xu. *Nat Cell Biol* **2002**, *4*, 658–665.

79 S. S. Lau, T. J. Monks, J. I. Everitt, E. Kleymenova, C. L. Walker. *Chem Res Toxicol* **2001**, *14*, 25–33.

80 H. Ohta, A. Sawada, J. Y. Kim, S. Tokimasa, S. Nishiguchi, R. K. Humphries, J. Hara, Y. Takihara. *J Exp Med* **2002**, *195*, 759–770.

81 T. Reya, M. O'Riordan, R. Okamura, E. Devaney, K. Willert, R. Nusse, R. Grosschedl. *Immunity* **2000**, *13*, 15–24.

82 T. Y. Ho, G. Witz. *Carcinogenesi* **1997**, *18*, 739–744.

83. A. Bhattacharjee, W. G. Richards, J. Staunton, C. Li, S. Monti, P. Vasa, C. Ladd, J. Beheshti, R. Bueno, M. Gillette, M. Loda, G. Weber, E. J. Mark, E. S. Lander, W. Wong, B. E. Johnson, T. R. Golub, D. J. Sugarbaker, M. Meyerson. *Proc Natl Acad Sci USA* **2001**, *98*, 13790–13795.

84. S. Ramaswamy, K. N. Ross, E. S. Lander, T. R. Golub. *Nat Genet* **2003**, *33*, 49–54.

The National Toxicogenomic Program / Initiatives

Handbook of Toxicogenomics: Strategies and Applications. Edited by Jürgen Borlak

ISBN: 3-527-30342-1

25
The National Toxicogenomics Program

James K. Selkirk, Michael D. Waters and Raymond W. Tennant

25.1
Introduction: The National Center for Toxicogenomics

Since the industrial revolution mankind has produced huge numbers of new chemicals, industrial and consumer products, and materials. Many of these substances or their derivatives and degradation products have found their way into the air, soil, and water supply. Governments have long recognized the potential public health danger, and many state and federal programs have been put in place to study the public health effects of these substances and to develop procedures to eliminate these hazardous materials as well as to prevent their continued release into the environment.

As a result of numerous routes of environmental contamination, all individuals are continually exposed to hazardous agents, suggesting that there is a certain probability that each individual will suffer an adverse effect. This process has been conceptualized by environmental health researchers and expressed as a paradigm that describes the continuum between exposure and disease. In addition to environmental exposures derived from external sources, an individual's diet or chemical components specific to an individual's workplace, occupation, or lifestyle can contribute to an adverse effect via inhalation, oral intake, or dermal exposure. The concentration of hazardous compounds in the environment can also vary over time, so that an individual may receive a finite internal dose of a compound and the effect would be determined by the individual's relative susceptibility. Intrinsically biologically active agents may have a much higher probability of causing an adverse effect in one or more target tissues in the human body (i. e., liver, skin, intestine, lung, blood, bone), since they do not require metabolic activation. In fact, many environmental agents do require metabolic activation, which frequently occurs in the target tissues. In any event, the amount of a compound that actually reaches the target tissue is described as the biologically effective dose. The reality is that a compound can reach a target tissue at a significant concentration and still have no biological consequences if the compound is efficiently removed or detoxified by cellular defence systems before cellular damage occurs. However, if cellular damage occurs, the damage can have a biological effect that leads to sustained or permanent changes in biological structures or

Handbook of Toxicogenomics: Strategies and Applications. Edited by Jürgen Borlak

ISBN: 3-527-30342-1

functions. Often, when no treatment or intervention is introduced, disease may develop and progress in substantially exposed individuals.

The application of gene expression technology to understanding the actions of chemicals and other environmental stressors on biological systems has been catalyzed by the rapid development of genome-based technology [1–3]. New molecular technologies, such as DNA microarray analysis and protein chips, can simultaneously measure the expression of hundreds to thousands of genes and proteins, providing the potential to accelerate discovery of toxicant pathways and specific chemical and drug targets. The power and potential of these new toxicogenomics methods are capable of revolutionizing the field of toxicology. In recognition of this fact, the National Institute of Environmental Health Sciences has created the National Center for Toxicogenomics (NCT) (http://www.niehs.nih.gov/nct/concept.htm), which has five major goals:

- to facilitate the application of gene and protein expression technology,
- to understand the relationship between environmental exposures and human disease susceptibility,
- to identify useful biomarkers of disease and exposure to toxic substances,
- to improve computational methods for understanding the biological consequences of exposure and responses to exposure,
- to create a public database of environmental effects of toxic substances in biological systems.

The NCT was formally established in September 2000 and is working to implement a strategy through which these goals can be achieved. The NCT and other organizations [4–6] are performing experiments to validate the concept of gene expression profiles as 'signatures' of toxicant classes, disease subtypes, or other biological endpoints. Initial studies indicate that classes of toxicants and toxic responses can be recognized as gene expression signatures by using microarray technology [7, 8]. Such experiments have begun to correlate gene expression profiles with other well defined parameters, including toxicant class, chemical structure, pathological or physiological response, and other validated indices of toxicity. For example, experiments have been designed to correlate gene expression patterns with liver pathologies such as necrosis, apoptosis, fibrosis, or inflammation. It is also possible to look for correlative patterns in surrogate tissues, such as blood. Changes in serum enzymes may provide diagnostic markers of organ function that are routinely used in medicine and in toxicology. Such 'phenotypic anchoring' of gene expression data using conventional indices will distinguish the toxicological signal from other gene expression changes that may be unrelated to toxicity, such as the adaptive, pharmacological, or therapeutic effects of a compound [9]. The capacity to array large numbers of individual gene fragments on small matrices that can be hybridized to mRNA or cDNA has made it possible to synchronously assess the variety of effects that specific chemicals can cause. These effects must be characterized in progressively greater depth for us to understand the biochemical and genetic complexity of the cells in which adverse effects are manifested. Thus, toxicology will progressively develop from predominantly individual chemical studies into a knowledge-based science in which experimental data from genomic, proteomic, and clinical data are compiled and in which new computational and informatics tools will play a significant role in deriving a new understanding of toxicant-related disease [9]. Such a knowledge base has been described [10]. Its development will require efforts at achieving a consensus on content and data-quality standards so that data from many sources can be reliably entered into the system.

25.2 Risk Assessment

The International Programme for Chemical Safety (IPCS) has produced [7] a generic Framework for Risk Assessment using many of the concepts presented in the April 1996 Proposed US Environmental Protection Agency (EPA) Cancer Risk Assessment Guidelines [4–6]. The ten elements of the framework are listed below:

- toxicological or disease endpoint,
- postulated mode of action,
- key events – measurable events related to the mode of action (biomarkers),
- dose–response relationship for the key events,
- temporal association/sequence of events,
- strength, consistency, and specificity of association of response with key events,
- biological plausibility and coherence,
- other modes of action,
- assessment of postulated mode of action,
- uncertainties, inconsistencies, and data gaps.

Collectively, these elements give an idea of how molecular studies of exposure and effect can be used in risk assessment.

The framework is applicable to all endpoints – to cancer as well as noncancer effects. It places major emphasis on understanding the mode of action of the agent in question. It assigns a central role to 'key events', such as molecular biomarkers and how they are related to the mode of action of the chemical. These key events should ideally display a dose–response relationship, as well as a temporal association of the key events with the disease of concern, and the sequence of events should be consistent with the hypothesized mode of action.

Clearly, this framework will require substantial basic and applied research to provide the information needed for risk assessment. It also provides a useful construct for our consideration of applications and impacts of toxicogenomics in human population studies, with subsequent impacts on human health and risk assessment. Using the results of human studies and animal data, risk assessors define the levels of environmental exposures that may lead to disease in a portion of the population. These decisions on potential health risks are frequently based on the use of default assumptions that reflect limitations in our scientific knowledge [8]. An important immediate goal of toxicogenomics, including proteomics, is to offer the possibility of making decisions affecting public health based on detailed toxicity, mechanism-of-action, and exposure data in which many of the uncertainties have been eliminated.

25.3 The NCT Strategy

An overarching strategy of the NCT is to identify and validate signatures of impending toxicological damage that can serve as biomarkers of effect. Current NCT research aims to formally discriminate between 'chemical signatures', reflecting early adaptive or pharmacological responses with no ensuing pathology, and 'effects signatures', which entail altered tissue steady state, toxicity, histopathology, or disease [26]. Collaborative research by scientists at the NCT Microarray Center (NMC) and Boehringer-Ingelheim Pharmaceuticals has shown that global gene expression profiles for chemicals from different mode-of-action classes can provide gene expression signatures of chemical exposures in male rats [7, 8]. These studies were performed on acutely exposed animals, and the expression patterns appear to be representative of the adaptive or pharmacologic activity of the chemicals. Using a small training set, Hamadeh et al. [8] were able to correctly ascertain chemical class signatures based on pattern recognition of genes induced acutely. The Toxicology/Pathology Group within the NCT has begun to conduct further proof-of-concept experiments designed to distinguish between the pharmacologic and toxicological effects of chemicals and to develop a learning set of responses that are linked to conventional phenotypic parameters of toxicity (i.e., hepatomegaly, hepatocellular necrosis, inflammation, etc.) [11]. These studies will take us one step closer to being able to address an issue that is of prime importance to the National Toxicology Program (NTP): the use of toxicogenomic approaches for understanding the biochemical processes associated with chronic chemical exposures. This is a particularly difficult problem but an important component of our strategy. To address this issue, it is important to determine whether or not serum/blood cells can be used as an alternative to specific target organ tissue, that is, can an informative subset of the pharmacologic and toxic parameters of acute chemical exposure seen in target tissues also be seen in blood. We are now testing this hypothesis, and if blood components can be used as a surrogate for tissue-specific chemical effects, this will open the door for comparative studies with exposed human populations. We are also in the process of developing learning sets of genomic profiling data for various classes of agents, with doses ranging from those that are pharmacologic to those that are toxic.

Key priorities for NCT intramural toxicogenomics studies are the profiling of specific compounds and disease processes that lead to target organ toxicities (e.g., hepato- and nephrotoxicity). These studies will entertain the following considerations, and emphasis will be placed on the early steps in the disease processes. Multiple compounds that elicit a particular hepato- or nephrotoxicity will be studied at multiple sampling times following exposure. Subtoxic as well as toxic doses will be used, and nontoxic isomers and related compounds will be included to assess the specificity of effects observed.

Drugs and chemicals will be selected for study based on criteria such as human exposure and recent toxicology studies demonstrating consistent cross-species effects. Ideally, a drug will show a therapeutic effect and chemicals will display mechanism(s) of toxicity that are prototypical for other agents, including those in our proof-of-concept studies. For example, acetaminophen (paracetamol) was the first agent to be studied comprehensively by the NCT. Its selection was based on an extensive literature [12] showing that liver toxicity is a common occurrence in rodents and in humans, its metabolism is similar in rodents and in humans, it displays both therapeutic and toxic effects, and there are opportunities for clinical investigation. Furthermore, it has been studied using toxicogenomic methods by several laboratories [13–16], offering the possibility of comparative assessment of observed molecular expression, toxicology, and pathology.

We also intend to perform comparative studies that address cross-species differences in toxicological responses as well as susceptibility differences in human subgroups. The combined and integrated data on gene/protein/metabolite changes collected in the context of dose, time, target tissue, and phenotypic severity across species will provide the interpretive information needed to define the molecular basis for chemical toxicity and to model the resulting toxicological and pathological outcomes [17]. It should then be feasible to search for evidence of exposure or injury prior to any clinical or pathological manifestation, facilitating identification of early biomarkers of exposure, toxic injury, or susceptibility. It is anticipated that toxicogenomics research will lead to the identification, measurement, and evaluation of biomarkers that are more accurate, quantitative, and specific.

Biomarkers recognized as important factors in a sequence of key events will help to define the way in which specific chemicals or environmental exposures cause disease. In other words, toxicogenomics should help to delineate the mode of action of various classes of agents and the unique attributes of certain species and population subgroups that make them more susceptible to toxicants as an important step in comparatively assessing potential human health risks [18].

Future NCT studies will define molecular perturbations caused by environmental chemicals in terms of phenotypic severity, dose, and time [19]. We are exploring quantitative or absolute gene expression profiling [20] and will consider combining such an approach with physiologically based pharmacokinetic (PB/PK) and pharmacodynamic modelling. PB/PK modelling can be used to derive a quantitative estimate of target tissue dose at any time after treatment, thus creating the possibility of anchoring molecular expression profiles in internal dose, as well as in time and phenotypic severity. Relationships among gene, protein, and metabolite expression may then be described as a function of the applied dose of an agent and the ensuing kinetic and dynamic dose–response behaviour in various tissue compartments. In addition, the species under study and interspecies and interindividual differences must be taken into account.

25.4 Toxicogenomics Broadly Defined

We define toxicogenomics as the study of the response of a genome to environmental stressors and toxicants. The response analysis combines perturbations of genetics, genome-scale mRNA expression (transcriptomics), cell and tissue-wide protein expression (proteomics), metabolite profiling (metabonomics), and bioinformatics with conventional toxicology in an effort to understand the role of gene–environment interactions in disease. Toxicogenomics seeks to identify and characterize mechanisms of action of known and suspected toxicants [21–32]. The analysis of gene expression patterns for different chemicals under different doses or times of exposure is used to gain a clearer understanding of genes that are mechanistically linked to a toxicological response. This process, including the development, perturbation, and reassessment of models that relate gene expression profiles to toxic outcomes, is referred to as systems toxicology [33, 34]. An important immediate goal of toxicogenomics is to offer the possibility of making decisions affecting public health based on detailed toxicity, mechanistic, and exposure data in which many of the uncertainties have been eliminated.

It will be important to determine how many and which genes should be required to characterize a toxic response and distinguish it from physiologically adaptive responses that are not linked to toxicity. The use of global gene expression data in hazard identification in the absence of a correct interpretation of the toxicological significance of the data would be unfortunate, since it might not implicate the correct genetic and biochemical pathways.

Using a combination of laboratory and field studies, comparison of chemicals from different mode-of-action classes (for example, cytotoxic chemicals, peroxisome proliferators, or estrogenic chemicals) will allow the identification of groups of genes whose expression at multiple doses and times is consistently linked to specific exposures and disease outcomes and will determine whether there are unique gene expression patterns for a given chemical toxicant.

The outcome of environmental exposures is clearly influenced by the function of many human genes, since all biochemical pathways are connected to some degree, either spatially or chronologically. Not all of these genes or their functions are known at present, but there is a continuous stream of new gene knowledge strengthening the known pathways and filling in the missing steps along the important metabolic grid. However, many genes have been identified that are likely to be important factors in genetic susceptibility to environmentally induced disease. These genes tend to fall into the following categories: cell cycle control, DNA repair, regulation of cell division, cell signalling, cell structure, apoptosis, and metabolism. Several genes whose expression controls metabolic pathways are crucial determinants of the outcome of exposure. Often, a compound enters a biological system in an inert form that is metabolically converted into a reactive species that causes cellular damage. The converse is also true: some metabolic pathways destroy toxic compounds by changing their chemical structure, thereby reducing the toxicity and transforming them into more water-soluble forms that are easier to excrete. Genes related to cell cycle and cell division regulate the ability of a cell to proliferate, grow, and differentiate. Changes in the progression of a cell through the cell cycle can increase the cell's ability to survive stress; usually, a proliferating cell exposed to stress enhances its survival by delaying the cell cycle so that cellular damage can be repaired prior to cell division. Cell signalling and gene expression pathways have profound effects on all cellular functions, including cell proliferation and differentiation. Some exogenous agents can activate these pathways in aberrant and deleterious ways (i. e., agents that mimic a biological component), which can disrupt or alter normal cellular function. DNA repair genes influence the outcome of exposure to environmental agents that cause DNA damage. Individuals with higher or lower capacity for DNA repair have decreased or increased risk, respectively, of certain types of environmentally induced disease. Heavily damaged cells often die by a process known as programmed cell death or apoptosis. This process protects the organism by removing aberrant cells and damaged structures.

To obtain the most relevant data from gene expression studies with microarrays requires that experiments be performed at multiple doses and varied exposure durations to identify those genes clearly linked to a toxic response. To develop approaches that will maximize the likelihood of detecting true positives for human exposure and minimize false negatives, a substantial matrix of data on chemicals with known exposure–disease outcomes must be obtained. This will require evaluation of the gene expression profiles of chemicals not causing health effects as well as those known to cause disease and chemicals with varying potency for causing disease. When the database on known chemicals becomes comprehensive enough, the fingerprints of new chemicals with unknown toxic properties can be compared to well characterized gene expression profiles, allowing the new chemical to be provisionally placed into one or more mode-of-action classes. Then more directed studies can be undertaken to confirm or refute the predicted mode of action and toxic outcome for the new chemical.

As with any new science, experience must be gained in toxicogenomics before its promise can be fulfilled. This experience will necessitate the assembly of massive amounts of data from many known toxicants as learning sets before the system can become predictive. The difficulty is that each of the new technological approaches being applied in genome and proteome analysis can overwhelm the current information infrastructure. The challenge is not simply managing the flow of data that will be generated by these new approaches. New models will be needed to manipulate the data rapidly, and new analytic strategies will be required to interpret it.

25.5 The Chemical Effects in Biological Systems (CEBS) Knowledge Base

The NCT is working to help the field of environmental health research evolve into a knowledge-based science in which experimental toxicogenomics and clinical data are compiled. The NCT, its university-based Toxicogenomics Research Consortium (http://www.niehs.nih.gov/nct/trc.htm), and resource contracts are engaged in the development, application, and standardization of the science upon which to build such a knowledge base, called Chemical Effects in Biological Systems (CEBS) (http://www.niehs.nih.gov/nct/cebs.htm). CEBS [34] will be created as a high-quality publicly accessible relational database that is compatible with standard laboratory output platforms. Database development will be integrated with strategic toxicogenomics experimental design and conduct. Standardized procedures, protocols, data formats, and assessment methods will be used to assure that data meet a uniform high level of quality. Raw datasets from NCT experiments will be available in their entirety. Relational and descriptive compendia will be included on toxicologically important genes, groups of genes, SNPs, and mutants and their functional phenotypes. Information about the biological effects of chemicals and other agents and their mechanism of action will be collected from the literature and stored. CEBS will be fully searchable by compound, structure, toxicity, pathology, gene, gene group, SNP, pathway, and network. Dictionaries and explanatory text will guide researchers in understanding toxicogenomics datasets. CEBS will be linked extensively to other databases and to Internet genomics and proteomics resources, providing users the suite of information and tools needed to fully interpret toxicogenomics data. Computational and informatics tools will play a significant role in improving our understanding of toxicant-related disease by creating a system of predictive toxicology.

25.6 Conclusions

Although genome-wide alterations in mRNA, proteins, or metabolites in tissue extracts may be useful in identifying signature gene changes, a critical step in verifying that the gene product(s) plays a role in a toxic process requires localization of the target genes and their products in specific cell types. This requires the use of in situ hybridization, immunohistochemistry, laser capture microdissection, and other techniques to identify the cells expressing the gene(s). Other techniques, such as Northern or Western blotting or real-time polymerase chain reaction, are used to verify the expressed genes or to selectively analyze their expression over time or dose parameters. It will also become more important to analyze expression in specific cell populations in order to profile the alterations in gene expression involved in chronic chemical exposure that lead to tumour development. The capability to focus on limited cell populations depends on cell-separation methods that will minimize the opportunity for cells to alter the patterns of genes expressed in situ. Methods that prolong the isolation and separation of target cells will induce adaptive responses in the cells that are not related to chemical exposure. This capability also depends on high-fidelity linear amplification of mRNA, the use of array platforms that require minimal amounts of cDNA, or proteomic methods that are highly sensitive.

At the present state of development of the field of toxicogenomics, the major advances in understanding toxic effects are largely made one chemical, agent, or mechanism at a time. However, the promise of this new technology is that it can be used to generate data on large numbers of chemicals under varying exposure conditions, thereby developing an unprecedented knowledge base that can be used to guide future research, improve environmental health, and aid in regulatory decisions. The development of the knowledge base will proceed incrementally and will require the collective efforts of many individuals and institutions to populate CEBS with data. However, as the database expands to include structurally or functionally related agents and as gene identity, functional genomics, and annotation progress, it will be possible to search in a comprehensive way for common, critical, or causal changes. It will become possible to create pathway maps of common cellular processes, and it will be possible to map partial genome arrays to pathways and to link such changes to known phenotypic markers of toxicity. The proposed databases and relational linkages must grow incrementally, and developers and users must have the patience and dedication to remain on course. Such incremental growth will eventually become exponential growth, and the field of toxicology will be profoundly changed. Given the vast numbers and diversity of drugs, chemicals, and environmental stressors, the diversity of species in which they act, the time and dose factors that are critical to the induction of beneficial and adverse effects, and the diversity of phenotypic consequences of exposures, it is only through the development of a rich knowledge base and its availability to the entire scientific community that toxicology and environmental health can rapidly advance. Concomitant with development of the data/knowledge base must be the evolution of informatics (computational and statistical) and data-mining tools (query algorithms, relational interfaces, etc.), and the training of individuals to apply them [35–38].

The NCT has committed itself to the national effort to develop the CEBS knowledge base as a long-range goal. The magnitude of the effort required to populate the databases that will comprise the knowledge base requires a collective will and collaborative efforts. We will continue to develop additional partnerships with scientists in academia, the private sector, and other governmental organizations to create a public knowledge base that will be a lasting resource for the scientific community. The efforts of the NCT can be followed at the NCT website [39].

References

1. R.J. Albertini: Biomarker responses in human populations: towards a worldwide map, Mutat Res 428 (1999) 217–226.
2. R.J. Albertini, J.A. Nicklas and J.P. O'Neill: Future research directions for evaluating human genetic and cancer risk from environmental exposures, Environ Health Perspect 104, Suppl 3 (1996) 503–510.
3. D.A. Bennett and M.D. Waters: Applying biomarker research, Environ Health Perspect 108 (2000) 907–910.
4. W.H. Farland: Cancer risk assessment: evolution of the process, Prev Med 25 (1996) 24–25.
5. V.L. Dellarco and J.A. Wiltse: US Environmental Protection Agency's revised guidelines for carcinogen risk assessment: incorporating mode of action data, Mutat Res 405 (1998) 273–277.
6. M. Andersen, D. Brusick, S. Cohen, Y. Dragan, C. Frederick, J.I. Goodman, G. Hard, B. Meek and E.J. O'Flaherty: U.S. Environmental Protection Agency's revised cancer guidelines for carcinogen risk assessment, Toxicol Appl Pharmacol 153 (1998) 133–136.
7. C. Sonich-Mullin, R. Fielder, J. Wiltse, K. Baetcke, J. Dempsey, P. Fenner-Crisp, D. Grant, M. Hartley, A. Knaap, D. Kroese, I. Mangelsdorf, E. Meek, J.M. Rice and M. Younes: IPCS conceptual framework for evaluating a mode of action for chemical carcinogenesis, Regul Toxicol Pharmacol 34 (2001) 146–152.
8. M.E. Andersen, M.E. Meek, G.A. Boorman, D.J. Brusick, S.M. Cohen, Y.P. Dragan, C.B. Frederick, J.I. Goodman, G.C. Hard, E.J. O'Flaherty and D.E. Robinson: Lessons

learned in applying the U.S. EPA proposed cancer guidelines to specific compounds, Toxicol Sci 53 (2000) 159–172.

9. P. Vos, R. Hogers, M. Bleeker, M. Reijans, T. van de Lee, M. Hornes, A. Frijters, J. Pot, J. Peleman, M. Kuiper et al.: AFLP: a new technique for DNA fingerprinting, Nucleic Acids Res 23 (1995) 4407–4414.

10. T. Money, S. Reader, L.J. Qu, R.P. Dunford and G. Moore: AFLP-based mRNA fingerprinting, Nucleic Acids Res 24 (1996) 2616–2617.

11. Y. Kiyozuka, H. Miyazaki, K. Yoshizawa, H. Senzaki, D. Yamamoto, K. Inoue, K. Bessho, Y. Okubo, K. Kusumoto and A. Tsubura: An autopsy case of malignant mesothelioma with osseous and cartilaginous differentiation: bone morphogenetic protein-2 in mesothelial cells and its tumor, Dig Dis Sci 44 (1999) 1626–1631.

12. D.C. Cross, J.P. Munoz, P. Hernandez and R.B. Maccioni: Nuclear and cytoplasmic tau proteins from human nonneuronal cells share common structural and functional features with brain tau, J Cell Biochem 78 (2000) 305–317.

13. C.G. Carlotti Jr., J.M. Drake, J.P. Hladky, I. Teshima, L.E. Becker and J.T. Rutka: Primary Ewing's sarcoma of the skull in children: utility of molecular diagnostics, surgery and adjuvant therapies, Pediatr Neurosurg 31 (1999) 307–315.

14. R. Leemans, B. Egger, T. Loop, L. Kammermeier, H. He, B. Hartmann, U. Certa, F. Hirth and H. Reichert: Quantitative transcript imaging in normal and heat-shocked *Drosophila* embryos by using high-density oligonucleotide arrays, Proc Natl Acad Sci USA 97 (2000) 12138–12143.

15. M.J. O'Sullivan, E.J. Perlman, J. Furman, P.A. Humphrey, L.P. Dehner and J.D. Pfeifer: Visceral primitive peripheral neuroectodermal tumors: a clinicopathologic and molecular study, Hum Pathol 32 (2001) 1109–1115.

16. D.K. Graham, L.C. Stork, Q. Wei, J.D. Ingram, F.M. Karrer, G.W. Mierau and M.A. Lovell: Molecular genetic analysis of a small bowel primitive neuroectodermal tumor, Pediatr Dev Pathol 5 (2002) 86–90.

17. M.C. Rissoan, T. Duhen, J.M. Bridon, N. Bendriss-Vermare, C. Peronne, B. de Saint Vis, F. Briere and E.E. Bates: Subtractive hybridization reveals the expression of immunoglobulin-like transcript 7, Eph-B1, granzyme B, and 3 novel transcripts in human plasmacytoid dendritic cells, Blood 100 (2002) 3295–3303.

18. A. Borchert, N.E. Savaskan and H. Kuhn: Regulation of expression of the phospholipid hydroperoxide/sperm nucleus glutathione peroxidase gene: tissue-specific expression pattern and identification of functional cis- and trans-regulatory elements, J Biol Chem 278 (2003) 2571–2580.

19. V.E. Velculescu, L. Zhang, B. Vogelstein and K.W. Kinzler: Serial analysis of gene expression, Science 270 (1995) 484–487.

20. S.L. Madden, E.A. Galella, J. Zhu, A.H. Bertelsen and G.A. Beaudry: SAGE transcript profiles for p53-dependent growth regulation, Oncogene 15 (1997) 1079–1085.

21. M.J. Aardema and J.T. MacGregor: Toxicology and genetic toxicology in the new era of 'toxicogenomics': impact of '-omics' technologies, Mutat Res 499 (2002) 13–25.

22. G.A. Boorman, S.P. Anderson, W.M. Casey, R.H. Brown, L.M. Crosby, K. Gottschalk, M. Easton, H. Ni and K.T. Morgan: Toxicogenomics, drug discovery, and the pathologist, Toxicol Pathol 30 (2002) 15–27.

23. H.K. Hamadeh, R.P. Amin, R.S. Paules and C.A. Afshari: An overview of toxicogenomics, Curr Issues Mol Biol 4 (2002) 45–56.

24. H.K. Hamadeh, P. Bushel, R. Paules and C.A. Afshari: Discovery in toxicology: mediation by gene expression array technology, J Biochem Mol Toxicol 15 (2001) 231–242.

25. Y. Hirabayashi and T. Inoue: [Toxicogenomics: a new paradigm of toxicology and birth of reverse toxicology], Kokuritsu Iyakuhin Shokuhin Eisei Kenkyusho Hokoku (2002) 39–52.

26. E.F. Nuwaysir, M. Bittner, J. Trent, J.C. Barrett and C.A. Afshari: Microarrays and toxicology: the advent of toxi-

cogenomics, Mol Carcinog 24 (1999) 153–159.

27. W.D. Pennie and I. Kimber: Toxicogenomics: transcript profiling and potential application to chemical allergy, Toxicol In Vitro 16 (2002) 319–326.

28. J.C. Rockett and D.J. Dix: Application of DNA arrays to toxicology, Environ Health Perspect 107 (1999) 681–685.

29. T. Storck, M.C. von Brevern, C.K. Behrens, J. Scheel and A. Bach: Transcriptomics in predictive toxicology, Curr Opin Drug Discov Dev 5 (2002) 90–97.

30. R.W. Tennant: The National Center for Toxicogenomics: using new technologies to inform mechanistic toxicology, Environ Health Perspect 110 (2002) A8–10.

31. R. Ulrich and S.H. Friend: Toxicogenomics and drug discovery: will new technologies help us produce better drugs?, Nat Rev Drug Discov 1 (2002) 84–88.

32. A.L. Castle, M.P. Carver and D.L. Mendrick: Toxicogenomics: a new revolution in drug safety, Drug Discov Today 7 (2002) 728–736.

33. T. Ideker, T. Galitski and L. Hood: A new approach to decoding life: systems biology, Annu Rev Genomics Hum Genet 2 (2001) 343–372.

34. M.D. Waters, G. Boorman, P. Bushel, M. Cunningham, R. Irwin, A. Merrick, K. Olden, R. Paules, J. Selkirk, S. Stasiewicz, B. Weis, B. Van Houten, N. Walker and R. Tennant: Systems toxicology and the chemical effects in biological systems knowledge base, Environ Health Perspect 111 (2003) 15–28.

35. M.B. Eisen, P.T. Spellman, D.B. Brown, D. Botstein: Cluster analysis and display of genome-wide expression patterns, Proc Natl Acad Sci USA 95: (1998) 14863–14868.

36. O. Ermolaeva, M. Rastogi, K.D. Pruitt, G.D. Schuler, M.L. Bittner, Y. Chen, R. Simon, P. Meltzer, J.M. Trent, M.S. Boguski: Data management and analysis for gene expression arrays, Nat Genet 20 (1998) 19–23.

37. P. Tamayo, D. Slonim, J. Mesirov, Q. Zhu, S. Kitareewn, E. Dmitrovsky, E. S. Lander, T.R. Golub: Interpreting patterns of gene expression with self-organizing maps: methods and application to hemapoetic differentiation, Proc Natl Acad Sci USA 96 (1999) 2907–2912.

38. J. Quackinbush: Computational analysis of microarray data. Nat Rev Genet 2 (2001) 418–427.

39. National Center for Toxicogenomics: http://www.niehs.nih.gov/nct/home.htm.

26
Toxicogenomics: Japanese Initiative

Tetsuro Urushidani and Taku Nagao

26.1
The Present State of Drug Development Genome Science

The human genome project, which started in 1990, was a great milestone in the history of science that revealed the entire genetic blueprint of the human being [1]. Simultaneously, it is said that it activated the economy of the U.S.A. and saved it from economic crisis. People outside the U.S.A. missed their chance to join the game earlier, when it was unrecognized that the gene itself would become a business opportunity. The Japanese government started its 'millennium plan' in 2000 to support and promote gene research, especially as related to five serious diseases – dementia, cancer, hypertension, diabetes, and allergy. However, it was somewhat too late.

In addition to support by the government, participation of private capital is indispensable for the development of scientific research. Although attention has only recently been directed to business based on genome science, presently, the movement of investors is slow and investment is not well focused. There was optimism at the beginning of the human genome project that development of remedies would immediately be possible when genomic information related to a certain disease was revealed. Today, however, everybody realizes that that was an illusion. However, every time a disease-related gene is identified or assigned, the news is always released with a comment that a medication for the disease will soon appear. This is a great misunderstanding. Even in the days when the human genome was barely sequenced, a large number of diseases caused by genes had already been identified. For example, in 1989 the causal gene of cystic fibrosis was found to be CFTR [2], and this fact in itself brought about no change in the therapy of this disease, and of course, cystic fibrosis is still incurable today. Similarly, it could be said that the analysis of familial Alzheimer's disease did not contribute to the clinical development of donepedil at all. However, it is not true that elucidation of the human genome contributes little to drug development. On the contrary, it is a powerful and efficient tool for producing a candidate compound in combination with high-throughput chemical synthesis and screening systems, once a target molecule is decided upon. This is why drug manufacturers around the world compete for the use of genome information. Will this strategy really accelerate drug discovery?

Handbook of Toxicogenomics: Strategies and Applications. Edited by Jürgen Borlak

ISBN: 3-527-30342-1

In the worldwide pharmaceutical market, as well as in Japan, the entry of new chemicals tends to be decreasing, in spite of the progress of technology in finding candidates for new drugs. Some reasons for this are that medical requirements have matured in certain fields and clinical trials are more difficult to perform, but the main reason appears to be discrepancies between preclinical and clinical results, which needs to be worked on. The possibility for a newly found chemical to be successfully developed as a medicine is quite low, even if it is perfectly aimed at its molecular target. According to the ex-president of GlaxoSmithKline, the success rate is lower than 1 in 10 000 [3]. Figure 26.1 displays the success rate of new chemical compounds as investigated by a committee of the Pharmaceutical Manufacturers Association in Japan [4], showing a very low success rate (63 out of 238) even for chemicals that were selected from among more than 400 000 candidates. If the number of chemical compounds that succeed as a medicine is proportional to the number of developed chemicals times a reasonable factor, a small number of large manufacturers with a huge scale of development should be able to monopolize the worldwide medical market. Even if the chance of success is too low to keep many projects going at once, there nevertheless is a chance for medium-scale companies, like those in Japan, to create a 'big' product. It is necessary for the pharmaceutical companies in Japan to figure out how they can successfully develop candidate chemicals into medicines so that they can survive in the 21st-century world market.

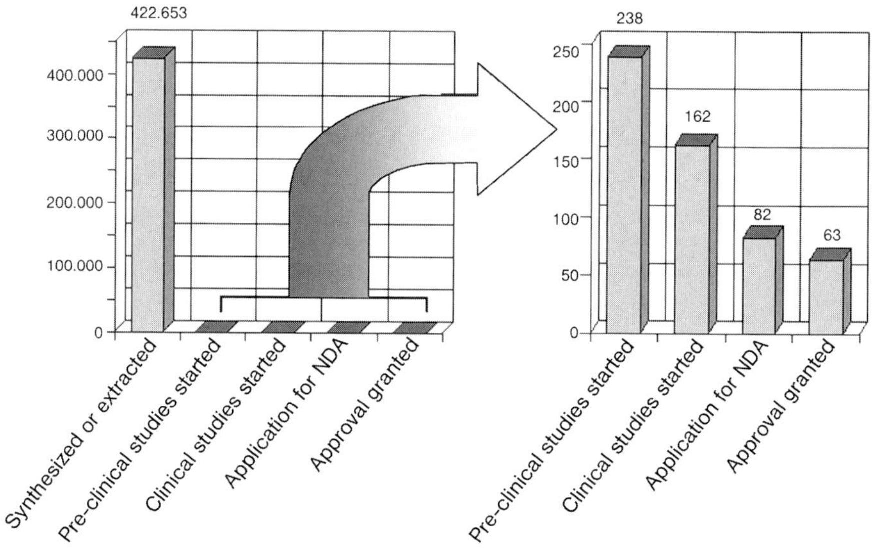

Fig. 26.1 Success rate of drug development in Japan (1996–2000). Data are taken from the report by the research and development working group of the Japan Pharmaceutical Manufacturers Association [4]. *Left panel:* Among 422 653 synthesized or extracted chemicals, fewer than 250 were examined in preclinical studies. *Right panel:* Expanded view of the last four bars in the left panel. Note that the success rate was 26.5% (63 out of 238), even for chemicals selected from the 422 653 starting chemicals and that the overall success rate was only 1 in 6709 or 0.015%.

26.2 The Necessity of Toxicogenomics

Many candidate drugs drop out in the stage of preclinical and clinical testing. A considerable proportion of the dropouts are related to toxicity (Figure 26.2), even in the statistics of 1997 [5]. Today, it is common sense that the appropriate molecular target to select is the human type. For example, in development of a drug acting on a 7-transmembrane receptor, cloned human-type receptor is used for screening. Previously, when preclinical screening was performed in laboratory animals, ineffectiveness due to species differences in the structure of the target molecule often emerged during clinical trials, but today, such an event does not happen. However, 'nonpredictable' deleterious effects or toxicity cannot be overcome by this strategy. In contrast to pharmacological effects, drug toxicity effectively happens in a black box and cannot be satisfactorily predicted in preclinical experiments. In some extreme cases, serious adverse effects emerge even after the drugs are widely distributed on the world market. A top priority should be the solution of this paradox, i. e., how to predict 'nonpredictable' toxicity. To do this, toxicogenomics is considered to be one of the most powerful strategies.

In classical toxicology, toxicity was mainly designated and assessed according to pathological changes observed in a certain organ as a result of a chemical administered in an excessive amount. In the clinical field, serious adverse effects in humans cannot be allowed, even they occur rarely. For this kind of situation, biostatistics, based on the incidence of a certain phenotype observed in limited numbers of animals that received a clinically meaningful dose, is useless because, to see reasonable numbers from toxic effects it is necessary to increase the animal dose to much higher than the clinical dose range. In preclinical tests, therefore, toxicologists have been obliged to extrapolate from data based on pathological changes observed in laboratory animals that received high, sometimes unreasonable, doses to the toxicity found with low incidence at the clinical dosage. There is, however, no assurance that these two phenomena are biologically related. The response of an or-

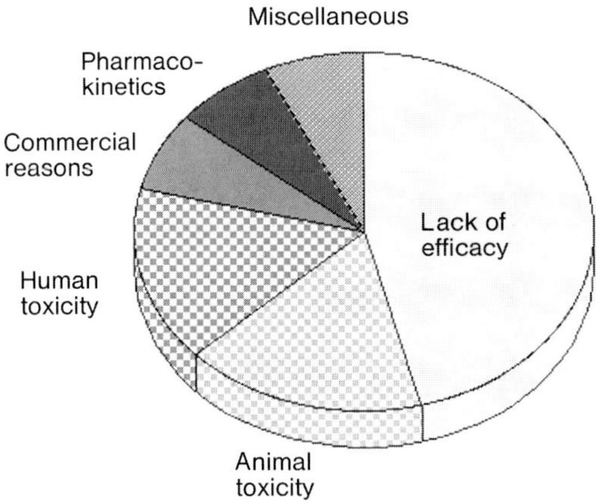

Fig. 26.2 Reasons for failure of 121 new chemicals in clinical development. Data published by the Center for Medicines Research were taken from the review by Kennedy [5]. Of 198 compounds, 77 anti-infective drugs were excluded since most of them were terminated because of unsatisfactory pharmacokinetics.

ganism to a toxicant at low dose that subsequently causes pathological changes in certain organs should be detectable as changes in gene expression, protein synthesis, metabolism, etc. Of these, the expression of genes, or the amount of mRNA, is the most sensitive measure and is one of the greatest advantages of the technology of genomics.

Although genomics, which comprehensively analyzes all the expressed genes, and proteomics, which comprehensively analyzes all the existing proteins, are powerful techniques, they have limitations. Especially when they are used for elucidating the causal factor(s) in a certain disease or for estimating the pharmacological effects of a certain drug, one often encounters a difficulty in extracting meaning from the enormous amount of information. In contrast, this 'omic' analysis is rather suitable to forecasting the 'unpredictable' response of a black box. For example, an 'omic' analysis of a certain disease starts with a comprehensive analysis, but the aim is to find biomarker(s) specific for the disease; in other words, the ideal goal is that the symptoms of the disease become explainable by one or a few changes in genes or proteins. On the other hand, it is theoretically unlikely that predicting the toxicity of various chemical substances can be based on a few biomarkers. Of course, one may expect that a small number of gene clusters that represent the property of a group with a common toxicological mechanism can be identified, and in fact, some successes have been reported [6]. However, needless to say, one should start with a comprehensive analysis, especially when predicting the toxicity of a new chemical entity.

26.3 Toxicogenomics Project 2002–2007

26.3.1 Planning Process and the Present Organization

As described in the previous section, the Japanese pharmaceutical industry and the Japanese government both recognized that predicting toxicity in the early stage of drug development is indispensable and that the construction of a database based on toxicogenomics technology and its use with bioinformatics technology seemed to be the most effective strategy. However, for the size of the drug manufacturing concerns in our country, the economic load was too heavy, in contrast with the huge enterprises in Europe and the U.S., which can construct their own databases. In this situation, the Ministry of Health, Labour and Welfare, the National Institute of Health Sciences (NIHS), and a working group of the Japan Pharmaceutical Manufacturers Association began to draft a research project in which both the government and private companies joined. Preliminary examination was carried out mainly in the Cellular and Molecular Toxicology Division, Biological Safety Research Center of the NIHS in 2000 to 2001 [7], and the project "Construction of a forecasting system for drug safety based on the toxicogenomics technique and related basic studies" for the five years from March 2002 to March 2007 was started. Half of the entire budget,

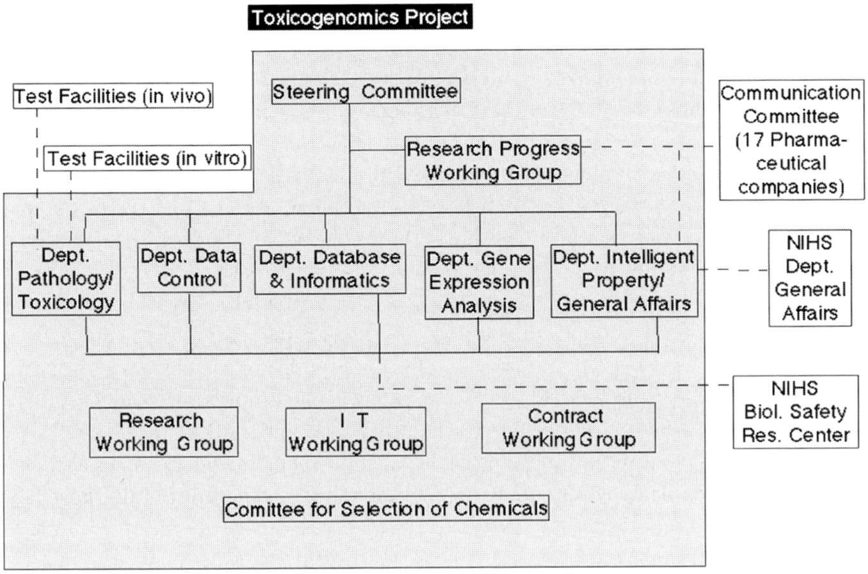

Fig. 26.3 Schematic map of the Toxicogenomics Project. The shadowed area is within the project.

about five billion yen, comes from the national budget, and the remaining half is contributed by the 17 companies that participated in the project within the Japan Pharmaceutical Manufacturers Association. Hitherto in Japan, cooperative research projects between national and private organizations have not been very active, especially in the field of pharmaceutical science. This project thus attracts attention from various quarters as a model case for the near future.

The schematic map of the project is shown in Figure 26.3. The project leader is the Director General of the NIHS, and researchers from the NIHS as well as those from the 17 drug companies participate in each department. The final goal of the project is to construct a large-scale toxicology database of chemicals and to develop a system for forecasting the toxicity of new chemicals. Due to the nature of this project, it is intended that distribution of the contents of the database and forecasting system will be limited to the project members until three years after the end of the project, and thereafter it will be opened to the public. Therefore, we would like to ask the readers' understanding that a detailed description of actual data is not possible in this paper.

26.3.2
Contents of the Project

To begin with, about 150 chemical compounds are selected, and the following are examined for each.

1) In-vivo tests using the rat
The species selected for analysis was the rat, which is very frequently used in preclinical examinations and for which much toxicological information has been accumulated. The facilities and experimental protocol coincide with the GLP. The test consists of a single-administration test (multiple time points with multiple dose levels) and a repeated-administration test (multiple length with various dose levels), and data on body weight, general symptoms, histopathological examination of liver and kidney, and blood biochemistry are obtained from each animal. Gene expression in liver and kidney is comprehensively analyzed.

2) In-vitro tests using rat hepatocytes
For rat liver primary cultured cells, comprehensive gene expression analysis is carried out at various time points after treatment with various concentrations of each of the 150 compounds.

3) In-vitro tests using human hepatocytes
Using human liver primary cultured cells, experiments equivalent to the above are carried out.

Before starting the project, preliminary examinations (especially for the acquisition of gene expression data with absolute values) were carried out in the Cellular and Molecular Toxicology Division, Biological Safety Research Center, NIHS. In the course of examination, various problems became evident when various microarray methods were compared. For comprehensive analysis of gene expression using a microarray, two commercial methods were evaluated, i. e., the Affymetrix system and the Stanford system. Although the Stanford system is excellent in view of the cost, the Affymetrix system is superior in specificity and quantification. It was felt that meaningful toxicological changes could not be detected by a simple semiquantitative comparison like the two-colour method, since the purpose is expression analysis in the organ that is damaged by a chemical substance. Furthermore, it is necessary to measure the absolute value of gene expression so as to evaluate the time course and dose–response to the chemicals.

With the Affymetrix system, some quantification of the expression level based on the total amount of mRNA in the sample is assured. However, when a damaged organ is compared with a normal one, the observed change in gene expression can be masked by various noise, such as a change in the total gene expression level. In this regard, the desired measure is the absolute content of mRNA per cell. Based on this requirement, a system that determines the gene expression quantity per cell was developed utilizing the spike included in the Affymetrix GeneChip (Kanno et al., submitted for publication). With this system, it became possible for virtually all genes on the GeneChip to be detected as a change or no change in the absolute contents. In the Toxicogenomics Project, this system has been adopted and the data are now being accumulated.

26.3.3
Advantage and Originality of the Project

A number of toxicogenomics projects with various scales and objectives, national or private, are now being performed worldwide. Here, the advantages and originality of our project are listed:

1) The project is specialized for drug development.
   The database constructed in this project is expected to estimate the possibility of potential side effects in the earliest stage of drug development, to enable selection of the candidate with the smallest risk in clinical trials. To achieve this purpose, the project employs a unique strategy. That is, the drug selection committee selects a "drug for which a clinical trial was terminated or whose marketing was ceased because human toxicity emerged, even though the potential for toxicity was undetected or neglected during preclinical tests", mainly from the 17 companies participating in the project. At present, selection is done with the aim of having a group of about 50 such drugs, which will be subjected to the tests described above.

2) Various types of high-quality data are linked to the gene expression database.
   It is sometimes seen in a gene expression database that some data are from different sources or some or all data lack related biochemical or histopathological information. Our project aims at the construction of a database with a perfect dataset. That is, the gene expression data from each individual animal is always linked to its biochemical data, pathological evaluation, images of the histopathology and their interpretation, chemical structure of administered drug, and relevant literature. The database includes not only the basis of the toxicity-forecasting system but also functions as a standard large-scale archive of hepato- and nephrotoxicity.

3) The database contains absolute values for gene expression levels.
   As described above, gene expression data accumulated in this project are in the form of absolute values per cell. Circadian variations in the expression of each gene can be detected in the solvent-control population, meaning that the drug effect becomes observable. Furthermore, this may enable us to analyze the pharmacological action, i.e., pharmacogenomics, by analyzing the gene expression pattern at lower doses, at which toxicity does not emerge, since most of the chemicals tested are intended as medicines.
   Although this database is unique, comparison with existing databases or with the usual nonquantitative analysis in the laboratory is also possible. According to this principle, it is easy to convert the absolute expression values into relative values, and thus qualitative comparison with other databases can be carried out.

4) Interspecies bridging is considered.
   Development of the system is aimed at the prediction of human toxicity. Since human experimenttation is impossible in any event, a laboratory animal must be used and subsequently the problem of species differences cannot be avoided. In this project, a full set of experiments, i.e., *in vivo* rat tests, tests on rat primary cul-

tured hepatocytes, and tests on human primary cultured hepatocytes will be completed for all chemical compounds with a controlled protocol. In this system, extrapolating from rat to human may be possible through comparing the gene expression profiles of the cultured cells. Of course, we realize that many problems remain, e.g., it may be possible that differences between *in vitro* and *in vivo* tests is stronger than the species differences. We are now optimistic concerning this issue and hope that data accumulation will allow other outcomes, such as identification of a specific group of genes that enables interpretation and bridging the species.

26.4 Future Perspectives and Conclusions

When this chapter was written, in the summer of 2003, the project had just started on animal experiments. At present, about 50 standard drugs with typical hepatic toxicities have been listed, and for some of them, including acetaminophen, carbon tetrachloride, and isoniazid, data acquisition has already been completed. Although practical evaluation of the project is a matter for the future, it should be useful to describe the future view based on the present situation.

As recent advances in the 'omics' technology are rapid, it sometimes happens that an expensive facility becomes out of date only half a year after its inauguration. This means that the quality and quantity of data are being vigorously improved, but it also means that standardization of methodology is never achieved. Especially in the field of toxicology, data validation between each facility is important. It would not be extreme to argue that integrating databases without methodological standardization is useless. The technique and strategy adopted by our project have significance in that they supply the platform for standardization of the toxicogenomics technology. In the present situation, there is still an objection as to whether this approach can be used in the field of regulation. However, once standardization is achieved, and the reliability and predictability of the data become superior to the toxicological index produced by the old approach, it should lead to large innovations in the regulatory scientific field.

At present, changes in the expression of various interesting genes are being found to participate in the toxic response. The problem facing us is that considerable numbers of such genes on a GeneChip are functionally unknown ESTs, and that, even for the known genes, their functions and functional partners are little understood. It might be possible to construct a forecasting system in ignorance of the physiological, pharmacological, or toxicological facts, but this does not seem promising. When the future of this technology is considered, it is important to bring the significance of gene expression changes into the system, by active collection of the ever-progressing information of the genome. In this connection, it is necessary to periodically update and improve the database during and after the project, to create a perfect database. It will be also fruitful to connect it with other types of databases, such as proteomics, metabonomics, etc., databases, creating a giant network of toxicology databases. In fact, another project of toxicogenomics has been just started with the initiative of the Cellular and Molecular Toxicology Division, Biological Safety Research Center, NIHS for the three years from 2003 to 2006. In this project, about 100 compounds, most of which are industrial and environmental chemicals, are to be tested for their effects on the gene expression profile of the mouse. The purpose of this project is also to create a database of chemical hazards based on absolute gene expression values per cell type. The greatest advantage of this project is that highly informative data for analyzing the mechanism of toxicity will be accumulated, since mouse genome information is nearly complete and various gene-modified mice are available. This would be a dream, but we hope that the integrated system will enable elucidation of the mechanisms of toxicity and prediction of human toxicity, in spite of species or individual differences, for any type of compound.

After this database and toxicity-prediction system are complete, it will be widely utilized in the basic technology of drug development. This will accelerate the early stages of preclinical trials by enabling wise choice of drug candidates and will subsequently decrease the rate of failure in clinical trials. This, we hope, will ultimately contribute to human welfare through the rapid supply of much safer and more useful drugs.

Acknowledgments

The project is supported in part by Health and Labour Sciences Research Grants, Research on Advanced Medical Technology in Japan.

References

1. Dennis, C., Gallagher, R. Campbell, P. Everyone's genome. Nature 2001, 409, 813.
2. Riordan J.R., Rommens J.M., Kerem B., Alon N., Rozmahel R., Grzelczak Z., Zielenski J., Lok S., Plavsic N., Chou J.L. Identification of the cystic fibrosis gene: cloning and characterization of complementary DNA. Science 1989, 245, 1066–1073.
3. Laurence, R.N. Sir Richard Sykes contemplates the future of the pharma industry. Drug Discovery Today 2002, 7, 645–648.
4. Japan Pharmaceutical Manufacturers Association (2002). Success Rate of Developing New Drugs. http://www.jpma.or.jp/12english/index09.html.
5. Kennedy, T. Managing the drug discovery/development interface. Drug Discovery Today 1997, 2, 436–444.
6. Kanno, J. Reverse toxicology as a future predictive toxicology. In: Inoue T. and Pennie, W.D. (Eds.) *Toxicogenomics*. Springer-Verlag, Berlin, Heidelberg, New York, 2003, 213–218.

Point of View from Regulatory Authorities

Handbook of Toxicogenomics: Strategies and Applications. Edited by Jürgen Borlak

ISBN: 3-527-30342-1

27
Toxicogenomics in Need of an ICH Guideline? Experiences from the Past

Frauke Meyer and Gerd Bode

27.1
Introduction

Toxicogenomics is defined as the "application of the knowledge of genes associated with disease states to study the toxicology of chemical and physical agents" [1]. The simultaneous determination of the expression of thousands of genes (transcriptomics) or proteins (proteomics) in a single experiment offers a great opportunity to revolutionize the drug development process but also poses the threat of serious misinterpretations. The positive options that these technologies offer for lead selection as well as for monitoring drug efficacy and safety in preclinical and clinical studies can best be developed within of a cooperative framework among regulators, industry, and academia. Such a framework could be crucially important for accelerating the process of data availability and final acceptance of these techniques as useful tools by the international scientific community.

All regulatory authorities of Europe, Japan, and the United States, as well as scientific experts from the pharmaceutical industry in these regions, support the International Conferences on Harmonization of Technical Requirements for the Registration of Pharmaceuticals for Human Use (ICH). The objectives of these conferences are:

- To discuss technical and scientific aspects and recommendations for pharmaceutical development and marketing authorisation.
- To reduce or obviate the need to duplicate preclinical or clinical studies carried out during the research and development of new medicines in different regions [2].
- To achieve a more economical use of human, animal, and material resources.
- To eliminate unnecessary delay in the global development and availability of new medicines for patients.
- To maintain quality, safety, and efficacy.
- To protect patients and public health.

At present, no recommendations from the ICH exist for the field of toxicogenomics, nor are there any regulatory requirements. Past experience with the ICH process

Handbook of Toxicogenomics: Strategies and Applications. Edited by Jürgen Borlak

ISBN: 3-527-30342-1

could offer an answer as to the benefits of technical recommendations for toxicogenomics in the light of present knowledge and the state of scientific development.

27.2
Application Options for Toxicogenomics

Functional or organ toxicity is often preceded by changes in gene expression. These changes can be far more sensitive and specific than organ toxicity and furthermore, are readily measurable endpoints. Additionally, the analyses require less time, money, animals, and resources than classical animal toxicity studies [3, 4].

Gene expression can help in the identification of substances with toxicological potential, the elucidation of their mechanisms of action, the definition of 'no-effect levels', and the identification of susceptible tissues and cell types. Additionally, the difficult extrapolation from one species to another might be facilitated [5]. Novel approaches integrate the expression analysis of thousands of genes with classical toxicological methods: effects at the molecular level are correlated with pathophysiological changes in the organism, enabling a detailed comparison of mechanisms and early detection and prediction of toxicity [6].

27.2.1
Comparative/Predictive Toxicogenomics

Although there is a limit to the number of cellular and organ manifestations of toxicity induced by pharmaceuticals or chemicals, the possible number of gene expression patterns for encoding these manifestations is enormous. Nonetheless, only about 2% of the human genome is involved in stress responses, representing a relatively small number of differentially expressed 'tox-genes' [7].

Comparative and predictive toxicogenomics tries to link specific patterns of gene expression (fingerprints) with toxicological reactions, which may include pathological changes [8, 9]. These fingerprints may play an important role in selecting and giving priority to compounds for more traditional stages of toxicity testing in industrial settings. They furthermore facilitate the monitoring of toxic responses at early exposure times before any pathomorphological manifestation of drug-induced toxicity occurs [3].

Predictive modelling can be seen as a multistage process of:

1. Data collection.
2. Model development (comparison and ranking of substance-related gene expression patterns).
3. Utility development (rigorous computation and data mining) [9].

Therefore, it will be necessary to categorize multiple classes of agents with well characterized toxicity profiles and related gene expression changes so as to represent the diversity of modes of actions of toxic agents. Establishing a solid database will be time-consuming and will require intense collaboration among toxicologists from industry, regulatory agencies, and academic institutions [10]. A harmonized consensus of the value and expressiveness of such data is desirable.

27.2.2
Mechanistic Studies (Mode of Action)

Many substances possess multiple mechanisms of actions, which depend on dose, time, and duration of exposure, as well as on the target cell phenotype. Besides the toxic effect of each individual mechanism, combinations of different mechanisms may cause cell injury as well as death [1, 6]. Microarray technology combines numerous experiments, pathways, and mechanisms at the same time [10], as toxicity generally is not only a result of changes in one or a few genes, but is often the final outcome of a cascade of gene interactions. Analysis of the cascade is not only time-saving but also leads to a better understanding of the sequence of events involving complex regulatory networks [3]. However, whether all cellular mechanisms can be identified at the mRNA level is unclear. Additionally, not all genes change their expression profile after exposure to a toxicant, as genes are subject to normal biological expression variability or repair mechanisms [11].

27.2.3
Risk Assessment

Risk assessment is a process by which scientific data pertaining to the toxicity of a chemical or pharmaceutical drug are evaluated so as to reach decisions concerning the release of that chemical into the environment or exposure of patients to a pharmaceutical compound. This process includes hazard identification, risk assessment in the model used, extrapolation of experimental data to human conditions, and risk management by identifying biomarkers for optimal monitoring [1]. Currently, simplified assays and models are used to monitor treatment efficacy and safety [8]. These assays and models often underestimate the biological complexity underlying toxic effects. In the coming years, risk assessment certainly will develop into a process that incorporates more scientific understanding of mechanistic data and biologically based models, in order to better characterize potential hazards in humans. In this regard, toxicogenomics provides a profound basis for an improved understanding of toxicity. The linkage of changes in the gene or protein profile after exposure to chemicals with an ultimate outcome of a disease provides information on:

- Identification of new mechanisms, pathways, and biomarkers.
- Assessment of the relevance of surrogate models for predicting human risk.
- Disease diagnosis and treatment (prediction of incipient toxicity).
- Profound insights on toxicity by compiling many potential toxicants and adverse effects in many biological systems and by searching for previously unrecognised correlations.
- Relationship of specific susceptibility factors to environmental disease risk.

- Account of functional variations that affect the bioavailability of a chemical, target organ damage, and/or other response to exposure and adverse outcome (e.g., genetic polymorphism).

Therefore, toxicogenomics, toxicoproteomics, metabonomics, and sophisticated bioinformatics will provide scientific information for risk assessment for the protection of human health [12, 13].

27.2.4 Dose-dependent Toxicity

Traditionally, animal toxicity studies are conducted with several dose levels, including a high dose inducing toxicity. Various extrapolation methods are used to estimate the effect at low doses in humans. It is expected that chemically induced changes in gene expression occur at doses below those required for induction of classical toxic endpoints (subpathological doses). Thus, analysis of changes in gene expression has the potential to provide useful information regarding biological effects at low exposures [14]. This might lead to improved extrapolations and to the identification of threshold concentrations representing a minimal health risk [1]. However, some changes in gene expression are adaptive, reversible, beneficial, and/or unrelated to pathological outcomes. To avoid over interpretation, it is prudent not to classify every gene expression change as a clear sign of an adverse effect [10].

27.2.5 Interspecies Extrapolation

For the evaluation of risk, results from animal studies are traditionally extrapolated to humans. Although a wide variety of useful laboratory animal models for the study of toxicological effects are available, quantitative differences in dose–response relationships or even qualitative differences in biological responses between humans and model species exist and contribute to the complexity of extrapolation in risk assessment [10]. An increased understanding of cellular mechanisms combined with genomic technologies offers the opportunity to find 'bridging biomarkers' that can be used to compare toxic responses among species, including humans. The degree of similarity in gene expression patterns between different species will provide a new tool for selecting the most appropriate animal model and for extrapolating from *in vitro* test systems to animal models [14]. Thus, toxicogenomics might improve the predictive accuracy of the human risk assessment process [1].

27.2.6 Human Biomarkers of Exposure

Within the pharmaceutical industry there is a rapidly growing effort to identify new biomarkers that will optimise the therapeutic benefit of drugs while minimizing their undesirable adverse effects by optimised methods of monitoring. Biomarkers are defined as biological molecules associated with a pathological process or pharmacological response to drug therapy [15]. Classically, compounds under study are chemically analysed (biomarkers of exposure) and functionally characterised by assessing pharmacological, toxic, or genotoxic effects on body fluids (biomarkers of effect) [16]. Changes in gene expression, protein, or metabolite profiles should improve the measurement of the extent of human exposure to a hazardous chemical or drug. To systematically identify and validate biomarkers, specific well characterized pathologies of genes, proteins, or small molecules within the cell need to be characterized, determining the relationship between these potential markers and specific types of target organ damage. 'Fingerprints' of cellular responses to chemical classes with known biological effects have to be identified to develop a library of chemical-class–specific cellular changes [1, 10]. Finally, these new biomarkers need to be validated for their applicability, reliability, and predictivity before they can be used as surrogates for evaluating safety or as decision-making tools [16]. These approaches will lead to a new system of biological classification of chemicals based on similarities of toxicant-induced gene expression profiles.

27.2.7
Regulatory Acceptance: Current Status

It is estimated that most of the top 20 pharmaceutical companies worldwide are now collecting genetic data during clinical trials to determine the drug response rather than exploring adverse drug reactions [17]. However, until now there have been no significant analyses of ethical, legal policy, and regulatory implications for the application of genetic information and technologies to hazard identification, risk assessment, risk management, and environmental regulation [13]. The main reasons are substantial concerns, as well as the uncertainty of regulatory positions on how to use genomics data. For regulatory applications, genomic technologies require careful evaluation and validation. The combination of the endpoints measured with pathological outcomes, accuracy and reproducibility of the data, and potential for false positive and false negative results with respect to the proposed objective of each measurement must be understood [11]. It is imperative that the results of gene expression analysis be transparent to those who will ultimately use these data for the protection of human health in the regulatory arena. To achieve a dialogue on the incorporation of genomic data in the regulatory process, a Society of Toxicology Task Force to Improve the Scientific Basis of Risk Assessment was formed [13] and regulatory agencies, such as the U.S. Food and Drug Administration (FDA) and the U.S. Environmental Protection Agency (EPA), are providing a discussion forum on this important issue [18]. The EPA believes that genomics will have an enormous impact on the ability to assess risks from exposure to stressors. For this reason, the EPA is interested in applying DNA array technologies to ongoing toxicological studies. In 2002, an Interim Policy on Genomics was released, encouraging prudent and beneficial uses of genomics information on a case-by-case basis [19]. A library of human and mouse genes that were previously implicated in responses to toxicological stimuli (transcriptomes) is still under development by the EPA MicroArray Consortium

(EPAMAC) [20]. To learn from industry how to use and interpret toxicogenomics-derived data, the FDA allows companies seeking drug approvals to submit these data without fear of regulatory reprisal. In the form of a 'safe harbour' policy, the FDA guarantees no regulatory action based on voluntarily supplied toxicogenomics information [21, 22] with one exception: if 'omics' data are used to support a safety decision for a drug, the data will be used in regulatory decision making [23].

27.3 ICH Process for Harmonization of Guidelines: Experience from the Past

27.3.1 Overview

In 1990, the International Conference on Harmonization of technical requirements for registration of pharmaceuticals for human use (ICH) was founded as a discussion forum to bring together regulatory authorities and experts from the pharmaceutical industries of Europe, Japan, and the United States in order to achieve greater harmonization in the interpretation and application of technical guidelines and requirements for product registration, to avoid duplicate testing carried out during drug development [2].

Establishment of globally harmonized guidelines requires implementation of three basic principles, which have been the cornerstones of ICH work:

- Development of scientific consensus through discussion among regulatory and industry experts.
- Wide consultation of draft consensus documents, through normal regulatory channels (e.g., FDA Federal Register), before final harmonized text is adopted.
- Commitment by regulatory parties to implement the ICH harmonized guidelines in their regions.
- Monitoring the implementation of the guidelines in different regions.

Thus, the adoption of ICH guidelines has led and will lead to more economical use of human, animal, and material resources and to the elimination of unnecessary delay, whilst maintaining safeguards [2, 24]. The ICH has been successful in issuing guidelines. There are altogether 14 guidelines providing recommendations to establish 'safety'. These guidelines focus on the potential for carcinogenesis, genotoxicity, toxicokinetics, duration of non-rodent repeat dose studies, reproductive toxicology, safety testing of biotechnology-derived products, and safety pharmacology issues.

An outline of the ICH harmonization process is given in Figure 27.1. More detailed information about the ICH and the ICH harmonization process for guidelines can be found on the Internet (http://www.ifpma.org/).

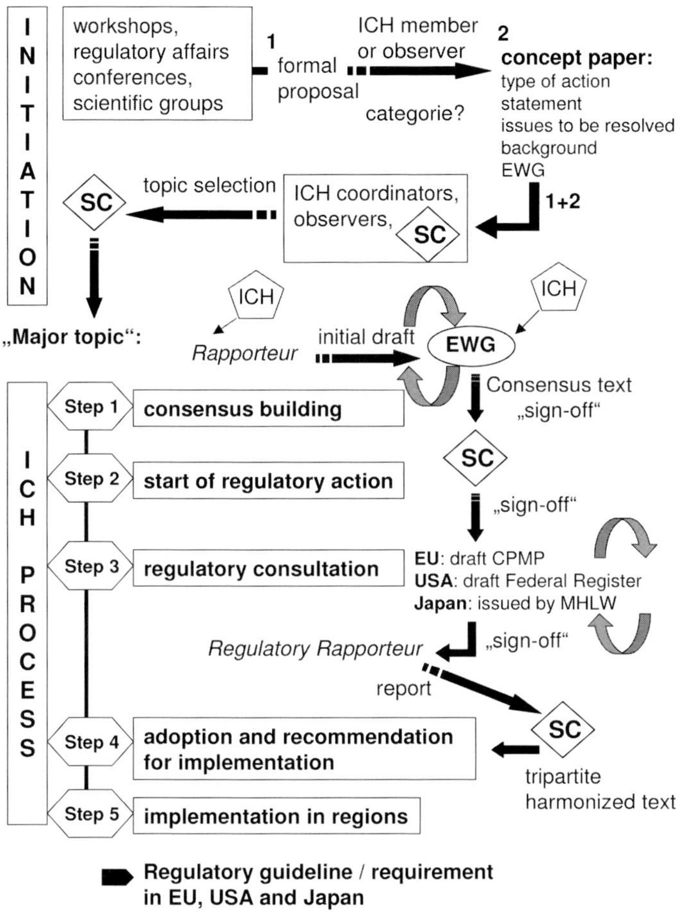

Fig. 27.1 Mechanism of harmonizing new technical requirements (initiation and full ICH process). SC = steering committee; EWG = expert working group; CPMP = Committee for Proprietary Medicinal Products; MHLW = Ministry of Health, Labour and Welfare.

27.3.2
ICH Carcinogenicity Guidelines as a Case Study: Experience with the Implementation of Alternative Models in Cancer Risk Assessment

Conventional testing to assess the potential of human carcinogenic risk from pharmaceutical or chemical compounds today traditionally includes two-year bioassays in rats and mice of both sexes; standard protocols are widely accepted. These main studies are usually preceded by tests for genetic toxicity and repeat-dose toxicology studies. Usually the dose levels for these long-term studies are selected on the basis of data from three-month dose-range–finding studies [25, 26]. However, lifetime rodent bioassays carry several issues: Selection of species, strains, dose, routes of exposure, and time course of exposure need to be justified. Mechanisms of action are seldom investigated routinely in the standard bioassays. The interpretation of results depends on subjective pathomorphological evaluation and on statistical criteria, and qualitative judgement is based on quantitative criteria. High-dose results in animals have to be extrapolated to low-dose exposures in humans (interspecies and dose extrapolation), sometimes over an enormous dose range. The relevance of rodent tumours obtained at the maximum tolerated dose (MTD) to humans is debatable. Tumour induction in rodents may be species-specific, and some tumours in rodents seem to have no counterpart in humans. The results for chemical carcinogenicity testing are concordant in only 70% of the comparisons between rats and mice [27]. It is therefore unlikely that the concordance between rodents and humans would be higher. Assays are time-consuming (approximately three years are required to design, conduct, analyse, and interpret these assays). These studies are expensive (about $1–1.5 million per study), and large numbers of animals (often more than 500) are killed. Finally, a number of compounds that test positive in standard carcinogenicity assays have turned out to be of no concern for humans [27–29]. Thus, using lifetime rodent bioassays in risk assessment may not always correctly predict human risk for developing tumours.

To improve extrapolation to humans, alternative short-term assays were recommended, among them transgenic or knockout mouse models. On the premise that the genetic modifications in these models are related to human cancer development, that the genetic event itself is insufficient to induce cancer, and that there is a potential to predispose animals to tumour development upon exposure to carcinogens, testing of the potential for tumorigenicity in these models may be more meaningful in assessing risk to humans [25, 26, 29].

Transgenic mouse strains are considered to be promising *in vivo* alternatives to the commonly used two-year rodent studies. These mice are bred with genetic predispositions that increase their susceptibility to insults from carcinogens and to the rapid development of tumours. These strains also offer the opportunity to gain important insights into how carcinogens produce tumours. Therefore, using transgenic animals when appropriate would result in a considerable reduction in the duration of the assays and a reduction in the number of animals needed. In addition, these models seem to generate results that are more reliable for assessments of risk in humans [24, 28, 29].

27.3.2.1 **Results from an ILSI-HESI Study**

Owing to the limitations of standard two-year rodent bioassays (see Section 27.3.2), the questions arise of (1) whether alternative approaches, such as transgenic or knockout mouse models, may obviate the necessity for routinely conducting two long-term rodent studies and (2) whether the use of rats and mice alone can provide enough information on carcinogenicity relevant to human risk assessment. The relative individual contribution of rat and mouse carcinogenicity studies in assessing human cancer risk has been addressed in six surveys, conducted by the International Agency for Research on Cancer (IARC), the U.S. Food and Drug Administration (FDA), the U.S. Physicians' Desk Reference (PDR), the Japan Pharmaceutical Manufacturers Association (JPMA), the EU Committee for Proprietary Medicinal Products (CPMP), and the U.K. Centre for Medicines Research (CMR). As a result of these analyses and of the discussions of the Expert Safety Working group of the International Conference on Harmonization in 1995, it was concluded that, in general, information from a second species (usually the mouse) was not conclusive and that data from short-term assays may provide more useful information [25].

However, at that time, very little information was available and none of the newer transgenic and knockout mouse models had been validated or evaluated. Moreover, the two-year bioassays have been accepted for carcinogenic risk assessment for more than 30 years. For the short-term assays, a research consortium was established under the auspices of the Health and Environmental Science Institute (HESI) of the International Life Science Institute (ILSI). The aim of the Committee on the Evaluation of Alternative Models on Carcinogenicity Testing, comprising experts from industry, government, and academia, was to undertake a collaborative study to evaluate a series of prototype compounds in several alternative models and to improve animal models used in cancer risk assessment [25, 27]. Over a period of six years (1996–2001), 21 compounds covering a broad range of activity from nongenotoxic to genotoxic human carcinogens (Table 27.1) were tested in five *in vivo* and one *in vitro* assay (Table 27.2) [28].

Tab. 27.1 Compounds that were tested in alternative carcinogenicity assays and their possible modes of action.

Class	*Compound*
Genotoxic human carcinogens	Cyclophosphamide, melphalan, phenacetin
Immunosuppressant human carcinogen	Cyclosporin A
Hormonal human carcinogens	Diethylstilbestrol, estradiol
Rodent carcinogens/putative human noncarcinogens (based on human data)	Phenobarbital, clofibrate, reserpine, dieldrin, methapyrilene
Rodent carcinogens/putative human noncarcinogens (by mechanism)	Haloperidol, chlorpromazine, chloroform, metaprotenerol, WY-14643, DEHP, sulfamethoxazole
Noncarcinogens	Ampicillin, D-mannitol, sulfisoxazole

Tab. 27.2 Alternative carcinogenicity assays that were evaluated.

Model	*Characteristic*
p53$^{+/-}$ knockout mouse	Deletion of one allele of the *p53* tumour-suppressor gene
Tg.AC transgenic mouse	Insertion of multiple copies of the *v-Ha-ras* oncogene
Tg.rasH2 transgenic mouse	Insertion of multiple copies of the human *c-Ha-ras* gene
XPA$^{-/-}$ knockout mouse	Deletion of both alleles of nucleotide excision-repair genes
XPA$^{-/-}$/*p53*$^{+/-}$ double knockout	Deletion of one allele of the *p53* tumour-suppressor gene and of both alleles of nucleotide-excision repair genes
SHE assay	In-vitro model: Syrian hamster embryo (SHE) assay

For all selected compounds, data were available from conventional two-year rodent bioassays, genotoxic evaluations, an established toxicology database of *in vitro* and *in vivo* modes of action, and data related to human exposure and effect [27].

The data generated over this period led to several conclusions. First, these models are sensitive but not overly responsive in regard to tumorigenesis. Second, four of the alternative models, the $p53^{+/-}$, $XPA^{-/-}$, *Tg.AC*, and the *Tg.rasH2* mice, are considered genetically stable and able to produce a wide spectrum of tumours depending upon the type of chemical exposure. These transgenic rodent models seem to be an adequate substitute for the two-year mouse bioassay [27]. The SHE assay is not appropriate for regulatory purposes regarding tumorigenicity, but might be employed for screening and ranking activities and is sometimes used by the FDA to clarify unexpected concerns during clinical trials [30]. Third, these transgenic models have the advantage of requiring less time, fewer animals, and possibly less expense, although these mice are expensive. Nevertheless, their use also has limitations, as do other animal bioassays, especially with respect to the issue of interspecies extrapolation, in trying to predict the potential hazards to humans [31]. Taken together, these models are not designed as stand-alone assays or as proof of human cancer risk, but they provide a useful addition to the process of assessing human tumour risk. They can play an important part of the overall 'weight of evidence'.

The effort to optimise testing procedures for determining the carcinogenicity of pharmaceuticals without jeopardising safety resulted in an ICH-harmonised tripartite guideline, ICH-S1 B. All ICH S1 (carcinogenicity) guidelines were recommended for adoption at step 4 of the ICH process (Figure 27.1) in 1997 by the ICH steering committee. In September 1997 the guidelines were implemented by the EU CPMP (see CPMP/ICH/299/95), in February 1998 by the FDA (Federal Register, vol. 63, p. 8983), and in July 1998 by the MHLW (PMSB/ELD Notification No. 548). Given the complexity of the process of carcinogenesis, no single experimental approach can be expected to predict human cancer risk correctly. Flexibility and critical judgment are recommended in choosing an optimal strategy for testing the carcinogenic potential of a pharmaceutical.

27.3.2.2 **Regulatory Acceptance of Transgenic Animals as Alternatives: Current Status**

The usefulness of transgenic rodents in assessing human cancer risk will principally depend on the orientation of specific agencies [31]. As a result of the harmonization efforts of the ICH in 1995, regulatory agencies evaluating pharmaceuticals have started, as of 1997, to accept data from transgenic models when considering new drug applications. Despite this uniform regulatory acceptance, broader experience and scientific acceptance within the pharmaceutical industry is needed. Studies utilizing these models are being submitted to regulatory agencies as part of a data package with greater frequency. In 2001, the FDA received approximately 60 alternative or transgenic-model protocols for review. In contrast, in Japan many companies are reluctant to submit transgenic model data to the government because of uncertainty. Japan prefers the *Tg.rasH2* mouse, which was for years subject to unclear patent conditions. This legal condition has contributed to delay of the use of transgenic mice in Japan as part of a new testing strategy. The Committee for Proprietary Medicinal Products

(CPMP) has to date not received many requests to review protocols for the new models [32]. This paucity of EU requests can partially be explained by the slightly more difficult access to regulatory advice, which is readily available from the FDA. However, transgenic models can be of great value as a part of a comprehensive weight-of-evidence approach to assessing human carcinogenic risk from chemical exposure [25].

27.3.2.3 Future Perspectives

The recommendation of the ICH to utilize one rodent bioassay, preferably in rat, together with one alternative approach to assess the carcinogenic potential of pharmaceuticals, is a step in the right direction [28]. In conjunction with the ILSI-HESI, this collaborative process by which these alternative models were evaluated may represent a prototype for assessing and introducing new methods to the regulatory scene in the future [29]. Nevertheless, the process of evaluating transgenic models as accelerated carcinogenicity bioassay models is still ongoing. Recommendations to optimise these models (e.g., increase animal numbers) have been published. Robust positive controls or rather a standard list of calibration chemicals, optimised group size, and exposure periods, as well as suitable statistical methods need to be defined and harmonized to ensure more consistent protocols [32, 33]. Finally, current understanding of carcinogenesis should be integrated into testing strategies. A combination of the results of transgenic or knockout mouse models with the results of the conventional rodent bioassays, as well as with toxicokinetics, pharmacodynamics, genetic variations, and structure–activity relationships will further reduce the need for rodent lifetime assays in coming years [28]. At the moment, the regulatory scene is in a period of transition during which the results of short-term tests, in combination with the results of the conventional two-year rodent bioassays, will provide an opportunity to evaluate the performance of carcinogenesis assays [26]. In conclusion, an ongoing discussion of the evaluation and application framework is needed for the use of remaining data and for the interpretation of these data for successful integration of alternative models into the risk assessment process. This case study reveals that the regulatory process is a long-term process, which focuses on the one hand on the drafting of guidelines and on the other hand on more carefully analysing older data and on stimulating the creation of new data, which then drives further recommendations on the basis of internationally accepted data.

27.4 Incorporation of Toxicogenomics into Drug Development, Evaluation, and Regulation: Benefits versus Risks

27.4.1 General Criteria for Successful Exploitation

Over the coming years, it is expected that drug development will benefit from genomic and proteomic technologies. For example, genome-wide expression analyses will provide insights into the pathways and mechanisms of toxicity. Drug-related toxicity could be characterized leading to better exposure and improved human risk assessment. New toxicity screens and biomarkers will be developed. Candidate molecules with lower toxicity could be identified and selected earlier, reducing cycle time in drug discovery and development [13, 34]. However, some of these technologies are still in their infancy, and many barriers and limitations must be overcome. Inconsistency in study design and sampling strategies (e.g., selection of model systems, dose, duration of exposure, temporal nature of gene expression), the lack of quantitative or qualitative correlations of exposure, dose, and adverse effect, as well as the lack of bioinformatics tools and analytical methods necessary to manage the volume of research findings and the lack of publicly available databases lead to results that may not be interpretable and may be difficult, if not impossible, to use in risk assessment [13, 16, 35, 36].

The success of fully exploiting these new technologies depends on several criteria:

- Accurate selection, amplification, and location of probe molecules.
- Accurate reference sequence information.
- Identification of a unique oligonucleotide.
- Accurate distinction among multiple products of a single gene.
- Accurate reconstruction of expressed sample nucleotide sequences.
- Accurate and reproducible transformation of image files to numerical data.
- Precise image scanning.
- Standardized methods.
- Harmonized gene nomenclature.

(At the moment many different annotations for the same gene are used, e.g., one gene in the mouse has 59 appellations [22]).

Besides these criteria, many challenges – technical, regulatory, ethical, and in communications – are evident before these new technologies become a standard tool in drug development and medical practice. The scientific community has to demonstrate the strength of the linkage of genomic (and proteomic) measurements to associated biological outcomes. The acceptable sensitivity, specificity, reproducibility, robustness, reliability, accuracy, precision, and clinical relevance of a chosen microarray platform application must be demonstrated.

Human variability and susceptibility also have to be taken into account. An individual's privacy and rights have to be protected. Finally, regulatory agencies have to develop early working relations with stockholders to provide reasonable and appropriate context-specific expectations. Fair, consistent, and critical risk–benefit analyses of the value and impact of new multiparametric genomic (and proteomic) technologies on both product development and patient care will have to be developed [35, 37]. Therefore, it might be appropriate to divide the process of incorporating toxicogenomics-derived data into drug development into two phases. Phase one should focus on the harmonization of standards, practices, precision of data, and quality control, whereas phase two should focus on the development of a gene expression database including data from a series of known toxicants [34].

27.4.1.1 Objectives-driven Approaches

Toxicogenomics can be utilized at any stage of the drug development process. Gene expression profiling is widely used, for example, in molecular screenings for candidate selection, in the development of short-term biomarkers for subchronic or chronic toxicities and of robust predictive biomarkers for drug-related effects in humans (surrogates of safety [4]), and in the field of issue management, comparing the mechanisms of target-organ pathologies between animals and humans [38]. The benefits or rather risks of incorporating toxicogenomics into drug development, evaluation, and regulation will be highly dependent on context. According to Petricoin et.al. [37], the drug development process can be divided into six main fields in which microarrays can be applied:

1. Assessing RNA and protein alterations in early drug screening.
2. Assessing RNA and protein alterations in nonclinical toxicology.
3. Assessing quality control of cells for manufacturing biologicals.
4. Assessing RNA and protein alterations in clinical samples as diagnostic biomarkers.
5. Assessing critical regions of a pathogen's nucleic acid sequence in clinical studies.
6. Assessing critical regions of inherited somatic cell DNA sequences in clinical studies and patient-tailored therapy.

From a regulatory point of view, microarray data will be scrutinized depending on whether these data are used for early drug discovery and hypothesis generation (fields 1 and 2) or as a clinical device to make diagnostic, therapeutic, or prognostic decisions regarding patients (fields 4–6).

27.4.1.2 Technical Prerequisites

The success of fully exploiting these new technologies depends on several technical prerequisites: mRNA processing, hybridisation parameters (e. g., base composition, temperature, concentration of monovalent and divalent ions, sequence complexity), use of inbred strains to reduce the potentially confusing effects of individual variations, clones (nonredundant, noncontaminated, sequence verified, species-, cell-, tissue-, and/or field-specific), and probes (e. g., large amounts of RNA are needed, limiting the type of sample).

To avoid artefacts resulting from prolonged manipulation, sample handling must be standardized. The quality of RNA is critical for efficient labelling and optimal signal. Even the methodology of RNA extraction can influence the proportion of different RNA species isolated [39].

Data Interpretation

Genome-wide expression patterns are analysed and interpreted using a specific hypothesis based on the current understanding of gene function and gene product interactions. This process requires data-reduction applications that fine-tune and filter the raw data and data output (see Section 27.4.1.3). As the biological understanding of gene products evolves, gene expression data may be reanalysed and reinterpreted by others, leading to alternative assessments. Therefore, fundamental knowledge, reliable data, accumulated experience, and excellent judgement are essential to avoid raising false concerns or over interpreting data, to evaluate links between gene expression changes and biological outcome, and to recognize legitimate toxicological responses [37].

Variable Imprecision

The ability to collect multiparametric datasets from a single sample leads to numerous views on the interpretations of biological meaning. Because a single sample results in a multiparametric dataset, a very small error rate applied across such large datasets can lead to a significant number of false positive or false negative signals. Individual measurements from a single microarray platform do not share the same precision, sensitivity, and specificity [37]. This imprecision can be reduced by numerous means to optimise data quality. For example, to assess sample quality, multiple replicates of the same sequence have to be placed on a single array; to assess background hybridisations, negative controls (sequences of bacterial genes) have to be included; to assess assay performance, positive controls and sample spikes have to be added; to assess cross hybridisations, probe sequences have to be optimised and mismatch probes have to be used; to enhance interlaboratory reproducibility, standard operating procedures have to be developed and regularly updated. In addition, bioinformatics tools have to be optimised (see Section 27.4.1.3). It is crucial to employ statistical methods for microarray analysis (e.g., replicates, standardization). Standards will ensure that results are credible, that full datasets and annotations are usable, and that data from repositories are accessible and permanently available [10, 40]. These standards and new statistical methods for establishing the significance of linking gene expression analyses to more conventional diagnostic endpoints or outcomes have to be developed and accepted [37].

Platform and Data Maturity

As the field of microarray technology is rapidly evolving and as this process is still ongoing, difficulties abound in standardization and consensus development. At the moment there are no 'gold standards'. Numerous platforms are available, and protocols and programs are modified often. Probes are designed from different gene sequences for targets with the same names, and the absence or presence of a specific gene depends on the array platform used [37]. A list of alternatives is given in Table 27.3.

Besides these alternatives, various analysis settings (e.g., image capture, image analysis options) and analytical tools (e.g., principal components analysis, hierarchical clustering, support vector machines, relevance networks) [41] play a pivotal role in data maturity and quality.

27.4.1.3 Bioinformatics and Data Interpretation

To use microarrays in risk assessment or disease diagnosis, large amounts of genomic data have to be mined for hidden patterns by bioinformatics tools. Bioinformatics is defined as the application of computing and mathematics to the manage-

Tab. 27.3 Alternative microarray technologies (platforms and protocols).

Method A		***Method B***
cDNA microarrays	versus	Oligonucleotide microarrays
High-density arrays	versus	Low-density arrays
Spotting	versus	In-situ synthesis or other
Single-dye hybridisations	versus	Dual-dye hybridizations
Fluorescent dye-labelled	versus	Biotin-labelled nucleotides
Single	versus	Two-step dye labelling
Amplification	versus	Direct labelling

ment and analysis of biological datasets to aid the solution of biological problems. These datasets are usually stored and managed in large databases. Computational procedures (i.e., algorithms) are used to explore the relationships among the members of datasets [15]. Transferred to toxicogenomics: raw hybridisation data are simplified to a table of gene/clone identity, expression value or ratio and then integrated with databases that contain genomic data, functional information, or literature references [39]. Among the central technical issues that need to be resolved before microarrays can realize their full potential in toxicology (see Section 27.4.1.2) are further development of computer science and bioinformatics. Especially database design and maintenance will be crucial and intricate details must be understood. First, any set of microarray measurements can be analysed and reanalysed in many different ways. Before multiple microarray measurements can be integrated into a single analysis, the reported measurements need to be normalized or modified to make them comparable. Distinct experimental design, intra- and inter-microarray variations, artefacts, heterogeneity of expression in cell subpopulations in most organs, or differences between the most commonly used microarray technologies are substantial sources of noise in the experiments [41]. Second, biologically function generally results from complex interactions between many components and features such as feedback, feed-forward, error checking, and redundancy. Transcriptional regulation is more sophisticated than the traditional view of gene expression being a simple on–off event [39]. Erroneous data (false positives), undetected gene expressions (false negatives), conflicting data, and biological variation limitations also need to be eliminated [42]. Finally, common databases, which combine information on different toxicological pathways and particular gene expression profiles, have to be created [9]. Genomics-derived data need to be stored in a standardized format that is easily accessible [3]. Correct statistical analysis and tools that link genes to known biological pathways, as well as discovery of new pathways, are in their infancy. Often the official gene name, predicted protein names, or gene-ontology classifications are not available. To reduce post-analytical work, tools that can automatically indicate the importance of particular findings have to be invented [41].

The National Center for Toxicogenomics (NCT) is developing the first public toxicogenomics database, Chemical Effects in Biological Systems (CEBS) (see Chapters

10 and 25). This database combines molecular expression datasets from transcriptomics, proteomics, metabonomics, and conventional toxicology with metabolic, toxicological pathway, and gene regulatory network information relevant to environmental toxicology and human disease [14]. Members of the Microarray Gene Expression Data Society (MGED) have solicited community input in developing standards for the publication of DNA microarray data. In 2001, a commentary was published describing the Minimal Information About a Microarray Experiment (MIAME), a proposed checklist of variables that should be included in every publication of array data to make cross-publication comparisons possible [43, 44]. More detailed information about MGED and MIAME can be found on the Internet (http://www.mged.org/).

27.4.1.4 Good Laboratory Practice: Compliance with FDA 21 CFR Part 11

All regulations under which the FDA considers electronic records, electronic signatures, and handwritten signatures attached thereon to be trustworthy, reliable, and generally equivalent to paper records are subsumed under 21 CFR Part 11 (Code of Federal Regulations) [45–47]. In the near future, all hardware, software controls, and documentation must be available for FDA inspection, and in consequence, GxP audit trails including quality assurance, quality control, information technologies as well as laboratory management and company data management have to be fundamentally changed.

Applied to toxicogenomics, external and internal annotation resources and all systems used in data generation, management, and analysis will be audited. The ability to apply 21 CFR Part 11 to toxicogenomics offers multiple advantages. First, all systems are validated, ensuring accuracy, reliability, and performance consistency, as well as the ability to discern invalid or altered records. Second, data integrity, authenticity, and reproducibility are ensured. Finally, compliance with FDA 21 CFR Part 11 might be a prerequisite for acceptance of 'omics' data by regulatory authorities. However, today the need for application of 21 CFR Part 11 to the new field of toxicogenomics remains unclear. A Regulated Array Information Management System (RAIMAN) is under development by Affymetrix in conjunction with the pharmaceutical industry [47], whereas GeneLogic takes the view that at the moment there is no need for such an implementation [51]. Discussions are still ongoing among regulators, industry, and academia concerning the question of how soon we need compliance with FDA 21 CFR Part 11.

Nevertheless, to promote scientific and regulatory acceptance of microarray data, to stimulate the use of these data during the human risk assessment process, and to achieve greater harmonization, toxicogenomics studies should be conducted in a GLP-compliant manner. Adequately trained study personnel, standard operating procedures (SOP) stipulating the conditions under which studies are planned, performed, monitored, recorded, reported, and archived, and suitable standards and controls are needed to ensure quality data and to minimize sources of variability.

However, certain additions and/or modifications of the current OECD (Organisation for Economic Cooperation and Development) principles are required to meet the current state-of-the-art for toxicogenomics and to assure the quality of the generated data. Standards of practice (e.g., functional performance, pass/fail measures, reference and/or control items) need to be formalized, and acceptance criteria (e. g., range values, predefined limits) and GMP (good manufactory practice) for microarrays need to be established.

27.4.2
Evaluation Process: Current Status

Molecular technologies including the field of genomics are already widely used in toxicology:

- to develop new screening strategies and biomarkers of toxicity,
- to determine mechanisms of cellular and molecular dysfunctions,
- to identify genetic variations that determine responses to chemical exposure and sensitivity to toxicity outcomes (pharmacogenetics/pharmacogenomics),
- to monitor alterations in key biochemical pathways [11].

There is basic work underlying the rapid progress in toxicogenomics, such as the development of microchip arrays, which is being done by academic, governmental, nonprofit, and corporate groups. A few of the groups involved are the NCBI, Celera Genomics (Rockville, MD, USA), the Institute for Genomic Research (Rockville, MD, USA), the Department of Biochemistry at Stanford University (Stanford, California), the Department of Molecular Genetics at Max-Planck Institute (Berlin, Germany), and the Fraunhofer Institute ITEM (Hannover, Germany) [49].

The National Institute of Environmental Health Science (NIEHS) in the U.S. has established a centre of excellence for cDNA microarray technology in predictive toxicology (see Chapter 25). The mission of this National Center for Toxicogenomics (NCT) is to promote the evolution and coordinated use of gene expression technologies and to apply them to the assessment of toxicological effects in humans. For this reason, experiments were performed to explore whether specific toxicities carry signature profiles, which can be recognized within certain dose and time parameters [50]. To provide a worldwide reference system, the NCT is developing an 'encyclopaedia' of tissue-specific gene expression signatures. This first publicly available toxicogenomics knowledge base, called Chemical Effects in Biological Systems (CEBS), combines molecular expression data sets from transcriptomics, proteomics, metabonomics (metabolic profiling), and conventional toxicology with metabolic and toxicological pathways, and gene regulatory network information relevant to environmental toxicology and human diseases (see Chapter 10) [51]. In addition, the NCBI has developed programs such as the Gene Expression Omnibus to support the public use and dissemination of gene expression data as well as to build a gene expression data repository and to provide an online resource for the retrieval of gene expression data from any organism or artificial source [49]. More details about the NCT and the national toxicogenomic programs in the U.S. can be found on the Internet (http://www.niehs.nih.gov/nct/). Trade associations have established committees to help with the validation of microarray analysis. One example, the initiative of ILSI-HESI, is discussed in Section 27.4.2.1.

27.4.2.1 ILSI-HESI Initiative

The committee for the Application of Genomics in Mechanism Based Risk Assessment was formed in 1999 as a non-profit international forum among government, academia, and industry, to advance the scientific basis for development and application of genomic methodologies to mechanism-based risk assessment. The use of toxicogenomics-derived data in risk assessment requires the implementation of three key issues:

- Evaluation of experimental methods for measuring changes in gene expression.
- Development of publicly international available databases linking gene expression data and key biological parameters.
- Determining if known mechanisms and pathways of toxicity can be associated with characteristic gene expression profiles (fingerprints).

To deal with these key issues, toxicity working groups were established, covering hepatotoxicity, nephrotoxicity, and genotoxicity, as well as a database working group collaborating with the European Bioinformatics Institute (EBI). Well studied drugs and chemicals with known mechanism of toxicity were used as test compounds in *in vitro* and *in vivo* studies to investigate temporal and low- versus high-dose response relationships and to analyse cross-platform and inter- and intra-laboratory variability. An overview of the common experimental design features is given in Figure 27.2.

At the beginning of 2003 all *in vivo* studies, *in vitro* work, and microarray readings were largely and successfully completed and data analysis was ongoing. The out-

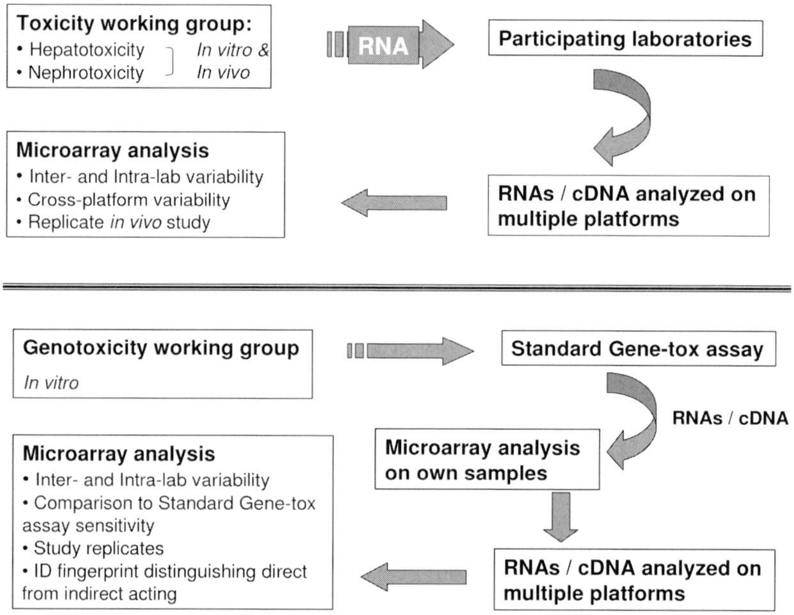

Fig. 27.2 ILSI-HESI Technical Committee on the Application of Genomics to Mechanism Based Risk Assessment: Experimental Program.

comes of this initiative have revealed and been used to characterize multiple potential and actual sources of variability, including expected sources of biological variability, operating procedures in the isolation and labelling of mRNA samples, non-standard settings on hardware and analysis software, microarray lot number, and differences in gene coverage and/or annotation across different technical platforms. Nevertheless, it could be shown that gene expression patterns relating to biological pathways are robust enough to allow mechanistic insights, that gene expression data can provide strong information on topographic specificity, that dose-dependent changes can be observed, and that concerns regarding oversensitivity of the technology may be unreasonable. Additionally, the importance of standardized microarray formats and public repository databases as a tool by which microarray data can be compared and interpreted by the scientific community at large has been recognized. In view of this, a database is under development in collaboration with the European Bioinformatics Institute (EBI). This database, linking gene array data with toxicological information (dose, histopathology, clinical chemistry), will improve the assessment of the potential utility of genomic data in risk assessment.

To summarize, the outcome of this initiative should provide, not only a new window into the use of genomics in toxicology, but also a model for toxicogenomic study design, data collection, and data storage [36].

27.5 Summary and Outlook

Toxicogenomics has the potential to improve the predictability and speed of preclinical safety assessments. Published results so far show that genome-wide expression analysis can be used for candidate selection, hypothesis generation, mechanistic investigation, and discovery of potential biomarker linkages. It is expected that in the near future, regulatory authorities will evaluate toxicogenomics data as supplementary information for efficacy and safety alongside classical preclinical and clinical studies for supporting new drug applications. However, before guidelines for microarray studies can be developed, scientific agreement on outlining a set of best practices for industry on an international basis (e.g., descriptions of experimental conditions and data quality), need to be established [35, 37]. Combining conventional toxicology and pathology with molecular genetics, biochemistry, cell biology, and computational bioinformatics will likely improve regulatory toxicological practice [11]. Microarray data generated today may become more informative and relevant to risk assessment as databases increase, comparability improves, and scientific knowledge expands. Over time, expression profiles will increase our understanding of mechanisms of toxicity through the identification of relationships between chemical drug exposure and changes in genome-wide expression patterns. Molecular interaction maps coupled with mechanistic models might represent the complex molecular interactions in a pathway in a meaningful manner [1, 39]. Use of toxicogenomics data from standard animal toxicity studies as well as from clinical trials could help:

- to minimize the number of variables in study design,
- to design therapeutic drugs with greater precision,
- to increase the sensitivity for detecting potentially toxic chemicals,
- to improve the efficiency of these studies,
- to increase the quality of drug pipelines,
- to define essential sets of biomarkers,
- to facilitate the development of more relevant *in vitro* systems,
- to affect the number of laboratory animals used [42, 50].

Therefore, there is an excellent opportunity to further apply the 'three Rs' of conscientious animal research: replacement, refinement, and reduction [52, 53].

Nevertheless, a consensus is needed among industry and regulators to clarify some basic questions:

- How can results of toxicogenomic studies be reliably interpreted?
- What are the 'gold standards' for toxicogenomics (e.g., reference RNA, reference data analysis)?
- How will the generated data be stored?
- How can validation for a standardized methodology be achieved?
- How will toxicogenomics reduce the necessity of animal testing (e.g., species selection)?
- How many and which genes should be measured to distinguish a toxic response from pharmacologic or physiologically adaptive responses?
- How can toxicogenomics data be incorporated in a more accurate risk assessment?
- How can gene-expression–derived data be used in legal matters, such as toxic chemical torts, workplace safety assessments, and patent cases? [1, 22]

Guidance, guidelines, and regulations will then emanate from such consensus [13].

In view of this, the ILSI-HESI initiative on the application of genomics in mechanism-based risk assessment is a step in the right direction because, increasingly, international harmonization (like that of ICH) is driven by accepted scientific data. Based on the principles and processes of the ICH, facilitating the integration of toxicogenomics-derived data into risk assessment for regulatory purposes should be critically discussed. Toxicogenomics should be proposed as a new ICH topic when:

- Genomic data are reliable and conclusive.
- International acceptance of such data for decision-making processes in industry and regulation exists.
- A concept paper has outlined the usefulness and benefits for regulations.
- A time schedule can be agreed upon for drafting the objectives, scope, general principals, methods applied, and safety strategy scheme for such new guidelines. The opportunities outlined should be used to provide the benefits of the new techniques for regulatory purposes and to the well-being of patients and people in general.

Acknowledgements

We thank Dr. Thorsten Meyer, Dr. Beate Hess, and Deborah Ockert for their review of this manuscript and for their helpful suggestions.

References

1. P.T. Simmons, C.J. Portier, *Carcinogenesis* **2002**, 23, 903–905
2. ICH website: http://www.ich.org/
3. R. Corvi, *ATLA* **2002**, 30 (Suppl. 2), 129–131
4. E.F. Nuwaysir, M. Bittner, J. Trent, J.C. Barrett, C.A. Afshari, *Molecular Carcinogenesis* **1999**, 24, 153–159
5. J.F. Medlin, *Environ. Health Perspect.* **1999**, 107, A256–258
6. W.H.M. Heijne, R.H. Stierum, M. Slijper, P.J. Van Bladeren, B. van Ommen, *Biochem. Pharmacol.* **2003**, 65, 857–875
7. S. Farr, R.T. Dunn, *Toxicological Science* **1999**, 50, 1–9
8. S. Steiner, N.L. Anderson, *Toxicol. Lett.* **2000**, 112–113, 467–471
9. H.K. Hamadeh, R.P. Amin, R.S. Paules, C.A. Afshari, *Curr. Issues Mol. Biol.* **2002**, 4, 45–56
10. M.J. Aardema, J.T. MacGregor, *Mut. Res.* **2002**, 499, 13–25
11. J.T. MacGregor, *Toxicological Science* **2003**, 73, 207–208
12. R.W. Tennant, ILSI-HESI Meeting (Toxicogenomics in risk assessment) **2003** (http://hesi.ilsi.org/publications/)
13. M.L. Cunningham, M.S. Bogdanffy, T.R. Zacharewski, R.N. Hines, *Toxicological Science* **2003**, 73, 209–215
14. A. Oberemm, U. Gundert-Remy, *Mitteilungen der Fachgruppe Umweltchemie und Ökotoxikologie*, **2003**, 1
15. M. Waters et al., *Environ. Health Perspect.* **2003**, 111, 811–824
16. Eisenbrand et al., *Food and Chemical Toxicology* **2002**, 40, 193–236
17. C. Güzey, O. Spigset, *Drug Safety* **2002**, 25(8), 553–560
18. Lesko et al., *J. Clin. Pharmacol.* **2003**, 43(4), 342–358
19. P. Gilman, EPA Interim Genomics Policy **2002** (http://www.epa.gov/)
20. J.C. Rocket, D.J. Dix, *Environ. Health Persp.* **1999**, 107(8), 681–685
21. T.W. Gant, *Trends in Pharmacol. Sci.* **2002**, 23(8), 388–393
22. C. Hogue, *Chemical & Engineering News* **2003**, 2, 1–5
23. R.E. Osterberg, personal communication **2003**
24. R.E. Osterberg, abstract for TestSmart Pharmaceuticals **2001** (http://caat.jhsph.edu/programs/workshops/testsmart/pharm-proc.htm)
25. D. Robinson, abstract for TestSmart Pharmaceuticals **2001** (http://caat.jhsph.edu/programs/workshops/testsmart/pharm-proc.htm)
26. H. Spielmann, *Toxicol. Pathol.* **2003**, 31(1), 54–59
27. G.S. Omenn, *Toxicol. Pathol.* **2001**, 29 (Suppl.), 5–12
28. C.W. Schmidt, *Environ. Health Persp.* **2002**, 110(5)
29. D.E. Robinson, J.S. MacDonald, *Toxicol. Pathol.* **2001**, 29 (Suppl.), 13–19
30. J.I. Goodman, *Toxicol. Pathol.* **2001**, 29 (Suppl.), 173–176
31. S.M. Cohen, *Toxicol. Pathol.* **2001**, 29 (Suppl.), 183–190
32. S.D. Pettit, *Toxicol. Pathol.* **2001**, 29 (Suppl.), 191–195
33. J. Ashby, *Toxicol. Pathol.* **2001**, 29 (Suppl.), 177–182
34. D. Gershon, *Naturejobs* **2002**, 17, 4–5
35. C.J. Henry, *Intern. J. Toxicol.* **2003**, 22, 3–7
36. S.D. Pettit, *ILSI/HESI Statusbericht*, **2003** (http://hesi.ilsi.org/publications/)
37. E. F. Petricoin III et al., *Nature Genetics* **2002**, 32, 474–479
38. A.L. Castle, M.P. Carver, D.L. Mendrick, *DDT* **2002**, 7, 728–736
39. P.A. Clarke, R. te Poele, R. Wooster, P. Workman, *Biochem. Pharmacol*, **2001**, 62, 1311–1336

40. J. Wakefield, *Environ. Health Perspect.* **2003**, 111(6), A334

41. A. Butte, *Nature Reviews* **2002**, 1, 951–960

42. G.M. Charles, *MURJ* **2001**, 5, 25–28

43. Ball et. al., *Science* **2002**, 298, 539

44. Ball et. al., *Nature* **2002**, 419, 323

45. F. von Gottschalk, *Transkript* **2003**, 5, 58

46. V. Lander, *Laborwelt* **2003**, 2, 16–18

47. S. Jokerst, *Preliminary Compliance Proposal* **2003** (http://www.affymetrix.com/)

48. M. Cavanaugh, personal communication **2003**

49. R.R. Young, *Toxicology* **2002**, 173, 103–121

50. R.W. Tennant, *Environ. Health Persp.* **2002**, 110, A8–10

51. R.A. Lovett, *Science* **2000**, 289, 536–537

52. M. Waters, G. Boorman, P. Bushel, M. Cunningham, R. Irwin, K. Merreic Olden, R. Paules, J. Selkirk, S. Stasiewicz, B. Weis, B. V. Houten, N. Wa and R. Tennant, *Environ. Health Persp.* **2003**, 111, 811–24

53. E.S. Jenkins, C. Broadhead, R.D. Combes, *ATLA* **2002**, 30, 459–465

Subject Index

Handbook of Toxicogenomics: Strategies and Applications. Edited by Jürgen Borlak

ISBN: 3-527-30342-1

d

n